Stiffness of the Elbow, Wrist and Related Pathologies

Luigi Pederzini • Toshiyasu Nakamura
Andrea Celli • Gregory I. Bain
Editors

Stiffness of the Elbow, Wrist and Related Pathologies

ISAKOS
International Society of Arthroscopy, Knee Surgery and Orthopaedic Sports Medicine

Springer

Editors
Luigi Pederzini
Department of Orthopedics
Hesperia Hospital
Modena, Italy

Andrea Celli
Department of Orthopaedic
and Traumatology Surgery Shoulder
and Elbow Unit
Hesperia Hospital
Modena, Italy

Toshiyasu Nakamura
Department of Orthopaedic
Surgery, School of Medicine
International University of Health
and Welfare
Tokyo, Japan

Gregory I. Bain
Department of Orthopedic Surgery
Flinders University of South Australia
and Flinders Medical Centre
Adelaide, Australia

ISBN 978-3-031-81380-1 ISBN 978-3-031-81381-8 (eBook)
https://doi.org/10.1007/978-3-031-81381-8

This Springer imprint is published by the registered company Springer Nature Switzerland AG
The registered company address is: Gewerbestrasse 11, 6330 Cham, Switzerland

Foreword

For most of orthopedics, minimally invasive surgery has become the standard of care. This demands a clear vision of the anatomy, often visualized with a telescope. Because of the small size of the wrist and elbow, exact portal placement with small instruments is needed. Arthroscopy of the wrist and elbow with standard joint space needs experienced providers. Loss of that joint space demands advanced techniques.

This book is a collaborative effort that deals with a very challenging situation where the wrist or elbow is filled with scar, preventing normal range of motion and severely impaired function. Currently, there are few effective treatments available for these conditions. International world-class editors and authors share their collective experience in identifying and classifying the various types of stiffness in the wrist and elbow. They present their indications and contraindications for therapeutic protocols to regain upper extremity function. The authors also share how bracing and postoperative rehabilitation are integrated into their treatment plan.

Once diagnosed, the authors share their knowledge with cutting-edge procedures. Many of these procedures may not yet be the standard of care, but they serve as a beacon for dealing with challenging problems and disabling functions, guiding the future of orthopedic practices.

We have all witnessed the rapid evolution in our approach to orthopedic problems. With its excellent anatomy and diagrams, this book elucidates why the newer methods are invaluable in treating these severely debilitating conditions. "In the middle of difficulty lies opportunity." This quote underscores that challenges can present hidden opportunities for growth and learning. John F. Kennedy said, "Change is the law of life. And those who look only to the past or present are certain to miss the future." With its wealth of knowledge, this book offers hope and optimism for the future of orthopedic care in patients with stiffness of the wrist and elbow.

Gary G. Poehling
Emeritus Chair of Orthopedics,
Atrium Wake Forest Baptist,
Winston Salem, NC, USA

Preface

The human elbow and wrist are complex structures essential for performing everyday tasks, from the simplest motions to intricate activities requiring precision. Stiffness in these joints can significantly impact an individual's quality of life, limiting mobility and function. Addressing these conditions requires a comprehensive understanding of the underlying pathophysiology, diagnostic approaches, and the latest treatment modalities.

This book is designed to be a comprehensive and practical resource for orthopaedic surgeons, physiotherapists, rehabilitation specialists, and other healthcare professionals involved in the management of elbow and wrist stiffness. By combining evidence-based insights, clinical expertise, and the latest advancements in both surgical and non-surgical treatments, we provide a structured approach to assessment and intervention.

Each chapter is written by experts in the field, bringing together extensive experience and evidence-based approaches to treatment. We have also highlighted emerging trends, including arthroscopic procedures and new surgical techniques that are shaping the future of treatment of these two joints.

We extend our gratitude to all the contributors whose expertise and dedication have made this work possible. Their collective efforts have enriched the content, ensuring that it remains a valuable tool for years to come. We also acknowledge the patients who inspire ongoing advancements in this field, reminding us of the importance of restoring function and improving lives.

Modena, Italy — Luigi Pederzini
Tokyo, Japan — Toshiyasu Nakamura
Modena, Italy — Andrea Celli
Adelaide, Australia — Greg Bain

Contents

Part I

Elbow: General and Diagnostic Considerations

Stiffness of the Elbow Joint

1

Sang-Hun Ko

1.1 Introduction

The function of the elbow joint is to precisely position the hand in three-dimensional space. It extremely increases the function of the hand. The functional range of motion of the elbow joint spans 30–130 degrees of flexion-extension, 50 degrees of pronation, and 50 degrees of supination. More than 90% of daily activities occur within those degrees. For this reason, if the range of motion of the joint is lower than the functional range of motion, it is diagnosed as stiffness. Anatomically, the elbow joint has a high joint conformity, and the soft tissues, such as the surrounding joint membrane, readily tend toward fibrosis due to the injury of the joint. Fibrotic contracture is known to happen well in elbow joint. The most common cause of elbow joint stiffness is trauma, and it can also result from long-term splint immobilization, ectopic ossification due to head injuries and burns, inflammatory arthritis, osteoarthritis, congenital or developmental diseases, and so on.

Because the reasonable plan for elbow joint stiffness differs depending on the cause, it is important to determine the precise cause and the degree of elbow joint stiffness. The causes of joint stiffness can be classified as traumatic and nontraumatic depending on the patient's trauma history. And it can be classified as intra-articular and extra-articular depending on the location of the lesion.

First, the cause of elbow stiffness is intrinsic. Elbow stiffness due to intrinsic causes usually affects patients who have primary arthritis, rheumatoid arthritis, and post-traumatic intra-articular fractures that have not been properly managed. If the articular cartilage has previously been intensely injured, regenerating the articular cartilage until it returns to normal would not be good. So, intrinsic stiffness is harder to manage than extrinsic stiffness, and the outcomes are frequently poorer than extrinsic stiffness.

The second cause of elbow stiffness is extrinsic. Extrinsic causes of elbow stiffness are the most common: Extrinsic causes of motion limitation can occur in all the soft structures of the elbow joint. The lesions are mostly contractures of the joint capsule and collateral ligaments and are due to heterotopic ossification. The contracture of the bilateral collateral ligament is a main factor leading to the stiffness of the elbow, and especially, the consecutive flexion limitation of elbow motion is reported to be an important cause of the contracture of the posterior band of the medial collateral ligament. Ectopic ossification develops outside the bone structure, and the exact cause and pathological mechanism have not yet been elucidated. It should be distinguished from calcifications of the elbow. Long-term

S.-H. Ko (✉)
Ulsan University Hospital, University of Ulsan College of Medicine, Ulsan, South Korea
e-mail: jaeyun@uuh.ulsan.kr

L. Pederzini et al. (eds.), *Stiffness of the Elbow, Wrist and Related Pathologies*,
https://doi.org/10.1007/978-3-031-81381-8_1

immobilization due to a fracture is also considered a major cause of extrinsic stiffness. Risk factors include trauma (dislocation with fracture, radial head fracture surgery 24 h after injury, open elbow dislocation), surgery (distal bicep tendon suture), burns (third degree burns of more than 20% of the entire body, over the elbow joint), central nervous system injury (traumatic brain damage or elbow joint trauma followed by brain damage), and a history of heterotopic ossification and systemic illnesses, including progressive fibrodysplasia. Taking a nonsteroidal anti-inflammatory drug (NSAIDs), like diclofenac or indomethacin, and a selective cycloxygenase-2 inhibitor is recommended as an effective treatment.

The third cause of elbow stiffness is multifaceted. In most clinical findings, elbow joint stiffness has multiple causes rather than just one. In this case, plain X-ray and computed tomography (CT) images are needed to identify the stiffness of the elbow joint. Plain radiographs are taken of the anterior, posterior, and lateral sides of the elbow joint to support joint alignment, healing state of the initial trauma, and narrowing the joint gap and to detect the presence of heterotopic ossification and loose bodies in the elbow joint. The lateral-side X-ray view is needed to identify the ulna-humeral joint surface and the anterior and posterior osteophytes of the elbow joint. It could be the cause of intra-articular contracture. CT is more precise than simple radiographs in identifying the exact location and size of osteophytes, ectopic ossification, and loose bodies. Planning operations via 3D-CT modalities can be extremely useful.

The purpose of management for elbow stiffness is to regenerate a stable elbow joint and re-establish the functional range of motion with a pain-free joint. For most patients, mild elbow stiffness could be managed nonoperatively. In patients who have mild flexion contracture caused by long-term immobilization after simple dislocation especially, good to excellent outcomes on their range of motion can be expected through active exercises.

The rule for conservative management is active-assisted passive range of motion using the contralateral arm. Sometimes the braces for dynamic or static exercises are used. Conservative immobilization management is expected to yield good to excellent outcomes in elbow stiffness owing to moderate iatrogenic causes with a short morbidity period. A surgeon must decide which surgical approach they will use before surgery, and the main points for consideration in this decision are the direction and severity of stiffness, scars from former operations, the presence of ulnar neuropathy, and the location of heterotopic ossification.

Surgery is indicated when the range of motion of the joint remains limited enough to interfere with the patient's daily life in spite of an appropriate period of physical therapy aiming to restore the range of motion of the joint. When restoring consecutive flexion after surgery owing to severe flexion limitation, prophylactic decompressive surgery is recommended because internal trauma to the ulnar nerve and posterior distraction injury could occur.

Surgical management of elbow joint stiffness can be classified mostly into open or arthroscopic joint capsule release and elbow arthroplasty. Approaches to open arthroplasty are classified into the following according to the skin incision and the surgical approach: the anterior approach, the medial approach, the lateral approach, and the internal and external parallel approach. The release of the posterior part of the medial collateral ligament is required. It could improve the consecutive flexion during resection in post-traumatic elbow joint contractures. Outerbridge–Kashiwagi arthroplasty (O–K arthroplasty), debridement arthroplasty, interposition arthroplasty, resection arthroplasty, and artificial joint arthroplasty for degenerative arthritis or severe elbow joint stiffness and total elbow replacement can sometimes be useful.

2 Anatomical Considerations in Elbow Stiffness

Andrea Celli, Cheli Andrea, Prandini Mauro, and Luigi Pederzini

2.1 Anatomical Considerations

The elbow joint consists of the articulations of the distal humerus, proximal ulna, and proximal radius (Fig. 2.1). It is a complex structure serving as a mechanical link between hand, wrist, and shoulder. Its main function is to position the hand in space. Its impairment can cause significant disability in the activities of daily living.

2.1.1 Bone Anatomy

The humeral metaphysis is a triangular bone fragment that is extremely narrow on the sagittal plane. Its base forms the articular surface of the trochlea; the sides consist of a medial and a lateral column bordering a flatter central area and forming a 40–45° angle on the frontal plane. The columns are separated by the olecranon fossa posteriorly and the shallower radial fossa and

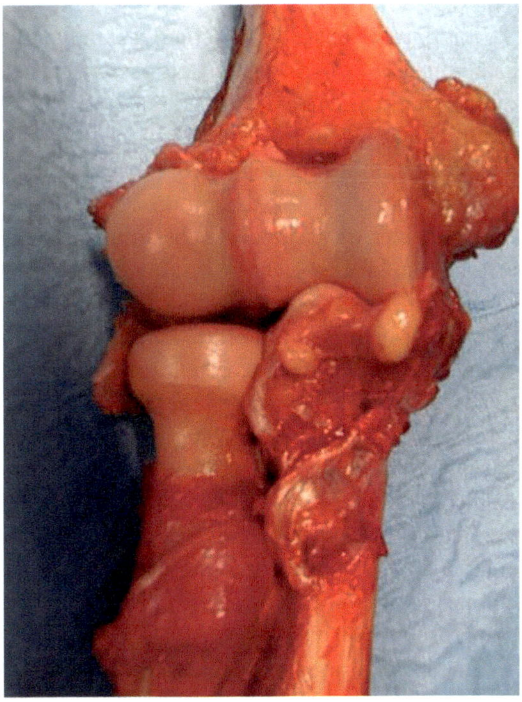

Fig. 2.1 The anatomical articular surface of the elbow joint is characterized by: (1) the intrinsic stability of the trochlea and coronoid process; (2) a high congruence between the concave radial head and the spherical capitulum; (3) the deep trochlear groove, which accommodates the prominent margin of the sigmoid notch; (4) the coronoid process, which is made more prominent by the 30° anterior tilt of the distal humerus; and (5) the height and congruence of the radial head with the lesser sigmoid notch, the capitulum, and the capitellotrochlear groove

A. Celli (✉)
Department of Orthopaedic and Traumatology Surgery, Shoulder and Elbow Unit, Hesperia Hospital, Modena, Italy

C. Andrea · P. Mauro
Department of Orthopaedic, Traumatology and Arthroscopic Surgeries, Nuovo Ospedale di Sassuolo, Modena, Italy

L. Pederzini
Department of Orthopedics, Hesperia Hospital, Modena, Italy

L. Pederzini et al. (eds.), *Stiffness of the Elbow, Wrist and Related Pathologies*,
https://doi.org/10.1007/978-3-031-81381-8_2

coronoid fossa anteriorly. A thin plate of cortical bone separates the olecranon fossa from the coronoid fossa (Fig. 2.2a, b).

From the lateral side of the distal humerus, the lateral epicondyle appears more anterior than the medial epicondyle and the radial column larger than the ulnar column.

The contours of the distal humerus are complex. In the lateral plane, the articular surfaces of the trochlea and capitellum show a forward angle of ca. 30° in relation to the long axis of the humeral shaft.

The elbow axis of motion in flexion and extension (rotation axis) is not a line passing through the midportion of the two epicondyles; rather, the anatomical flexion–extension axis passes through the geometrical center of the capitellum and of the trochlear sulcus. The plane of the sulcus is neither parallel to the long axis of the humerus nor perpendicular to the axis of the epicondyles.

The center of rotation can be found through external landmarks. London et al. [1] have used true lateral X-ray views to identify the elbow rotation axis, which is in the center of the three concentric arcs formed by the capitellum, the trochlear sulcus, and the medial facet of the trochlea.

The rotation axis of the distal humerus is usually tilted internally by 3–5° in relation to the plane of the epicondyles; it has a 4–8° valgus tilt in relation to the long axis of the humerus and is anterior to the humeral midline on a line that is collinear with the anterior cortex of the distal humerus.

The angle formed in the coronal plane by the longitudinal axes of the humerus and the ulna with the elbow extended (carrying angle) can only be assessed with the elbow fully extended. The normal carrying angle shows an interindividual variation of 10–15° in men and 15–20° in women, due partly to the oblique axis of the distal humerus and partly to the shape of the proximal ulna.

The relationship between the axis of the distal humeral medullary canal and the flexion–extension axis as defined by the geometrical center of the trochlea and the capitellum is called anterior offset and has major implications in the design and implantation of elbow prostheses.

The olecranon is a large, curved eminence that together with the proximal portion of the coronoid process forms the greater sigmoid notch of the ulna (Fig. 2.3a, b).

It is a deep depression that enables articulation with the trochlea. By allowing motion only in the anteroposterior plane, it provides joint stability. The cartilage on the greater sigmoid notch is usually discontinuous and forms two discrete articular facets, anterior and posterior. The articular facets of the olecranon and the coronoid process are separated by a cartilage-free area (bare area).

The greater sigmoid notch has a posterior angulation of 30°, matching the 30° anterior tilt of the distal articular surface of the humerus [2].

With respect to the greater sigmoid notch, the proximal ulnar shaft shows a proximal ulna dorsal angulation (PUDA) in the sagittal plane and a proximal ulna varus angulation in the frontal plane. In lateral view, the PUDA (4–5° [3] to 5–7°; range, 0–14°) is determined by measuring the intersection angle between lines tangent to the dorsal aspect of the olecranon and the dorsal margin of the ulnar shaft [4]. The mean distance

Fig. 2.2 (**a**) Two bone columns bordering a flatter central area are separated by the radial fossa and the coronoid fossa. The articular condyles of the distal humerus are the trochlea and the capitulum. The articular surface of the trochlea has a pulley-like shape and extends from the coronoid fossa to the posterior olecranon fossa. The medial lip is larger and more prominent than the lateral. A central groove oriented slightly laterally articulates with the olecranon notch. The capitulum is seen only from the anterior side of the distal humerus. It has a spheroid shape and articulates with the fovea of the radial head. The capitellotrochlear groove is covered with hyaline cartilage and is in permanent contact with the peripheral margin of the radial head. (**b**) The deep olecranon fossa separates the lateral and medial column. A thin plate of cortical bone separates the olecranon fossa posteriorly from the coronoid fossa anteriorly. The posterior aspect of the lateral column is flatter than that of the medial column, enabling easy application of precontoured plates on the posterolateral humerus. A key goal in the treatment of distal humeral fractures is to restore the shape and size of the olecranon fossa, trochlea, and olecranon and their relationships as well as anterior trochlea rotation, carefully avoiding malalignment of the lateral and medial column. The medial and lateral columns form a triangular, spool-shaped structure

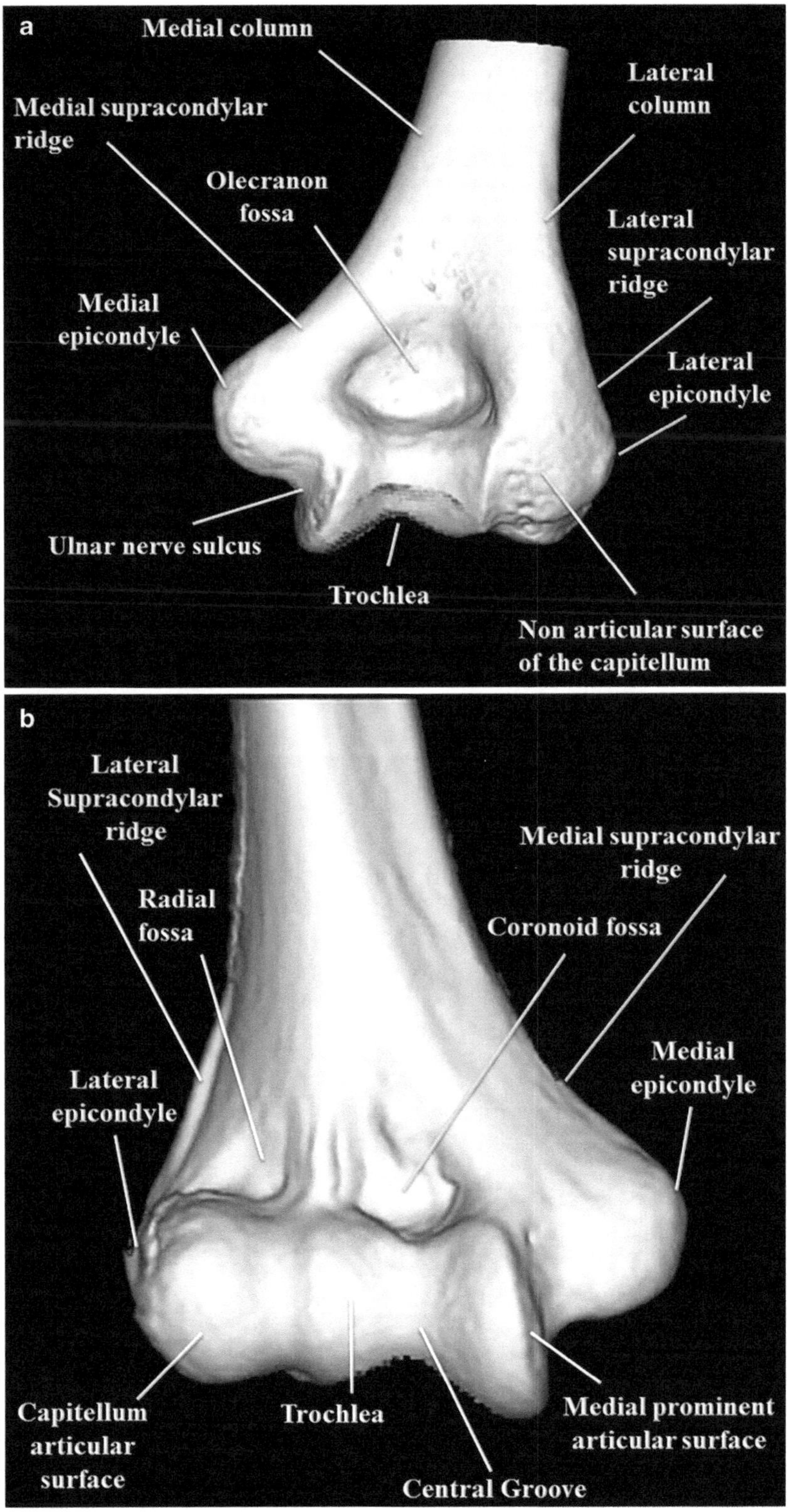
a
Medial column
Lateral column
Medial supracondylar ridge
Olecranon fossa
Lateral supracondylar ridge
Medial epicondyle
Lateral epicondyle
Ulnar nerve sulcus
Trochlea
Non articular surface of the capitellum
b
Lateral Supracondylar ridge
Medial supracondylar ridge
Radial fossa
Coronoid fossa
Medial epicondyle
Lateral epicondyle
Capitellum articular surface
Trochlea
Medial prominent articular surface
Central Groove

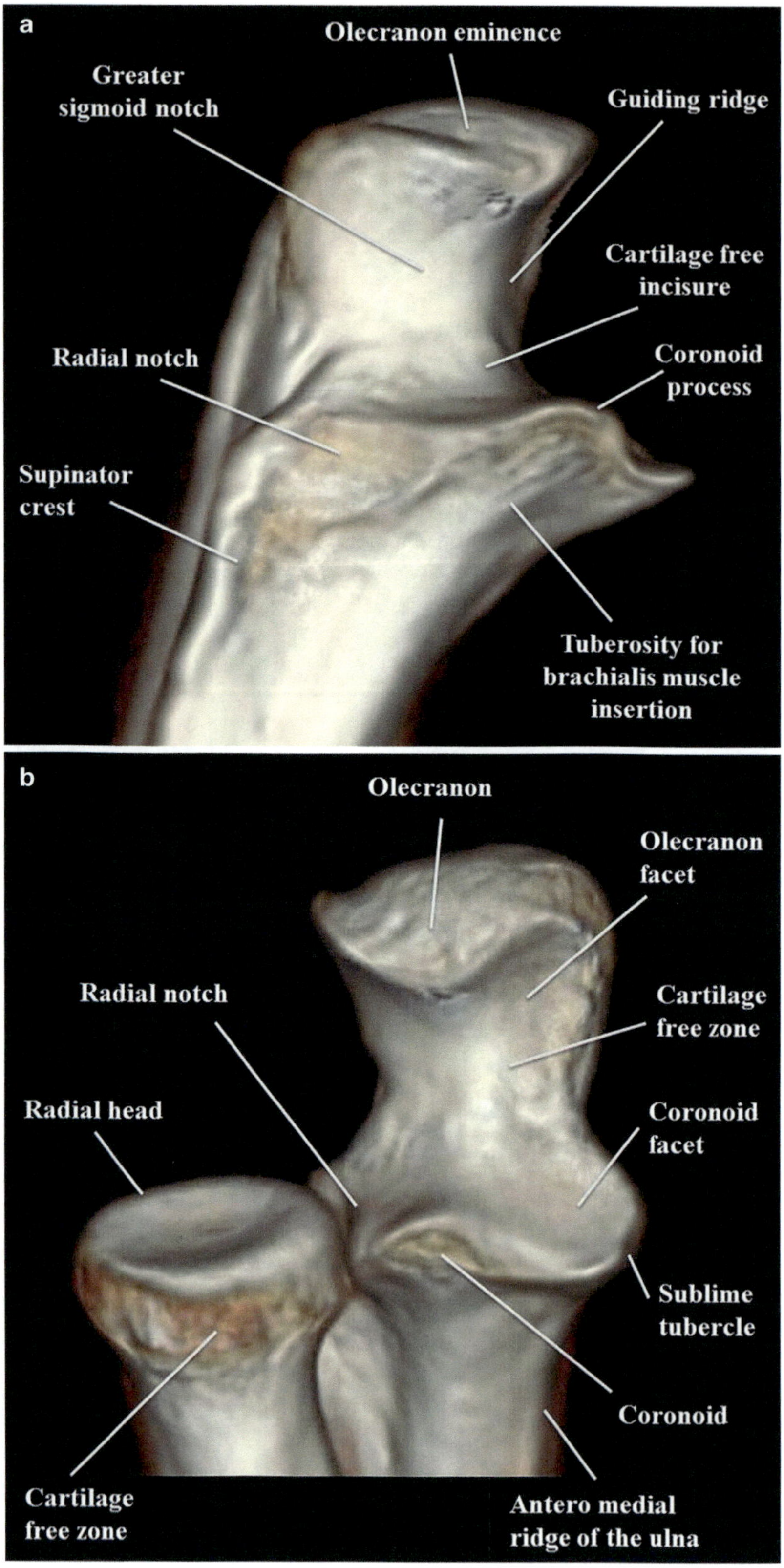

Fig. 2.3 (**a, b**) The olecranon and the coronoid process form the greater sigmoid notch of the ulna. The articular facets of the coronoid and the olecranon are linked by the cartilage-free area. The diameter of the medial flange of the coronoid facet is larger than that of the lateral flange. In surgical reductions of olecranon and coronoid fractures, it is crucial to preserve the full dimension of the greater sigmoid notch and the anatomical position of the facets in relation to the trochlea. Failure to do so may result in elbow stiffness or instability. The radial head articulates with the capitulum, forming the radiocapitellar joint, and with the lesser sigmoid notch of the proximal ulna, forming the proximal radioulnar joint. An important bony landmark is the insertion of the anterior bundle of the medial collateral ligament on the sublime tubercle, which is found on the medial border of the coronoid facet, at the proximal end of the anteromedial ridge of the ulna. The term "sublime" is due to the insertion of the flexor digitorum sublimis tendon (flexor digitorum superficialis)

from the olecranon tip to the apex of the PUDA is 47 mm [4].

The proximal end of the radius consists of the disk-shaped head, the neck, and the radial tuberosity (Fig. 2.3b). The head and part of the neck are intra-articular.

The radial head (RH) is a disk-shaped structure ca. 3.5 mm in thickness. It is not round but rather ovoid and is longer in the anteroposterior (ca. 2.5 cm) than in the coronal plane (ca. 2.2 cm).

A shallow proximal depression covered with hyaline cartilage on the RH articulates with the capitellum. Of the RH circumference, 250° articulate with the ulna, allowing for ca. 180° of pronation and supination. The remaining 120° are not covered with cartilage; they are those most prone to fracture and constitute the safe zone for the implantation of internal fixation devices [5].

The RH is eccentric relative to the longitudinal axis of the radius, with an offset angle of 15°.

2.2 Joint Stability

2.2.1 Elbow Stability in Flexion-Extension

Elbow stability is ensured by joint congruence and by static (capsuloligamentous) and dynamic (musculotendinous) constraints. Bone and soft-tissue structures contribute equally to intrinsic stability of the joint.

The primary static constraints are the medial collateral ligament (MCL) (Fig. 2.4a–d) and lateral collateral ligament (LCL) complex (Fig. 2.5a, b) and the humeroulnar joint; secondary constraints are the RH, the joint capsule, and the muscles that cross the elbow joint.

The coronoid process is a key contributor to elbow stability, ensuring varus stability and providing the main constraint against posterior forearm subluxation.

The olecranon also provides a major contribution to elbow stability. Its support to loadbearing depends on the amount of proximal ulna that remains after a fracture. Stability requires preservation of at least 30% of the articular surface of the ulna, since it also bears the insertion of the ulnar collateral ligament.

The elbow is supported by the MCL and LCL complex, which forms a fan-shaped thickening of the capsule on its medial and lateral aspects.

The MCLs consist of three bundles: anterior, posterior, and transverse.

The LCLs comprise several components: lateral radial collateral ligament, annular ligament, lateral ulnar collateral ligament, and accessory lateral collateral ligament, the latter being not consistently present.

The capsule origin is proximal to the radial and coronoid fossae and to the olecranon.

The capsule is attached distally to the anterior border of the coronoid process and the annular ligament and posteriorly to the articular margin of the sigmoid notch of the olecranon.

The forearm muscles, on the medial and lateral sides of the elbow, contribute to static and dynamic stability.

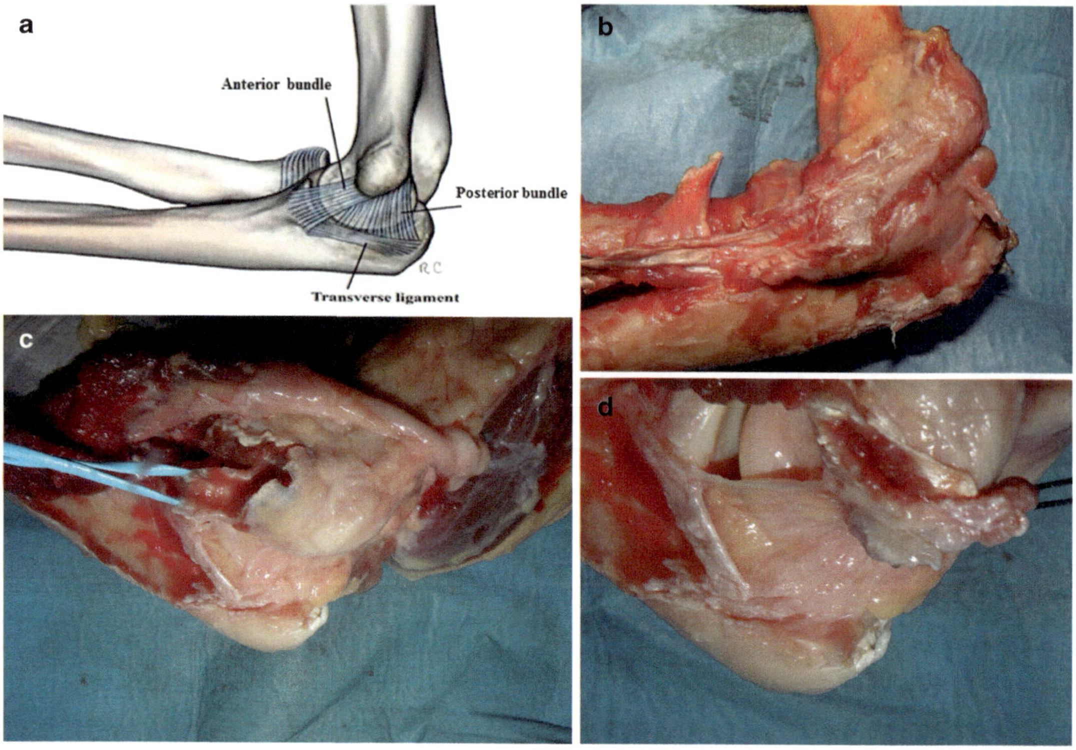

Fig. 2.4 The medial collateral ligament complex is made up of three components: the anterior and posterior bundles and the transverse ligament (**a**, **b**). The anterior and posterior bundles are tensed differentially by valgus loading through the arc of elbow flexion. The anterior bundle is most important in resistance from mid-flexion to full extension (**c**), whereas the posterior bundle plays a larger part in full joint flexion (**d**). The anterior bundle can be subdivided into an anterior and a posterior band. The anterior band provides the primary constraint to valgus load from 30° to 90° of flexion, whereas the posterior band becomes taut from 90° to 120° of flexion. The posterior band and posterior bundle provide the secondary and tertiary constraints. The transverse ligament appears to have no role in elbow stability

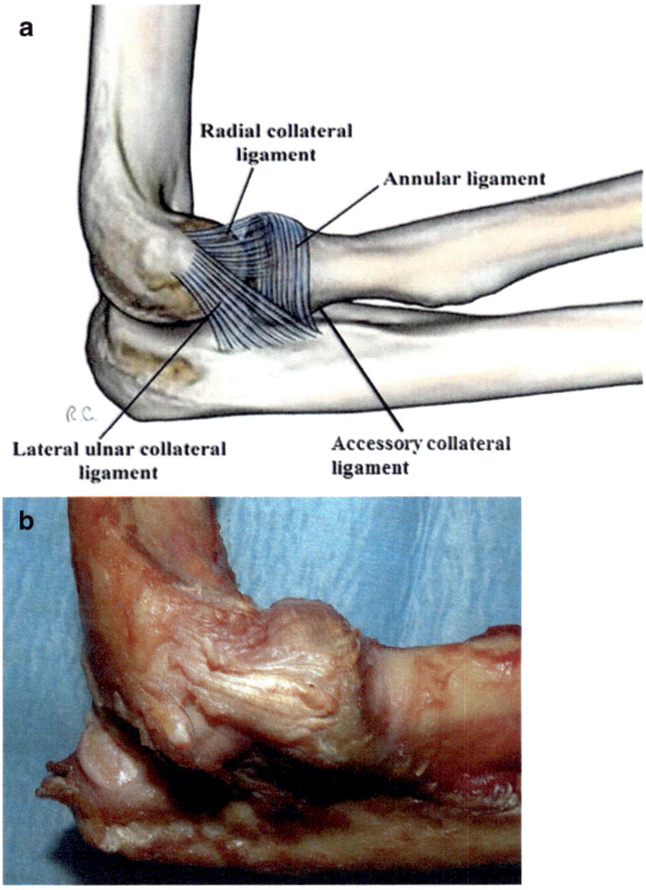

Fig. 2.5 (**a**, **b**) The major components of the lateral ligament complex are the lateral ulnar collateral ligament, the annular ligament, and the accessory lateral collateral ligament. The lateral ulnar collateral ligament is the key stabilizer involved in resistance to varus stress and in posterolateral stability. Its origin is close to the geometrical center of the elbow rotation axis in the center of the isometric point of the capitulum. The radial collateral ligament also plays an important part in posterolateral rotatory instability through its attachment to the annular ligament. The annular ligament encircles the radial head, attaching to the lesser sigmoid notch of the ulna, and plays a major role in preventing anterior and posterior radial head subluxation. The accessory lateral collateral ligament helps stabilize the annular ligament

2.3 Etiology of Elbow Stiffness

The preoperative assessment of a stiff elbow should identify the articular and periarticular tissues involved and, especially, determine the degree of preservation of the articular surfaces and osteoarticular congruence.

A logical surgical planning requires an extensive knowledge of the anatomical obstacles and associated lesions, namely:

- Periarticular soft-tissue contractures
- Osteoarticular incongruence

2.4 Periarticular Soft-Tissue Contractures

2.4.1 Skin Contracture

Severe skin burns, post-traumatic contracting wounds, and hypertrophic scars often cause skin retraction on the anterior surface of the elbow.

Full-thickness eschar excision can release the elbow, while the large exposed areas of the deep structures (especially the tendons) can be covered with skin grafts or local and regional island flaps.

In patients with burn injuries, an aggressive passive motion therapy is believed to contribute to the development of heterotopic ossification (HO) and should be avoided [6, 7], particularly in patients with an altered level of consciousness. This late painful and functionally limiting sequela of burn injuries is quite common in the elbow joint.

2.4.2 Contracture Due to Muscle Imbalance

Spastic flexion deformity of the elbow is often a sequela of cerebral vascular accidents in adults or of spastic hemiplegia in children. In patients with severe deformity, correction of joint flexion may be achieved by lengthening the biceps and brachial muscle tendons.

Neurological lesions (e.g., poliomyelitis or obstetrical palsy in children and brachial plexus lesion in adults) may involve chronic static paresis of the elbow. Paresis of the flexor muscles is often associated with extensor muscle contracture whereas contracture of the flexor muscles is associated with paresis of the elbow extensor muscles.

Before restoring elbow flexion and extension with muscle–tendon transfer, triceps or biceps tendon lengthening is required to recover the passive range of motion (ROM). Capsule release is often necessary, too.

2.4.3 Capsule and Ligament Contracture

The most common cause of extrinsic contracture without osteoarticular damage is simple elbow dislocation.

Josefsson [8] has described the relationship between joint stiffness and long immobilization after reduction. In a retrospective study, Melhoff et al. [9] found the relationship between length of immobilization and capsule contracture in patients without degenerative joint disease.

The soft-tissue structures surrounding the elbow joint react in a unique way after injury, inducing significant capsule, ligament, and muscle disruption.

Significant bleeding from the capsule and the highly vascularized brachialis muscle, which lies directly on the capsule, is seen in the first few hours after the trauma.

In the first few weeks, edema and early scar tissue formation are the main causes of stiffness.

In the absence of motion, capsule or ligament scar tissue often becomes organized. Tissue fibrosis and retraction lead to HO development in muscle or tendon. Early gentle motion helps to prevent elbow stiffness.

During development of elbow stiffness, the MCLs and LCLs, which are often injured, tend to contract and undergo a process of calcification.

In 110 dislocated elbows, Linscheid and Wheeler [10] described true HO in 4.5% and collateral ligament calcification in more than 25%.

Damage to the collateral ligaments is not frequently recognized until the onset of post-traumatic ossification at the humeroulnar insertion. Secondary shortening of the MCL can be the cause of significant elbow stiffness: a retracted MCL posterior band can induce flexion contracture greater than 60° whereas a tauter anterior part can induce extension contracture greater than 80°.

LCL scarring and retraction (with or without ossification) gradually reduce elbow flexion and extension and eventually lead to ankylosis, due to the fact that the LCLs (radial and ulnar band) are taut throughout flexion and extension [11].

2.5 Heterotopic Ossification

Para-articular ectopic ossification is a sequela of a traumatic event involving formation of highly organized bone, which replaces the surrounding injured soft tissue (Fig. 2.6a, b). Its etiology is still to be elucidated. After the trauma, in presence of bone morphogenic protein, mesenchymal cells and fibroblasts probably differentiate and proliferate into cartilage and osteoblasts [12, 13]. Direct trauma is the most frequent cause of HO, whose incidence is a function of trauma severity. Thompson and Garcia [14] found a 3% incidence

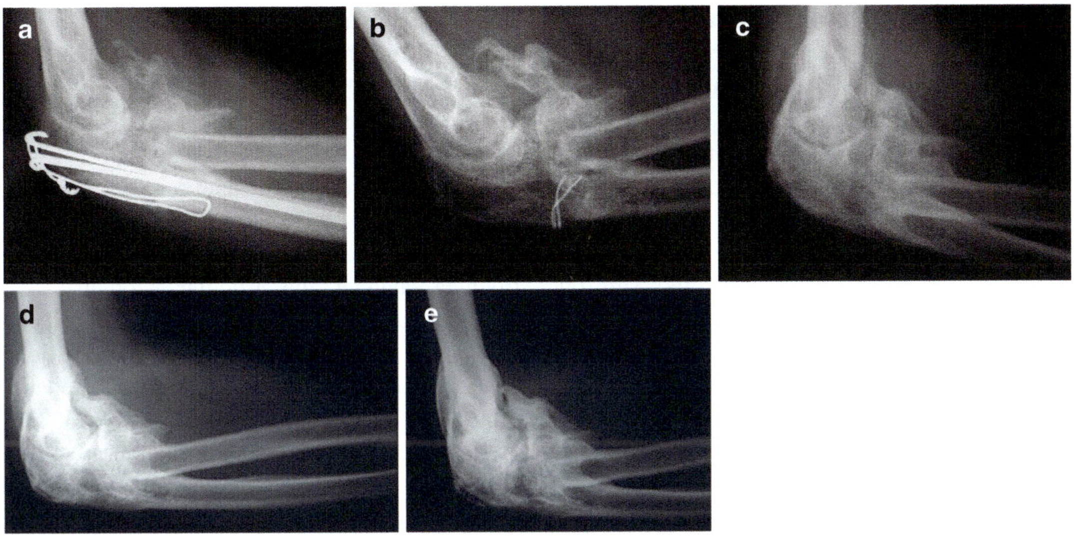

Fig. 2.6 (**a-e**) The heterotopic ossification is defined mature when linear trabeculation is present and the margin separating from the surrounding soft tissue with cortical borders

in simple dislocation and a 15–20% incidence in patients with complex instability and RH fracture.

Bromberg and Morrey [15] described a 9% HO incidence after delayed excision of the fractured RH. Patients with elbow trauma and central nervous system injury are more prone to HO development. In head-injured patients with elbow and forearm trauma, HO incidence has been reported to range from 76% [10] to 33% [16].

HO typically develops where the tissue is swollen and hyperemic. Its formation is hastened by the progressive loss of ROM associated with immobility or muscle contraction due to neurological lesions [17]. HO onset usually begins 2–3 weeks after surgery or the neurological insult, when aggressive manipulation is performed to avoid the progressive loss of joint motion.

Hastings and Graham [18] have proposed a radiographic and clinical classification of elbow HO:

- **Class I**: HO involving no functional limitation
- **Class II**: HO involving:
  - IIA, limited flexion–extension
  - IIB, limited pronation–supination
  - IIC, limited flexion–extension and pronation–supination
- **Class III**: ankylosis

Garland has identified two HO sites (anterior and posterior) [19], while Hastings and Graham [18] have described it in anterior, posterior, and lateral sites of the elbow joint. In each area any tissue can be involved and HO can arise from:

1. Anterior elbow:
   - Coronoid
   - Humeroulnar joint
   - Humeroradial joint
   - Peri-articular soft tissue such as capsule or brachial muscle
2. Posterior elbow:
   - Olecranon
   - Humeroulnar joint
   - Olecranon fossa
3. Lateral elbow:
   - MCLs
   - LCLs

2.6 Osteoarticular Incongruence

Inadequate reduction and internal fixation are frequent complications after joint fracture. Osteoarticular deformity due to mechanical limitations is often associated with loss of motion, capsular contracture, and HO.

The complex bone anatomy of the elbow joint must be restored in the coronal, sagittal, and horizontal planes. In the distal humerus, the medial and lateral columns form a triangular spool-shaped construct on the articular surface [20].

Fracture treatment aims to restore normal anatomical shape and relationships between:

- The size of the trochlea and the capitellum, which should be adequate to the size of the olecranon notch and to the proximal concavity of the RH
- The anatomical axis of the ulnotrochlear and radiocapitellar articulations in the sagittal, coronal, and transverse planes

The axis of the articular condyles in relation to the long axis of the humerus presents:

- A 30° anterior rotation in the sagittal plane
- A 5–7° internal rotation in the transverse plane
- A 6–8° valgus inclination in the frontal plane
- A 4–8° anterior offset of the flexion–extension axis (the distance between the flexion–extension axis and the long axis of the humerus).

In this way, the semilunar notch of the proximal ulna, which has a 30° posterior orientation, matches the trochlea. The medial column of the distal humerus diverges by about 45° from the sagittal axis and the lateral column by about 20°, projecting anteriorly and becoming the capitellar articular surface. Anatomical reconstruction of the column enables easy recovery of the correct position of the articular surfaces.

The main causes of elbow ROM reduction after articular fractures are:

- Malunion and non-union
- HO
- Contracture of periarticular soft tissues

2.7 Supracondylar and Intercondylar Fractures

2.7.1 Malunion

In the sagittal plane, anterior or posterior malalignment of the lateral column and capitellum with respect to the medial column and the trochlea changes the articular geometry. The alteration of the anatomical axis of elbow rotation is due to changes in the ulnotrochlear joint axis and to malalignment of the radiocapitellar joint.

In supracondylar fracture malunion, elbow stiffness is often due to the loss of anterior rotation of the articular condyles.

The loss of condyle anteversion (10–20°), is well tolerated and does not reduce elbow ROM; when it exceeds 30°, the elbow loses about 30–40° flexion (Fig. 2.7).

In the frontal plane, the loss of the elbow valgus tilt often induces cubitus varus deformity in children with limited elbow ROM; in particular, limited extension is due to olecranon impingement in the olecranon fossa. In these patients, secondary posterolateral rotatory instability can arise later [21]. Elbow stiffness can develop when displaced condylar fractures are not reduced. The common radiological aspect of unreduced condylar fractures is an inverted V-shaped angular deformity. The anatomical deformity of the trochlea implies a secondary loss of flexion–extension. In children, the condition is compatible with a full elbow ROM in adult age.

The exuberant callus of HO can occlude the coronoid or olecranon fossae, limiting elbow ROM.

2.7.2 Non-union

Supracondylar non-union is a rare complication, but this is a typical HO site in distal humeral fractures. Non-union is due to the failure to combine stable rigid fixation and early mobilization.

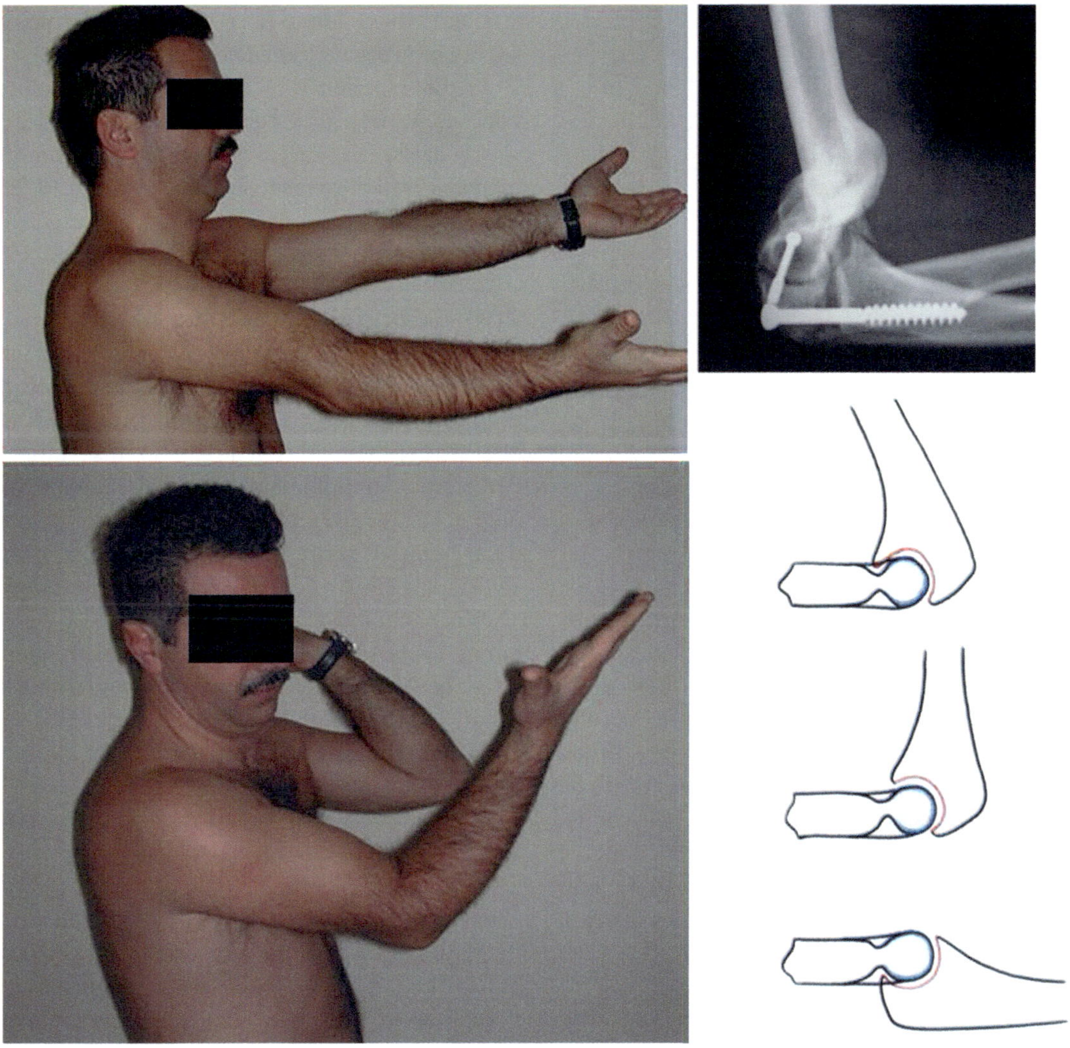

Fig. 2.7 The loss of the condyle anteversion, more than 30 degrees, is not tolerated and the elbow loses its flexion with over extension

2.8 Intra-articular Comminuted Fractures

2.8.1 Malunion

Failed repositioning of the articular bone fragments yields a distorted anatomy of the trochlea and capitellum. The humeral joint loses the congruent bone interfaces of the ulnotrochlear and radiocapitellar joints. Failure to restore trochlear anatomy and the relationship to the olecranon and coronoid surfaces involves significant disability.

Care must be taken not to reduce the size of the trochlea or alter the anatomical position of the capitellum because this may prevent proper seating of the articular surfaces of the olecranon and the RH (Fig. 2.8).

In comminuted fractures, bone is often missing or an articular fragment bone does not allow recovery of correct trochlear size and shape. In such cases, a cortico-cancellous bone graft or an interposition bicortical graft from the iliac crest can restore the intercondylar anatomical relationships.

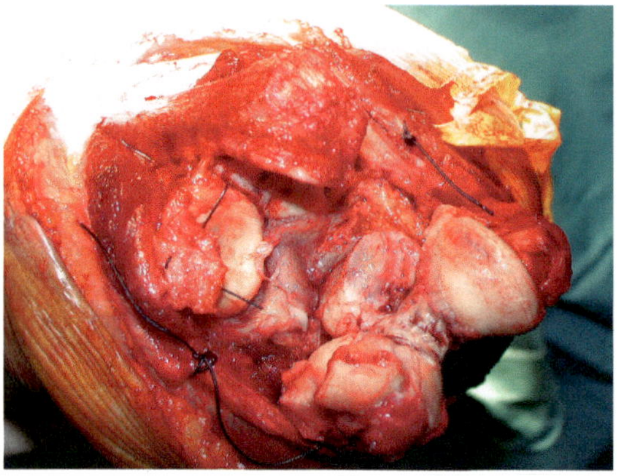

Fig. 2.8 The anatomical position of the capitellum and the correct size and shape of the trochlea must be recovered in the fracture of the distal humerus to prevent the proper seating of the articular surface of the olecranon and radial head

Malunion of the distal articular surfaces produces a mechanical obstacle to ulnotrochlear motion and a secondary limitation of flexion and extension. These patients are likely to develop osteoarthritis and more severe elbow stiffness and pain. In the postoperative assessment, the surgeon evaluates the anatomical state of the articular surfaces, because forced motion and manipulation under anesthesia can increase joint damage, soft-tissue fibrosis, or HO. In this way ROM is lost, not gained.

2.8.2 Non-union

Non-union is the result of fracture comminution or inappropriate initial management. In addition, the surgical trauma and the presence of intra-articular synovial fluid can compromise the blood supply of the bone fragments [22].

In the experience of the Mayo Clinic, most non-unions are extra-articular and only 7% lead to pseudarthrosis [23]. Patients often complain of pain and instability and very often present ROM loss [24].

2.9 Condylar Fractures

Malunion or non-union of one column can lead to elbow deformity. Displaced fractures of the lateral condyle may cause cubitus valgus deformity and ulnar nerve entrapment, whereas displaced fractures of the medial condyle produce cubitus varus deformity and a loss of ROM.

When condylar fracture malunion or non-union occur in children, the deformed adult elbow has often excellent function. These patients usually develop arthritis with pain and loss of motion in the sixth or seventh decade [25].

2.10 Capitellar Fractures

Capitellar malunion often depends on missed diagnosis of the fracture. Anteroposterior radiographs and low-quality lateral views often do not allow detecting the fracture when the small fragments lie in the upper part of the joint. Capitellar fractures in this non-anatomical position can lead to elbow stiffness at 90° of flexion due to RH impingement and capitellar malunion (Fig. 2.9).

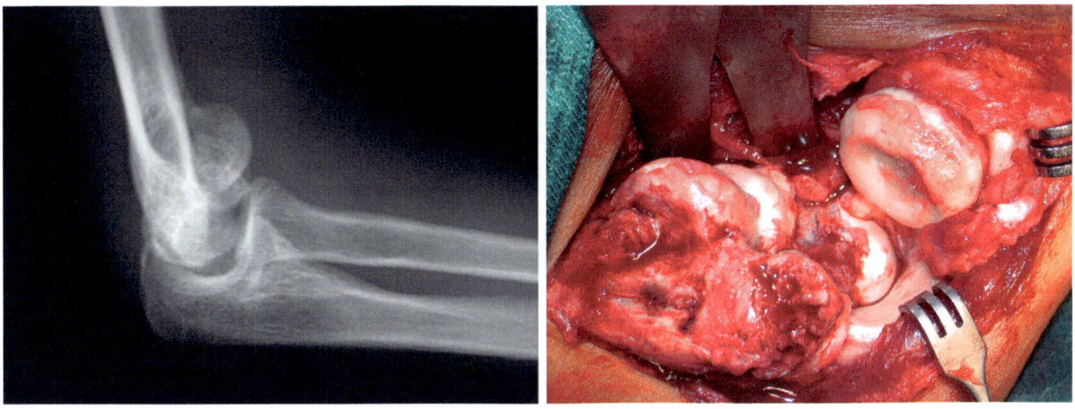

Fig. 2.9 The capitellum fracture can lead to an elbow stiffness for impingement of the radial head with the capitellum malunion

2.11 Olecranon Fractures

Elbow stiffness after surgical reduction and internal fixation is often caused by an inadequate understanding of the anatomy of the articular surface of the olecranon. After fracture reduction, the surgeon should evaluate the alterations in the shape and size of the articular anatomy and the presence of any bone impingement between olecranon and trochlea in flexion–extension.

In a different way, in comminuted fractures it is useful to set in line the posterior cortex of the ulna (length, size, and shape), whereas the articular cartilage often presents fragments that are difficult to set in a correct anatomical position, especially in the mid-portion of the sigmoid notch.

Reduction and internal fixation with K-wires and a tension-band reduce the olecranon–coronoid joint space, thus reducing olecranon–trochlea movement. The loss of elbow extension is often about 30° whereas flexion is rarely affected. This occurs in 50–75% of patients [26]. Inadequate fracture reduction is the main cause of post-traumatic degenerative arthritis, whose long-term incidence ranges from 2% [27] to 20% [28].

The main predisposing factors for olecranon non-union are inadequate fixation and early motion; the patient preserves a false motion between the bone ends with less pain. After surgical treatment of olecranon non-union with bone grafting and osteosynthesis of the avulsed fragment, postoperative active motion must be limited if the fragment is osteoporotic. When rigid internal fixation is achieved with a plate, the main complication is necrosis of the injured skin overlying the olecranon.

2.12 Radial Head Fracture

The most common complications of RH fractures are:

- Malunion or non-union of the displaced or comminuted fractures:
  - The distorted RH anatomy can lead to incongruence with the lesser sigmoid notch of the ulna and the capitellum (Fig. 2.10).
  - The angular deviation of the RH with subluxation of the proximal radioulnar joint will lead to a mechanical block.
- Heterotopic ossification:
  - It is frequent in case of serious injury of periarticular soft tissues or delayed treatment.

Patients with malunion, non-union, or HO lose forearm pronation–supination and elbow flexion–extension with pain and radiographic degenerative arthritis.

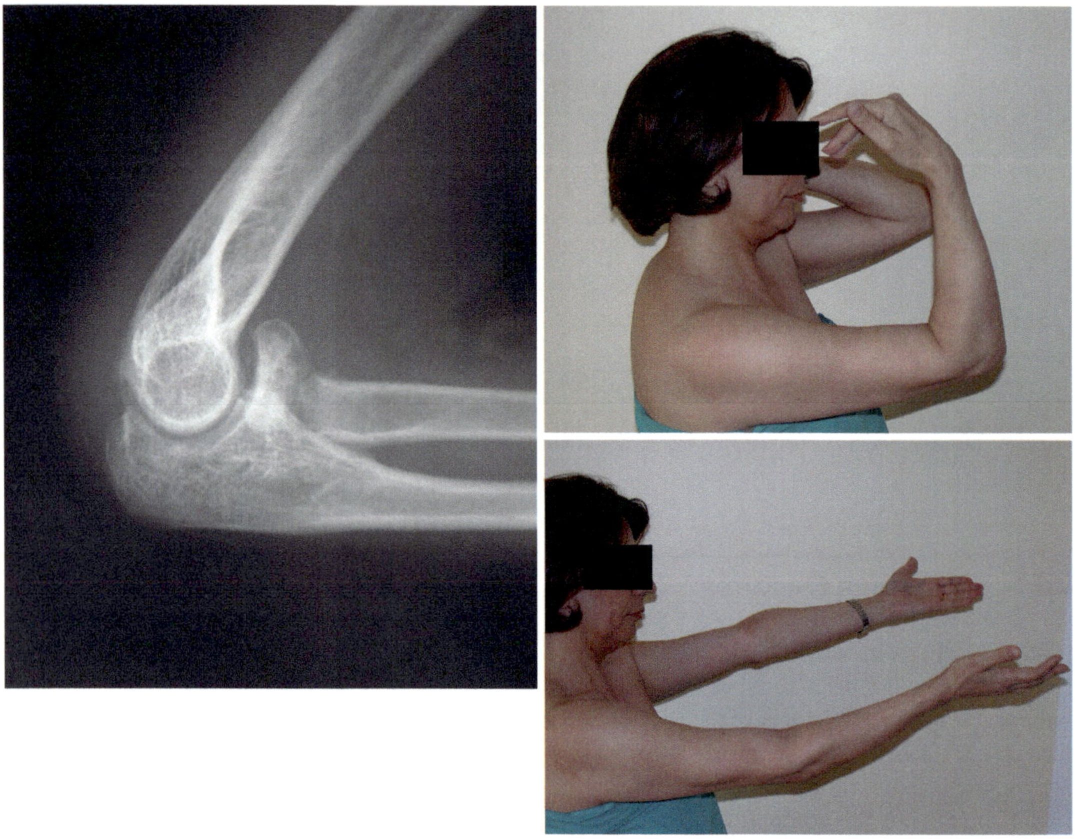

Fig. 2.10 The malunion or non-union of the radial head fractures can lead to an incongruity with the lesser sigmoid notch and with the capitellum producing a mechanical block

2.13 Classification of the Anatomical Damage

Morrey et al. [29] have classified post-traumatic stiffness into extrinsic, intrinsic, and mixed contracture.

2.13.1 Extrinsic Contracture

It involves contracture of soft tissues (posterior and anterior capsule and ligaments and muscles surrounding the joint). Another cause of extrinsic contracture is a bone bridge across the joint due to HO.

2.13.2 Intrinsic Contracture

It is found in patients with intra-articular fracture in presence of intra-articular adhesion due to articular cartilage damage or distorted articular surface anatomy.

2.13.3 Mixed Contracture

These patients present intrinsic and extrinsic contractures.

This classification clearly identifies the causes of elbow stiffness. However, it should be stressed that:

- Extrinsic contracture can lead to intra-articular adhesion or secondary osteoarthritis.
- Intrinsic contracture is always associated with extrinsic contracture.

In the preoperative clinical assessment, we know that stiff elbow always involves capsule contracture and that the combination of two major factors can modify patient prognosis and surgical management:

1. Presence of HO
2. State of the bone joint anatomy

Based on these considerations, after comparing the preoperative clinical diagnosis and the intraoperative anatomopathological findings we propose a classification of three types of elbow stiffness:

Type 1. Contracture of the capsular ligaments and periarticular muscle–tendons with preserved osteoarticular anatomy and absence of HO.

Type 2. Soft-tissue contracture associated with HO without osteoarticular damage. In this type, "HO is surgically more demanding than the soft-tissue contracture" [29].

Type 3. Soft-tissue contracture with or without HO associated with osteoarticular damage. The joint loses articular surface congruence and the bone is distorted such as in:

(a) Malunion or non-union of intra-articular fractures
(b) Chronic unreduced subluxation

In this type, "the articular surface incongruence and articular bone distortion is surgically more demanding than HO or tissue contracture" [29].

References

1. London ST. Kinematics of the elbow. J Bone Joint Surg Am. 1981;63:529–32.
2. Shiba R, Sorhie C, Sin DW, Bryout T. Geometry of the humeral ulnar joint. J Orthop Res. 1988;6:897–906.
3. Grechenig W, Clement H, Pichler W, Tesch NP, Windisch G. The influence of lateral and anterior angulation of the proximal ulna and the treatment of a Monteggia fracture: an anatomical cadaver study. J Bone Joint Surg Br. 2007;89:836–8.
4. Rouleau DM, Faber KJ, Athwal GS. The proximal ulna dorsal angulation: a radiographic study. J Shoulder Elbow Surg. 2010;19:26–30.
5. Smith GR, Hotchkiss RN. Radial head and neck fractures: anatomic guidelines for proper placement of internal fixation. J Shoulder Elbow Surg. 1996;5:113–7.
6. Demling RH, Lalonde C. Rehabilitation and wound remodelling. In: Burn trauma. New York: Thieme; 1989. p. 209–13.
7. Peterson SL, Mani MM, Crawford CM, et al. Post burn heterotopic ossification: in sights for management decision making. J Trauma. 1989;29:365–9.
8. Josefsson PO, Johnell O, Gentz CF. Long term sequelae of simple dislocation of the elbow. J Bone Joint Surg. 1984;66A:927–30.
9. Mehlhoff TL, Noble PL, Bennet JB, et al. Simple dislocation of the elbow in the adults. Results after closed treatment. J Bone Joint Surg. 1988;70A:244–9.
10. Linscheid RL, Wheelee DK. Elbow dislocation. JAMA. 1965;184:171.
11. Joseffson PO, Gentz CF, Johnell O, et al. Surgical versus nonsurgical treatment of ligamentous injuries following dislocation of the elbow joint: a prospective randomized study. J Bone Joint Surg. 1987;69A:605–8.
12. Buring K. On the origin of cells in heterotopic bone formation. Clin Orthop. 1975;110:293.
13. Urist MR, De Longo RJ, Finerman S. Bone cells differentiation and growth factors. Science. 1989;220:680.
14. Thompson HC III, Garcia A. Myositis ossificans: aftermath of elbow injuries. Clin Orthop. 1967;50:129.
15. Bromberg MA, Morrey BF. Results of delayed excision of the radial head after fracture. J Bone Joint Surg. 1973;55A:1629.
16. Sazbon L, Najenson T, et al. Widespread periarticular new-bone formation in long term comatose patients. J Bone Joint Surg. 1981;63-B:120.
17. Garland DE, Dowling V. Forearm fractures in the head-injured adult. Clin Orthop. 1983;176:190.
18. Hastings H II, Graham TJ. The classification and treatment of heterotopic ossification about the elbow and forearm. Hand Clin. 1994;10:417–37.
19. Garland DE, Blum C, Waters RL. Periarticular heterotopic ossification in head injured adults: incidence and location. J Bone Joint Surg. 1985;67A:1261.
20. Jupiter JB. Complex fractures of the distal part of the humerus and associated complications. J Bone Joint Surg. 1994;76-A:1252–64.
21. O'Driscoll SW, Morrey BF, Karinek S, et al. Elbow subluxation and dislocation: a spectrum of instability. Clin Orthop. 1992;74A:1235–41.
22. Jupiter JB, Goodmann LJ. The management of complex distal humerus non unions in the elderly by elbow capsulotomy, triple platting and ulnar nerve neurolysis. J Shoulder Elbow Surg. 1992;1:37.
23. Bryan RS, Bickel WH. "T" condylar fractures of the distal humerus. J Trauma. 1971;11:830.

24. Ackerman G, Jupiter JB. Non union of fractures of the distal end of the humerus. J Bone Joint Surg. 1988;70A:75.
25. Kolenak A. Ununited fracture of the lateral condyle of the humerus. A 50 years follow-up. Clin Orthop. 1977;124:181.
26. Heldsworth BJ, Mossad MM. Elbow function following tension band fixation of displaced fractures of the olecranon. Injury. 1984;16:182–7.
27. Helm RH, Hornshy R, Miller SWM. The complication of surgical treatment of displaced fractures of the olecranon. Injury. 1987;18:48–50.
28. Kiviluoto O, Santavirta S. Fractures of the olecranon. Acta Orthop Scand. 1978;49:28–31.
29. Morrey BF. Posttraumatic contracture of the elbow. J. Bone Joint Surg. 1990;72A:601–18.

Physical Examination of the Stiff Elbow

3

Victor Greco, Alexus M. Cooper, Taylor R. Wood, and Benjamin R. Graves

3.1 Background

Elbow stiffness is a relatively common condition that may affect patients of all ages and can result from a multitude of instigating events. Additionally, elbow stiffness can impact any or all of the four directions of movement of the elbow. For example, the elbow contractures seen with the congenital condition arthrogryposis produce a characteristic fixed extension deformity, whereas the elbow arthritis that follows an intra-articular fracture may produce a block to terminal flexion and/or extension. Regardless of etiology, the examination of the stiff elbow requires careful evaluation for optimal planning and treatment.

3.1.1 Anatomy of the Elbow

The brachium and forearm join to form the elbow joint, which is made up of articulations between the humerus, ulna, and radius bones. These three bones adjoin to form the ulnohumeral, radiocapitellar, and proximal radioulnar (PRUJ) joints of the elbow. The elbow joint is relatively complex due to the interconnections of three bones to produce flexion, extension, and forearm rotation. The elbow is a highly constrained joint with static and dynamic stabilization, which makes it prone to stiffness. Thorough knowledge of the elbow's complex anatomy is essential when performing an effective physical examination of the stiff elbow, and when combined with a detailed patient history, helps guide the clinician toward an appropriate plan for treatment.

The three articulations of the elbow joint are as follows: (1) the ulnohumeral joint, which forms where the trochlear groove of the proximal ulna meets the trochlea of the medial distal humerus; (2) the radiocapitellar joint, which forms where the articulating disk of the proximal radius (the radial head) meets the capitellum of the lateral distal humerus; and (3) the proximal radioulnar joint (PRUJ), which forms where the radial head and sigmoid notch of the proximal ulna meet. The PRUJ and radiocapitellar joints allow for approximately 180 degrees of forearm rotation, and the radiocapitellar joint and ulnohumeral joints allow for elbow flexion and extension in the sagittal plane [1–3]. The articular congruency of the radius, ulna, and humerus bones imparts an inherent stability to the elbow joint in flexion and extension in the sagittal plane; however, stability in the coronal plane requires both static and dynamic contributions from collateral ligaments and muscle/tendon units that cross the elbow, respectively.

Immediately surrounding the articulating bones that make up the elbow joint is the joint

V. Greco · A. M. Cooper · T. R. Wood
B. R. Graves (✉)
Department of Orthopaedic Surgery, Atrium Wake Forest Baptist Health, Winston Salem, NC, USA

L. Pederzini et al. (eds.), *Stiffness of the Elbow, Wrist and Related Pathologies*,
https://doi.org/10.1007/978-3-031-81381-8_3

capsule. Lined by synovial cells, the joint capsule produces the lubricating and nourishing synovial fluid contained within the joint. The joint capsule is thin anteriorly, but provides some contribution to varus–valgus stability during elbow extension [4].

Thickenings in the capsule make up the primary static ligamentous restraints to varus and valgus forces across the elbow. As the capsule is incorporated into the collateral ligaments of the medial and lateral elbow, the medial ulnar collateral ligament (MUCL) and lateral collateral ligament (LCL) are formed [4]. Spanning from the medial epicondyle of the humerus to the sublime tubercle of the medial ulna is the medial ulnar collateral ligament (MUCL), which contains distinct anterior, posterior, and transverse bands. The posterior band is thin and does not play a major role in stress resistance [4]. The transverse band is located just anterior to the posterior band and is often difficult to discern from the capsule [4]. The anterior band is the most important portion of the MUCL for resistance to valgus stress across the elbow [2–4].

The lateral collateral ligament (LCL) originates from the lateral epicondyle of the humerus and inserts onto the supinator crest of the lateral ulna. The radial collateral ligament (RCL) complex, also known as the lateral collateral ligament, has three components as well: the radial collateral ligament "proper," the lateral ulnar collateral ligament (LUCL), and the annular ligament [2, 3]. The annular ligament and the radial collateral ligament provide stability to forearm rotation through stabilization of the PRUJ and the radiocapitellar joint, with the radial collateral ligament proper contributing to a lesser degree [2, 4]. The LUCL is an important stabilizer of the lateral elbow, helping to resist posterolateral rotatory and varus stresses across the elbow [2–4].

Dynamic stability comes from the muscles that control active elbow range of motion (ROM), which belong to one of the four quadrants: anterior, lateral, medial, and posterior [2, 3]. Anteriorly, the distal tendon of the biceps brachii inserts onto the radial tuberosity. Just posterior to the biceps brachii, the broad and strong brachialis is found adjacent to the anterior joint capsule and inserts on the cubital tuberosity of the proximal ulna [2, 4]. The muscle group that originates laterally is termed the common extensor tendon and is made up of wrist and digit extensors. This muscle group includes the extensor carpi radialis longus (ECRL), extensor carpi radialis brevis (ECRB), extensor digitorum communis (EDC), and extensor carpi ulnaris (ECU) [2, 4]. Medially, the flexor/pronator mass is made up of the muscles and tendons that produce wrist/digit flexion and forearm pronation, and is comprised of the pronator teres, flexor carpi radialis (FCR), palmaris longus, flexor carpi ulnaris (FCU), and flexor digitorum superficialis (FDS), all originating from the medial epicondyle of the humerus [2, 4]. The triceps brachii is the only posterior muscle group and inserts on the olecranon process of the ulna and the anconeus muscle [2, 4]. Additionally, the supinator muscle attaches to the lateral supracondylar ridge near the triceps brachii [2].

The three main motor/sensory nerves that cross the elbow are the ulnar, median, and radial nerves. The ulnar nerve is located anterior and medial to the medial head of triceps and posterior to the medial humeral epicondyle within the cubital tunnel [2, 4]. Osborne's fascia forms the roof of the cubital tunnel and continues distally with the arcuate ligament to hold the ulnar nerve in place during elbow flexion and extension. After exiting the cubital tunnel, the ulnar nerve travels between the humeral and ulnar heads of the FCU distally [2, 4]. At the level of the elbow, the radial nerve travels laterally between the brachialis and brachioradialis muscles before it passes anteriorly over the radiocapitellar joint [2, 4]. Just distal to the joint, it divides into the posterior interosseous nerve (PIN), which provides motor innervation to the wrist and digit extensors, and the superficial radial nerve, which provides sensation to the dorsal–radial wrist and hand [3]. Proximal to the elbow joint, the median nerve follows the fascial plane between the biceps brachii and brachialis muscles, and distally the nerve is found in the plane between the pronator teres and brachialis, perforating the two heads of the pronator teres on its way to the hand [4].

3.1.2 Normal Range of Motion of the Elbow

There are two degrees of freedom within the elbow, which produce four vectors of movement: flexion, extension, pronation, and supination [6]. Normal range of motion of the elbow is approximately 0–145° of flexion/extension and 90–90° of pronation/supination [5]. To have an elbow that functions adequately for day-to-day life, one needs to have approximately 30–130° flexion and 50° of both pronation and supination [2, 6].

3.2 Etiologies of the Stiff Elbow

An elbow is considered to be "stiff" with any loss of range of motion greater than 30° of extension and less than 120° in flexion [1, 6, 7]. Thickening of soft tissues, especially of the elbow joint capsule, may produce a loss of arc of motion due to inflammatory cytokines and fibroblast infiltration that produce a disorganized cellular matrix [6, 8, 9]. Compared to elbows without contracture, it has been shown that in stiff elbows there is an increase in collagen cross-linking leading to decreased proteoglycans and water, all of which have been associated with changes in transforming growth factor beta (TGF-b) levels [6, 10].

Contracture etiology is categorized into intrinsic, extrinsic, or mixed. Intrinsic contracture may result from intra-articular pathology, including joint surface incongruity, osteophytes, synovitis, joint capsule stiffness, and/or ligamentous contracture. Extrinsic contractures are produced by extra-articular causes, which may include stiffness or other abnormalities of the muscles, tendons, fascia, or skin that cross the elbow joint [5, 11].

Causes of elbow stiffness can be traumatic and/or atraumatic, congenital or acquired. Examples of congenital etiologies of elbow stiffness are arthrogryposis or congenital dislocation of the radial head [1]. Atraumatic, acquired etiologies of elbow stiffness can include osteoarthritis, inflammatory arthritis, and post-septic arthritis that lead to degeneration of the articular surface, causing pain and eventual stiffness [1]. Osteophyte formation, as seen in osteoarthritis, can decrease elbow range of motion as well through mechanical blockade, typically at terminal elbow flexion and/or extension [1].

Traumatic causes of elbow stiffness include burns, fractures, nervous system pathology, heterotopic ossification (HO), or myositis ossificans [6]. Burns can decrease the elasticity of the skin, therefore impeding mobility [1]. Fractures and/or dislocations of any or all of the three articulations of the elbow can alter the articular architecture of the elbow, leading to decreased range of motion [1, 9]. For example, in the normal elbow the distal humerus is anteriorly translated with respect to the shaft, creating a 30–40° angle between the central humeral axis and articular segment [5, 9]. If this angle is altered, there is less room for the coronoid and soft tissues during flexion [5]. The coronoid and olecranon fossae can also be disrupted due to malunion, fibrosis, implant impedance after surgical intervention, myositis, or callous formation, which would limit flexion and extension [5]. If the articular congruency of the PRUJ is altered, pronation and supination may be limited [5]. Maximal extension can be limited by the impaction of the olecranon into the fossa's anterior capsule and ligaments [2, 3]. Maximal flexion can be limited by anterior muscle bulk or by the impaction of the radial head and coronoid process into their respective fossae [2, 3]. Tight flexor muscles and a tight triceps can also limit maximal extension or flexion, respectively [2, 3]. Additionally, trauma can lead to osteochondral defects and eventual osteophyte formation that prevents smooth motion or a mechanical block at the articular surface, especially if associated with loose body [1, 9]. In the acute phase of trauma, it has been shown that there are increased myofibroblasts that are highly contractible as well as increased extracellular matrix that can lead to soft tissue contracture; however, this pathology is not seen in chronically stiff elbows [9]. Increased alpha smooth muscle actin and higher joint capsule matrix turnover may also play roles in the lack of ROM in the post-traumatic elbow [1, 12].

Heterotopic ossification (HO) is the abnormal formation of lamellar bone in non-skeletal tissue, often occurring after trauma, and occurs when pluripotent mesenchymal cells differentiate into osteoblasts to produce bone typically in muscle tissue [9]. This process is typically seen 2–12 weeks following a traumatic event or even after surgical intervention in the elbow, as it produces a mechanical block to joint motion [1, 9]. Head injury patients have a higher incidence of HO, which is thought to be related to increased circulation of osteoblastic growth factors after trauma [1].

3.3 Physical Exam

Physical examination of the stiff elbow begins with a thorough patient history and a detailed visual inspection with comparison to the unaffected side. A general physical examination of the elbow evaluating the skin, nerves, and myotendinous and bony anatomy is then performed. Lastly, multiple conditions may produce a painful and stiff elbow. As such, specific special examination maneuvers should be employed to help aid in diagnosis of these conditions and are detailed in this section.

3.3.1 History

Obtaining a thorough history is paramount to understand the acute and/or chronic changes that lead to the development of stiffness in the elbow for a particular patient. Key information is gathered by asking specific questions regarding a history of congenital musculoskeletal deformity/disorders, autoimmune/inflammatory disease, trauma, associated symptoms, and overall timeline of events preceding the development of a stiff elbow [1]. History of other comorbid conditions such as prior surgical/non-surgical treatment, infection, hemarthrosis, or spasticity should also be obtained [1]. Failure to ask these questions of patients and/or caregivers may lead to an incorrect diagnosis and a low likelihood of improved symptoms. In addition, an understanding of the patient's current vocational and recreational requirements is critical for establishing achievable treatment goals and realistic patient expectations.

3.3.2 Inspection

The affected elbow should be visually inspected for readily observable factors that may be contributing to limited elbow range of motion including wounds and/or scars from current or prior trauma, burns, or surgical intervention [1, 13]. In the case of unilateral elbow stiffness, the contralateral elbow should be inspected to establish a "baseline" for a particular patient.

Sweat and hair patterns of the skin of the upper extremity should be inspected carefully. Hand temperature and skin tone differences may be indicators of underlying complex regional pain syndrome (CRPS), which would likely produce stiffness and pain in the forearm and hand as well as in the elbow [14, 15]. CRPS is most common in middle-aged women, especially after trauma to the affected area, and the upper extremity is most often affected with distal extremity being more common than proximal. Signs and symptoms of CRPS, including hyperesthesia, allodynia, skin color/temperature asymmetry, edema, sweating asymmetry, weakness, tremor, dystonia, and/or trophic changes, should be documented carefully [14]. As listed in the Budapest Criteria for CRPS (Table 3.1), if all four criteria are met, a diagnosis of CRPS is made based on these signs and symptoms [14].

3.3.3 Range of Motion

A thorough examination of the elbow should begin with an examination of the joints proximal and distal, which includes the ipsilateral shoulder and wrist. Abnormalities in either or both of these joints may produce abnormal elbow mechanics and may affect elbow range of motion. Subsequently, examination of the stiff elbow should include comparison to the unaffected, normal elbow if possible.

Table 3.1 Budapest Criteria for Complex Regional Pain Syndrome (CRPS): at least all four criteria must be met in order to establish a diagnosis

Criteria	Description			
1	Continuous pain disproportionate to inciting event			
2	At least one symptom in greater than or equal to three in the following categories:			
	Sensory	Vasomotor	Sudomotor/edema	Motor/trophic
	Hyperesthesia, allodynia	Asymmetric temperature/ skin color changes	Asymmetric edema/sweating	Decreased range of motion, weakness, tremor, dystonia, and trophic changes to skin, nails, and hair
3	At least one sign present in greater than or equal to two of the following:			
	Sensory	Vasomotor	Sudomotor/edema	Motor/trophic
	Hyperalgesia ± allodynia	Evidence of asymmetric temperature ± skin color changes	Evidence of asymmetric edema/ sweating	Evidence of decreased range of motion, weakness, tremor, dystonia, and trophic changes to skin, nails, and hair
4	Absence of another diagnosis			

Reproduced with permission from: Harden et al. [38]

The elbow functions primarily as a loose hinge joint with flexion and extension occurring at the articulation of the radiocapitellar joint and ulnocapitellar joints [13]. Under normal circumstances, a patient should be able to touch the back of their head without flexing their neck to accommodate; however, this action can be affected by stiffness of the glenohumeral joint. It is helpful to document if the patient is able to touch the back of their head, touch their ear, and touch their mouth as this can help establish reasonable patient expectations for postoperative range of motion gains. An arc of elbow flexion/extension of 100° (from 30° to 130°) is required for most daily activities [7]. Ideally, patients should be able to range from 0–10° of hyperextension to 145° of flexion. Careful scrutiny of a patient's range of motion through flexion and extension is important to assess and document given that a loss of 50° in the arc of motion may lead to an 80% loss of function [7]. Stiffness in pronation and supination can greatly affect daily function and can be challenging to treat as it may include the wrist and elbow joint as well as the interosseous membrane of the forearm. The normal range of forearm rotation is 180° with pronation of 80–90° and supination of approximately 90° [13]. Goniometric measurement may be used to accurately and reproducibly quantify range of motion measurements in these planes [16].

There are multiple annotation styles commonly employed to denote the arc of motion of the elbow. Regardless of how motion is documented, a consistent system that includes maximum elbow flexion, extension, pronation, and supination should be employed. The Authors' preferred annotation style is captured by the acronym FEPS, which stands for Flexion, Extension, Pronation, and Supination. The numerical value assigned to flexion and extension is based on the right angle formed when the elbow is flexed to 90°. Flexion is documented as the maximum angle achieved while bending (e.g., 140°), and extension is documented as the maximum angle achieved by straightening the elbow (e.g., 0°). An elbow that extends to neutral would be denoted as 0, whereas an elbow that hyperextends 10° would be documented as +10°. As shown in Fig. 3.1, the patient flexes to 140° and lacks 35° of terminal extension, which would be documented as 140/35. Pronation and supination are recorded from neutral forearm rotation, and a typical forearm rotation ranges from 90–95° of pronation to 85–90° of supination (Fig. 3.2). Using the FEPS annotation acronym, the patient in Fig. 3.1 would have elbow range of motion documented as 140/35/90/85. Comparison to the unaffected limb is strongly recommended to establish a relative baseline for the patient (Fig. 3.3).

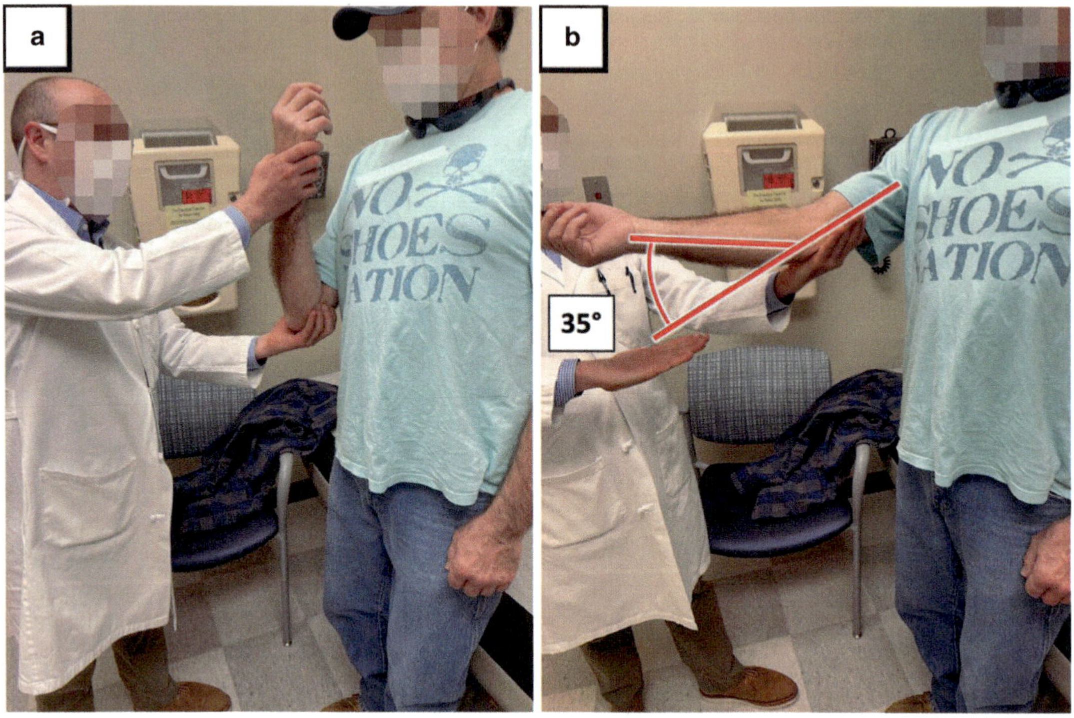

Fig. 3.1 Examining a patient's elbow flexion (**a**), and extension (**b**). Note the 35 lack of terminal extension

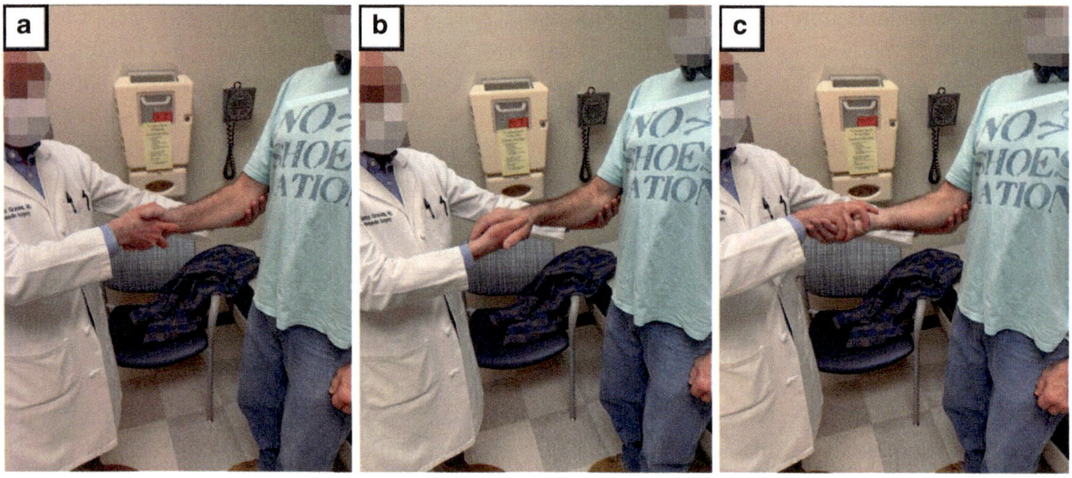

Fig. 3.2 Examining a patient's forearm rotation, starting from neutral (**a**), maximum pronation (**b**), and maximum supination (**c**)

3.3.4 Carrying Angle

It is important to document the carrying angle of the elbow, also termed the varus/valgus angle, as this can indicate the presence of congenital/developmental dysplasia and/or remote trauma, including chronic dislocation and malunion. The carrying angle of the elbow is the angle made between lines drawn through the median axis of the arm and the median axis of the fore-

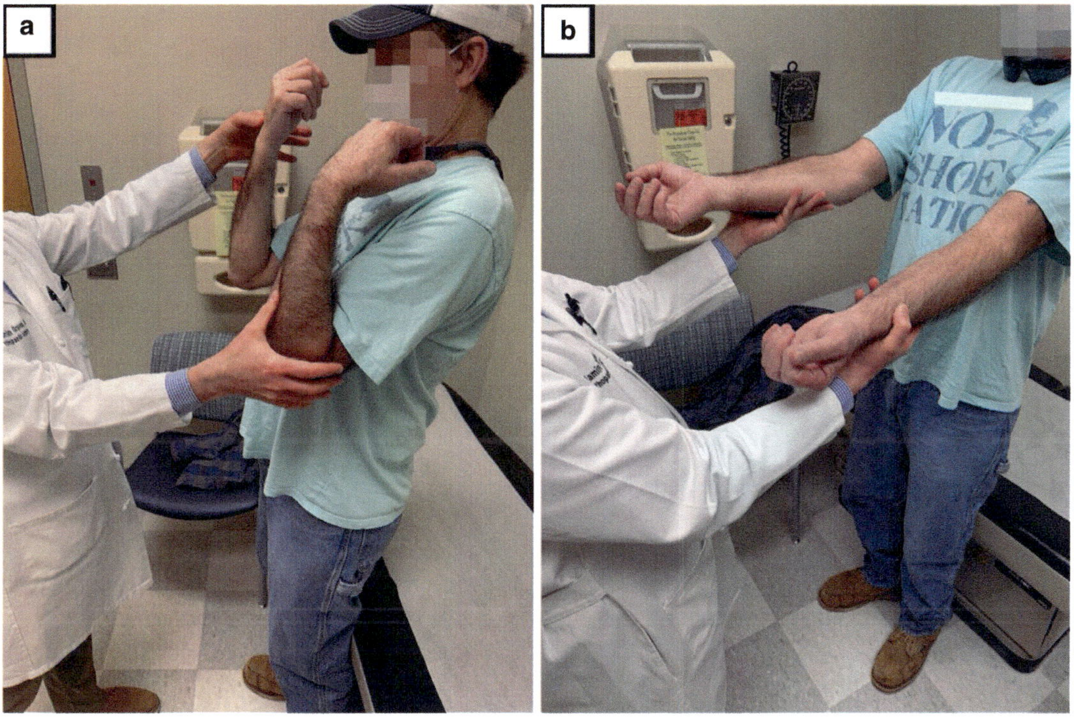

Fig. 3.3 Comparing a stiff elbow with the normal, unaffected side will help establish a baseline in flexion (**a**), and extension (**b**). Note that this patient's right elbow lacks the deep flexion and terminal extension when compared to his left elbow

arm in full extension and supination [17]. In *Homo sapiens*, the carrying angle has been theorized to accommodate clearance of the hips with the forearms while walking [18, 19]. Assessment of the carrying angle in the stiff elbow may help to further characterize functional impairment caused by stiffness (Fig. 3.4).

A multitude of techniques have been proposed for carrying angle assessment including radiographic measurements, goniometry, and electromagnetic tracking to name a few [19, 20]. Goniometric measurement may once again be used to obtain this given its low cost and accessibility. In the event surrounding soft tissues interfere with this process, identification of bony landmarks on the acromion, medial and lateral epicondyles of the humerus, and the distal radial and ulnar styloid processes may be helpful. Typical carrying angle is noted to be on average 11° for men and 14° for women and can vary based on age, sex, and hand dominance [18].

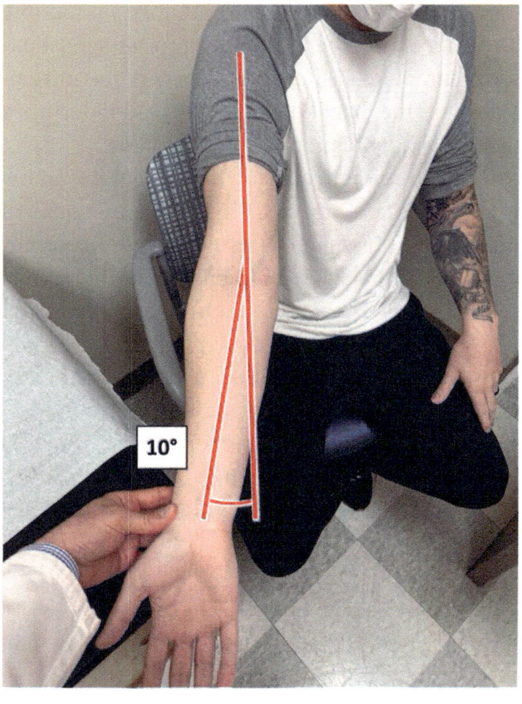

Fig. 3.4 A right elbow with an approximate carrying angle of 10 degrees

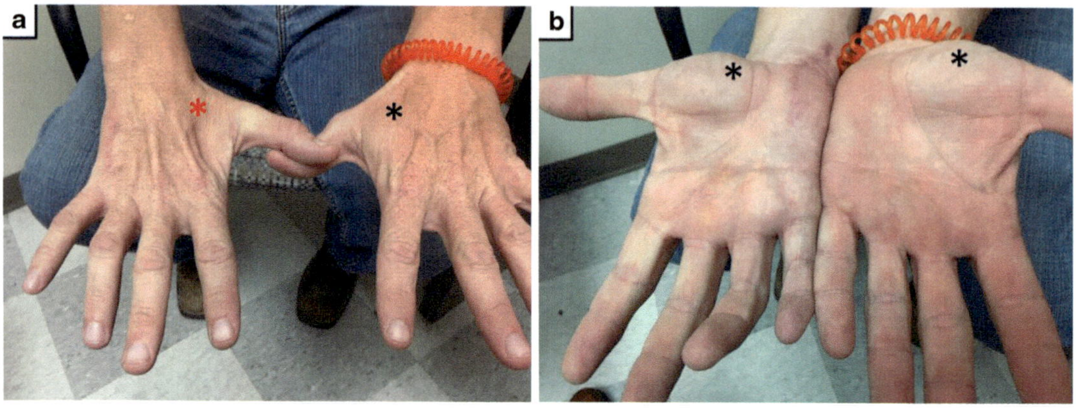

Fig. 3.5 (**a**) Comparison between a normal first dorsal interosseous muscle (left hand, black asterisk), and severe atrophy (right hand, red asterisk). Examination of the palmar right and left hands (**b**) reveals thenar muscles with similar bulk and tone

3.3.5 Muscle Bulk/Strength

The bulk and tone of the muscles of the hand, forearm, and brachium can provide insight into chronic neurologic pathology, most commonly affecting the intrinsic muscles of the hand (ulnar nerve) and the thenar mass (median nerve) (Fig. 3.5). The ulnar nerve is highly susceptible to compressive neuropathy with prolonged flexion contracture of the elbow; as such, the musculature of the hand must be assessed during a thorough examination of the stiff elbow.

Muscle strength and stiffness about the elbow joint may be impacted by pain, mechanical obstruction, or underlying neurovascular compromise to muscles that enact on the elbow joint. **The Medical Research Council Manual Muscle Testing Scale** is used to grade the muscle strength about the elbow joint [6]. Although technically a full range of motion is required to achieve a strength grade higher than 1 using this scale, muscles are assessed against the examiner's manual resistance and are graded as follows:

0 = No muscle activation
1 = Trace muscle activation, such as a twitch, without achieving full range of motion
2 = Muscle activation with gravity eliminated, achieving full range of motion
3 = Muscle activation against gravity, full range of motion
4 = Muscle activation against some resistance, full range of motion
5 = Muscle activation against examiner's full resistance, full range of motion.

3.4 Osseous Exam

3.4.1 Radiocapitellar Pathology

When determining arthritic or intra-articular pathology, patients generally will have pain with range of motion, elbow effusion, and tenderness over bony landmarks. With radiocapitellar arthritis, tenderness over the radiocapitellar articulation is common. Loss of terminal extension can be present as well due to effusion or swelling within the joint. The radiocapitellar compression test is performed by ranging the patient's elbow in passive pronation and supination while applying an axial load to the lateral elbow. Pain or palpable crepitus is considered a positive test, which may be present in osteochondritis dissecans as well as arthrosis of the radiocapitellar joint [21].

3.4.2 Ulnohumeral Arthritis/Valgus Extension Overload (VEO)

Repetitive stress due to throwing or pitching can produce excessive shear forces over the posteromedial olecranon and compression of the radiocapitellar joint. This, in turn, may lead to chondrolysis, posteromedial olecranon osteophyte formation, and loose bodies and may contribute to the development of osteochondritis dissecans of the radiocapitellar joint. This condition is generally found in younger patients that are throwing athletes or gymnasts [22]. Pain at terminal flexion or extension over the posteromedial olecranon may be indicative of osteophyte formation or arthritic changes related to valgus extension overload (VEO). Tenderness may be elicited by palpating the posteromedial olecranon with the elbow in full extension. Loss of terminal extension is common. Assessing for VEO can also be performed by the VEO impingement test, "arm bar test," "and bounce test."

During the VEO impingement test, the examiner places a valgus stress across the elbow in 20–30° of flexion and quickly extends it. The examiner then repeats this test without the valgus stress and palpates over the posteromedial olecranon. Attention should be directed posterior to the medial collateral ligament (MCL) insertion as patients with this condition may have a concomitant MCL injury. The "arm bar test" is highly sensitive for posterior impingement. This is performed with the patient's elbow extended, shoulder internally rotated. The examiner then places their hand over the elbow and simulates forced elbow extension. Pain associated with this may be indicative of posteromedial impingement. Finally, the "bounce test" is a similar test that involves repeated elbow terminal extension. Pain with this maneuver may be useful in determining posteromedial impingement [23].

3.5 Ligament and Tendon Exam

3.5.1 Posterolateral Rotatory Instability (PLRI)

Many examination maneuvers exist to aid in diagnosis of PLRI or LUCL injury including the lateral pivot shift test, the posterolateral rotatory drawer test, chair push-up test, table-top relocation test, and prone push-up test. The lateral pivot shift test may be performed with the patient awake in a clinic setting, or while anesthetized in the operating room. The patient is positioned supine with the affected extremity over the patient's head. The shoulder is fully externally rotated and the elbow is maximally supinated. The examiner then places one arm on the patient's proximal forearm and another on the wrist. A valgus and compressive force is elicited over the elbow while the forearm is held in maximal supination. Beginning from extension, the patient's elbow is slowly flexed. At approximately 20–40° of elbow flexion (with valgus, compression, and supination), the elbow is most vulnerable to posterolateral instability. In the awake patient, they may feel pain and apprehension. In the anesthetized patient, a palpable clunk may be felt or heard. This is indicative of PLRI. As the elbow is flexed past 40–50°, another clunk may be heard or felt, which is the reduction of the radiocapitellar joint [24, 25].

The posterolateral rotatory drawer test places the patient's elbow in 40° of flexion as the examiner performs an anterior-to-posterior drawer maneuver over the lateral elbow. With PLRI, a positive test is indicated by pain, apprehension, or palpable clunk over the lateral elbow [26]. In the chair push-up test, the patient is seated in a chair with arm-rests and is asked to push up from the chair while their forearms are supinated, with the elbows flexed to 90° and positioned wider than shoulder width. A positive test is indicated by pain or apprehension as the patient tries to rise from the chair. The table-top relocation test involves the patient standing in front of a table while the hand of the symptomatic extremity is placed on the lateral edge in a supinated position [27]. This exam involves three parts. First, the patient is asked to slowly flex the elbow while placing force through their arm into their hand. Pain and instability may be felt as the elbow flexes to 40°. Next, this maneuver is repeated with the examiner's hand or thumb over the radial head. Relief or improvement of symptoms here may be apparent if PLRI is present. Thirdly, the examiner then removes the thumb, again eliciting pain and apprehension if PLRI is present. Finally, the prone push-up test is relatively self-explanatory. The patient is asked to do a push-up with the elbows beginning at 90° with forearms supinated and arms abducted greater than shoulder-width. A positive test is indicated by pain and apprehension as the patient performs a push-up from extension of the elbows to flexion [27].

3.5.2 Medial Ulnar Collateral Ligament (MUCL)

As previously discussed, the MUCL is divided into the anterior, posterior, and transverse bundles. The integrity anterior bundle is the most important component as it provides the greatest stability against valgus forces across the elbow. Point tenderness just inferior to the medial epicondyle may be indicative of an MUCL injury as most of the ruptures occur from the medial epicondyle. Palpation is best assessed with the elbow at 50–70° of elbow flexion as this will move the flexor–pronator mass anterior to the MUCL [28]. The milking maneuver and moving valgus stress test are two focused tests that assess the integrity of the MCL. The milking maneuver consists of placing the patient's shoulder abducted 70–90° while the elbow is maximally flexed. The examiner then pulls the patient's thumb in supination as the shoulder is forward flexed and the elbow remains flexed past 90°. This simulates the stress point in a throwing athlete. The test is considered positive if the patient feels pain or instability as the examiner pulls the thumb. The moving valgus stress test, as described by O'Driscoll, was described to increase the sensitivity of MCL injuries. This is performed with the patient's elbow maximally flexed as the shoulder is abducted and maximally externally rotated. The examiner places a hand over the lateral elbow and applies a valgus force as the elbow is quickly extended to 30°. A positive test is concluded if the patient exhibits maximal pain from 120° to 70° as the elbow moves from flexion to extension, which reproduces the positions of late cocking and early acceleration, respectively [22].

3.5.3 Biceps Brachii

The distal biceps tendon can be assessed by visualization, palpation, and special testing as well. When inspecting for biceps pathology, the "reverse Popeye deformity" may be apparent when a ruptured biceps muscle has migrated proximally. Tenderness to palpation over the biceps tendon itself may indicate partial rupture if the biceps tendon can still be probed. Dynamically, greater loss of supination than forearm flexion may indicate biceps tendon pathology. Passive forearm pronation test observes the patient's biceps muscle in different positions. A normal exam will show that the biceps muscle moves proximally with forearm supination and distally with forearm pronation. Special tests such as the hook test, biceps squeeze test, and biceps crease interval (BCI) can also be utilized.

During the hook test, the patient actively flexes their elbow to 90° as the examiner probes and tries to "hook" the tendon from the lateral side of the elbow [29]. Ability to hook and pull a taut biceps tendon indicates that the biceps tendon is still attached distally. It is important that this exam be performed from lateral to medial. If performing from the medial side, an intact bicipital aponeurosis may fool the examiner, producing a false negative result [29]. If the biceps tendon can be hooked but still elicits a painful response, this may be indicative of a partial rupture.

The Ruland biceps squeeze test is performed with the patient's elbow flexed to 70° in slight pronation [30]. This relaxes the brachialis muscle. The examiner then squeezes both the myotendinous junction and the muscle belly itself. In normal anatomy, the forearm should supinate as the biceps muscle belly is moved away from the humerus. A lack of forearm supination during examiner squeeze is considered a positive test.

The biceps crease interval (BCI) measures distances between anatomic landmarks to determine if there is proximal migration of the biceps. The patient's elbow is brought from full flexion to full extension and the main crease in the antecubital fossa is first marked. Next, the location at which the biceps tendon turns most sharply toward the AC is marked. This is known as the "cusp." The distance between the crease and the cusp is the BCI. Values >6 cm or >1.2× the value of the contralateral arm are positive for biceps tendon rupture [31].

3.5.4 Triceps Brachii

If rupture of the triceps tendon occurs, localized swelling and pain may be present over the posterior elbow along with a palpable defect for full tears. The modified Thompson squeeze test is performed with the patient lying prone with the elbow at the end of the table and hand pointed toward the ground. The examiner then squeezes the triceps muscle belly. An intact triceps will cause some forearm extension with squeezing of the triceps. A test is considered positive if no forearm extension occurs with triceps squeeze [32].

3.6 Nerve/Compressive Neuropathies

3.6.1 Cubital Tunnel Syndrome/Ulnar Neuropathy

The most common pathologic neurologic condition about the elbow, which may directly produce pain and stiffness of the elbow, is compression and/or instability of the ulnar nerve as it crosses the medial elbow. Typical presentation is a patient with medial elbow pain with paresthesias over the small finger and ulnar ring finger; as this process worsens, patients may develop intrinsic hand weakness that patients may report as difficulty with fine motor tasks such as buttoning a shirt, or weakness with grip. A positive Tinel's sign is elicited when the patient feels pain with radiation into the fingers when the course of the ulnar nerve across the medial elbow is percussed. This should be performed in full extension along the course of the nerve from the medial intermuscular septum, cubital tunnel, and between the ulnar and humeral heads of the flexor carpi ulnaris (FCU) muscle [33]. The elbow flexion test is another test to assess for cubital tunnel. The patient is asked to flex their elbow. If symptoms are reproduced after >60 s of elbow flexion, this is considered a positive test.

Assessment of ulnar nerve position and stability is paramount, as subluxation and/or dislocation may produce elbow pain and stiffness. As the patient flexes and extends the elbow, the examiner palpates the medial elbow to ensure the ulnar nerve does not subluxate or dislocate anterior to the medial epicondyle [34]. Ulnar nerve location, position, and movement is important to ascertain prior to any surgical procedures that may be performed in the elbow as injury to the ulnar nerve may lead to catastrophic hand weakness, numbness, and lack of manual dexterity for fine motor tasks.

3.6.2 Radial Tunnel/Supinator Syndrome/PIN Syndrome

Radial nerve compression at the elbow is a rare condition and is considered a diagnosis of exclusion. Symptoms may be confused with lateral epicondylitis; however, key differences exist between these two entities. Radial tunnel syndrome is assessed through compression of the radial nerve along different points along its course, which may produce elbow pain, dorsal forearm pain, and/or weakness in the hand. Typically, maximal tenderness seen with radial tunnel syndrome will be 3–5 cm distal to the lateral epicondyle while lateral epicondylitis exhibits maximal tenderness just distal to the tip of the lateral epicondyle over the origin of the mobile wad/wrist extensors [35]. Both diagnoses may exhibit pain with resisted long finger or wrist extension.

3.6.3 Pronator Syndrome

Pronator syndrome, or proximal median nerve entrapment (PMNE), is characterized by pain and/or paresthesias in the thumb, index, and long and radial ring finger. This is similar to carpal tunnel syndrome; however, patients usually endorse worsening symptoms with prolonged periods of forearm rotation. A positive Tinel's sign may be produced with percussion proximal and lateral to the pronator teres muscle belly. Another common test used to delineate pronator syndrome is known as the pronator compression test. The pronator compression test is performed by applying pressure over the patient's proximal volar forearm proximal and lateral to the pronator teres muscle belly. A positive test is produced if the exam maneuver reproduces symptoms within 30 s of compression [36]. Pain and paresthesias with resisted elbow flexion and forearm supination indicate possible median nerve compression at the bicipital aponeurosis. Symptoms produced by resisted forearm pronation during elbow extension may indicate median nerve compression between the two heads of the pronator teres. Finally, symptoms reproduced by resisted contraction of the long finger flexor digitorum superficialis (FDS) may indicate median nerve compression at the FDS fibrous arch [37].

3.7 Conclusion

A stiff elbow can result from a multitude of soft tissue and/or bony causes. A detailed history and detailed physical examination will help the clinician reach the correct diagnosis. This, in turn, will help guide treatment with the goal of returning the patient's elbow to a more functional and painless range of motion.

References

1. Nandi S, Maschke S, Evans PJ, Lawton JN. The stiff elbow. Hand (New York, NY). 2009;4(4):368. https://doi.org/10.1007/s11552-009-9181-z.
2. Martin S, Sanchez E. Anatomy and biomechanics of the elbow joint. Semin Musculoskelet Radiol. 2013;17(5):429–36. https://doi.org/10.1055/s-0033-1361587.
3. Alcid JG, Ahmad CS, Lee TQ. Elbow anatomy and structural biomechanics. Clin Sports Med. 2004;23(4):503–17, vii. https://doi.org/10.1016/j.csm.2004.06.008.
4. Miyasaka KC. Anatomy of the elbow. Orthop Clin North Am. 1999;30(1):1–13. https://doi.org/10.1016/s0030-5898(05)70057-2.
5. Mittal R. Posttraumatic stiff elbow. Indian J Orthop. 2017;51(1):4–13. https://doi.org/10.4103/0019-5413.197514.
6. Masci G, Cazzato G, Milano G, et al. The stiff elbow: current concepts. Orthop Rev (Pavia). 2020;12(Suppl 1):8661. https://doi.org/10.4081/or.2020.8661.
7. Morrey BF, Askew LJ, Chao EY. A biomechanical study of normal functional elbow motion. JBJS. 1981;63(6):872.
8. Cohen MS, Schimmel DR, Masuda K, Hastings H, Muehleman C. Structural and biochemical evaluation of the elbow capsule after trauma. J Shoulder Elbow Surg. 2007;16(4):484–90. https://doi.org/10.1016/j.jse.2006.06.018.
9. Akhtar A, Hughes B, Watts AC. The post-traumatic stiff elbow: a review. J Clin Orthop Trauma. 2021;19:125–31. https://doi.org/10.1016/j.jcot.2021.05.006.
10. Filh GM, Galvão MV. Post-traumatic stiffness of the elbow. Rev Bras Ortop. 2015;45(4):347–54. https://doi.org/10.1016/S2255-4971(15)30380-3.
11. King GJ, Faber KJ. Posttraumatic elbow stiffness. Orthop Clin North Am. 2000;31(1):129–43. https://doi.org/10.1016/s0030-5898(05)70133-4.
12. Hildebrand KA, Zhang M, van Snellenberg W, King GJW, Hart DA. Myofibroblast numbers are elevated in human elbow capsules after trauma. Clin Orthop Relat Res. 2004;419:189–97.
13. Bryce CD, Armstrong AD. Anatomy and biomechanics of the elbow. Orthop Clin North Am. 2008;39(2):141–54, v. https://doi.org/10.1016/j.ocl.2007.12.001.
14. Misidou C, Papagoras C. Complex regional pain syndrome: an update. Mediterr J Rheumatol. 2019;30(1):16–25. https://doi.org/10.31138/mjr.30.1.16.
15. Dor A, Vatine JJ, Kalichman L. Proximal myofascial pain in patients with distal complex regional pain syndrome of the upper limb. J Bodyw Mov Ther. 2019;23(3):547–54. https://doi.org/10.1016/j.jbmt.2019.02.015.
16. van Rijn SF, Zwerus EL, Koenraadt KL, Jacobs WC, van den Bekerom MP, Eygendaal D. The reli-

ability and validity of goniometric elbow measurements in adults: a systematic review of the literature. Shoulder Elbow. 2018;10(4):274–84. https://doi.org/10.1177/1758573218774326.
17. Kumar B, Pai S, Ray B, et al. Radiographic study of carrying angle and morphometry of skeletal elements of human elbow. Rom J Morphol Embryol. 2010;51(3):521–6.
18. Sharma K, Mansur DI, Khanal K, Haque MK. Variation of carrying angle with age, sex, height and special reference to side. Kathmandu Univ Med J. 2013;11(44):315–8. https://doi.org/10.3126/kumj.v11i4.12540.
19. An KN, Morrey BF, Chao EY. Carrying angle of the human elbow joint. J Orthop Res. 1984;1(4):369–78. https://doi.org/10.1002/jor.1100010405.
20. Van Roy P, Baeyens JP, Fauvart D, Lanssiers R, Clarijs JP. Arthro-kinematics of the elbow: study of the carrying angle. Ergonomics. 2005;48(11–14):1645–56. https://doi.org/10.1080/00140130500101361.
21. Baumgarten TE. Osteochondritis dissecans of the capitellum. Sports Med Arthrosc Rev. 1995;3(3):219.
22. O'Driscoll SWM, Lawton RL, Smith AM. The "moving valgus stress test" for medial collateral ligament tears of the elbow. Am J Sports Med. 2005;33(2):231–9. https://doi.org/10.1177/0363546504267804.
23. Redler LH, Watling JP, Ahmad CS. Physical examination of the throwing athlete's elbow. Am J Orthop (Belle Mead NJ). 2015;44(1):13–8.
24. O'Driscoll SW, Bell DF, Morrey BF. Posterolateral rotatory instability of the elbow. JBJS. 1991;73(3):440.
25. Smith MV, Lamplot JD, Wright RW, Brophy RH. Comprehensive review of the elbow physical examination. J Am Acad Orthop Surgeons. 2018;26(19):678. https://doi.org/10.5435/JAAOS-D-16-00622.
26. Camp CL, Smith J, O'Driscoll SW. Posterolateral rotatory instability of the elbow: part I. Mechanism of injury and the posterolateral rotatory drawer test. arthroscopy. Techniques. 2017;6(2):e401–5. https://doi.org/10.1016/j.eats.2016.10.016.
27. Arvind CHV, Hargreaves DG. Table top relocation test—new clinical test for posterolateral rotatory instability of the elbow. J Shoulder Elbow Surg. 2006;15(4):500–1. https://doi.org/10.1016/j.jse.2005.11.014.
28. Chen FS, Rokito AS, Jobe FW. Medial elbow problems in the overhead-throwing athlete. J Am Acad Orthop Surg. 2001;9(2):99–113. https://doi.org/10.5435/00124635-200103000-00004.
29. O'Driscoll SW, Goncalves LBJ, Dietz P. The hook test for distal biceps tendon avulsion. Am J Sports Med. 2007;35(11):1865–9. https://doi.org/10.1177/0363546507305016.
30. Ruland RT, Dunbar RP, Bowen JD. The biceps squeeze test for diagnosis of distal biceps tendon ruptures. Clin Orthop Relat Res. 2005;437:128–31. https://doi.org/10.1097/01.blo.0000167668.18444.f5.
31. ElMaraghy A, Devereaux M, Tsoi K. The biceps crease interval for diagnosing complete distal biceps tendon ruptures. Clin Orthop Relat Res. 2008;466(9):2255–62. https://doi.org/10.1007/s11999-008-0334-0.
32. Viegas SF. Avulsion of the triceps tendon. Orthop Rev. 1990;19(6):533–6.
33. Elhassan B, Steinmann SP. Entrapment neuropathy of the ulnar nerve. J Am Acad Orthop Surg. 2007;15(11):672–81. https://doi.org/10.5435/00124635-200711000-00006.
34. Calfee RP, Manske PR, Gelberman RH, Van Steyn MO, Steffen J, Goldfarb CA. Clinical assessment of the ulnar nerve at the elbow: reliability of instability testing and the association of hypermobility with clinical symptoms. J Bone Joint Surg Am. 2010;92(17):2801–8. https://doi.org/10.2106/JBJS.J.00097.
35. Stanley J. Radial tunnel syndrome: a surgeon's perspective. J Hand Ther. 2006;19(2):180–4. https://doi.org/10.1197/j.jht.2006.02.005.
36. Rodner CM, Tinsley BA, O'Malley MP. Pronator syndrome and anterior interosseous nerve syndrome. J Am Acad Orthop Surg. 2013;21(5):268–75. https://doi.org/10.5435/JAAOS-21-05-268.
37. Hartz CR, Linscheid RL, Gramse RR, Daube JR. The pronator teres syndrome: compressive neuropathy of the median nerve. J Bone Joint Surg Am. 1981;63(6):885–90.
38. Harden RN, Bruehl S, Stanton-Hicks M, Wilson PR. Proposed new diagnostic criteria for complex regional pain syndrome. Pain Medicine. 2007;8(4):326–31. https://doi.org/10.1111/j.1526-4637.2006.00169.x.

Functional Evaluation of Stiff Elbow

4

Carina Cohen, Bernardo B. Terra, and Benno Ejnisman

Elbow stiffness can be a debilitating condition that significantly impacts a patient's ability to perform activities of daily living. The elbow joint is particularly susceptible to stiffness due to its highly congruent bony anatomy, relatively confined joint space tightly stabilizing collateral ligament complex, and the close relationship of the surrounding muscles acting as secondary stabilizers. While trauma, surgery, posttraumatic arthritis, and possible concomitant occurrence of heterotopic ossification (HO) are among the most common causes of stiffness, joint degeneration resulting from aging might also contribute [1–3].

Elbow stiffness can be caused by osseous impingement or deformity, soft tissue contracture, or a combination of both. Morrey et al. reported that most of our daily activities could be accomplished within a range of 30–100° of elbow flexion. However, more recent studies showed that a greater flexion arc is required for modern daily activities such as using a mobile cellular phone. Whether elbow stiffness is symptomatic is patient specific and depends on the patient's flexion arc required to perform work, sports, or hobbies. Therefore, the definition of elbow stiffness cannot be specified by precise values but is patient specific. Restoring adequate range of motion (ROM) can be challenging in some cases. For that reason, it is crucial that the proper treatment options are utilized and the right treatment workup is followed [4, 5].

4.1 Etiology of Elbow Stiffness

Multiple causes contribute to elbow stiffness, with trauma being the most common. Posttraumatic stiffness occurs as a result of four stages: bleeding, edema, granulation, and fibrosis. Regarding the latter, histopathologic studies show an increased number of myofibroblasts, collagen crosslink formation, and expression of transforming growth factor-beta, leading to excessive capsular scarring. Moreover, a decreased capsular content of proteoglycan and water leads to further contraction, additionally limiting the ROM. HO is another important factor for stiffness, induced by the upregulated expression of bone morphogenetic protein in response to inflammation. This leads to the formation of mature lamellar bone in the soft tissues around the joint, creating a mechanical block that restricts elbow motion [6, 7].

The incidence of HO ranges from 1.6% up to 56%, increasing with the extent of trauma, concomitant joint dislocation, surgery, prolonged immobilization, burns, or neurological injury. It is uncommon after elbow trauma but when associated with concomitant head trauma, the incidence increases substantially. Morrey et al.

C. Cohen (✉) · B. B. Terra · B. Ejnisman
Centro de Traumatologia do Esporte (CETE), Federal University of São Paulo, UNIFESP, São Paulo, Brazil

L. Pederzini et al. (eds.), *Stiffness of the Elbow, Wrist and Related Pathologies*,
https://doi.org/10.1007/978-3-031-81381-8_4

divided elbow stiffness into a classification consisting of intrinsic, extrinsic, and combined contractures. Herein, intrinsic contractures are associated with intra-articular (IA) injuries, such as IA adhesions or malunions, loss of articular cartilage, protruding metalwork, loose bodies, and infection [8–10].

Conversely, extrinsic contractures do not have a direct relation with the joint. These consist of capsular and ligamentous contractures, skin contractures following burns, HO, neural adhesion, extra-articular malunions, and extra-articular infection. Most posttraumatic contractures include both intrinsic and extrinsic factors, classifying them as mixed [11].

4.2 Clinical Evaluation

Elbow flexion and extension should be measured and compared to the contralateral side as maximal flexion ranges from 140° to 150° and maximal extension from −10° to 10° in healthy subjects and is dependent on sex and age. Despite elbow stiffness usually being relatively pain free, end-range tenderness can be found in most cases. Elbow stability is often not abnormal; however, it can be difficult to test in patients with limited ROM.

In stiff elbows, pathological changes of the posteromedial capsule, as well as tissue scarring or even protruding metalwork due to previous surgery, increase the likelihood of ulnar entrapment, especially in posttraumatic stiffness. Therefore, the ulnar nerve should be carefully examined for signs of either entrapment or instability, and the location in its sulcus should be carefully documented. Signs of ulnar entrapment or adhesion can be provoked during deep flexion [12, 13].

Elbow has two degrees of freedom, and the available movements in space are flexion, extension, pronation, and supination. Several studies on the ROM of the elbow assessed a variation from −21° to 12° in extension, and from 122° to −164° in flexion [7].

A functional joint must also guarantee stability, which depends both on the complex conformation of the articular surfaces, and on the capsule–ligament structures and muscle components. Morrey et al. defined the arc of movement of the functional elbow during the daily life activity of 100°, both for flexion–extension (30–130°) and for pronation–supination (50° in both directions). Elbow stiffness is defined as the loss of movement greater than 30° in extension and loss of flexion of less than 120° [12, 14].

A thorough history and physical examination complimented by imaging studies comprise the requisite evaluation for elbow stiffness. The history should include the onset, duration, character, and progression of symptoms. Inquiries should be made into elbow trauma or pathology, especially infection, and prior non-surgical or surgical treatments. Comorbid conditions should be investigated, as they may have implications on the elbow such as hemophilia with resulting hemarthroses or neurologic conditions involving spasticity [15, 16].

The patient's vocational and recreational pursuits should be established in order to determine the level of demand that will be placed on the elbow.

Physical examination should begin with a neurovascular exam with particular attention to ulnar nerve function. Not only is the ulnar nerve commonly involved in elbow trauma, but also if operative treatment for the elbow is necessary, preoperative ulnar nerve function should be known. Active and passive elbow range of motion, for both flexion–extension and pronation–supination, should be examined. The character of the endpoint at the extremes of motion should be noted. While a firm endpoint suggests a bony block to motion, a soft endpoint is indicative of a soft tissue contracture. Crepitus appreciated during elbow range of motion may signify degenerative changes, synovitis, or fracture [17, 18].

Patients rarely complain of symptoms at rest, and pain is often felt in cases of extreme movement, or in patients with underlying severe OA. Resting pain is suggestive of the presence of infection, especially in patients who underwent previous surgery. In these cases, the dosage of C-reactive protein (PCR) and the erythrocyte sedimentation rate (ESR) should be given. Sometimes the pain may be due to nerve compression paresthesia or scars with skin hypersensitivity. Clinical examination includes the evaluation of the shoulder, wrist, and hand because they inevitably affect the functionality of the elbow. It starts with an accurate inspection, aimed at recognizing any surgical scars or burns [19].

A severe joint limitation is suggestive of a bone block, while a gradual limitation is indicative of soft tissue blockage. The presence of crackles during mobilization is indicative of degenerative changes, synovitis, or fractures. Pain in cautious mobilization is indicative of intrinsic components of stiffness, while pain at the highest degrees of flexion–extension and prone–supination is prevalent in cases of impingement between the olecranon and the coronoid process, and in the distal part of the humerus, often being caused by osteophyte formations.

Particular attention must be paid to the evaluation of ulnar nerve function, which is often involved in traumatic and degenerative processes; in cases requiring surgical treatment (release and anterior transposition), the preoperative evaluation of the ulnar nerve should always be documented. Late ulnar neuropathy can arise due to its stretching, after the recovery of the elbow extension, in flexion contractures. In some cases, examination under anesthesia is indicated to distinguish true elbow stiffness from functional limitations on an antalgic basis. In most cases, an anteroposterior (AP) and lateral X-ray of the elbow are enough. Stiffnesses greater than 30° are often associated with distorted AP images, which renders oblique projections necessary [2].

Also, intra-articular bone fragments can be identified with radiographs. Computed tomography (CT) should be required when joint damage is associated and when HO needs to be studied. Magnetic resonance imaging (MRI) is not fundamental for this type of pathology, because it does not allow an in-depth study of bone structures, still providing good information on soft tissues. Electromyography (EMG) is necessary when there is clinical suspicion of neuropathy of the ulnar nerve [3].

4.3 Functional Evaluation

The current standard of treatment evaluation includes the use of clinical rating systems. These rating scales assess multiple areas of interest (such as pain, range of motion, severity of dysfunction, treatment effectiveness) and yield a summarized value that is supposed to correspond to the effect of the diseased joint on the patient. These scoring systems can be designed to be administered to patients or to the physician. Initially, the latter was mostly the focus of these scoring systems, but more recently, several scoring systems, based purely on the patient's perception of the functioning of the joint, have been developed [20]. Ideally, we should look for a single outcome evaluation system that is reliable, valid, and sensitive to changes of clinical importance, which takes into account both patients' and physicians' perspectives and which is short and practical to use.

Pain has a very strong influence on both physician-rated and patient-rated quantitative measures of elbow function. Consequently, these measures may be strongly influenced by the psychosocial aspects of illness that have a strong relationship with pain, and objective measures of elbow function such as mobility may be undervalued [21].

Also, to access elbow function, measuring strength is very important, especially in patients planning for elbow arthrolysis surgery, as reduced muscle strength is a common complication after this surgery. Most of the manual muscle testing is subjective and misleading. Therefore, measuring strength with a dynamometer would be a more objective and responsive measure and it could be measured over time and compared to normative data [22].

Using elbow-specific rating systems seems to be a sensible choice when handling conditions limited to the elbow. This can be expected to result in achieving better validity and responsiveness characteristics at least, and perhaps also higher reliability scores [23]. Capuano et al. showed that scoring systems used to evaluate 14 patients who had undergone elbow arthroscopy failed to correlate to patients' satisfaction comparing three different scoring scales [24].

Inappropriate use of a rating system might have great impact. Nowadays, it has become common practice to use rating scales as the primary endpoint in clinical studies. If a study fails to reveal the efficacy of a new intervention, it is of paramount importance that this cannot, for example, be ascribed to poor responsiveness of the rating scale [20, 25].

The validity, reliability, and responsiveness characteristics of a measurement tool are not solely inherent to the rating system itself but are more or less a product of the rating system properties and the characteristics of the population it is being used for. This means that an already validated outcome measurement tool might have to be validated more than once to justify its use in different populations. Although this perspective may be generally accepted, it is often neglected, and rating systems are used for pathophysiologic and surgical conditions or interventions for which they have never been properly validated. This may lead to incorrect results and is therefore not recommended either [20].

Many scoring systems have been used for elbow disorders. Longo et al. presented 18 elbow scoring systems in their characteristics, applications, and limitations but concluded that we are still far from a single outcome evaluation system that is reliable, valid, and sensitive to clinically relevant changes, takes into account both patients' and physicians' perspectives, and is short and practical to use [25].

Sun et al. presented the Liverpool Elbow Score (LES) as a valid elbow-specific scoring system that can be used to evaluate function in patients with elbow stiffness. It consists of a patient-rated questionnaire that assesses the elbow function, including a question about pain; and clinical data, which can be measured objectively, regarding the condition of the elbow. LES can be equally applied in different populations to evaluate joint function in patients with elbow stiffness, with better evaluation than others since it uses self-assessment questionnaires in addition to physician-assessment parameters, although it does not inquire about qualities of life [26].

Later in a review, The et al. concluded that currently, the only elbow-specific rating system that is validated using high-quality methodology is the Oxford Elbow Score, a patient-administered outcome measure tool that has been validated on heterogeneous study populations since other rating systems still have to be proven in the future to be as good as the Oxford Elbow Score for clinical or research purposes [20].

The elbow joint is critical to upper extremity function as it positions the hand in space. With a stiff elbow, the entire upper extremity range of motion is diminished and function suffers. While there are multiple non-operative and operative treatment options available to address the bony and/or soft tissue basis of elbow stiffness, prevention is of paramount importance, as this is a difficult condition to treat. Careful functional evaluation should be done although precise elbow scoring rating systems still need to be proven.

A 26-year-old patient who was the victim of a car accident was evolving with a comminuted fracture of the distal humerus, AO 13C3. He underwent open reduction and internal fixation with plates. He developed severe elbow stiffness (range of motion 70–90 degrees) with neuropraxia of the ulnar nerve. Three months after the initial surgery, he underwent open release of stiffness, posterior approach, associated with transposition of the ulnar nerve.

Postoperative period with good recovery of the patient's range of motion (Images 4.1, 4.2–4.3, 4.4–4.5, 4.6–4.7, 4.8–4.9, 4.10–4.12 and 4.13–4.14).

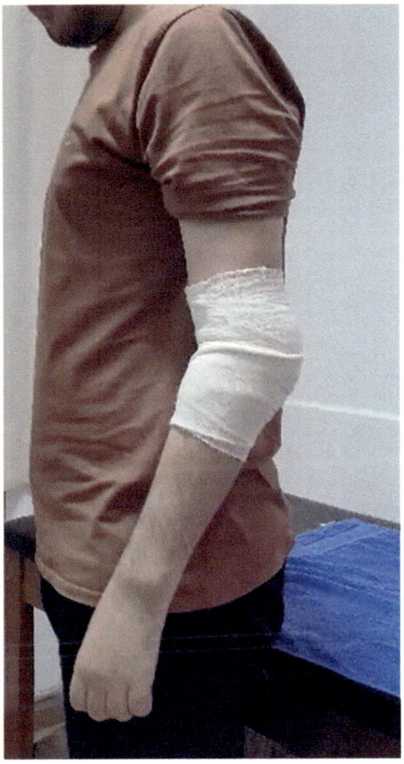

Image 4.1 The crashed car of the patient

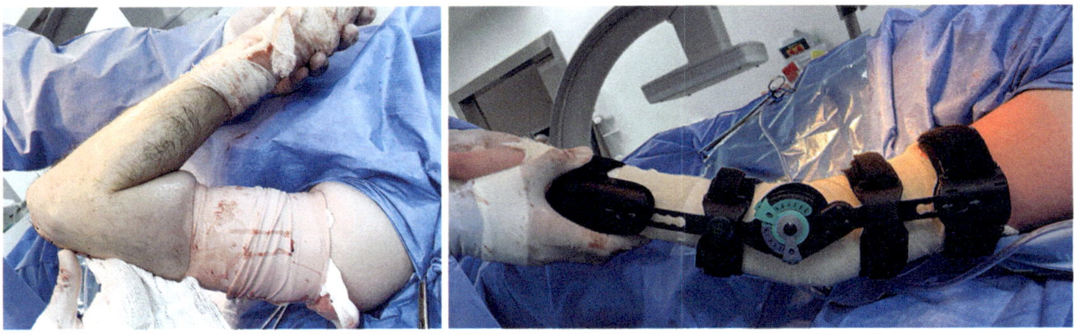

Images 4.2–4.3 X-ray and CT scan demonstrating the complex distal humerus fracture AO 13C3

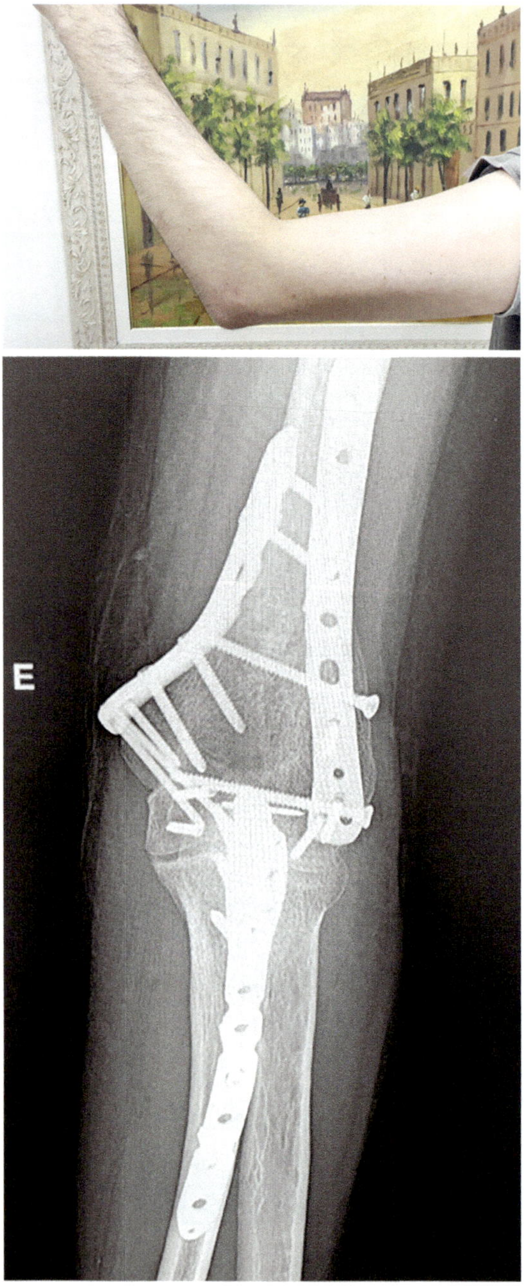

Images 4.4–4.5 Intraoperative, posterior access to the distal humerus

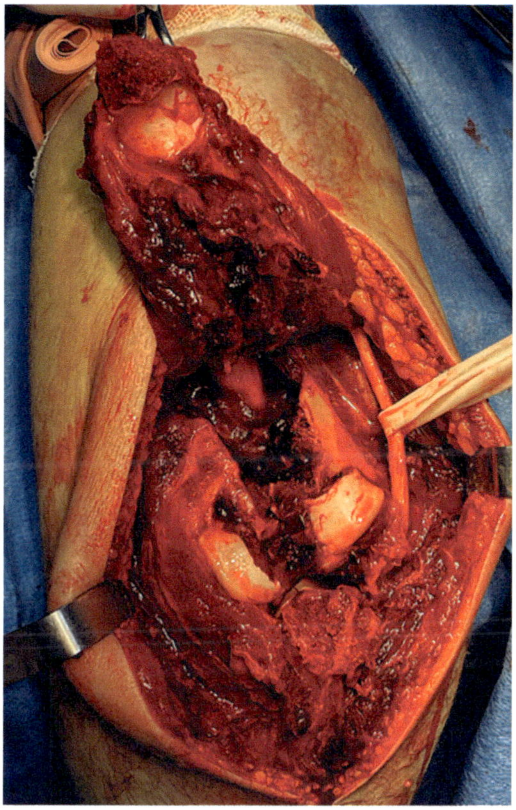
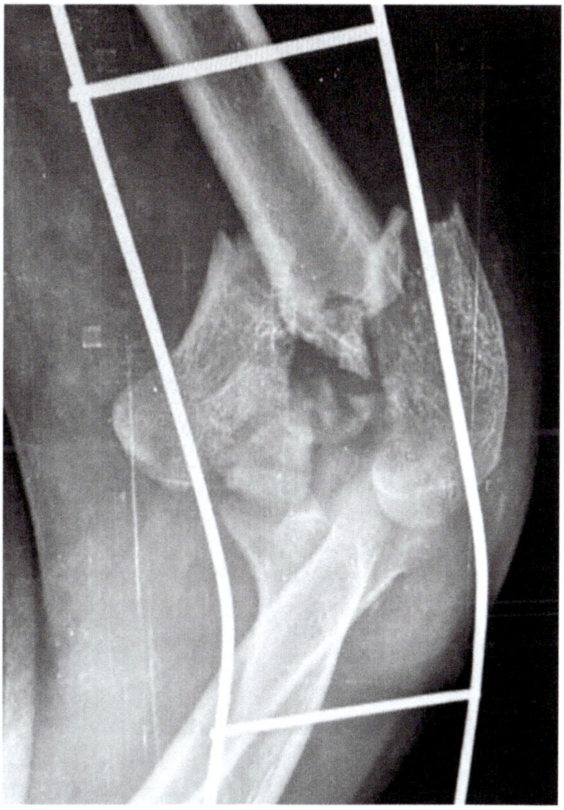

Images 4.6–4.7 Postoperative X-ray

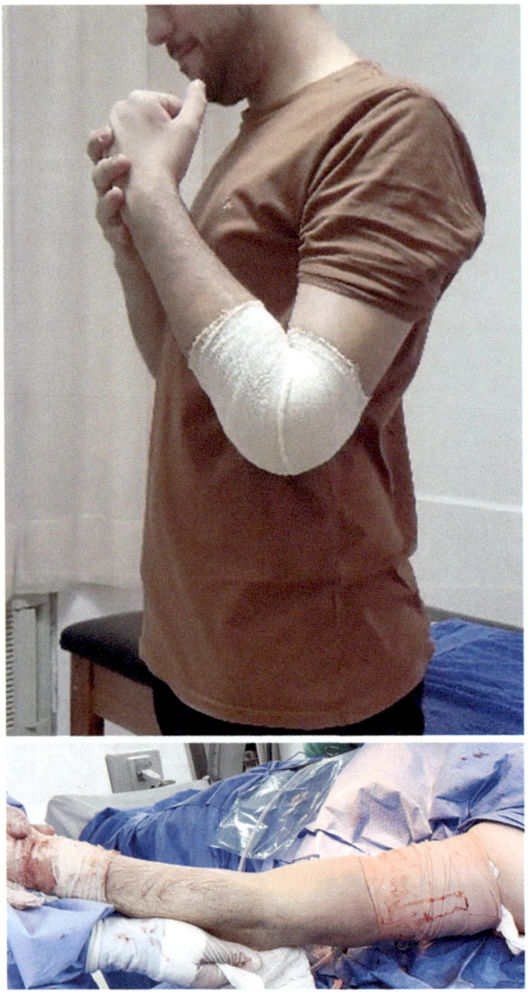

Images 4.8–4.9 The arc of the movement with severe limitation (90 flexion/−70 extension)

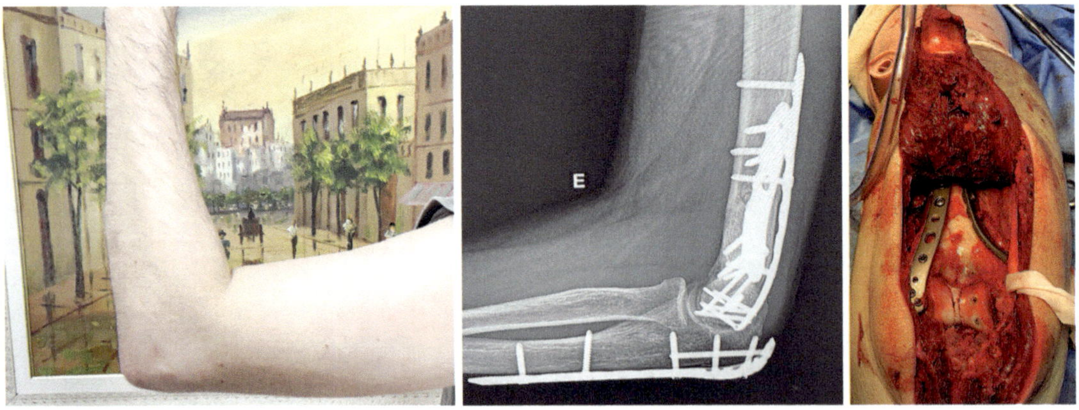

Images 4.10–4.12 Immediate postoperative images of the open liberation surgery of the rigid elbow and ulnar nerve neurolysis and transposition

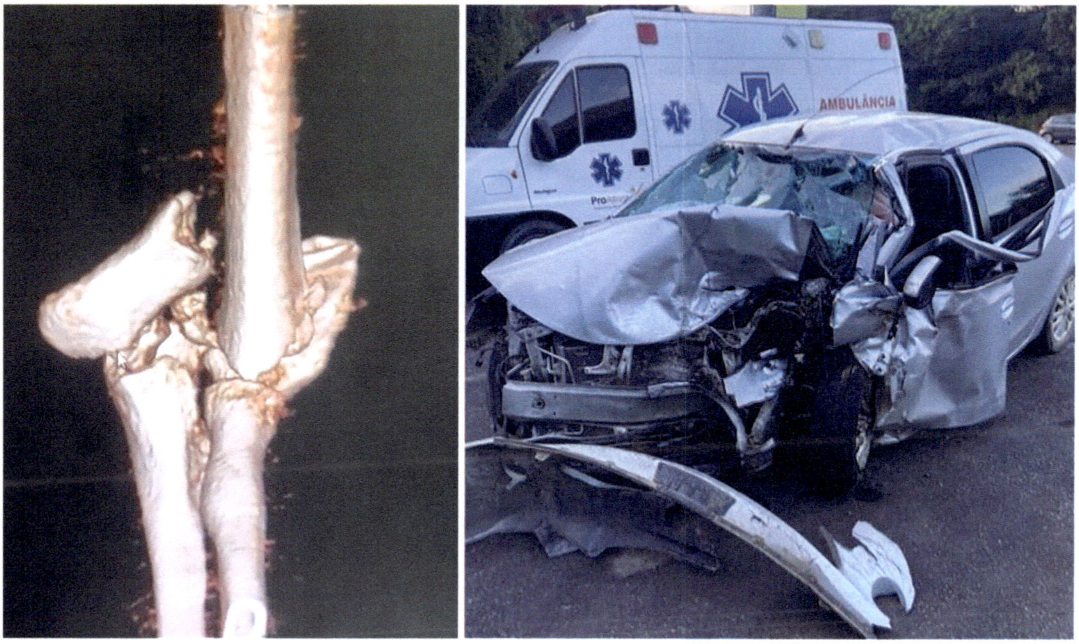

Images 4.13–4.14 Two weeks after the surgery, the patient presents with good function of the elbow

References

1. Müller AM, Sadoghi P, Lucas R, Audige L, Delaney R, Klein M, et al. Effectiveness of bracing in the treatment of nonosseous restriction of elbow mobility: a systematic review andmeta-analysis of 13 studies. J Shoulder Elb Surg. 2013;22(8):1146–52.
2. Siemensma MF, van der Windt AE, van Es EM, Colaris JW, Eygendaal D. Management of the stiff elbow: a literature review. EFORT Open Rev. 2023;8(5):351–60.
3. Liu S, Liu J j, Li X j, Ruan H j, Fan C y. Open arthrolysis and prosthetic replacement of the radial head for elbow stiffness associated with rotation limitation. J Shoulder Elb Surg. 2013;22(2):275–9. https://doi.org/10.1016/j.jse.2012.10.022.
4. Masci G, Cazzato G, Milano G, Ciolli G, Malerba G, Perisano C, et al. The stiff elbow: current concepts. Orthop Rev (Pavia). 2020;12(1S):36–41.
5. Morrey BF, Askew LJ, Chao EY. A biomechanical study of normal functional elbow motion. J Bone Joint Surg Am. 1981;63(6):872–7.
6. Morrey BF. Post-traumatic contracture of the elbow. Operative treatment, including distraction arthroplasty. J Bone Joint Surg Am. 1990;72(4):601–18.
7. Keschner MT, Paksima N. The stiff elbow. Bull NYU Hosp Jt Dis. 2007;65(1):24–8.
8. Lounev VY, Ramachandran R, Wosczyna MN, Yamamoto M, Maidment ADA, Shore EM, et al. Identification of progenitor cells that contribute to heterotopic skeletogenesis. J Bone Joint Surg Am. 2009;91(3):652–63.
9. Attum B, Obremskey W. Posttraumatic elbow stiffness: a critical analysis review. JBJS Rev. 2016;4(9):e1.
10. Bonniaud P, Margetts PJ, Ask K, Flanders K, Gauldie J, Kolb M. TGF-beta and Smad3 signaling link inflammation to chronic fibrogenesis. J Immunol. 2005;175(8):5390–5.
11. Myden C, Hildebrand K. Elbow joint contracture after traumatic injury. J shoulder Elb Surg. 2011;20(1):39–44.
12. O'Driscoll SW, Giori NJ. Continuous passive motion (CPM): theory and principles of clinical application. J Rehabil Res Dev. 2000;37(2):179–88.
13. Morrey ME, Abdel MP, Riester SM, Dudakovic A, van Wijnen AJ, Morrey BF, et al. Molecular landscape of arthrofibrosis: microarray and bioinformatic analysis of the temporal expression of 380 genes during contracture genesis. Gene. 2017;610:15–23.
14. Manocha RHK, Banayan S, Johnson JA, King GJW. Overhead arm positioning in the rehabilitation of elbow dislocations: an in vitro biomechanical study. J Hand Ther. 2022;35(2):245–53.
15. Tibbo ME, Limberg AK, Salib CG, Turner TW, McLaury AR, Jay AG, et al. Anti-fibrotic effects of the antihistamine ketotifen in a rabbit model of arthrofibrosis. Bone Joint Res. 2020;9(6):302–10.
16. Efird W, Kellam P, Yeazell S, Weinhold P, Dahners LE. An evaluation of prophylactic treatments to

prevent post traumatic joint stiffness. J Orthop Res. 2014;32(11):1520–4.
17. Spitler CA, Doty DH, Johnson MD, Nowotarski PJ, Kiner DW, Swafford RE, et al. Manipulation under anesthesia as a treatment of posttraumatic elbow stiffness. J Orthop Trauma. 2018;32(8):e304–8.
18. Sos C, Petit A, Brunet J, Rabarin F, Saint Cast Y, Raimbeau G, et al. Comparison of results of arthroscopic arthrolysis between traumatic and degenerative elbow stiffness. Orthop Traumatol Surg Res. 2023;109(2):103436.
19. Lanzerath F, Wegmann K, Hackl M, Uschok S, Ott N, Müller LP, et al. Surgical arthrolysis of the stiff elbow: a systematic review. Arch Orthop Trauma Surg. 2023;143(5):2383–93.
20. The B, Reininga IHF, El Moumni M, Eygendaal D. Elbow-specific clinical rating systems: extent of established validity, reliability, and responsiveness. J Shoulder Elb Surg. 2013;22(10):1380–94. https://doi.org/10.1016/j.jse.2013.04.013.
21. Doornberg JN, Ring D, Fabian LM, Malhotra L, Zurakowski D, Jupiter JB. Pain dominates measurements of elbow function and health status. J Bone Joint Surg Am. 2005;87(8):1725–31. https://doi.org/10.2106/JBJS.D.02745.
22. Cai J, Wang W, Yan H, Sun Y, Chen W, Chen S, Fan C. Complications of open elbow arthrolysis in post-traumatic elbow stiffness: a systematic review. PLoS One. 2015;10(9):e0138547. https://doi.org/10.1371/journal.pone.0138547.
23. Dawson J, Doll H, Boller I, Fitzpatrick R, Little C, Rees J, et al. The development and validation of a patient-reported questionnaire to assess outcomes of elbow surgery. J Bone Joint Surg Br. 2008;90(4):466–73.
24. Capuano L, Poulain S, Hardy P, Longo UG, Denaro V, Maffulli N. No correlation between physicians administered elbow rating systems and patient's satisfaction. J Sports Med Phys Fitness. 2011;51(2):255–9.
25. Longo UG, Franceschi F, Loppini M, Maffulli N, Denaro V. Rating systems for evaluation of the elbow. Br Med Bull. 2008;87(1):131–61.
26. Sun Z, Fan C. Validation of the Liverpool Elbow Score for evaluation of elbow stiffness. BMC Musculoskelet Disord. 2018;19(1):302. https://doi.org/10.1186/s12891-018-2226-0.

5 Diagnostic Imaging of the Stiff Elbow

Carina Cohen, Tatiane Cantarelli, Abdalla Skaf, and Benno Ejnisman

5.1 Introduction

Elbow stiffness is a debilitating condition characterized by limited range of motion and reduced flexibility in the elbow joint, where the etiology may or may not be associated with a traumatic event [1–5]. It can be due to abnormalities in bone, soft tissue, or a combination of both [2–4, 6]. The condition may result from various intra-articular and extra-articular factors, including posttraumatic arthritis, joint incongruity, ankylosis, osteoarthritis with bone spurs, and proliferative synovitis, such as synovial chondromatosis, as well as heterotopic bone formation, capsular thickening, and musculotendinous contracture [1, 6–10].

Traumatic events, burns, and head injuries have been identified as known contributors to elbow contractures, with the severity of the insult directly impacting the degree of stiffness experienced [2]. Elbow stiffness can also be attributed to atraumatic factors, which encompass a range of conditions such as osteoarthritis and inflammatory arthritis, postseptic arthritis, multiple hemarthroses in hemophiliacs, and congenital contractures observed in arthrogryposis and congenital radial head dislocation [2, 5].

Imaging plays a crucial role in confirming the etiology of elbow stiffness, determining the involved anatomic elements, and guiding treatment planning and procedures [11]. Soft tissue abnormalities are best assessed using ultrasound (US) or magnetic resonance imaging (MRI), while osseous abnormalities are commonly evaluated through radiography and computed tomography (CT) scans [6]. Accurate imaging assessment is essential for selecting the appropriate treatment strategy, whether it involves conservative approaches for soft tissue abnormalities or arthroscopy or open surgery for osseous abnormalities [6]. The effective diagnosis of elbow stiffness requires a multifaceted approach, involving a thorough medical history, physical examination, and appropriate imaging studies [5, 9]. Our objective is to present a comprehensive review of diagnostic imaging modalities for assessing elbow stiffness.

5.2 Diagnostic Imaging Modalities

The standard imaging workup for evaluating a stiff elbow should include the assessment of remaining bone stock, bone alignment, articular congruency, location and severity of osteoarthri-

C. Cohen (✉) · B. Ejnisman
Federal University of São Paulo (UNIFESP), São Paulo, SP, Brazil

T. Cantarelli · A. Skaf
Department of Radiology, Hcor- Hospital do Coração, São Paulo, SP, Brazil

ALTA Diagnostic Center (DASA Group), São Paulo, Brazil

L. Pederzini et al. (eds.), *Stiffness of the Elbow, Wrist and Related Pathologies*,
https://doi.org/10.1007/978-3-031-81381-8_5

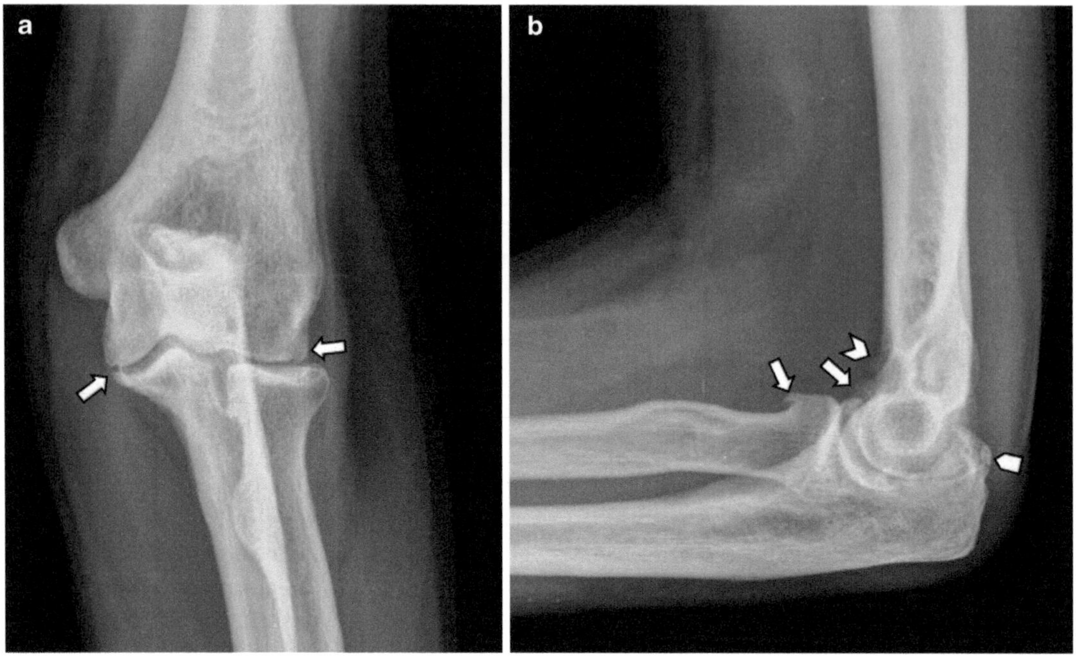

Fig. 5.1 Left elbow primary osteoarthritis in a 70-year-old man: (**a**) The anteroposterior (AP) radiography view shows mild degenerative changes characterized by osteophytes (arrows) and narrowing of the joint space. (**b**) The lateral view shows osteophytes (arrows), a bone spur at the anterior aspect of the distal humerus (arrowhead), and a loose body in the posterior recess (chevron)

tis, presence of osteophytes and their impact on articular mobility and relation to neurovascular structures, presence and location of loose bodies, surgical implants, and capsular and ligamentous injuries [11, 12]. Elbow stiffness can be evaluated using different imaging modalities, such as plain radiographs, CT and CT arthrography, MRI, and ultrasound (US).

5.2.1 Radiographs

Conventional radiography remains the primary step in evaluating elbow stiffness, and it should involve plain radiographs, including anterior–posterior, lateral, and two oblique views [2, 3, 5, 6, 9, 11]. If the elbow is unable to fully extend due to contracture, two anteroposterior views should be taken—one perpendicular to the distal humerus and another perpendicular to the proximal radius and ulna [11]. Although plain radiography is easily accessible, it frequently lacks accuracy [12].

During the radiographic evaluation of the elbow, several aspects should be examined, including malunion, malalignment, loose bodies, osteophytes, joint space narrowing, articular congruency, periarticular calcification, and heterotopic ossification [11] (Figs. 5.1 and 5.2). Fluoroscopy can be utilized to differentiate between a bony block and soft tissue contracture [2] and it is considered reliably to identify most free-floating loose bodies [13].

5.2.2 CT/CT Arthrography

In recent years, the use of CT in musculoskeletal radiology has significantly increased, primarily due to the availability of high-resolution reformations, and its utility is well-established [6, 9]. CT/CT arthrography studies should

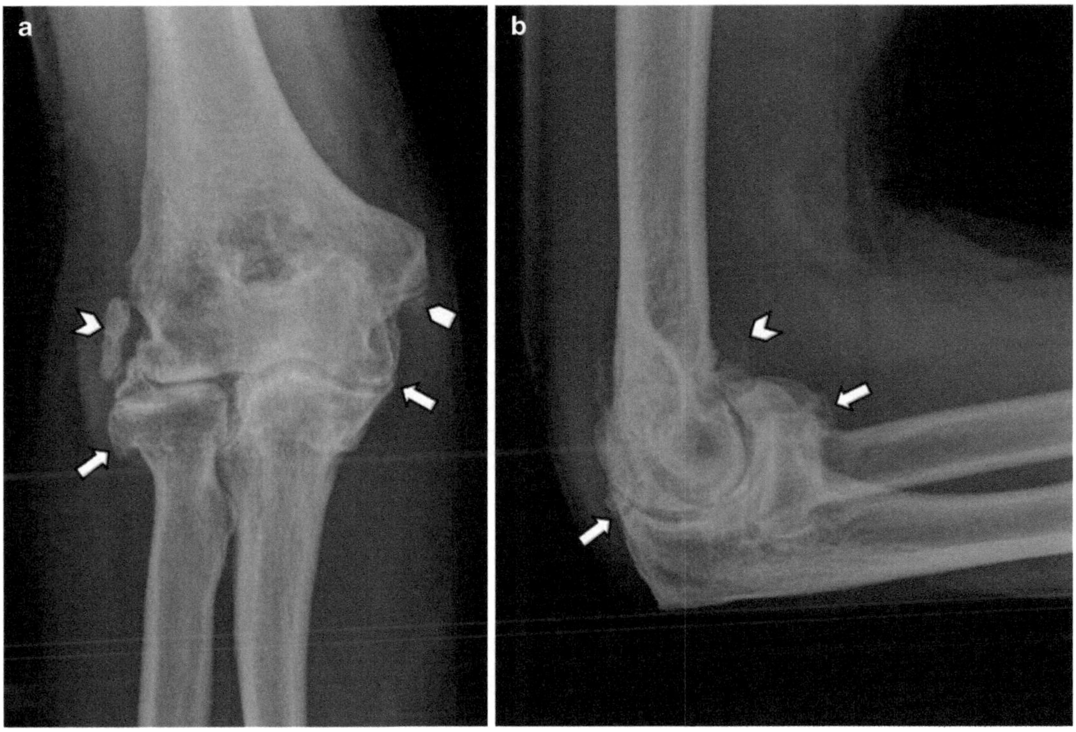

Fig. 5.2 Posttraumatic right elbow arthritis in a 51-year-old man: (**a**) The AP radiography view shows degenerative changes characterized by osteophytes (arrows), narrowing of the joint space, and subchondral sclerosis. There are also avulsed bone fragments resulting from previous trauma at the lateral epicondyle (chevron) and medial epicondyle (arrowhead). (**b**) The lateral view shows osteophytes (arrows) and a loose body at the anterior aspect of the elbow joint

encompass the evaluation of heterotopic ossification, synovitis, loose bodies, osteophytes, joint space narrowing, fibrosis, ankylosis, malunion, non-union, and posttraumatic sequela [4, 5, 9, 11]. For a more comprehensive assessment of the elbow joint, CT with multiplanar and three-dimensional reconstructions is recommended [2, 3, 11]. Among these, the sagittal reformations hold particular significance, as they allow for quantitative evaluation of the limitation of flexion and extension; as a result, patients with restricted extension can expect to gain the highest diagnostic information from CT imaging [6] (Fig. 5.3).

Loose bodies and osteophytes located in the anterior and posterior joint space, particularly in the fossa coronoidea and fossa olecrani, are frequently not visible on conventional radiography [6]. However, these osteophytes in the fossae may have significant biomechanical implications [6].

CT imaging provides a superior assessment of the diagnosis of osteoarthritis with precise delineation of the joint space and degree of joint space narrowing, and the characterization of osteophytes, which are nearly always present in the trochleoulnar compartment and are found in approximately 25% of cases in the radiocapitellar compartment [11]. CT or CT arthrography is considered superior to conventional radiography for evaluating loose bodies, offering higher accuracy [6, 14]. In a study comparing the two imaging modalities, CT had a detection accuracy of 79% for loose bodies, outperforming conventional radiography's accuracy of 67%. The sensitivity and specificity of CT were 93% and 66%, respectively, while those of conventional radiography were 86% and 48%.

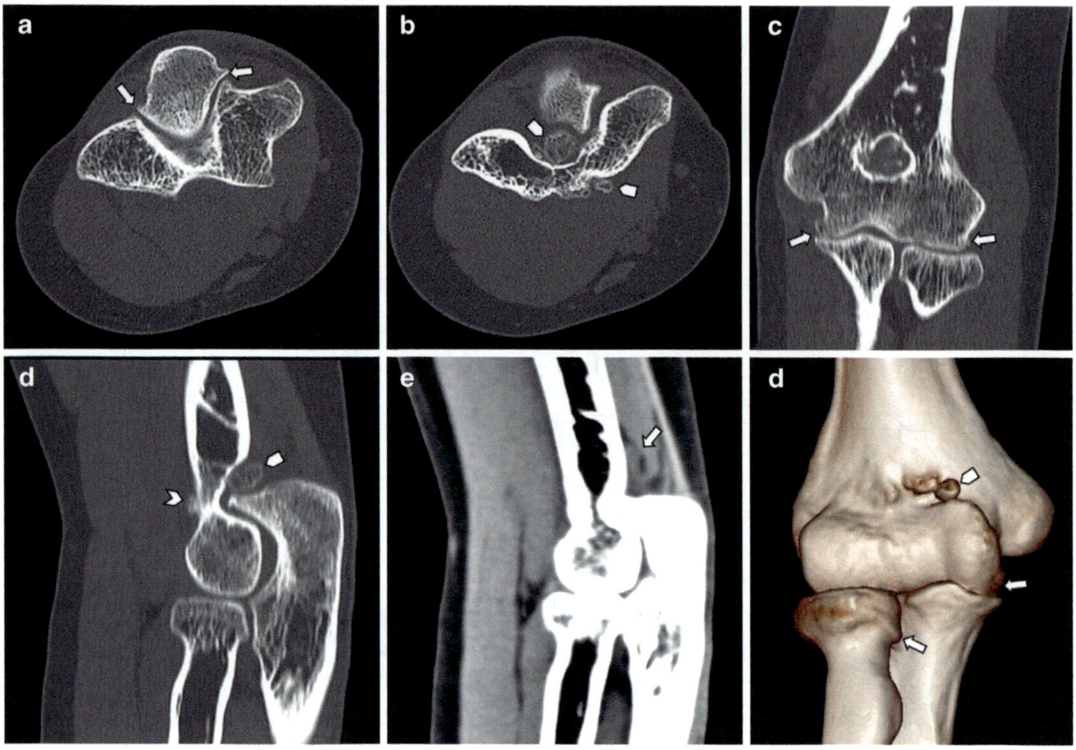

Fig. 5.3 Posttraumatic right elbow arthritis in a 37-year-old woman: (**a**) The axial plane CT scan provides detailed imaging of the joint, highlighting degenerative changes, such as osteophytes (arrows) and narrowing of the joint space. (**b**) It also demonstrates ossified loose bodies (arrowheads). (**c**) The reformatted coronal plane image reveals osteophytes (arrows) and narrowing of the joint space. (**d**, **e**) The reformatted sagittal-oblique plane shows bone spurs on the anterior aspect of the distal humerus (chevron), a loose body in the posterior recess (arrowhead), and joint effusion (arrow). (**f**) The volume rendering reformatting displays visible osteophytes on the radial head and trochlea (arrows) and an anterior loose body (arrowhead)

The differences in accuracy were particularly noticeable in detecting loose bodies in the dorsal joint space, where CT exhibited an accuracy of 79% compared to conventional radiography's 64%, sensitivity of 90% vs. 60%, and specificity of 74% vs. 66% [6].

CT arthrography is a minimally invasive technique that offers an excellent assessment of the cartilage articular surface [11]. CT arthrography can show osteochondral fragments as small as 3 mm in diameter [12]. In cases where cartilaginous lesions are present, relying solely on osteophyte treatment may not lead to a complete improvement in elbow function, and patients may experience persistent pain even after surgical management [11]. The superiority of CT arthrography over conventional CT for assessing loose bodies remains controversial [6]. CT arthrography is especially valuable in detecting non-ossified intra-articular loose bodies, such as cartilage fragments [11]. However, before performing CT arthrography, it is essential to obtain a non-contrast acquisition to identify calcified loose bodies that might be hidden or obscured by the intra-articular iodinated contrast [11]. Additionally, CT arthrography can aid in diagnosing capsular retraction when the articular capacity is reduced to approximately 6 ± 3 mL [11]. It can be combined with an intra-articular corticosteroid injection, serving as both a diagnostic and therapeutic test by reducing capsular inflammation [11].

5.2.3 US

Ultrasonography is a recommended imaging modality for evaluating ligamentous, tendinous, ulnar neuropathy, joint effusion, and synovitis [11]. The motion of loose bodies into the articular cavity can be enhanced by dynamic maneuvers during ultrasound [15]. However, it is not the preferred method for assessing loose bodies and osteochondral traumatic lesions, and should only be used for this purpose when other imaging methods are unavailable [11] (Fig. 5.4). Special attention should be given to the ulnar nerve, as it is frequently involved in traumatic or degenerative processes, while radial and median nerves are less susceptible to injury; they can be affected by scar formation, heterotopic ossification, or iatrogenic injury [11].

5.2.4 MRI

The advantages of using MRI include multiplanar imaging, avoiding radiation exposure, and the ability to diagnose primarily cartilaginous lesions and other conditions like osteochondritis dissecans [12, 16]. However, MRI's role in the assessment of elbow stiffness is limited, and it is typically performed when soft tissue involvement is suspected, such as synovitis, ligament dysfunction, or neuropathies [4, 5, 11, 17]. MR arthrography is also an option, enabling a combined evaluation of capsular and periarticular soft tissues, such as musculotendinous and capsuloligamentous scarring, cartilage articular surface, osteophytes, and intra-articular loose bodies [11]. Regarding loose body detection with MRI, Dubberley et al. reported relatively high sensitivity but relatively low specificities of 20% [12]. Some pathologies can present with multiple loose bodies within the joint, such as primary or secondary synovial chondromatosis, with large joints like the knee, elbow, and shoulder being commonly affected [15]. Typical symptoms include joint swelling, restricted motion, and later development of intermittent locking and pain [7, 15] (Fig. 5.5).

MRI can aid in identifying capsular and/or ligament thickening, indicated by low signal intensity in both T1- and T2-weighted images due to bleeding, edema, granulation tissue formation, and fibrosis [11, 17]. Additionally, non-fat-saturated T1-weighted sequences can be useful in identifying fibrotic changes in intra-articular fatpads, such as low signal intensity bands and peripheral thickening [11] (Fig. 5.6).

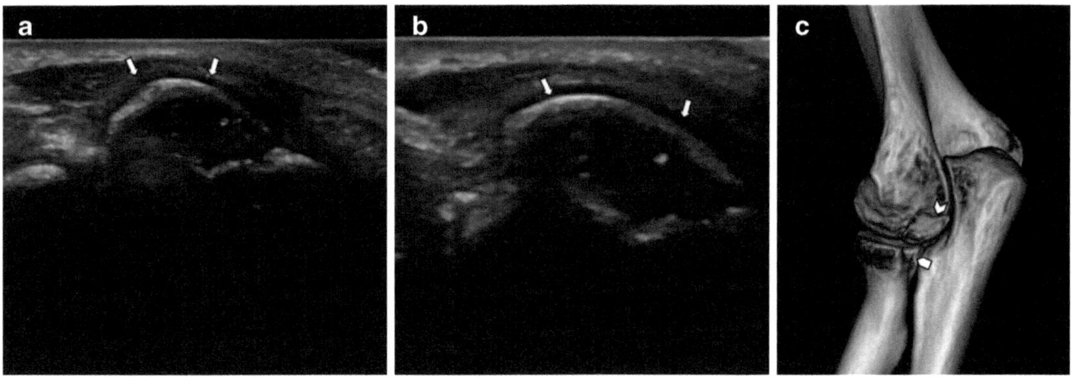

Fig. 5.4 Posttraumatic sequela in the right elbow of a 59-year-old woman: (**a**, **b**) Ultrasonography images at the transverse and longitudinal axes depict a bone fragment interposed into the radiocapitellar joint space (arrows). (**c**) The CT image with 3D volume reformatting displays the same bone fragment (chevron) interposed within the joint space, further confirming its presence. Additionally, the image reveals a sequela of a fracture with significant bone loss in the radial head (arrowhead)

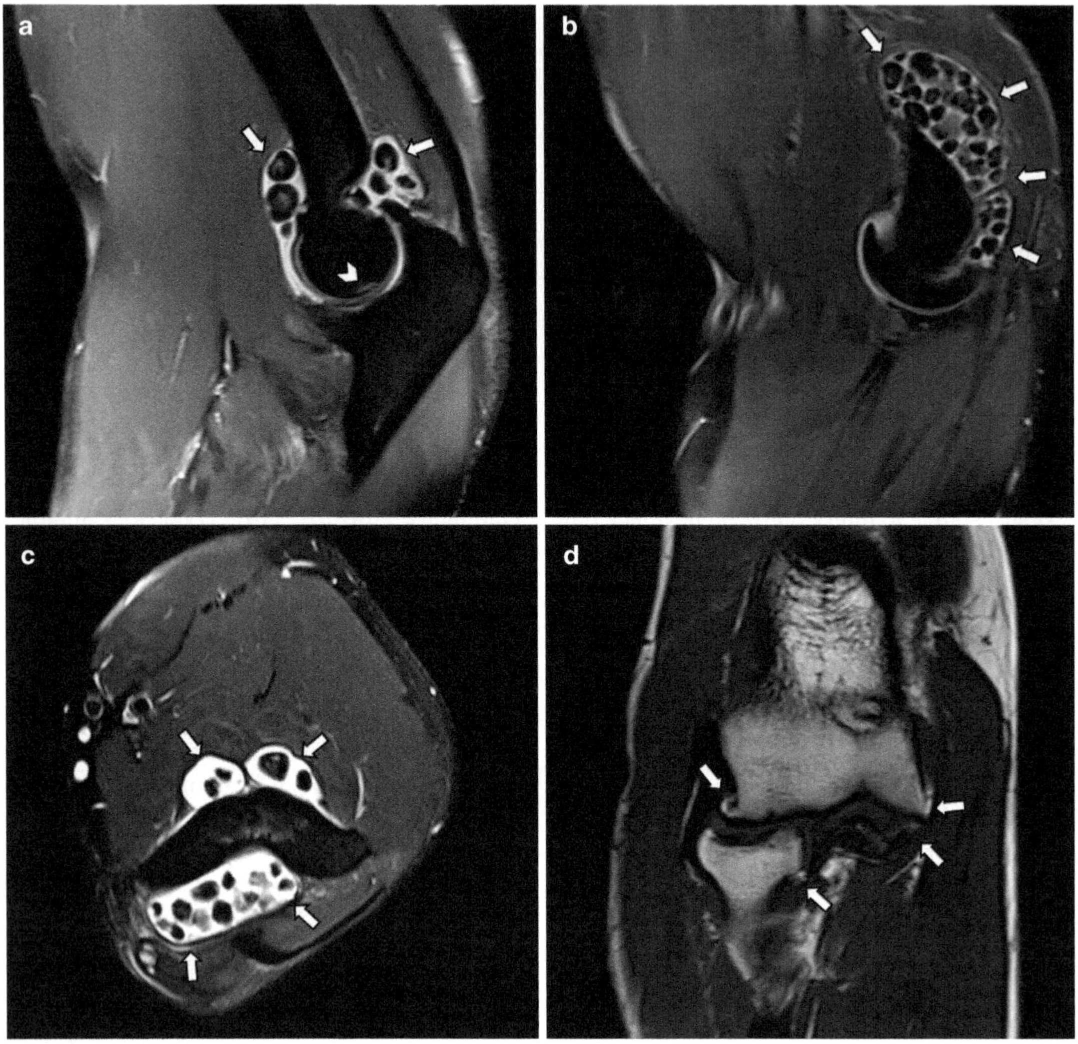

Fig. 5.5 Secondary synovial chondromatosis in the right elbow of a 46-year-old man: (**a**, **b**) The sagittal and (**c**) axial T2-weighted MRI images highlight the extent of synovial chondromatosis, demonstrating numerous cartilaginous nodules with varying sizes (arrows) within the synovial fluid-filled space, along with a cartilage defect (chevron). (**d**) The coronal T1-weighted MRI image provides detailed visualization of the joint structures, revealing degenerative changes with the presence of multiple osteophytes (arrows)

The superficial location of the ulnar nerve makes it susceptible to trauma and impingement due to degenerative joint changes [11, 18]. Furthermore, intra-articular space-occupying lesions, like ganglion cysts, might not be detectable on CT and can lead to neuropathies or elbow stiffness if located in the anterior joint compartment [11].

Atraumatic elbow contractures with negative radiographs might be related to soft tissue tumors, necessitating further evaluation with MRI [11, 17]. Additionally, patients with pain as their primary complaint after trauma, without osseous lesions on radiographs or CT, should be assessed for type 1 complex regional pain syndrome, as they may not respond to conventional therapeutic strategies [11].

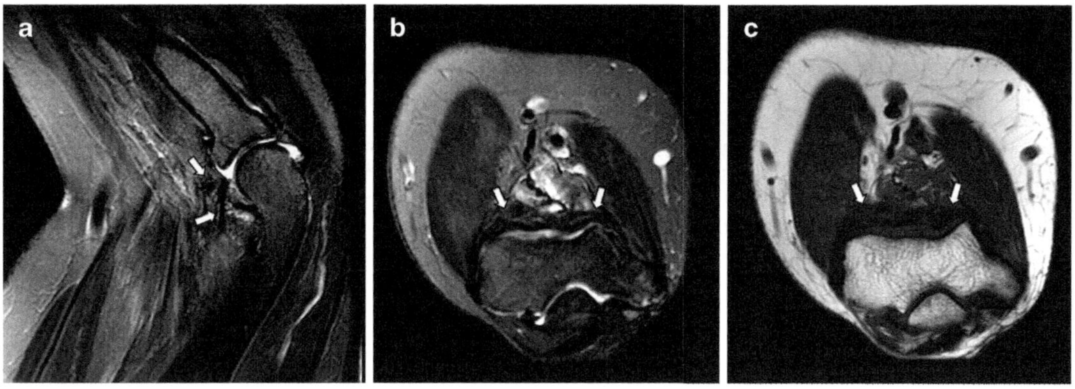

Fig. 5.6 Postoperative fibrotic changes in the left elbow of a 56-year-old woman: MRI images on T2 fat-suppressed weighted at the (**a**) sagittal and (**b**) axial planes, and (**c**) axial T1-weighted sequences show low signal intensity bands and thickening of the anterior joint capsule (arrows), indicative of fibrotic alterations

5.3 Conclusion

Considering the complexity of diagnosing elbow stiffness, the incorporation of medical imaging to the history and physical examination proves essential for optimal patient management. A study highlighted the superior effectiveness of CT over conventional radiography in evaluating the osseous causes of elbow stiffness, particularly due to improved detection of loose bodies and osteophytes. CT arthrography is a valuable preoperative tool for assessing the cartilage articular surface, while MRI can be recommended when conventional radiography and CT are inconclusive, especially for patients with atraumatic joint stiffness seeking potential soft tissue origins. Imaging plays an essential role in identifying the cause and extent of elbow stiffness, guiding treatment planning and procedures, and assisting in the formulation of effective treatment strategies.

References

1. Keschner MT, Paksima N. The stiff elbow. Bull NYU Hosp Jt Dis. 2007;65(1):24–8.
2. Nandi S, Maschke S, Evans PJ, Lawton JN. The stiff elbow. Hand (N Y). 2009;4(4):368–79.
3. Siemensma MF, Windt AEV, Es EMV, Colaris JW, Eygendaal D. Management of the stiff elbow: a literature review. EFORT Open Rev. 2023;8(5):351–60.
4. Akhtar A, Hughes B, Watts AC. The post-traumatic stiff elbow: a review. J Clin Orthop Trauma. 2021;19:125–31.
5. Masci G, Cazzato G, Milano G, Ciolli G, Malerba G, Perisano C, et al. The stiff elbow: current concepts. Orthop Rev (Pavia). 2020;12(Suppl 1):8661.
6. Zubler V, Saupe N, Jost B, Pfirrmann CW, Hodler J, Zanetti M. Elbow stiffness: effectiveness of conventional radiography and CT to explain osseous causes. AJR Am J Roentgenol. 2010;194(6):W515–20.
7. Griesser MJ, Harris JD, Likes RL, Jones GL. Synovial chondromatosis of the elbow causing a mechanical block to range of motion: a case report and review of the literature. Am J Orthop (Belle Mead NJ). 2011;40(5):253–6.
8. Adolfsson L. Post-traumatic stiff elbow. EFORT Open Rev. 2018;3(5):210–6.
9. Mellema JJ, Lindenhovius AL, Jupiter JB. The posttraumatic stiff elbow: an update. Curr Rev Musculoskelet Med. 2016;9(2):190–8.
10. Jupiter JB, O'Driscoll SW, Cohen MS. The assessment and management of the stiff elbow. Instr Course Lect. 2003;52:93–111.
11. Lombard C, Teixeira P, Germain E, Dodin G, Louis M, Blum A, et al. Elbow stiffness imaging: a practical diagnostic and pretherapeutic approach. J Clin Med. 2021;10(22):5348.
12. Dubberley JH, Faber KJ, Patterson SD, Garvin G, Bennett J, Romano W, et al. The detection of loose bodies in the elbow: the value of MRI and CT arthrography. J Bone Joint Surg Br. 2005;87(5):684–6.
13. Hudson TM. Joint fluoroscopy before arthrography: detection and evaluation of loose bodies. Skeletal Radiol. 1984;12(3):199–203.

14. Ward WG, Belhobek GH, Anderson TE. Arthroscopic elbow findings: correlation with preoperative radiographic studies. Arthroscopy. 1992;8(4):498–502.
15. Bianchi S, Martinoli C. Detection of loose bodies in joints. Radiol Clin North Am. 1999;37(4):679–90.
16. Seah RB, Mak WK, Bryant K, Korlaet M, Dwyer A, Bain GI. Four-dimensional computed tomography scan for dynamic elbow disorders: recommendations for clinical utility. JSES Int. 2022;6(1):182–6.
17. Fortier MV, Forster BB, Pinney S, Regan W. MR assessment of posttraumatic flexion contracture of the elbow. J Magn Reson Imaging. 1995;5(4):473–7.
18. Shuai C, Hede Y, Shen L, Yuanming O, Hongjiang R, Cunyi F. Is routine ulnar nerve transposition necessary in open release of stiff elbows? Our experience and a literature review. Int Orthop. 2014;38(11):2289–94.

Three-Dimensional Printing in the Treatment of Post-traumatic Stiff Elbow

6

Andrea Celli, Biagini Alessio, Cheli Andrea, and Luigi Pederzini

6.1 Introduction

The elbow is one of the most complex joints in the upper limb. Technological advances have brought surgical planning into the digital era and now enable selecting the most appropriate surgical strategy before the procedure [1]. However, accurate and effective planning of post-traumatic stiff elbow surgery is still challenging. Three-dimensional (3D) printing—a rapid prototyping technology that uses a 3D digital model to build a physical object layer by layer—holds considerable promise for orthopedic surgery applications [2, 3]. Before the procedure, examination of a 3D-printed model of the injured elbow supplies highly detailed information on the joint [4, 5] and allows to establish an accurate surgical plan, thus also improving doctor–patient communication.

Post-traumatic elbow stiffness is characterized by various levels of severity, from simple retraction of periarticular soft tissues (capsula, tendons, ligaments) to extensive bone deformity. A wide range of therapeutic options, from simple rehabilitation to prosthetic implantation, are available to manage such widely different presentations. In the preoperative planning stage, it is important to identify the most suitable treatment strategy based on injury assessment. We have examined a series of patients with post-traumatic elbow stiffness to understand where and how 3D printing provides an advantage in preoperative planning and the choice of treatment [6–11].

6.2 Materials

Source quality is a key element in the process of creating a 3D print from medical images. 3D models of objects can be created based on sequences of Digital imaging and communications in medicine (DICOM) images available in computed tomography (CT) devices. The greater the number of images acquired in the examination sequence, the higher the quality of the model, as it minimizes artifacts and irregularities. Internal fixation devices and metal components that may be present in a joint affect the 3D model and are not always easy to remove from the images. Therefore, where possible, the examination should be performed with instruments that can reduce their effects.

A. Celli (✉) · B. Alessio
Department of Orthopaedic and Traumatology Surgery, Shoulder and Elbow Unit, Hesperia Hospital, Modena, Italy

C. Andrea
Department of Orthopaedic, Traumatology and Arthroscopic Surgeries, Nuovo Ospedale di Sassuolo, Modena, Italy

L. Pederzini
Department of Orthopedics, Hesperia Hospital, Modena, Italy

L. Pederzini et al. (eds.), *Stiffness of the Elbow, Wrist and Related Pathologies*,
https://doi.org/10.1007/978-3-031-81381-8_6

6.3 Creation of 3D Models from Images

Inobitec Dicom Viewer, Materialize, and Slicer3D are some of several software products developed to obtain 3D models from medical images. We employed the software Inobitec Dicom Viewer Pro, which is simple to use and allows to view and reconstruct 3D models starting from CT and magnetic resonance imaging (MRI) scans. The software also allows performing several other operations, some based on artificial intelligence, on the image sequences. After importing an image sequence from CT or MRI, a preliminary 3D model can be obtained in a few clicks. The model is useful to understand the quality of the source and, on its basis, to perform all the operations required to create the file for 3D printing. First, the bony parts that are not disconnected from the segment involved in the reconstruction are eliminated; then, a check for artifacts is performed, to try and remove them by adjusting the contrast in the display. If this procedure fails to remove all artifacts and shows the bone portions clearly separated from each other, manual segmentation is required. This involves selecting the portions of interest by scrolling and analyzing the images of the sequence one by one in the sagittal, coronal, and axial views. After a 3D model that satisfies the surgeon's requirements has been obtained, it is made into a mesh, that is, a set of triangles that provides the mathematical geometry of the model.

6.4 3D Printing of the Final 3D Model

The model thus generated is then imported into the appropriate slicing software, which allows creating the machine language for the 3D printer. These models can be constructed using the main additive manufacturing technologies, that is, filament (FDM), resin (SLA/DLP), and powder (SLS) 3D printing. Some materials, mostly resins, mimic the strength and mechanical properties of bone. To ensure correct resolution of the 3D model it must be oriented in the best way, and support structures must be used to ensure that each undercut present can be created.

6.5 Methods

6.5.1 Case Series of Post-traumatic Stiff Elbow: Considerations of Four Elbow Surgeons

For a recent study of the value of 3D printing for post-traumatic elbow stiffness surgery, we recruited six patients with stiffness of varying severity, who underwent clinical evaluation with X-rays and CT with 3D reconstruction. We referred the cases to four upper-limb surgeons with at least 15-year experience in elbow surgery, who were not involved in the study. We asked them to evaluate the patients based on their surgical strategy (arthroscopic or open technique), to state the type of surgical approach, and to rate the scope for functional recovery and the risk of complications. Then we obtained 3D-printed models of the six stiff elbows and asked the surgeons to evaluate them using the same parameters.

6.5.1.1 Case 1

Patient: A 66-year-old right-handed woman

Trauma: Blunt trauma to the right elbow without fracture

Treatment: Half-cast for 15 days followed by physiotherapy

Range of motion (ROM) 12 months from the trauma: Flexion–extension, 100°–40°; pronation–supination, 80°–80°

Imaging: X-rays and CT, 3D printing (Fig. 6.1a–e)

Outcome: None of the surgeons changed surgical strategy after viewing the 3D-printed model; they found it useful only as a teaching aid with no advantage over CT with 3D reconstruction.

6.5.1.2 Case 2

Patient: A 33-year-old right-handed woman

Trauma: Undisplaced fracture of the radial head without elbow dislocation

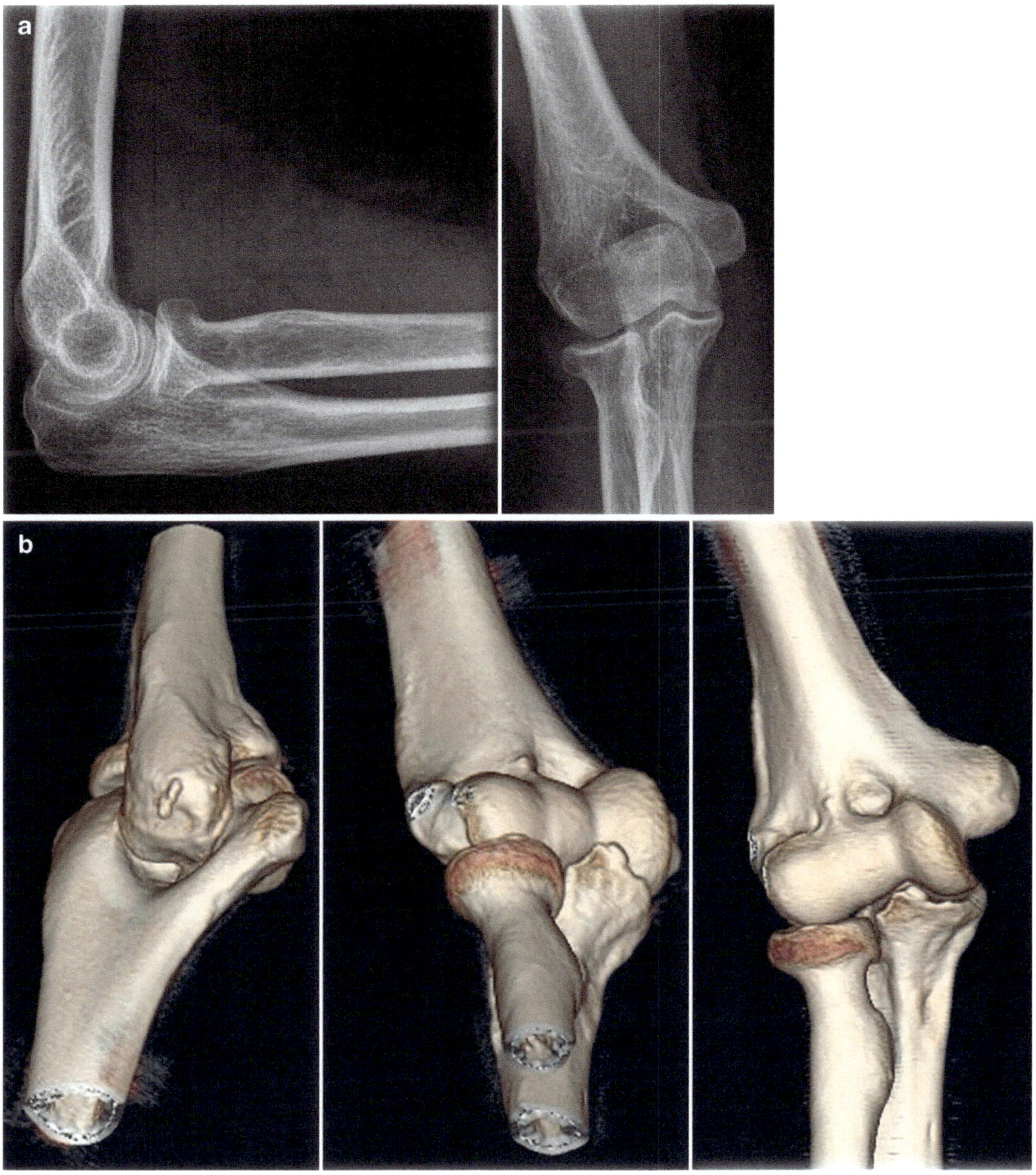

Fig. 6.1 (**a–e**) Case 1

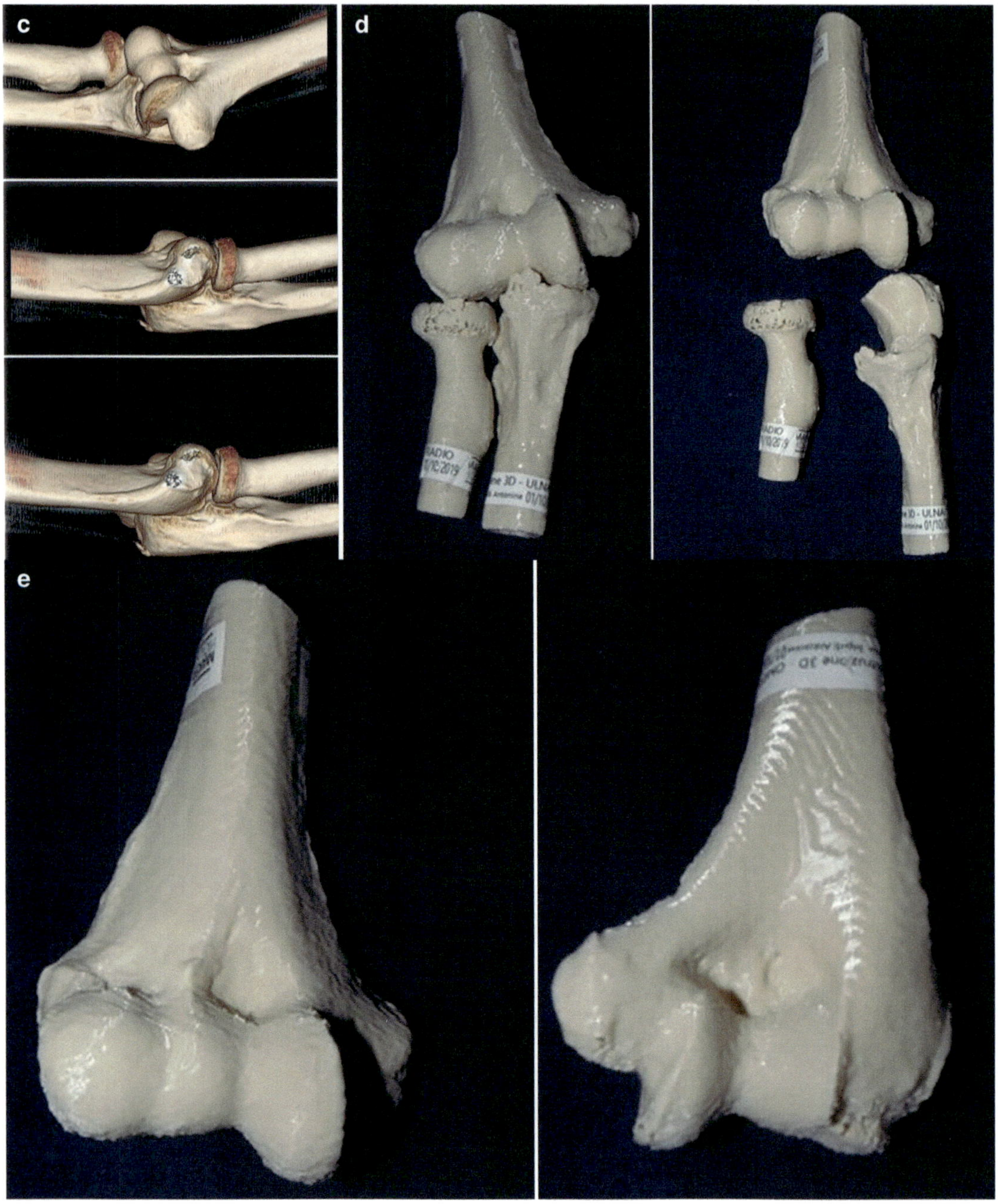

Fig. 6.1 (continued)

Treatment: Cast for 35 days followed by rehabilitation program

ROM 12 months from the trauma: Flexion–extension, 110°–60°; pronation–supination, 45°–45°

Imaging: X-rays and CT, 3D printing (Fig. 6.2a–f)

Outcome: None of the surgeons changed surgical strategy after viewing the 3D-printed model; they found it useful only as a teaching aid with no advantage over CT with 3D reconstruction.

6.5.1.3 Case 3

Patient: A 37-year-old right-handed man

Trauma: Undisplaced fracture of the radial head with elbow dislocation

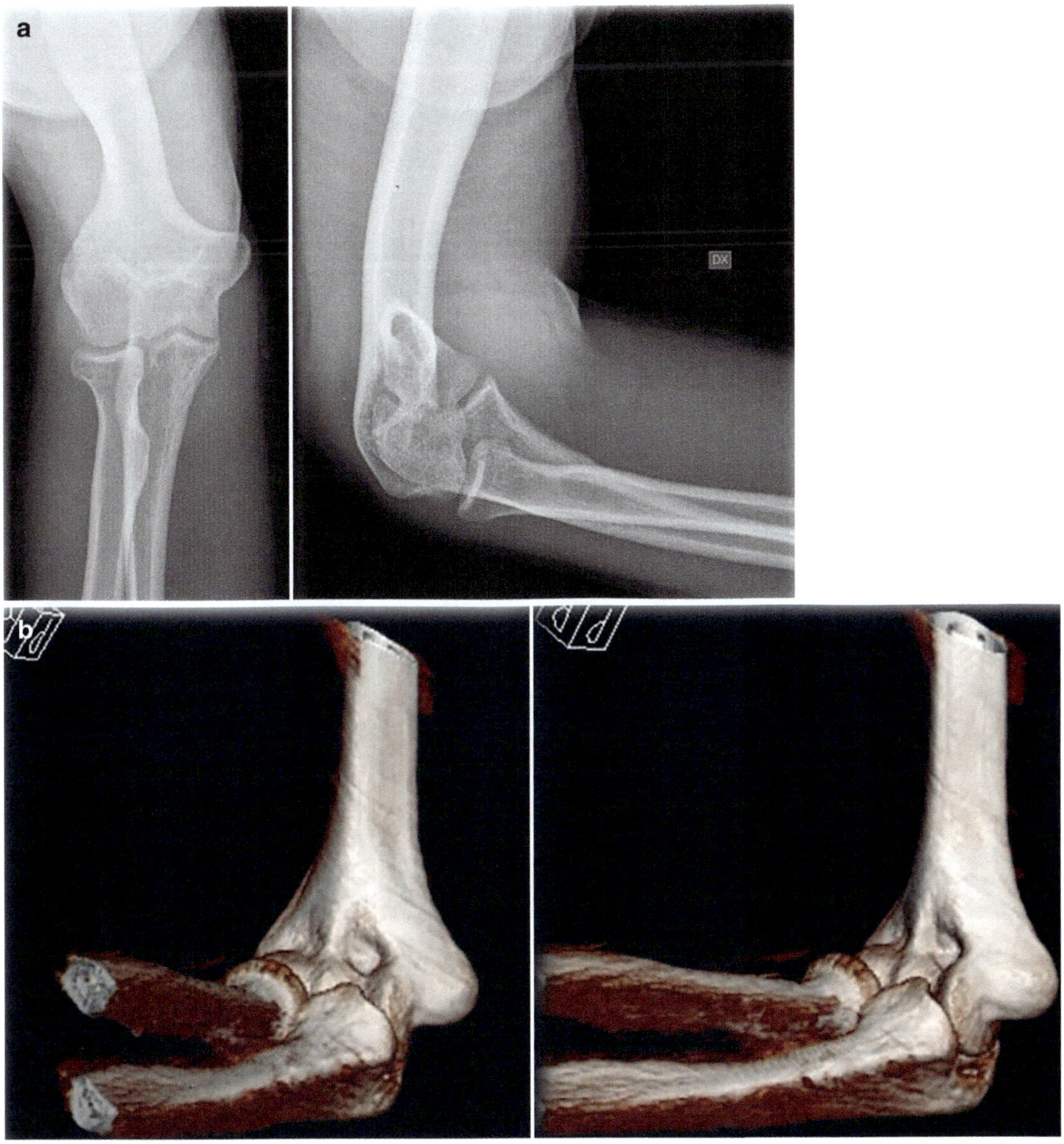

Fig. 6.2 (**a–f**) Case 2

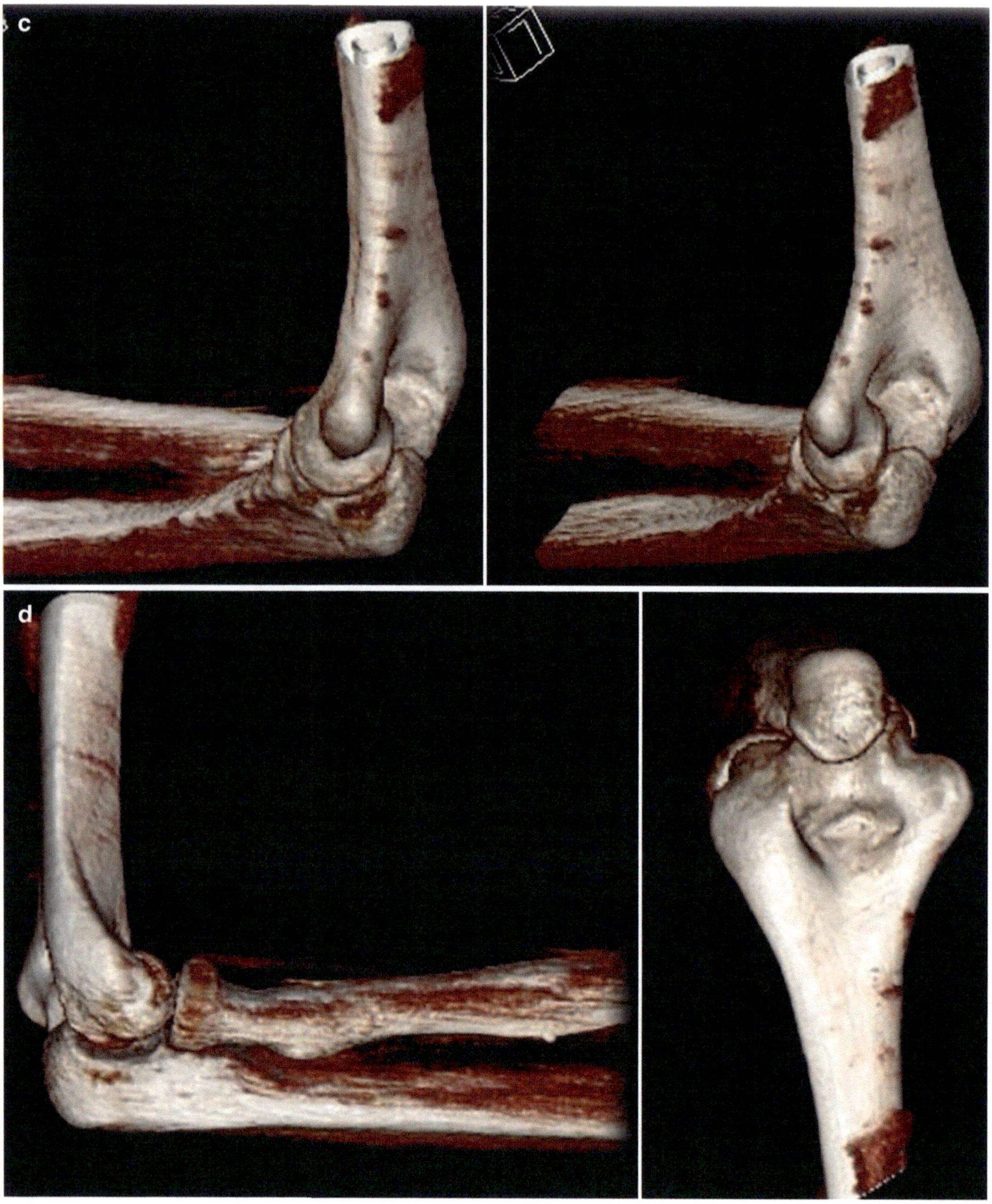

Fig. 6.2 (continued)

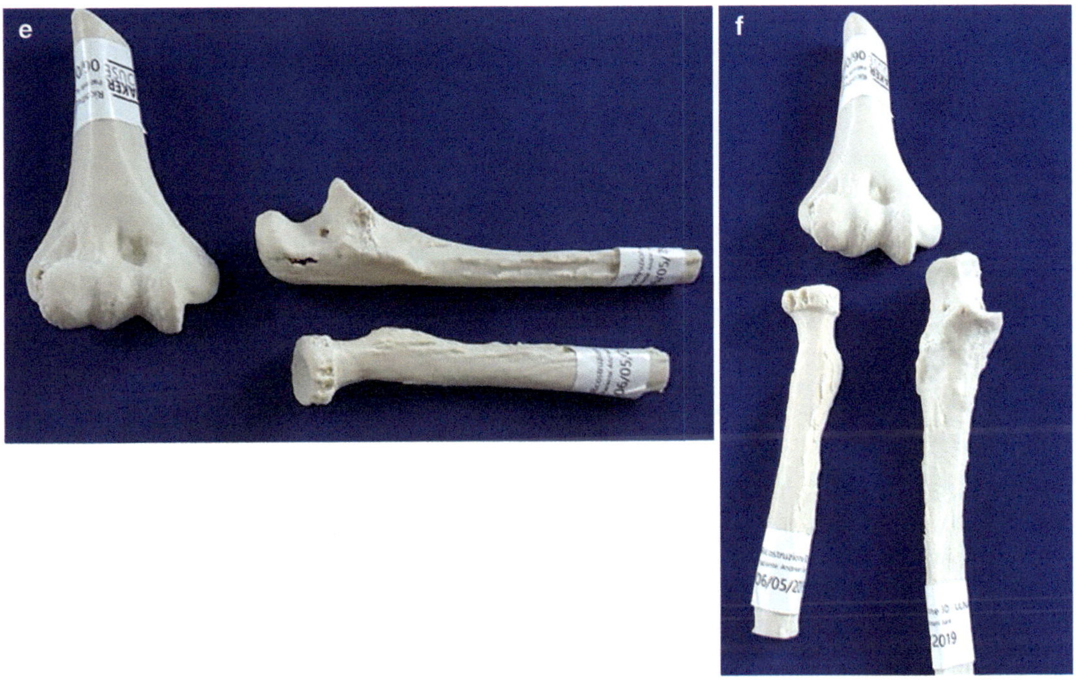

Fig. 6.2 (continued)

Treatment: Cast for 30 days followed by rehabilitation program

ROM 12 months from the trauma: Flexion–extension, 100°–60°; pronation–supination, 80°–80°

Imaging: X-rays and CT, 3D printing (Fig. 6.3a–d)

Outcome: One examiner changed surgical strategy after examination of the 3D-printed model. All surgeons found it more useful to choose the surgical strategy and rate the risk of complications than CT imaging with 3D reconstruction.

6.5.1.4 Case 4

Patient: A 36-year-old right-handed man

Trauma: Undisplaced fracture of the olecranon, left elbow

Treatment: Cast for 40 days followed by rehabilitation program

ROM 12 months from the trauma: Flexion–extension, 120°–80°; pronation–supination, 80°–80°

Imaging: X-rays and CT, 3D printing (Fig. 6.4a–d)

Outcome: Two examiners changed surgical strategy after examination of the 3D-printed model. All surgeons found it more useful to choose the surgical strategy and rate the risk of complications than CT imaging with 3D reconstruction.

6.5.1.5 Case 5

Patient: A 23-year-old right-handed man

Trauma: Displaced distal humeral fracture, left elbow

Treatment: Open reduction and internal fixation with K-wires, cast for 40 days followed by rehabilitation program

ROM 12 months from the trauma: Flexion–extension, 100°–80°; pronation–supination, 30°–30°

Imaging: X-rays and CT, 3D printing (Fig. 6.5a–c)

Outcome: Three examiners changed surgical strategy after examination of the 3D-printed model. All surgeons found it more useful to choose the surgical strategy and rate the risk of complications than CT imaging with 3D reconstruction.

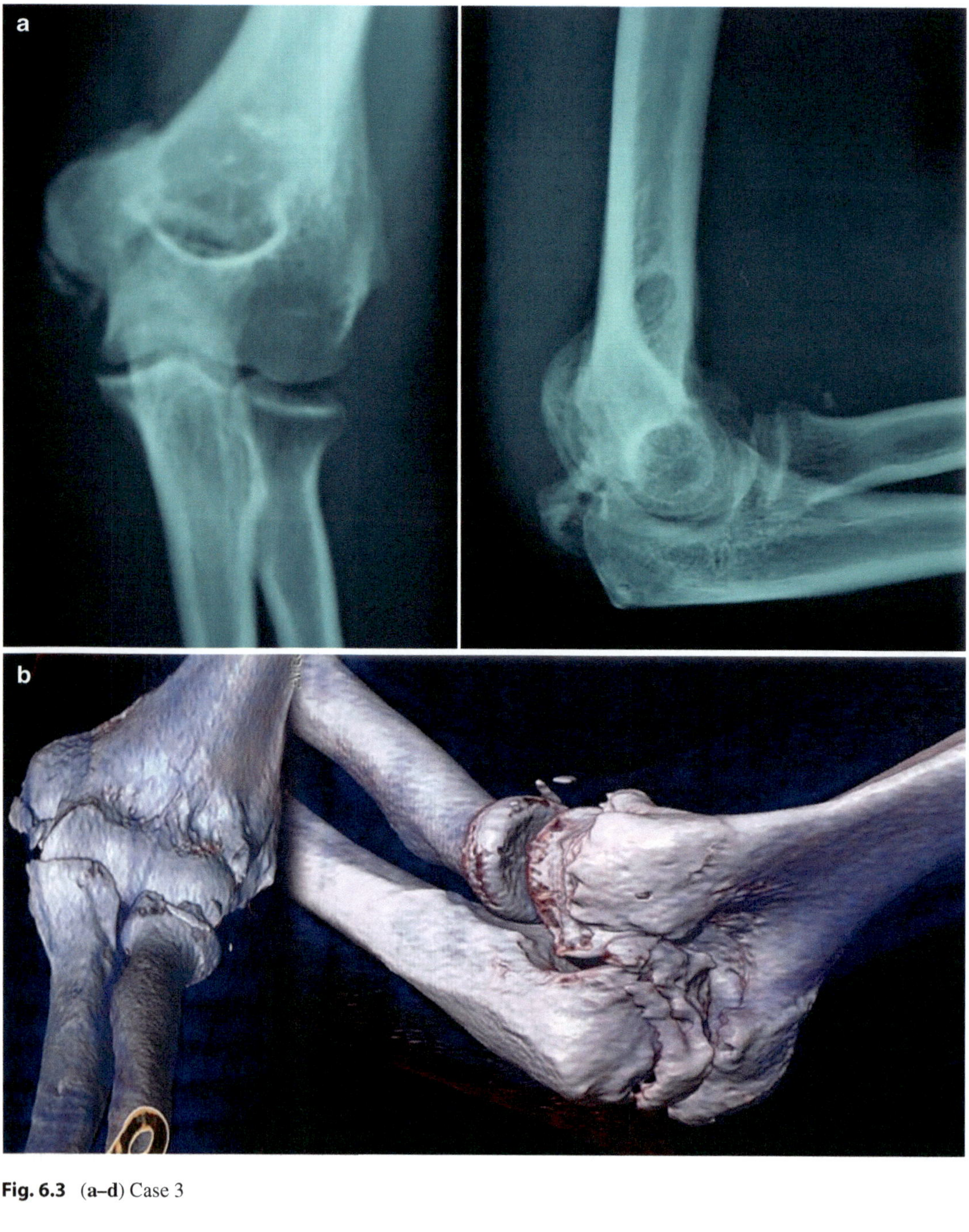

Fig. 6.3 (**a–d**) Case 3

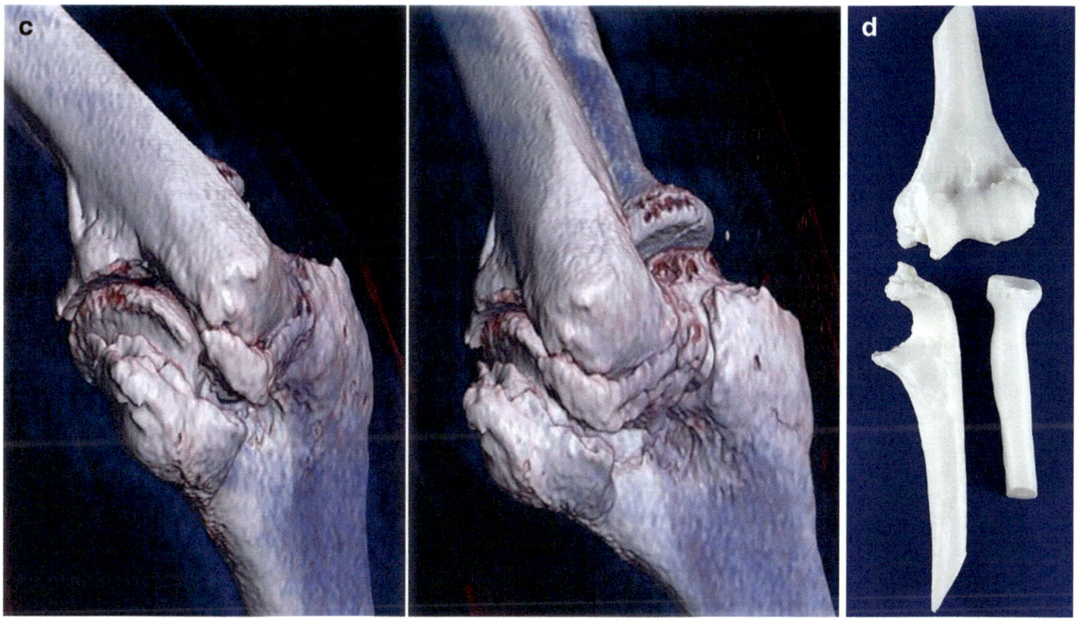

Fig. 6.3 (continued)

6.5.1.6 Case 6

Patient: A 26-year-old left-handed man

Trauma: Distal humeral fracture, left elbow

Treatment: Cast for 50 days followed by rehabilitation program

ROM 12 months from the trauma: Flexion–extension, 90°–80°; pronation–supination, 20°–10°

Imaging: X-rays and CT, 3D printing (Fig. 6.6a–d)

Outcome: All examiners changed surgical strategy after examination of the 3D-printed model and all found it more useful to choose the surgical strategy and rate the risk of complications than CT imaging with 3D reconstruction.

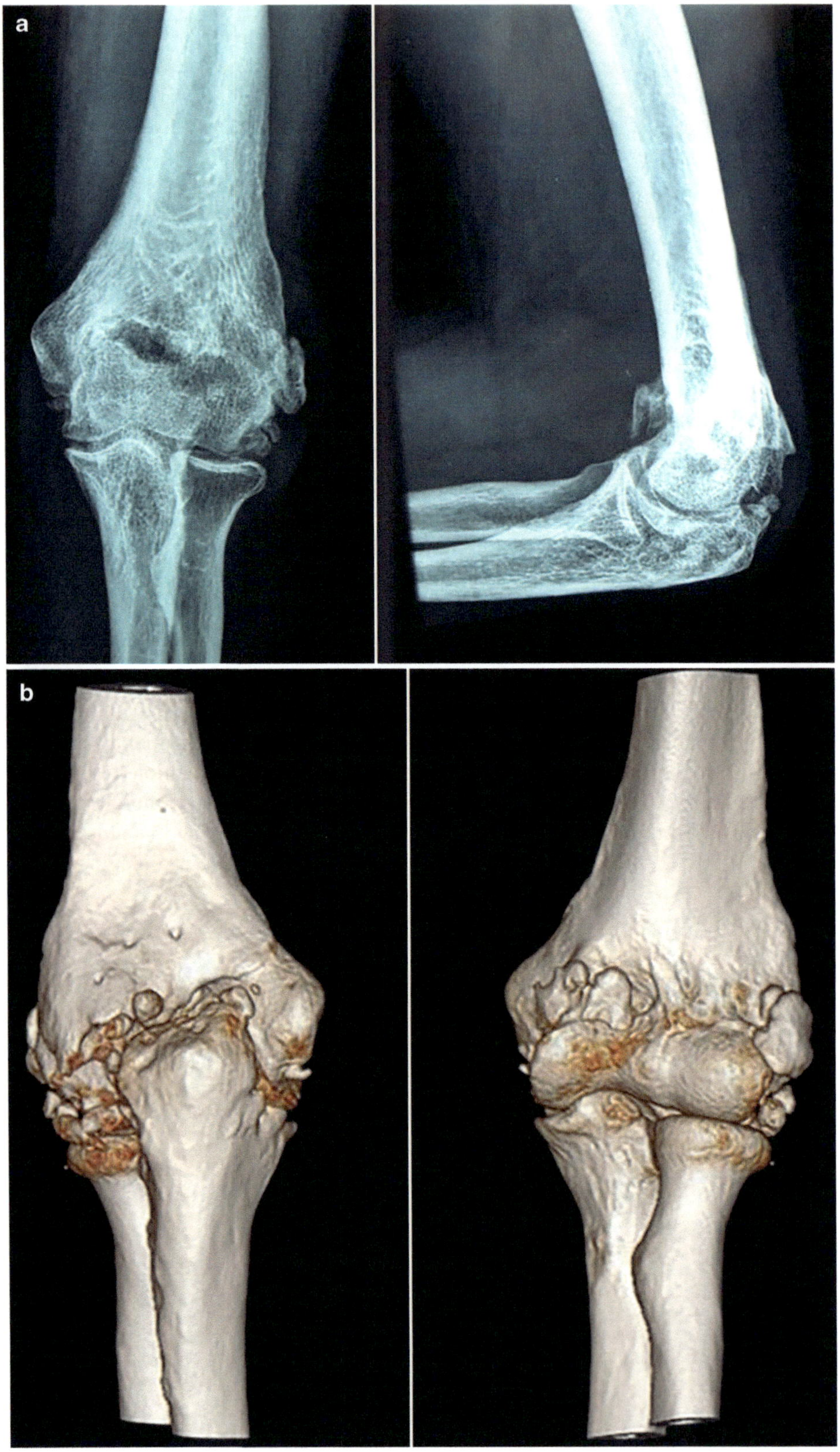

Fig. 6.4 (**a–d**) Case 4

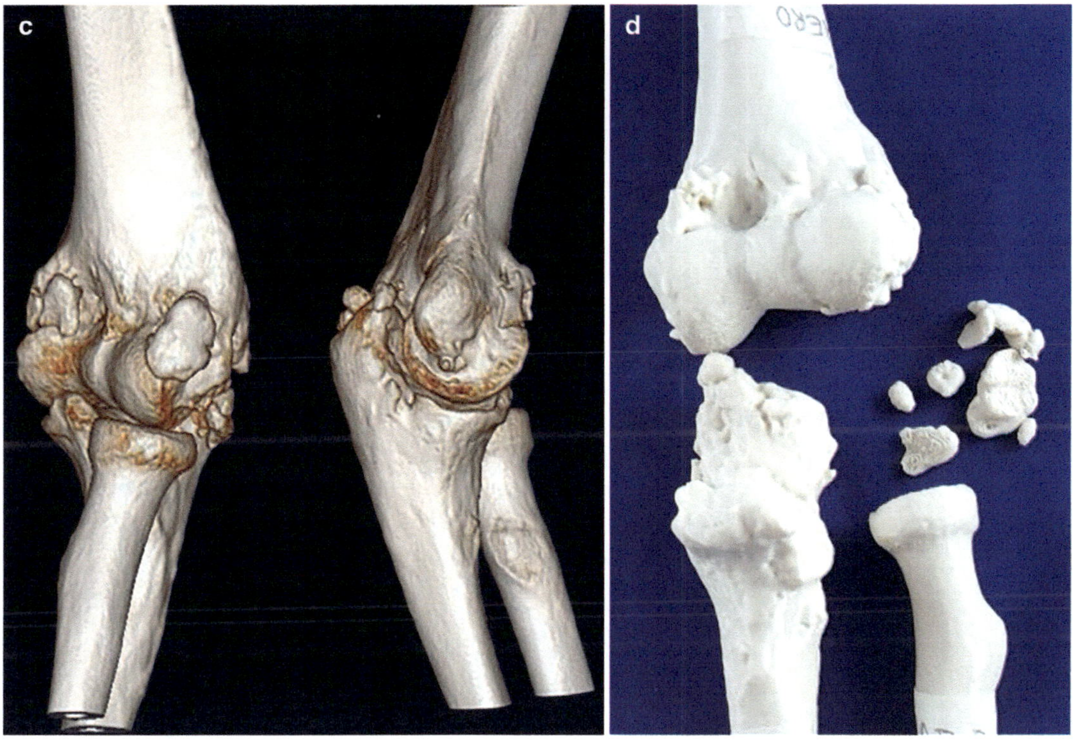

Fig. 6.4 (continued)

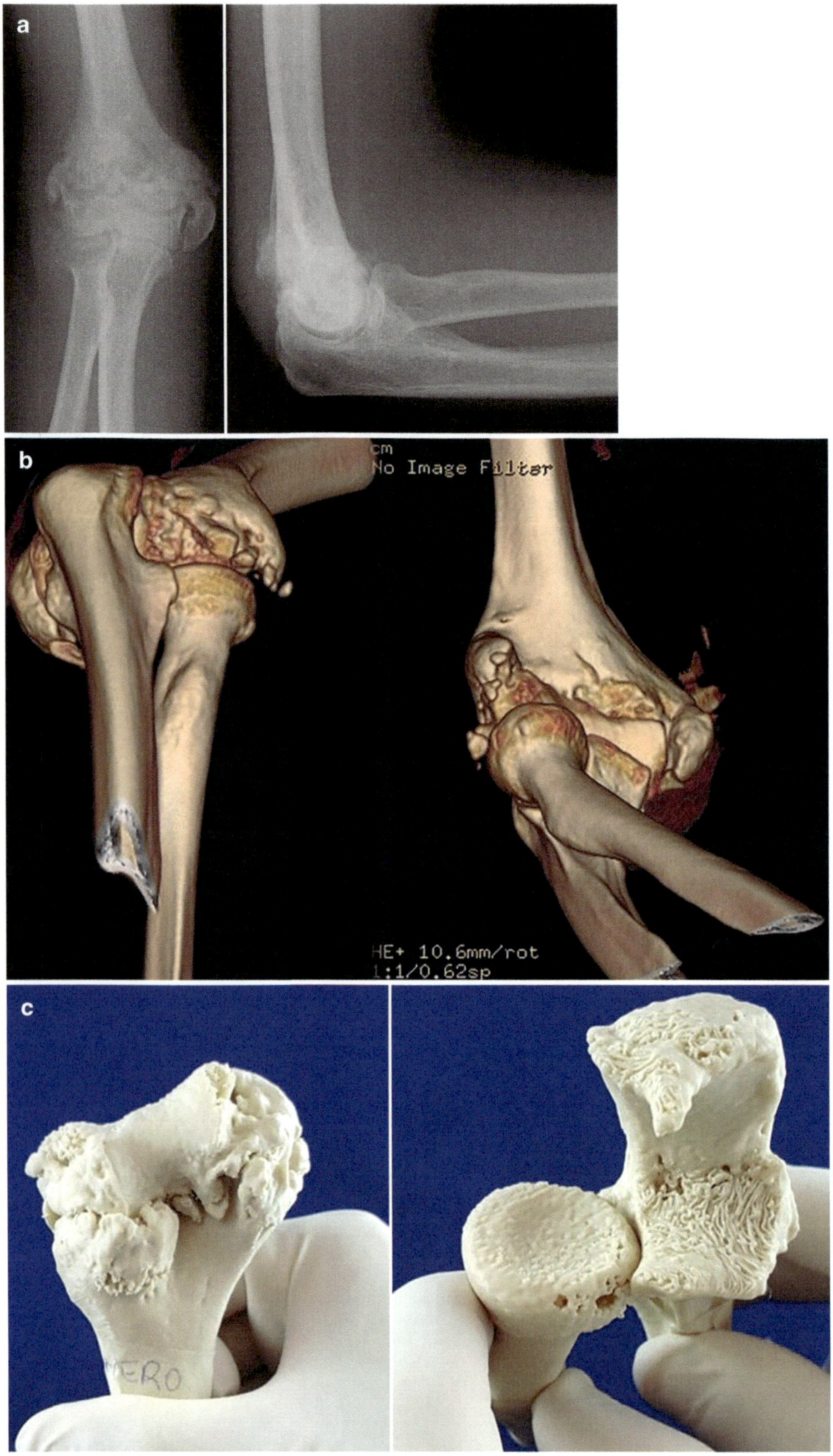

Fig. 6.5 (**a–c**) Case 5

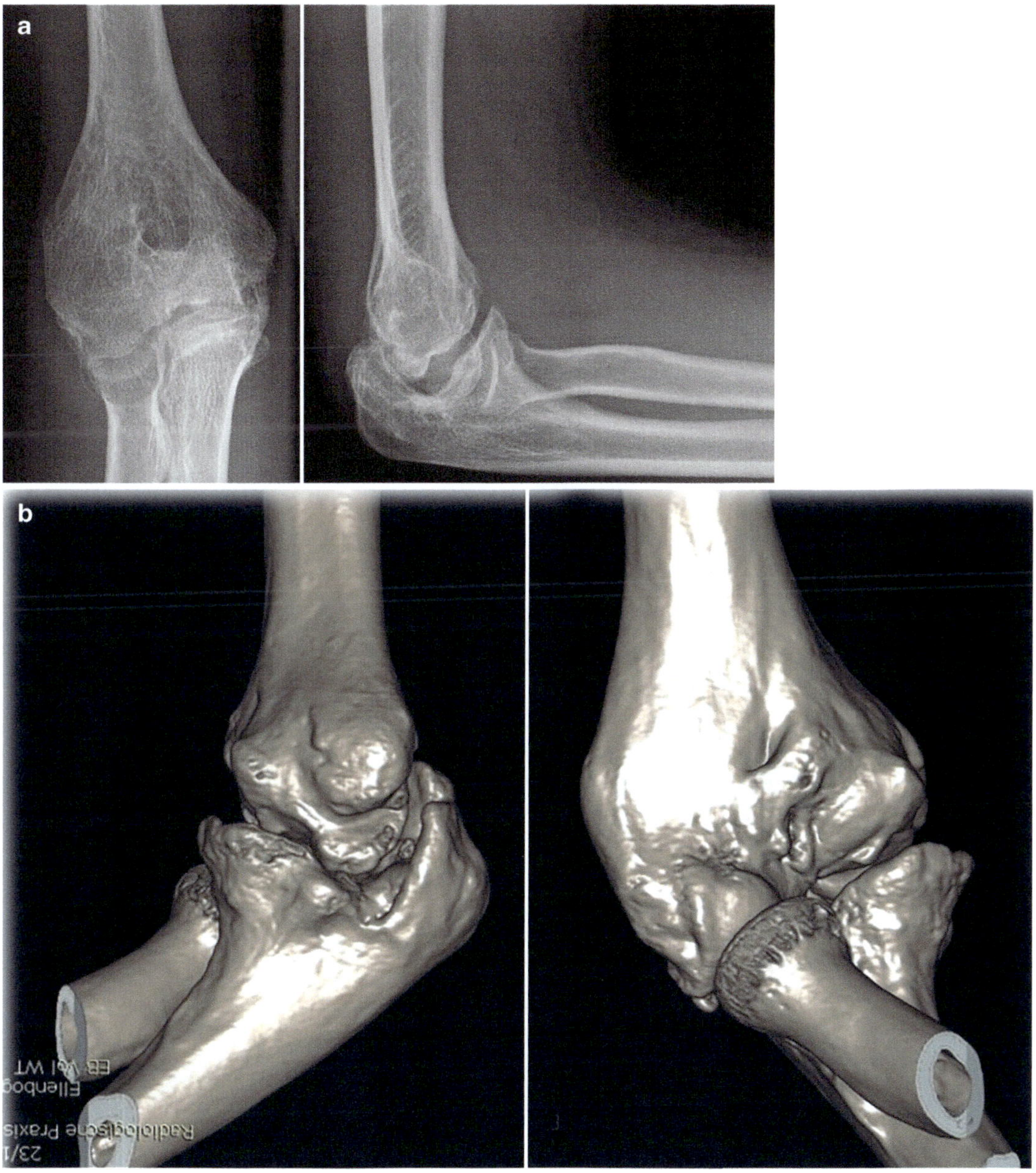

Fig. 6.6 (**a–d**) Case 6

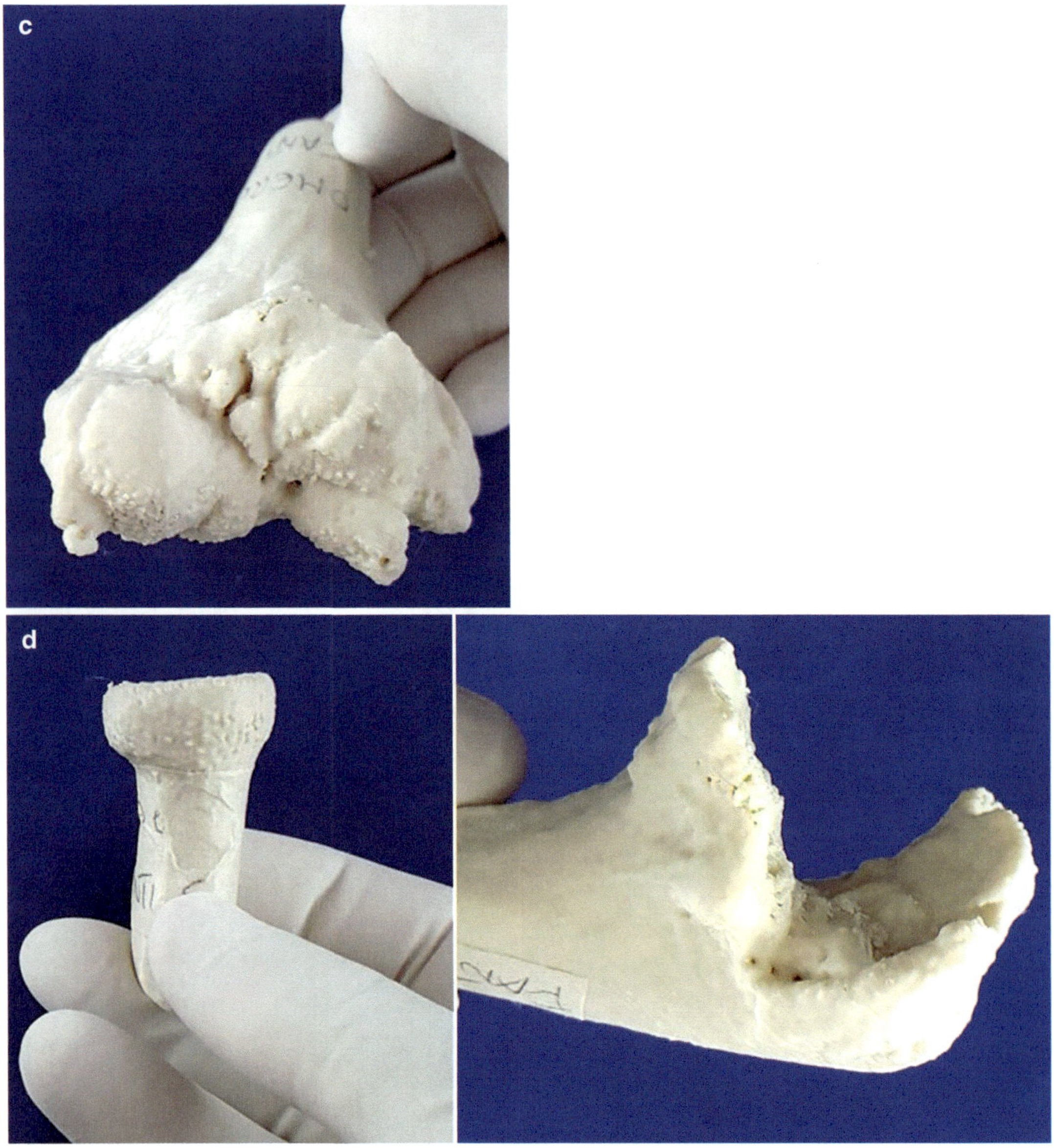

Fig. 6.6 (continued)

6.6 Considerations

We compared the results of two types of preoperative assessment, that is, X-rays and CT versus 3D-printed model, to gauge the added value provided by 3D-printed models. We found that in cases with more severe injury (complex lesions involving the articular surface of the elbow), the 3D-printed model was more informative than the traditional diagnostic approach to perform preoperative planning, to assess the possibility of motion recovery, and to rate potential complications.

Our report involves a small number of assessments and of surgeons. Though limited, its purpose is to describe the application of a new preoperative planning method to the treatment of post-traumatic elbow stiffness. Altogether, our data suggest that in complex lesions involving the joint surfaces, a 3D print of the stiff elbow affords a more accurate choice of surgical strategy and assessment of the possibility of functional recovery compared with radiographic and CT with 3D reconstruction. In simple lesions with minimal involvement of the articular surfaces, the method provided a marginal benefit limited to preoperative planning. In patients with preserved joint surfaces and periarticular heterotopic ossification, 3D printing helped to choose the most suitable surgical approach to the ossification, whereas in those with extensive joint deformity it also provided crucial information on the extension of the joint damage and the possibility of restoring adequate congruence and articular stability, which are key to the recovery of functional motion and obviate the need for joint replacement. 3D printing is of less use when joint stiffness is not associated with skeletal injury or minimal joint deformity, where the main cause of loss of motion is soft-tissue retraction. In our opinion, 3D printing will increasingly be applied to help surgeons in choosing the most appropriate treatment strategy in post-traumatic stiff elbow surgery, especially in patients with malunion or non-union of joint surfaces.

References

1. Qiao F, Li D, Jin Z, Hao D, Liao Y, Gong S. A novel combination of computer-assisted reduction technique and three dimensional printed patient-specific external fixator for treatment of tibial fractures. Int Orthop. 2016;40(4):835–41.
2. Mulford JS, Babazadeh S, Mackay N. Three-dimensional printing in orthopaedic surgery: review of current and future applications. ANZ J Surg. 2016;86(9):648–53.
3. Qiao F, Li D, Jin Z, et al. Application of 3D printed customized external fixator in fracture reduction. Injury. 2015;46(6):1150–5.
4. Li Z, Li Z, Xu R, et al. Three-dimensional printing models improve understanding of spinal fracture-a randomized controlled study in China. Sci Rep. 2015;5:11570.
5. Li C, Yang M, Xie Y, et al. Application of the polystyrene model made by 3-D printing rapid prototyping technology for operation planning in revision lumbar discectomy. J Orthop Sci. 2015;20:475–80.
6. Lal H, Patralekh MK. 3D printing and its applications in orthopaedic trauma: a technological marvel. J Clin Orthop Trauma. 2018;9(3):260–8.
7. Fleming ME, Waterman SS, Lewandowski LR, Chi BB. Use of 3-dimensional stereolithographic polymer models for heterotopic ossification surgical excision. Orthopedics. 2013;36(4):282–6.
8. Hoang D, Perrault D, Stevanovic M, Ghiassi A. Surgical applications of three-dimensional printing: a review of the current literature & how to get started. Ann Transl Med. 2016;4(23):456.
9. Wong KC. 3D-printed patient-specific applications in orthopedics. Orthop Res Rev. 2016;14(8):57–66.
10. Mendonça CJA, Guimarães RMDR, Pontim CE, Gasoto SC, Setti JAP, Soni JF, Schneider B Jr. An overview of 3D anatomical model printing in orthopedic trauma surgery. J Multidiscip Healthc. 2023;4(16):875–87.
11. Thomas CN, Mavrommatis S, Schroder LK, Cole PA. An overview of 3D printing and the orthopaedic application of patient-specific models in malunion surgery. Injury. 2022;53(3):977–83.

Classification of Elbow Stiffness

7

Alessandro Marinelli, Enrico Guerra,
and Gregory I. Bain

7.1 Introduction

Stiffness is a clinical disorder that affects the patient's function of the entire upper limb. It can be caused by a variety of elbow disorders. The most common cause is post-traumatic; this category also includes burns, head injuries, and elbow surgeries. However, elbow stiffness also can be caused by atraumatic etiologies, such as osteoarthritis, inflammatory joint disease, ulnar nerve entrapment, tumor, infection, metabolic disease (e.g., hemophilia), and congenital conditions (arthrogryposis). Being able to classify elbow stiffness is the first step to understand the etiology and to plan the treatment strategy.

The chapter content was already published in: A. Marinelli, E. Guerra, G. Bain. Classification of elbow stiffness, Journal of ISAKOS, Volume 9, Issue 2, 2024, 234–239, ISSN 2059-7754, https://doi.org/10.1016/j.jisako.2023.10.011. Reproduced with the permission of ISAKOS and Elsevier.

A. Marinelli (✉) · E. Guerra (✉)
Shoulder and Elbow Unit, Istituto Ortopedico Rizzoli, Bologna, Italy
e-mail: alessandro.marinelli@ior.it; enrico.guerra@ior.it

G. I. Bain
Department of Orthopedic Surgery, Flinders University of South Australia and Flinders Medical Centre, Adelaide, Australia
e-mail: greg@gregbain.com.au

7.2 Classification

Many classification systems have been developed for elbow stiffness.

7.2.1 Plane of Motion

Based on the involved plane of motion, we can evaluate if stiffness affects either flexion–extension or forearm rotation or both. This classification system is practical for evaluating patient impairment and for planning surgery (Fig. 7.1).

7.2.2 Severity

Stiffness can be classified on the basis of the arc of motion in flexion–extension or forearm rotation as: minimal (>91°), moderate (61°–90°), severe (31°–60°), or very severe (<30°). This classification is simple and practical for assessment, prognosis, and surgical decision-making. It can also be used to evaluate impairment and improvement.

7.2.3 Etiology

Elbow stiffness can be classified on the basis of etiology as post-traumatic, micro-traumatic, degenerative or inflammatory, neurogenic, and

L. Pederzini et al. (eds.), *Stiffness of the Elbow, Wrist and Related Pathologies*,
https://doi.org/10.1007/978-3-031-81381-8_7

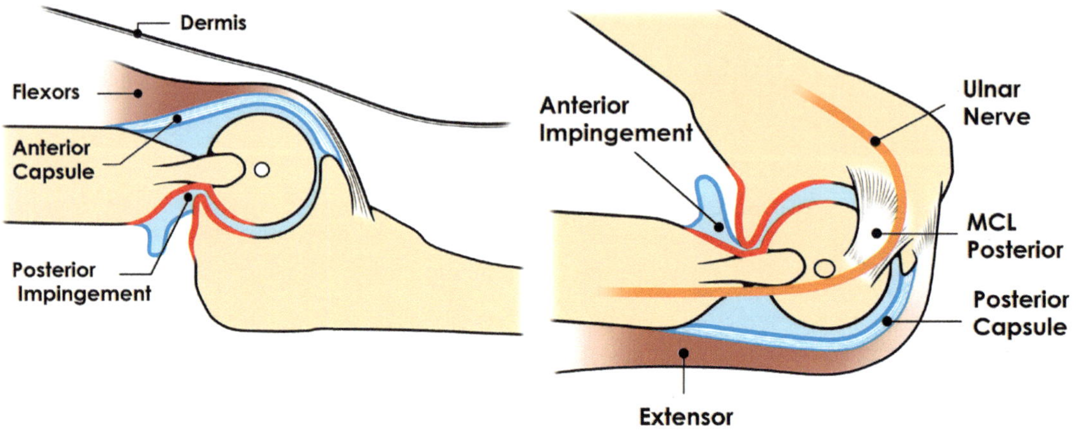

Fig. 7.1 This diagram illustrates how the various anatomical factors can restrict extension and flexion. (**a**) Elbow extension can be restricted anteriorly by skin contracture, flexor muscles, or the anterior capsule. Posteriorly it can be restricted by posterior bony impingement. (**b**) Elbow flexion can be restricted posteriorly by contracture of the triceps, posterior capsule, or posterior band of medial collateral ligament (MCL). Anteriorly the osseous impingement. Note the ulnar nerve can indirectly cause a contracture, as the pain will restrict the patient from mobilizing the elbow (neurogenic stiffness). (From: Alessandro Marinelli and Gregory Bain. The Stiff Elbow: classification and treatment algorithm. ISAKOS Newsletter. 2018; 2:18–21) [1]

others (congenital, tumor, burns, infection, etc.). This system is useful for evaluating treatment indication.

7.2.4 Prognosis

Jupiter et al. divided post-traumatic elbow stiffness into two categories: simple and complex [2]. Simple stiffness is characterized by mild to moderate contracture (motion >80°), no prior surgery, minimal heterotopic ossification, and a well-preserved osseous anatomy. Complex stiffness is associated with nerve dysfunction, prior nerve transposition, retained hardware, substantial heterotopic ossification, articular incongruity, and an arc of motion <80°. This system is useful for evaluating the risks and benefits of surgical treatment as the complex form is associated with a higher surgical complication rate and requires more expertise.

7.2.5 Anatomical Location

Among the most used classifications of joint stiffness, there is the classification proposed by Morrey, which divides into intrinsic, extrinsic, and mixed the etiologies limiting the joint motion [3].

- *Extrinsic factors* (i.e., extra-articular factors that spare the joint space) include capsular-ligament contracture, muscle/tendon retraction, ulnar nerve neuropathy, heterotopic ossification, and skin contracture.
- *Intrinsic factors* (i.e., intra-articular factors) include intra-articular adhesions and deformities, cartilage lesions, loose bodies, and impinging osteophytes.
- *Mixed*: are those that have both intrinsic and extrinsic elements.
- Watts and Bain proposed the capsule be considered a separate category, and to add neurological factors. This created a new classification, including all causes of elbow stiffness, not just the post-traumatic ones [1].

According to this classification, it is possible to classify the stiffness into four types, based on localization and etiology:

1. Intra-articular
2. Capsular
3. Extra-articular
4. Neurological

The reason why the capsular group should be separated is that it has a different etiology, treatment, and prognosis. Isolated capsular contracture can be caused by immobilization or hemarthrosis. The capsular contractures can be treated with an open or arthroscopic release or resection, usually with a good outcome. Capsular contractures are also common with the intra-articular pathologies. As Morrey noted, there are cases that have a mixed etiology [2].

Based to this classification, the elbow joint can be schematically considered as a machine that is mobilized by a nerve, which activates a muscle, which moves the articulation, that is stabilized by ligaments (Fig. 7.2).

We developed, in analogy with the ISAKOS shoulder stiffness classification [4], an all-inclusive pathoanatomical classification of elbow stiffness (Table 7.1).

With the correct identification of the pathological process, this classification system allows the surgeon to address each component and tailor the treatment appropriately.

Intra-articular pathologies (e.g., chondral flaps, loose bodies, intra-articular adhesion, impinging osteophytes, or synovitis) can be treated with arthroscopy. In advanced cases with severe joint involvement, a simple debridement is unlikely to be successful and a joint arthroplasty is required.

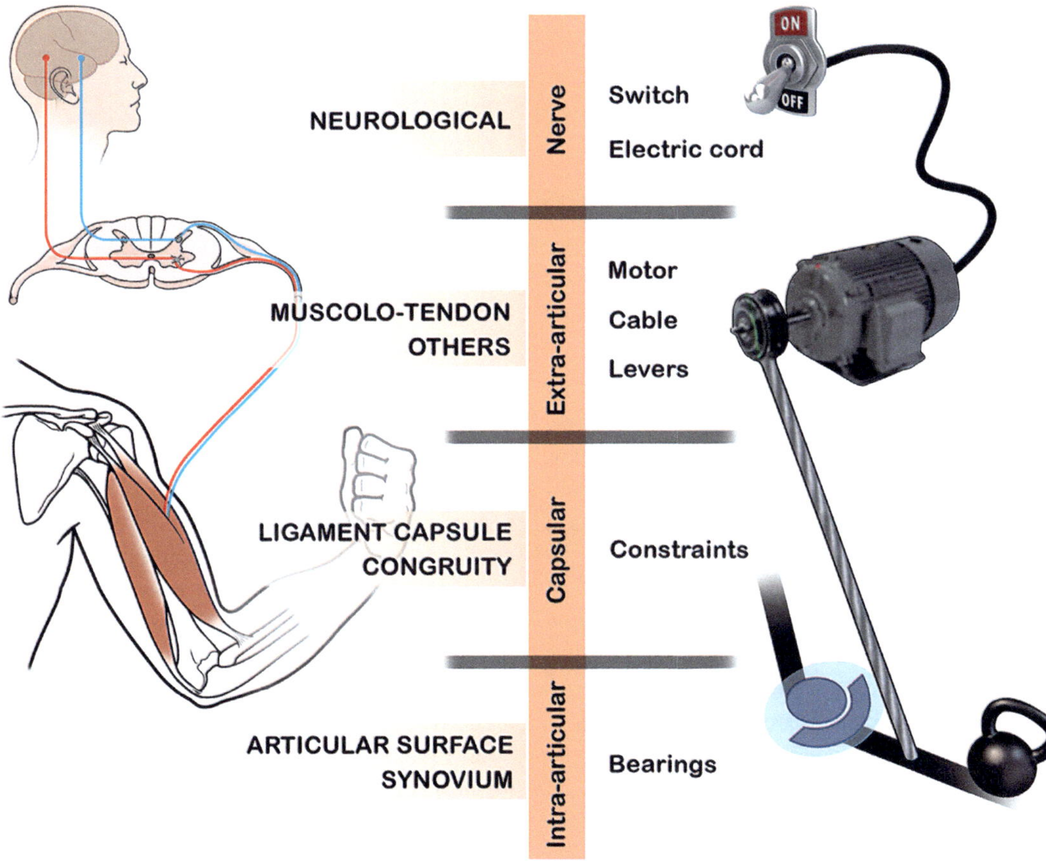

Fig. 7.2 The elbow machine demonstrates how the joint moves. It also highlights the four distinct anatomical areas where disorders may act to affect the elbow motion. (From: Alessandro Marinelli and Gregory Bain. The Stiff Elbow: classification and treatment algorithm. ISAKOS Newsletter. 2018; 2:18–21) [1]

Table 7.1 All-inclusive pathoanatomical classification of elbow stiffness

Intra-articular (bearings)	Capsular (constraints)	Extra-articular (motor, cable, levers)	Neurologic (control, electrics, sensors)
Articular surface	Ligaments	Muscles	Central nervous system
Osteochondral	Contracture	Myopathy	Behavioral dystonia
Degeneration	Calcifications	Fatty infiltration	Spasticity
Subchondral	Capsule	Tendons and bursa	Peripheral nervous system
Dysplasia, fractures	Contracture	Tear, calcifications	Ulnar, radial, medial nerves
Avascular necrosis	Calcifications	Bursitis	Cutaneous nerves
Synovium	Instability	Other	Sensory and autonomic
Inflammatory	Subluxation	Fracture, malignancy	Charcot joint
Crystal arthroplasty	Dislocation	HO, skin contracture	Chronic regional pain syndrome

From: Alessandro Marinelli and Gregory Bain. The Stiff Elbow: classification and treatment algorithm. ISAKOS Newsletter. 2018; 2:18–21 [1]

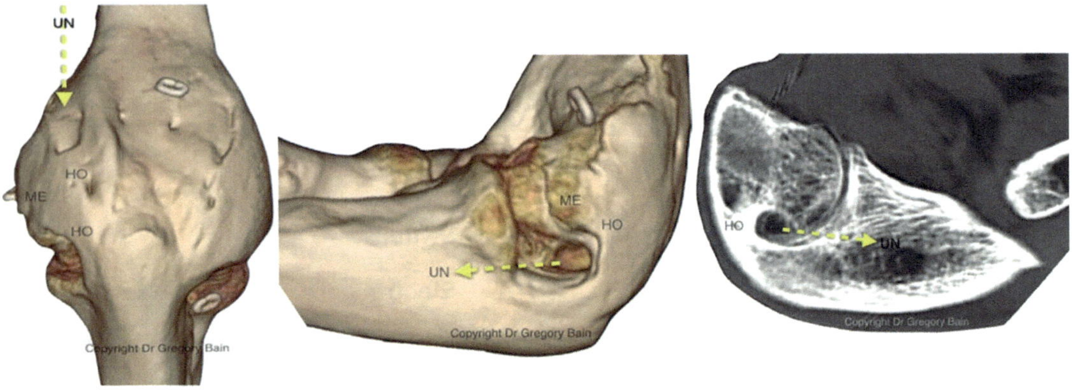

Fig. 7.3 Heterotopic Ossification after traumatic brain injury. CT scan images show how the ulnar nerve is completely wrapped in the new heterotopic ossifcation. (**a**, **b**) 3D CT scan images. (**c**) sagittal CT image

Extra-articular pathologies (e.g., heterotopic ossification [Fig. 7.3], muscle/tendon contractures, skin) are usually treated with an open procedure with resection or release of the offending structures. Endoscopic treatment for these conditions is possible but the technique is still evolving.

Capsular contractures (e.g., immobilization) can be treated with open or arthroscopic techniques. Arthroscopic release or resection of the capsule has a good outcome, especially if it is an isolated problem. Capsular contractures are also common in conjunction with intra-articular pathologies.

Neurological (e.g., spasticity, entrapment) (Table 7.2): The ulnar nerve and its involvement in elbow pathologies are very important. Post-traumatic ulnar nerve entrapment has a slow and insidious onset. It will present with medial elbow pain, with radiation to the ulnar side of the hand. The patient's presentation may be of elbow stiffness, with the elbow postured in about 20° of flexion, as extension will be uncomfortable. Percussion over the ulnar nerve will be uncomfortable. Associated MCL instability needs to be assessed, as this may be the cause of the ulnar nerve traction and pain. Non-operative modalities should be initially offered. However, surgical release of the ulnar nerve usually improves the pain. If the MCL is unstable, then MCL repair of reconstruction will also be required.

In 1998, Kay proposed a practical classification for post-traumatic stiffness of the elbow that was based on the presence, severity, and combination of the three most common factors causing stiffness (capsular contracture, articular fractures, heterotopic ossification), identifying the five clinical situations more frequent in the clinical practice [5].

Table 7.2 Neurological compression sites around the elbow

Ulnar nerve	Median nerve	Radial nerve and PIN
Arcade of Struthers	Ligament of Struthers	ECRB edge
Anconeus epitrochlearis	**Lacertus fibrosis**	**Arcade of Frohse**
Osborne's fascia	**Pronator teres**	Recurrent leash of Henry
Flexor pronator aponeurosis	FDS arch proximal free edge	Distal edge of supinator

From: Gregory Bain, Michel van den Bekerom, Janak A. Mehta. Clinical Anatomy of the Elbow Surgical Techniques for Trauma and Sports Related Injuries of the Elbow, 2019, Copyright ISAKOS [8]. https://doi.org/10.1007/978-3-662-58931-1
Causes from proximal to distal. Most common sites are in **bold**

7.3 S.T.I.F Classification

More recently, in collaboration with Shawn O'Driscoll the S.T.I.F. (**S**tiffness **T**ypes and **I**nfluencing **F**actors) classification has been developed (Table 7.3) [1, 6, 7]. This system highlights the five common disorders causing stiffness as well as the six influencing factors that often affect the treatment and clinical outcome.

The S.T.I.F. classification system highlights the importance to consider associated lesions as ulnar nerve symptoms, collateral ligament calcifications, skin contracture, or hardware presence as significant decision factors guiding the treatment strategy (Fig. 7.4).

Table 7.3 The S.T.I.F. system details the five common causes of stiffness and the six influencing factors

S.T.I.F. classification Stiffness types and influencing factors	
Prevalent type of stiffness	Treatment and prognosis influencing factors
1. Soft tissue contracture	(a) Ulnar nerve symptoms
2. Arthritis	(b) Hardware/prior surgery
3. HO.	(c) LCL/MCL calcification
4. Malunion/non-union	(d) Skin contracture
5. Persistent instability	(e) Articular pain
	(f) Loose bodies

From: Alessandro Marinelli and Gregory Bain. The Stiff Elbow: classification and treatment algorithm. ISAKOS Newsletter. 2018; 2:18–21 [1]
HO heterotopic ossification

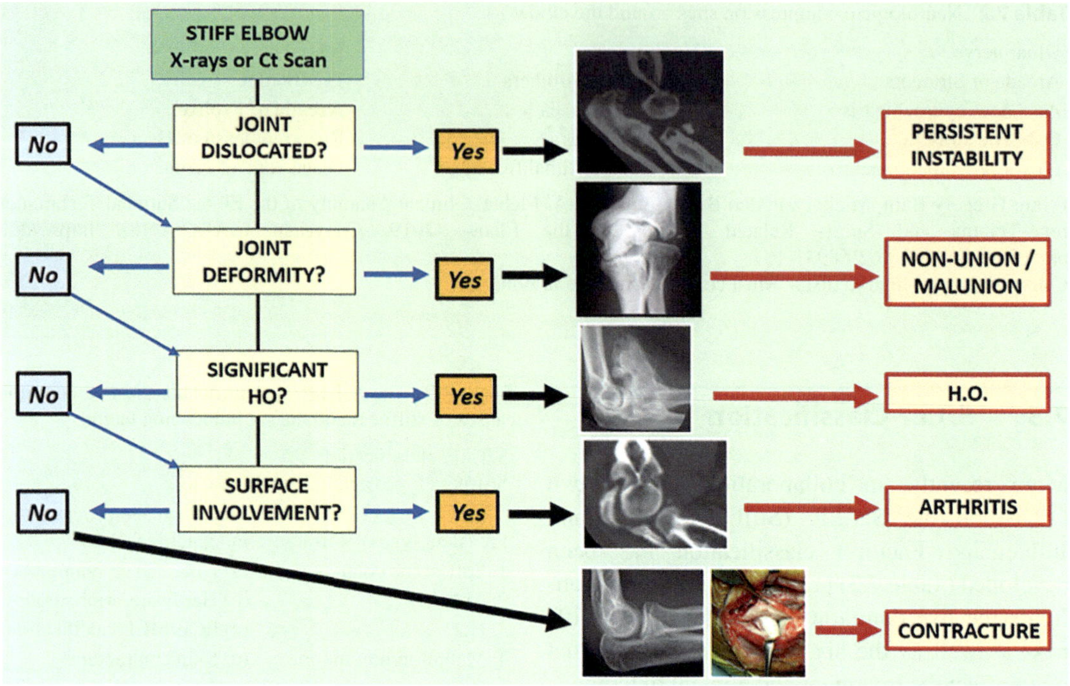

Fig. 7.4 Elbow stiffness diagnostic flow: The diagnostic flow of elbow stiffness summarizes the thinking process we follow to identify the prevalent type of stiffness looking at the X-rays or CT scan of a patient with a stiff elbow. Soon we will be able to use Artificial Intelligence of CT images to diagnose the cause of stiffness. Computational modeling will reveal the area of bony impingement, recommending the areas of osteophyte resection and predicting the clinical outcome. (From: Alessandro Marinelli and Gregory Bain. The Stiff Elbow: classification and treatment algorithm. ISAKOS Newsletter. 2018; 2:18–21) [1]

7.4 Treatment Algorithm

Based on the S.T.I.F. classification system, it is possible to propose a treatment algorithm that includes the severity of the disorders as a guide to surgical treatment and the preferred operative approach (open or scope) [1, 6, 7] (Table 7.4).

Table 7.4 The S.T.I.F. treatment algorithm for elbow stiffness: The type of stiffness, its severity, and the age of the patient are all factors that direct the preferred type of surgery

Decisional treatment algorithm for elbow stiffness release		
Prevalent type of stiffness	Surgery	Approach
1. Soft tissue contracture	– Release	Scope
	– Release (column procedure)	Open
2. Arthritis	**Mild or moderate arthritis**	Scope
	– Osteocapsular arthroplasty	Open
		Combined
	Severe arthritis	Open
	– Biologic interposition/distraction arthroplasty (external fixators)	
	– TEA (>70 years)	
3. HO	– Removal	Open
4. Malunion/non-union	– ORIF/osteotomy	Open
	– TEA (>70 years)	
5. Chronic subluxation	– Rad. Head/Coron. / Ligam. reconstr. / external fixators	Open
	– TEA (>70 years or not possible reconstruction)	

From: Alessandro Marinelli and Gregory Bain. The Stiff Elbow: classification and treatment algorithm. ISAKOS Newsletter. 2018; 2:18–21 [1]

H.O. heterotopic ossification, *TEA* total elbow arthroplasty, *ORIF* open reduction and internal fixation

7.5 Conclusion

Over the last 20 years, we have witnessed dramatic changes in the approach to elbow stiffness. With the progressive increase in the number of elbow release surgeries and improvement of our treatment ability, the need of new classifications has been felt. The new classifications system highlights the etiology of the stiffness and provides a framework to better understand the natural history, direct the surgical management, and interpret the likely clinical outcomes. Moreover, taking into consideration the influencing factors is of paramount importance in the surgical indication and prognosis. S.T.I.F. classification is also useful in research because, identifying homogenous pattern of stiffness allows a proper comparison among different treatments. All of these factors can help define the important questions for management of the elbow (Table 7.5).

Table 7.5 Elements to consider when assessing elbow stiffness

A. Patient
1. Age, comorbidities, needs, expectations, compliance
B. Elbow
1. Flexion/forearm rotation
2. Duration of stiffness
3. Improvements
4. Stability/congruency
5. Pain
6. Neurologic symptoms
7. Prior surgery/hardware presence
8. Skin condition
C. Adjacent joint
1. Hand, shoulder, neck function

From: Alessandro Marinelli and Gregory Bain. The Stiff Elbow: classification and treatment algorithm. ISAKOS Newsletter. 2018; 2:18–21 [1]

References

1. Watts AC, Bain GI. New techniques in elbow arthroscopy. In: Savoie FH, Field LD, editors. AANA advanced arthroscopy: the elbow and wrist. Philadelphia: Saunders-Elsevier; 2010. p. 124–31.
2. Jupiter JB, O'Driscoll SW, Cohen MS. The assessment and management of the stiff elbow. Instr Course Lect. 2003;52:93–111.
3. Morrey BF. The posttraumatic stiff elbow. Clin Orthop Relat Res. 2005;431:26–35.
4. Guerra E, Kelberine FM, Marinelli A, Rotini R, Bain G. The stiff elbow: classification and treatment algorithm. In: Bain G, Eygendaal D, van Riet R, editors. Surgical techniques for trauma and sports related injuries of the elbow. Heidelberg: Springer; 2020.
5. Kay NR. Arthrolysis of the post-traumatic stiff elbow. In: Stanley D, Kay NR, editors. Surgery of the elbow. London: Arnold; 1998. p. 228–34.
6. Marinelli A, Bain GI. The stiff elbow: classification and treatment algorithm. ISAKOS Newslett. 2018;2:18–21.
7. Marinelli A, Guerra E, Bain GI, Rotini R. Classification of elbow stiffness. In: Bhatia DN, Bain GI, Poehling GG, Graves BR, editors. Arthroscopy and endoscopy of the elbow, wrist and hand. Cham: Springer; 2022. https://doi.org/10.1007/978-3-030-79423-1_37.
8. Bain GI, Clitherow HDS. Shoulder stiffness: the pathogenesis and classification of shoulder stiffness. In: Itoi E, Bain G, et al., editors. Shoulder stiffness. Springer; 2015.

8 Elbow Stiffness in Pediatric Population is Rare

Sara Padovani, Marco Amadio, Fabrizio Marzano, Leo Massari, and Alessandra Colozza

8.1 Introduction

Elbow stiffness in pediatric population is rare frequent in comparison to adult population. Due to high grade of soft tissue elasticity, children and adolescent tend to recover elbow range of motion (ROM) remarkably well after a period of immobilization.

Elbow stiffness is defined as an arc of extension motion of less than 100 and/or a contracture of more than 30 in flexion. It may involve not only flexion-extension but also pronation–supination arc of movement. In adults, a minimum arc of movement of 100° (130/30 in flexion–extension and 50/50 in supination–pronation) is generally accepted as functional for daily activities [1]. The arc of flexion and consequently the ability to reach the face with hands are more important than a full terminal extension.

In paediatric population, there is not a functional range of movement defined. Children often participate in sports and competitive activities that require complete range of movement and full extension—and even hyperextension, such as gymnasts, baseball pitchers and overhead players.

Valone et al. demonstrated that the elbow functional arc of motion described for adults is sufficient to achieve most positional and functional tasks in children and adolescents but not for contemporary tasks. Specific contemporary tasks such as the use of a cellular phone and typing on a keyboard utilize more elbow flexion and pronation [2]. More in details, adolescents use more elbow flexion, more forearm pronation and less extension and supination to achieve tasks. The reason could be the different shoulder kinematics between adolescents and children and the differential growth of the humerus and radius/ulna as a child grows. The authors underlie the importance of a greater need for overall motion at the elbow and specifically flexion and pronation to achieve contemporary tasks, as it may help guide surgeons in the care of children and adolescents with elbow and forearm deformities and contractures [2].

There are many causes of elbow stiffness: post-traumatic, acquired and congenital diseases. Elbow stiffness must be correctly addressed especially in children that represent high demand patients.

S. Padovani · F. Marzano · A. Colozza (✉)
Department of Orthopedics and Traumatology, Ospedale degli Infermi di Faenza, Faenza, Italy

M. Amadio · L. Massari
Orthopedics and Traumatology Unit, Sant'Anna University Hospital of Ferrara, Ferrara, Italy
e-mail: msl@unife.it

L. Pederzini et al. (eds.), *Stiffness of the Elbow, Wrist and Related Pathologies*,
https://doi.org/10.1007/978-3-031-81381-8_8

8.2 Etiopathogenesis

Causes of elbow stiffness in paediatric population are numerous and can be classified into three main categories: *post-traumatic, congenital and acquired.*

The most common cause of stiffness is post-traumatic injury; it includes fractures and malunion, burns, head injury and elbow surgery. Atraumatic aetiologies include inflammatory joint disease, infection, metabolic disease, haemophilia and congenital conditions (arthrogryposis) [1, 3, 4].

8.3 Post-traumatic Causes

Elbow injuries in paediatric population that could evolve in joint stiffness are fractures and joint dislocations. Supracondylar fracture of humerus is the most common injury followed by the lateral humeral condyle fracture. Monteggia fracture dislocation, although not as common as supracondylar fracture, can be easily missed and liable to late presentation.

Long-term complications of supracondylar fracture and occasionally of lateral humeral condyle fractures are angular deformities of the elbow such as cubitus varus and valgus.

8.4 Fractures

8.4.1 Supracondylar Humerus Fracture

Supracondylar humerus fractures are the most common elbow injury in children. They account for approximately 50–70% of all elbow fractures in children (Fig. 8.1). This injury occurs most often in boys between the ages of 4 and 7 and most frequently occurs after a fall on an outstretched upper extremity. Supracondylar humerus fractures are usually divided into extension and flexion types with extension types being far more common (~97–99%).

Post-traumatic elbow stiffness is reported in 3–6% following supracondylar fracture due to soft tissue contracture, or heterotopic ossifications (HO). There are some predisposing fac-

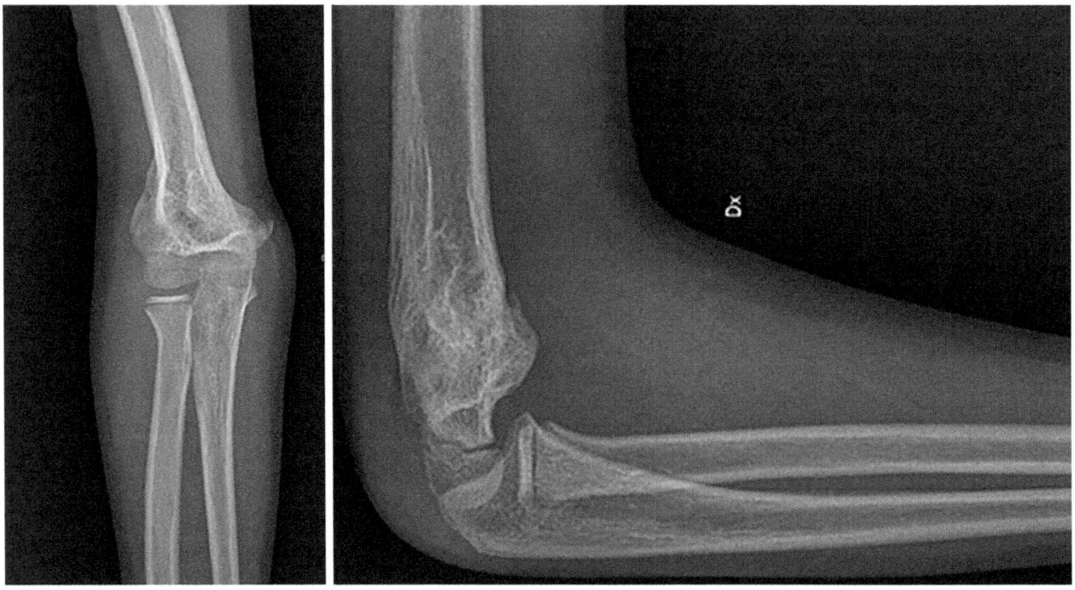

Fig. 8.1 AP and LL right elbow X-rays in a 12-year-old boy 3 months after supracondylar distal humerus fracture treated by K-wire pinning

tors: the open reduction, vigorous manipulation in closed reduction, strenuous rehabilitation protocols [1, 5].

8.4.2 Lateral Condyle Fracture

Lateral condyle fractures of the distal humerus involve physis and the articular surface. The diagnosis of condylar fractures can be very difficult in children because the distal immature humerus is still cartilaginous, and fractures could be missed on initial radiographs. This type of fracture commonly occurs in children between the ages of 4 and 10 with a peak incidence around 5–6 years of age.

Lateral condyle fractures had been classified in two types by Milch in 1964. In type 1, the fracture line traverses the capitellum and falls lateral to the trochlea, and in type 2, the fracture line extends further medially to the trochlear groove.

Rutherford in 1985 proposed a new classification based on the degree of displacement. Type 1 fractures are nondisplaced, type 2 fractures are displaced less than 2 mm, and type 3 fractures are displaced and malrotated.

The difficulty in treating lateral condyle fractures is in differentiating 'stable nondisplaced' fractures from potentially 'unstable, minimally displaced' fractures [6]. The treatment of lateral condyle fractures depends on the degree of fracture displacement.

The most common complications from lateral condyle fractures include delayed union, non-union, malunion, cubitus varus, stiffness and avascular necrosis of the lateral condyle. The most frequent problematic complication of lateral condyle fractures is delayed union or non-union.

Neglected lateral condyle fractures commonly cause stiffness and elbow instability and require careful evaluation (Fig. 8.2) [1, 6].

8.4.3 Medial Epicondyle Fracture

Medial epicondyle fractures account for approximately 10% of all paediatric elbow fractures and occur most commonly between the ages of 7 and

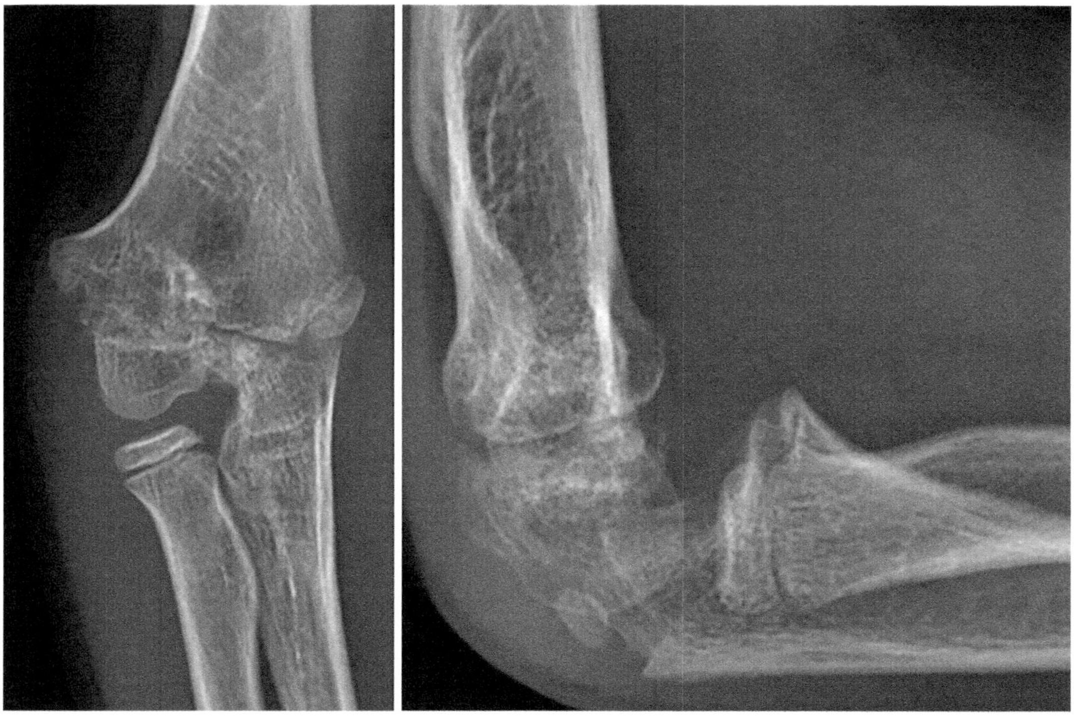

Fig. 8.2 A case of neglected lateral condyle fracture in a girl with post-traumatic stiff elbow

15 years. Approximately 50–60% of all medial epicondyle fractures are associated with a concurrent elbow dislocation. The mechanism of injury is usually excessive valgus stress which is why this fracture is often seen in baseball pitchers (significant valgus stress on their elbow with pitching). Stiffness is the most common complication associated with medial epicondyle fractures (Fig. 8.3). It is best avoided by decreased immobilization time and early gentle range-of-motion exercises [6].

8.4.4 Radial Neck Fracture

Fractures of the neck of the radius account for 5% of elbow injuries and 1% of all injuries in children. These fractures frequently affect children between the ages of 4 and 14 (Fig. 8.4). There are two anatomic types of radial neck fracture. The most common is by far the simple metaphyseal fracture of the radial neck with subsequent Salter type II epiphyseal separation. The other type of epiphyseal separation is rare and characterized by intra-articular fracture extension (Salter types III and IV). Stiffness and reduction in the arc of motion are the most common complications associated with radio-ulnar synostosis. Other complications are malunion and non-union, radial head overgrowth, avascular necrosis more often correlated to open reduction [6].

8.4.5 Dislocations

Ulno-humeral joint dislocation usually occurs in older children (10–15 years) and can be associated with elbow fractures such as medial epicondyle fractures. The annual rate of elbow dislocation is 3–6% of all elbow injuries in children; the most common causes are sports and trampoline jumping [6, 7]. Treatment is usually closed reduction followed by brief immobilization. Open reduction is indicated for dislocations

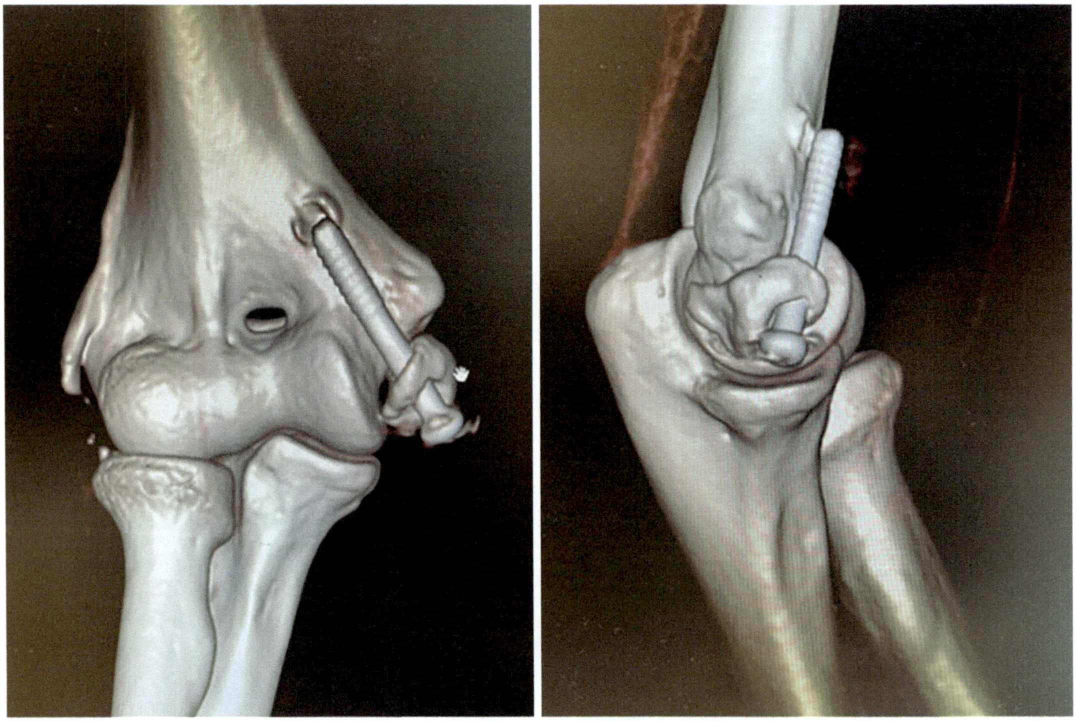

Fig. 8.3 A case of mal-union of medial epicondyle fracture treated by percutaneous screw

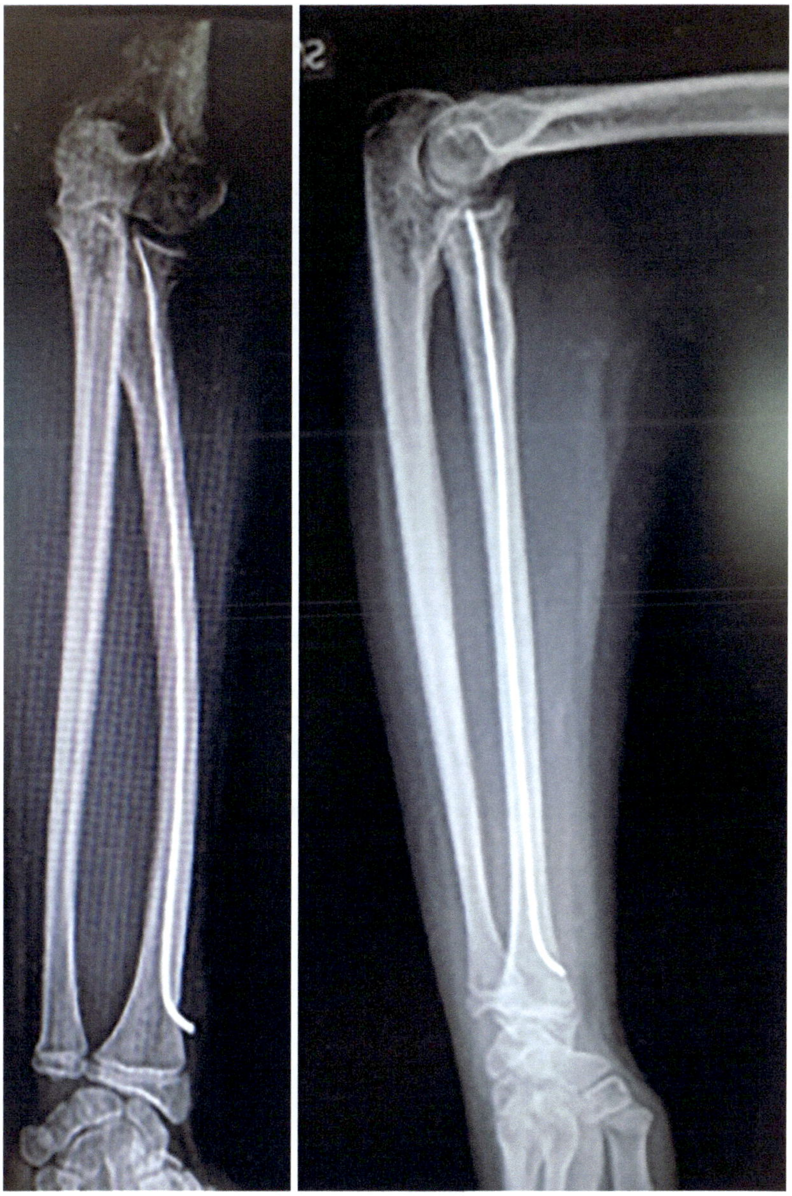

Fig. 8.4 A case of 14-year-old-girl radial neck fracture treated by Metaizeau technique

associated with a medial epicondyle fracture with an incarcerated fragment (Fig. 8.5).

Radio-humeral joint dislocation is often associated with a fracture of the ulna; this pattern of lesion is called Monteggia fracture and accounts for 0.4% of all forearm fractures in children. They typically occur in children between 4 and 10 years of age after a fall onto an outstretched hand. There have been described various injury mechanisms leading to different types of radial head dislocation (anterior, posterior or lateral) accompanied by ulnar fractures or bowing deformities (Fig. 8.6). Bado proposed a radiographic classification system which distinguishes four types of Monteggia injuries. It classifies the fracture–dislocation pattern according to the direction of the radial head dislocation. The apex of the ulna fracture or bowing deformity follows the direction of the radial head displacement. Letts et al. modified the Bado classification for

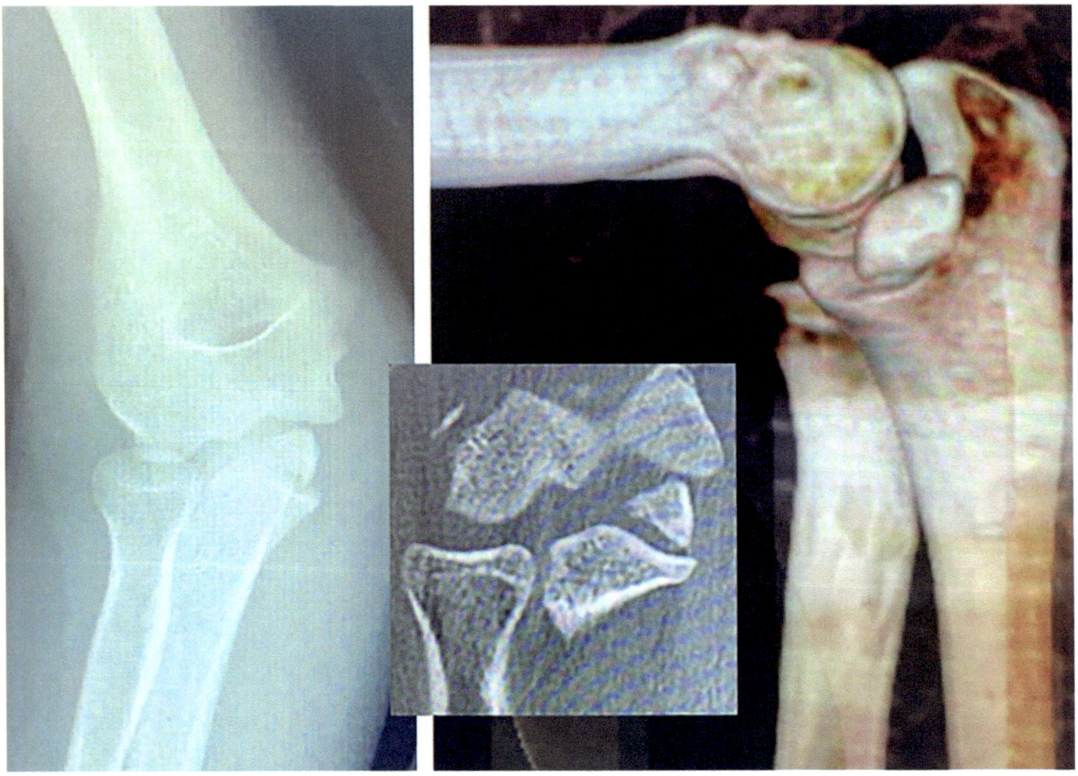

Fig. 8.5 A case of displaced intra-articular epitrochlear fragment after elbow joint dislocation in a 16 years old boy

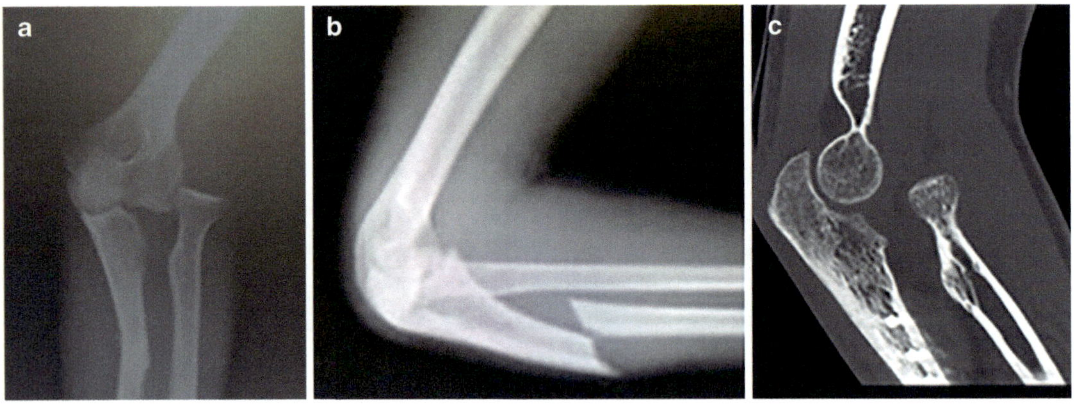

Fig. 8.6 A case of Monteggia fracture dislocation in a 17-year-old boy. (**a**) AP X-ray; (**b**) LL X-ray; (**c**) coronal view CT scan

paediatric patients by supplementing typical paediatric fracture patterns such as bony plastic deformations and greenstick type fractures to the anterior radial head displacement group (Bado type I) [6–7].

8.5 Early Complications

8.5.1 Heterotopic Ossification (HO)

Heterotopic ossification (HO) is the formation of bone in atypical, extraskeletal tissues that may occur following elbow trauma, brain injury or major burns. Location and size of HO can cause restriction of elbow range of motion and in the worst scenario joint ankylosis. There are a few conditions that are associated with spontaneous formation of heterotopic bone about the elbow. Injury to bone, ligament, muscle, tendon or joint capsule from the distal humerus to the proximal ulna or radius can incite local ectopic bone formation. Iatrogenic trauma, such as open surgery or elbow arthroscopy, has been reported to cause elbow heterotopic ossification. Alternatively, trauma to the central nervous system (including spinal cord injury) and debilitating burns have also been identified as risk factors for spontaneous formation of heterotopic bone about the elbow.

HOs are removed to allow joint motion. The consensus in the literature is that the safest time for excision of heterotopic ossification is after its complete maturation, which is 1–2 years after appearance [8]. Current trend reports that early excision associated with early exercise is effective for the treatment of HO aiming at a low recurrence rate and satisfactory function [9].

8.6 Late Complications

8.6.1 Cubitus Varus

Cubitus varus is a possible complication if supracondylar fractures are not reduced anatomically and properly fixed. Anatomically, the deformity results from the displacement of the distal fracture fragment in three dimenion: varus tilt, internal rotation and extension. Extension deformity presents as loss of terminal degrees of flexion. Although functional deficits are rare with these deformities, there may be slightly limited range of motion and unacceptable cosmesis. Cubitus varus can result in posterolateral rotatory instability (PLRI), tardy ulnar nerve palsy, snapping triceps, which may aggravate ulnar nerve symptoms and triceps tendon dislocation [10].

8.6.2 Cubitus Valgus

Cubitus valgus can be the result of medial epicondyle fracture or Milch fracture (Fig. 8.7). Non-union and malunion of the lateral humeral condyle fracture is a common cause of cubitus valgus. This deformity is often symptomatic and functionally disabling due to lateral instability and stiffness of elbow. It is also a common cause of tardy ulnar nerve palsy. The lateral condyle fragment is often enlarged due to the remodelling process; so, it does not fit well with the metaphysis. Furthermore, contracture of common extensor muscles can result in stiffness of the elbow. Correction of cubitus valgus with corrective osteotomy and anterior transposition of ulnar nerve is the treatment of choice [10].

8.6.3 Missed Monteggia Lesion

Failure to recognize a Monteggia fracture on initial consultation occurs in 20–50% of case (neglected Monteggia). Persistent dislocation of the radial head results in progressive dysplastic changes of the radiocapitellar joint: the radial head loses its concave articular surface and the humeral capitellum flattens, limiting the range of elbow flexion and extension. Restricted forearm pronation and supination, pain, palpable mass, progressive cubitus valgus deformity and osteoarthritis and occasionally tardy posterior interosseous nerve (PIN) palsy may occur as a consequence of untreated radial head dislocation.

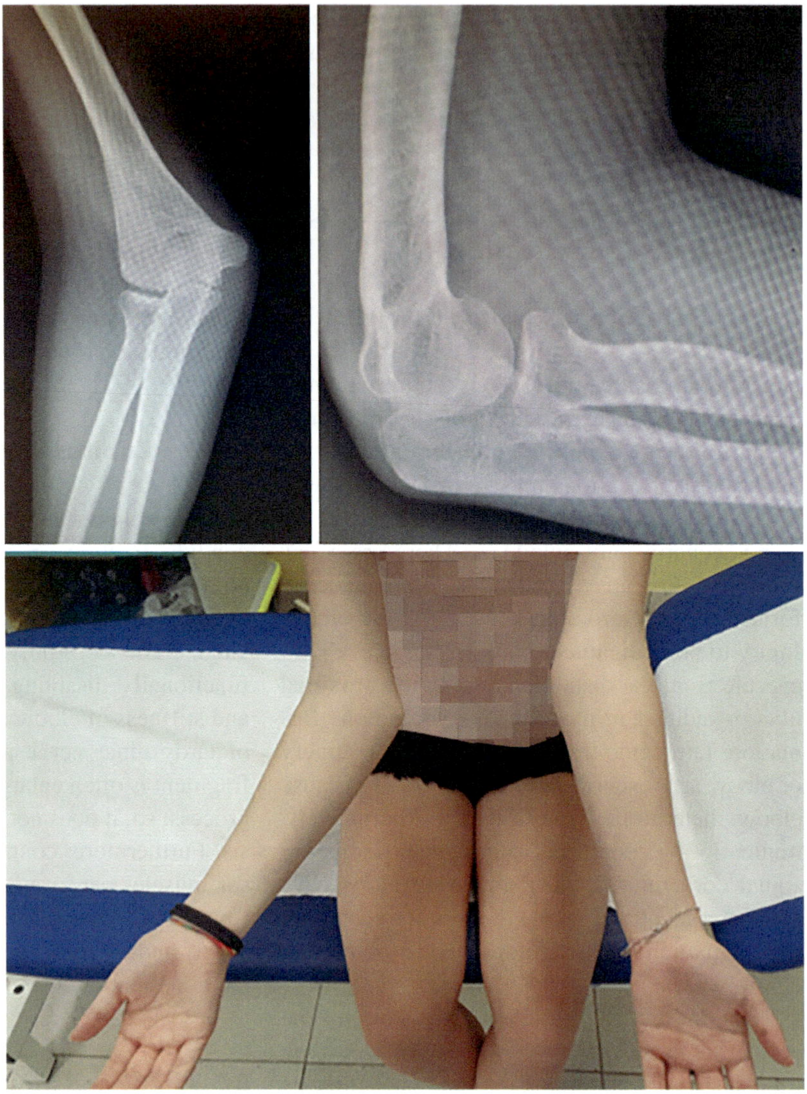

Fig. 8.7 An example of Cubitus valgus deformities in a 17 years old girl, AP and LL X-ray and clinical aspect

Current consensus is that these elbows deteriorate gradually; hence, many surgeons recommend intervention mainly to prevent further deterioration of the deformity and to reduce pain. The most popular treatment consists of ulnar osteotomy and radial head relocation with or without the repair of annular ligament [10].

8.7 Congenital Causes

Congenital causes of stiff elbow are rare disorders. It is important to knowing and suspecting congenital causes to recommend a genetic cousnselling is helpful for diagnose congenital disorder potentilally associated with stiff elbow. These deformities may lead to serious long-term complications [11].

8.7.1 Arthrogryposis Multiplex Congenita (AMC)

Arthrogryposis is a rare condition, occurring in 1 in 3000 live births. AMC is characterized by multiple joint contractures with deficient dysplastic musculo-tendinous units. In 72% of cases, upper limb is involved with a 32% affecting wrist, 26% hand, followed by the elbow [12].

The stiff elbow in arthrogryposis can be of two different types. Stiff in flexion: the elbow usually has a useful range around the functional position. Biceps is strong and triceps often weak or absent.

The second and more disabling type is the elbow stiff in extension. The joint is usually stiff in full extension, with only a rock of movement. The triceps is always strong and the biceps and brachialis are usually absent.

The association with wrist or shoulder contracture is common and bilateral presentation is frequent [3]. Treatment varies according to variability of phenotype, from splinting and stretching in mild cases to surgical treatment in severe deformities with different kind of transfers. Van Heest et al.[13] reported treatment recommendation for elbow flexion dysfunction: begin exercise at birth to obtain passive ROM. If at least 90 degree of elbow passive motion are not gained after 18-24 months of rehabilitation, surgery is reccomanded. i.e. capsulotomy with triceps lengthening provide passive ability for hand-to-mouth activities. After the child is 4 years old, tendon transfers for elbow flexion on the dominant arm are recommended, particularly the triceps to biceps transfer.

8.7.2 Beals Syndrome (CCA, Congenital Contractural Arachnodactyly)

This is an autosomal dominant connective tissue disorder, connected with fibrillin gene (FBN2) [14]. It involves commonly elbow, knee and fingers and it can be associated with kyphoscoliosis too.

8.7.3 Larsen Syndrome

It can be another cause of stiffness in paediatric elbow. This disorder is associated with mutations on FLNB gene (for the cytoplasmatic protein Filamin B) and clinical manifestations can involve congenital dislocations of the hip, knee or elbow (with stiffness) [15].

8.7.4 Congenital Radial Head Dislocation

It is a rare condition, often bilateral, with an incidence of 0.06–0.16%. It can be confused with traumatic dislocation of radial head—particularly when the child presents after a minor trauma. The radiological appearances are typical with hypoplastic dome-shaped radial head lacking normal concavity at the proximal end and hypoplastic capitellum. Posterior dislocation is more common. Elbow is generally held in 10–15° of flexion with forearm in pronation and severe restriction of supination. At wrist ulnar positive variance is common with restricted wrist movements. Typically, restrictions of the elbow and forearm movements are noted in the late childhood and remain unchanged. Patients commonly present with painful elbow, prominence of radial head and restriction of range of movement, particularly supination. Conventionally open reduction in radial head is not recommended because of the adaptive changes in the radial head and proximal radioulnar joint (PRUJ). Radial head excision is an option in adult patients, and it is known to improve pain and removes the bump, but rotational movements do not improve [10].

8.7.5 Congenital Radioulnar Synostosis (CRUS)

All synostosis forearms are fixed in pronation due to failure of cavitation affecting elbow during 7th foetal week. The CRUS is associated with other anomalies such as Apert syndrome (acrocephalosyndactyly), Carpenter syndrome (acropolysyndactyly), arthrogryposis and Klinefelter syndrome. It is bilateral in 60% and can be bony, cartilaginous or fibrous (Fig. 8.8). It is often painless but can be functionally disabling in bilateral cases. Treatment depends on the degree of fixed pronation and functional deficit. Rotational osteotomy is the preferred surgery than the excision of synostosis, but successful excision of synostosis has also been reported [10].

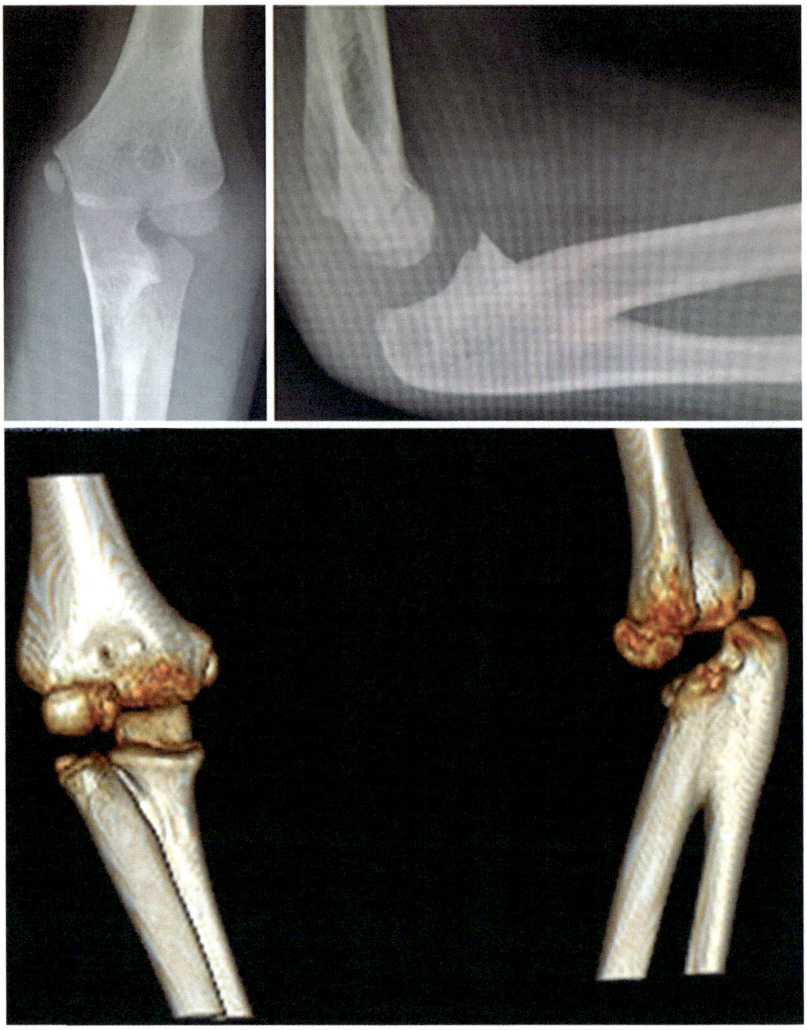

Fig. 8.8 X-rays and 3D CT scan of congenital bilateral radio-ulnar synostosis

8.7.6 Spastic Cerebral Palsy

Spasticity presents as muscular hypertonia and hyperexcitability of the stretch reflex, which are typical of upper motor neuron syndrome. It is due to a defect or lesion of the immature brain. The characteristic posture of the upper extremities in spastic cerebral palsy is the inward rotation of the shoulder, flexion of the elbow and pronated forearm, flexion of the wrist with ulnar deviation and the deformity of the fingers (flexion contracture, swan-neck, and thumbs-in-palm) [16]. Spastic elbow and forearm pathologies are spastic flection and extension contraction, supination and pronation spastic deformities. All these categories could be dynamic and static deformities [16, 17].

- *Spastic Flexion Contracture of the Elbow*: It is the most common. EMG helps confirm the presence of volitional capacity as well as abnormal synergy of each of the elbow flexors. The brachioradialis muscle most commonly shows continuous spastic activity as well as one or both heads of the biceps muscle. Selective elbow flexor lengthening techniques allow mobilization of the elbow in extension. More in details, when the deformity is primarily dynamic, the biceps should be lengthened at its proximal musculotendinous junction. If the static component of the deformity is predominant, a Z-plastic of the distal biceps tendon is advisable.

- *Elbow with static deformity and non-volitional control.* Persistent spasticity of the elbow flexors may induce a myostatic contracture and flexion deformity. This can result in skin maceration and a breakdown of the antecubital space. This position of severe elbow flexion also predisposes the ulnar nerve to compression neuropathy. If the elbow flexion contracture is severe and chronic, the brachialis muscle should be completely transected. In very severe contractures, it may be necessary to perform multiple Z-plastics of the antecubital skin or even sometimes flap coverage. If preoperative nerve conduction studies demonstrated an ulnar neuropathy at the level of the elbow, anterior transposition of the ulnar nerve should be performed. Postoperatively, the elbow is immobilized in extension at the point where there is no tension on the neurovascular structures or skin. Physical therapy, serial casting or dynamic splinting can be used later to improve extension range.
- *Spastic Extension:* It is less common. Patients have difficulties in reaching their face to perform activities of daily living. A surgical option is represented by lengthening of the triceps tendon, which allows improved flexion ROM. This procedure should be used with caution in patients who rely on their arms to assist with ambulation.
- *Spastic Pronation*: Pronation is more common than supination deformities of the forearm. Dynamic EMG shows varying degrees of volition and spasticity of the pronator teres, pronator quadratus and biceps. The clinical goal is to improve active supination function by reducing pronator dyssynergy. Fractional lengthening of the pronator teres is an accepted treatment.
- *Spastic Supination*: It is very uncommon. Dynamic EMG detects contribution of biceps and the supinator muscles. This deformity can be treated by rerouting the biceps tendon distally around the radius to reposition the forearm in neutral rotation. On rare occasions, supinator release is required.

8.8 Acquired Pathologies

8.8.1 Osteochondrosis of the Humeral Capitellum or Panner Disease

In 1927, a Danish orthopaedic surgeon, Dr. Dane Panner, first described radiographic changes of the entire capitellum. The average age of presentation is 9 years; boys are more affected. Repetitive stress or microtrauma over a period of time disrupts the chondrogenesis, and osteogenesis that occurs at the epiphysis and interference of the blood supply leads to sclerosis and frag-mentation of the capitellum. Claessen et al. in their review reported pain in 66%, swelling in 55% and limitation of elbow movement in 62% of patients in his review article [18]. Typically, there is a limitation of extension movement approximately by 20° rather than flexion movement deficit. The symptoms are exacerbated by activity and relieved by rest. The X-rays show changes in the morphology, contour irregularities, flattening of articular elbows in anteroposterior (AP) and lateral view. A characteristic radiographic and computed tomography (CT) scan is the subchondral vacuum phenomenon. It represents a gas accumulation within the subchondral cleft and it is a sign of bone ischemia. It may indicate avascular necrosis and impending articular collapse. The vacuum phenomenon disappears when repair and reossification eventually occurs [19]. Reduction in elbow activities that increase valgus stress may relieve pain and allow a return to normal elbow motion and function. Immobilization and anti-inflammatory medications provide marked relief in most cases. Panner disease is a self-limiting disease and the majority of patients heal without any morbidity.

8.8.2 Osteochondritis Dissecans (OCD)

Osteochondritis dissecans (OCD) is an acquired disorder of the articular cartilage and subchondral bone, resulting in separation of the subchondral bone and overlying cartilage [20]. It occurs most frequently in patients >10 years old, engaged in overhead throwing or weight-bearing sports (e.g., baseball, tennis, gymnastics). The OCD affects the humeral capitellum of the dominant arm (Fig. 8.9), but also the olecranon, radial head and trochlea. Bilateral OCD is reported in approximately 20%. OCD generally shows a lesion with a well-defined edge, whereas Panner disease typically presents as a more diffuse pathology of the capitellum. Patients complain pain or swelling of the elbow during or after activity, which subside with rest. In advanced stage, patients report loss of extension and catching or locking of the elbow. Imaging is useful to distinguish between stable or unstable lesions. CT scan is suitable for depicting the size and location of the OCD lesion, determining the properties of the bone fragment and is most sensitive in identifying intra-articular bodies. MRI is most useful for classification and to determine the stability of the lesion. On MRI, the cartilage can be visualized most clearly, including an assessment of the lateral cartilage margin of the capitellum, which is important in determining the course of treatment. The treatment options for OCD of the elbow include conservative treatment, arthroscopic surgery and open surgery (debridement, fragment fixation, graft). The choice of treatment depends on several aspects such as severity, stability, bone maturity, and the size, location and characteristics of the lesion [19].

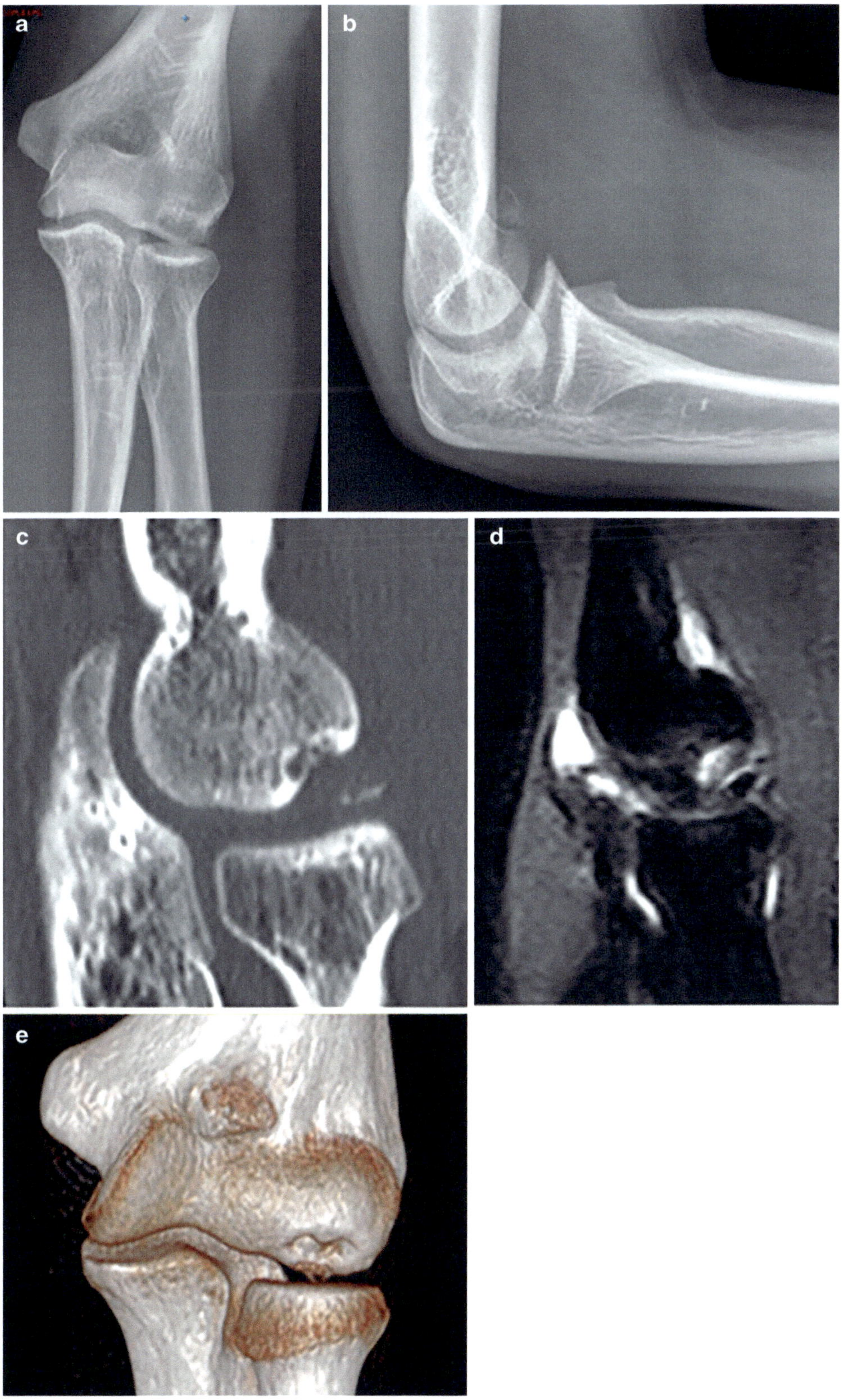

Fig. 8.9 A case of 17-year-old gymnast with humeral capitulum OCD. (**a, b**) AP and LL X-ray; (**c**) sagittal plane CT scan; (**d**) sagittal plane MRI; (**e**) 3D-CT scan

8.9 Classification

There are several classification systems reported in literature. In 2005, Morrey at al proposed a classification in three categories, extrinsic, intrinsic, and mixed, based on anatomical location and aetiology of the disorder [19].

Watts in 2010 and ISAKOS in 2015 described the all-inclusive pathoanatomical classification of elbow stiffness. They identified four causes of elbow stiffness: intra-articular, capsular, extra-articular, and neurological [21].

In 2017, the stiffness type and influencing factor classification (STIF) was proposed [22].

8.10 Clinical Presentation

Clinical examination of elbow in child can be challenging, especially in very young patients or new-born who are unable to describe their symptoms. Patient should be evaluated in a comfortable place with his/her parents.

Clinical history and previous elbow surgery, general physical exam and local examination of the upper extremity represent essential information to guide the correct diagnosis.

Elbow stiffness has a variety of aetiologies and it is mandatory to rule out each condition and differential diagnosis before reaching a definitive diagnosis. Information about upper arm trauma, previous elbow surgery, duration and type of immobilization and sport activities can lead to post-traumatic elbow stiffness problem. If there is no history of trauma, clinician should make a differential diagnosis between all acquired and congenital cause of elbow stiffness. Symptoms like fever associated with alteration of withe blood cell count should always be assessed as they could suggest inflammatory or infective causes of joint disease.

The degree and duration of contracture, and any symptoms of ulnar neuropathy, even if transient, can be predictive of ulnar traction neuropathy. If the patient has less than 90° of flexion or preoperative ulnar neuropathy, consideration should be given for ulnar nerve release and anterior transposition at the same time as the contracture release.

8.11 Physical Examination

Full examination of the involved upper extremity is essential, and measurements should be compared to the contralateral unaffected side. Inspection of the skin, previous wounds, surgical scars, muscle atrophy, and obvious bony deformity are investigated. Palpate for areas of tenderness and/or pain that could be indicative of a non-union or ligament injury. Assessment of active and passive ROM in flexion, extension, pronation and supination should be quantified using a goniometer, making note of hard or soft end-feel at terminal motion. Angular deformity in the coronal plane should be quantified with the elbow in full extension. The neurovascular exam should test any neuropathy or instability of the ulnar nerve, the radial and median nerve. Elbow stability should be tested by varus-valgus stress, the lateral pivot shift, and the chair raise test, the milking manoeuvre, and the moving valgus stress test when possible. These tests can also be performed under fluoroscopy to gain a better understanding of the joint's stability under stress [1, 4].

8.12 Imaging

The first step in diagnosis is the X-ray. Anteroposterior, lateral, radiocapitellar and oblique views of bilateral elbows should be included for comparison. These should be carefully inspected for evidence of prior fracture, malunion, non-union, prominent implants, joint subluxation or incongruence, joint degeneration and heterotopic ossification.

The elbow of a child is made predominantly of cartilage. Secondary ossification centres appear at different ages in a defined order: capitellum, radial head, medial epicondyle, trochlea, olecranon and lateral epicondyle. The capitellum is the first secondary ossification centre and is fully visible at 2 years of age. The ossification centres are used as a radiographic parameter at paediatric age. There are parameters to define the correct anatomical relationship: the anterior humeral line, the radiocapitellar line and Baumann's angle [21].

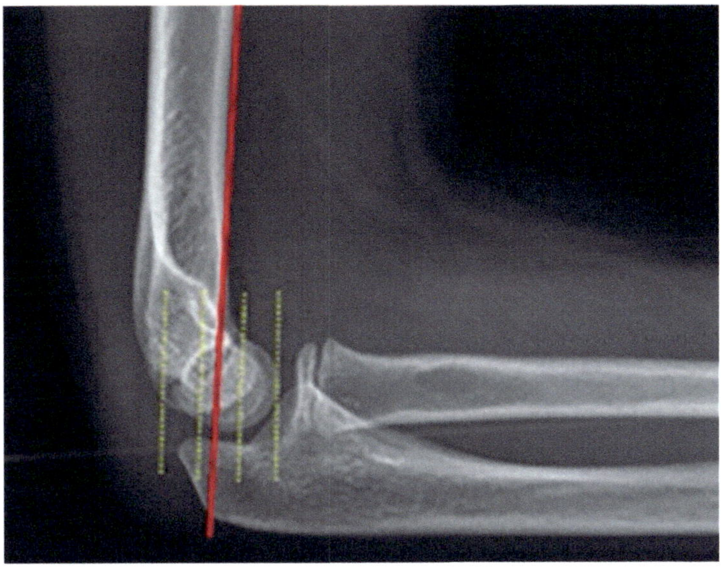

Fig. 8.10 Anterior humeral line on lateral X-ray view

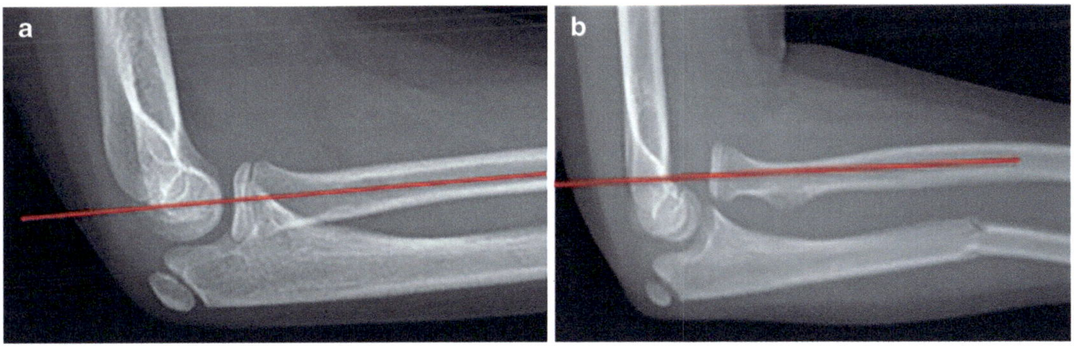

Fig. 8.11 Radiocapitellar line passes through the centre of the capitellum (**a**) normal condition; (**b**) radial head dislocation in a Monteggia fracture

- *The anterior humeral line:* It is drawn on a lateral X-ray view down the anterior surface of the humerus and normally crosses the middle third of the capitellar ossification centre (Fig. 8.10). It is used to assess sagittal displacement and the adequacy of reduction in supracondylar humerus fracture.
- *The radiocapitellar line:* It is drawn through diaphysis of the proximal radius and the centre of the radial neck and passes through the centre of the capitellum (Fig. 8.11). In case of dislocation of the radial head, this line will no longer pass through the centre of the capitellum (Fig. 8.11b). It is useful in case of Monteggia fracture dislocation, in particular when the ulna has a plastic deformity and cause subluxation of radial head.
- *The Baumann's angle*: It is the humeral-capitellar angle, which is measured on an AP radiograph between the long axis of the humerus and a line through the physis of the lateral condyle, and mean value is 75°–80°. It helps to detect cubitus varus malalignment.

There are a group of injuries around the elbow resulting from high energy trauma that is routinely missed at initial presentation because of normal X-rays. These kinds of injuries have been defined by Waters et al. as TRASH lesions (The Radiographic Appearance Seemed Harmless) (Fig. 8.12) [11]. These are a group of osteochondral injuries having poor outcomes if not treated adequately. Prompt diagnosis warrants a high index of suspicion even when a radiograph

Fig. 8.12 TRASH lesion

Pediatric Elbow TRASH Lesions
• Unossified medial condylar humerus fractures
• Unossified transphyseal distal humerus fractures
• Lateral condylar avulsion shear fractures
• Monteggia fracture dislocations
• Entrapped medial epicondylar fractures
• Complex osteochondral elbow fracture–dislocations below the age of 10 years
• Radial head anterior compression fractures with progressive radiocapitellar subluxation
• Osteochondral fractures with joint incongruity

appears to be normal with a disproportionately swollen elbow in a child. Magnetic resonance image (MRI) and ultrasound (US) help in reaching the right diagnosis and further management.

Computed tomography (CT) scan can be useful to understand complex fractures, location of heterotopic ossifications, ulno-humeral and radio-humeral congruency and articular morphology.

MRI is useful in adolescents in case of osteochondral lesion, Panner disease and OCD. MRI is the gold standard for ODC diagnosis; it provides information about size, location, presence of joint effusion, bone marrow change and loss of continuity of cartilage.

8.13 Non-surgical Treatment

Post-traumatic elbow arthrofibrosis (PEA) affects between 6% and 45% of children and is a well-known consequence of both intra- and extra-articular elbow joint trauma [23]. The treatment algorithm for PEA begins with ice, heat, supervised physical therapy, active ROM exercises, electrical stimulation and splinting. Physical therapy and bracing are the mainstays of non-operative management for paediatric elbow contracture. The protocol of exercise should not be strenuous or painful to maintain the patient compliance.

The use of botulinum toxin has become popular for orthopaedics as a treatment for spastic and dystonic muscle. Clostridium botulinum produces non-toxic proteins and a complex mixture of proteins containing botulinum neurotoxin. All these proteins can inhibit release of acetylcholine from nerve terminals. BTX-A reduces muscular activity in a dose-dependent manner. The dosage must be correlated with weight, size/volume, level of hypertonia, number of muscles to be injected and the underlying weakness. The injection of BTX could be administered under local or general anaesthesia or with conscious sedation. This depends on patient age, muscular districts, number of sites to be treated and underlying pathologies. The timing of the injections is controversial. Most clinicians agree that the earlier the spasticity is reduced, the better the outcome. Botulinum toxin can be injected as early as 18 months of age [24].

8.14 CMUA Closed Manipulation Under Anaesthesia

When conservative measures fail, closed manipulation under anaesthesia (CMUA) could be a valid option in paediatric population. CMUA for PEA appears to be a relatively simple and low-cost alternative procedure to open or arthroscopic surgical options.

Rane et al. in their study describe 13 patients younger than 18 years who underwent CMUA for PEA between 2005 and 2015 [23]. Median time to CMUA from initial surgery was 4.2 months. The authors report a significant improvement in elbow flexion of 22° ($p < 0.001$) and extension of 29° ($p < 0.001$). The average pre-manipulation motion arc of 60° significantly increased to 110° at final assessment ($p < 0.001$). In conclusion, CMUA appears to be a valuable alternative and reliable procedure for improving PEA in paediatric patients who appear to respond better than their adult counterparts. Despite its advantages, CMUA and aggressive manipulation are not without risks of iatrogenic injuries such as neurologic injuries, post-manipulation HO, physeal arrest, bony bar formation, fractures or other growth abnormalities.

8.15 Operative Management

Surgery should be considered when conservative treatment fails. Treatment should be planned in every case and differs according to different diagnosis (post-traumatic, acquired or congenital) and type of stiffness (intra-articular, capsular, extra-capsular or neurological) [1, 21, 22].

8.15.1 Intra-articular

Intra-articular pathologies with preserved articular joint anatomy/morphology, such as osteochondritis dissecans, loose bodies, impinging osteophytes, or synovitis can be treated by elbow arthroscopy.

Elbow arthroscopy is primarily performed in the paediatric population for osteochondritis dissecans (OCD) of the capitellum. However, recently there have been a growing number of indications for elbow arthroscopy in the younger population, including treatment of fractures, arthrofibrosis, posterior olecranon impingement syndrome and congenital disorders.

A recent literature review performed by Gouveia et al. [25] analysed indications, functional outcomes and complication rates of elbow arthroscopy in a paediatric population (<18 year of age). The authors find that elbow arthroscopy is an effective treatment option for paediatric patients with a variety of potential indications, although the majority of paediatric elbow arthroscopy is performed for OCD. The risk of neurovascular complications is greater in children, but they are tipically transient.

In younger patients, elbow joint size leads to choose smaller arthroscope (2.5–2.8 mm). In a case report, Colozza et al. reported a 6-year-old boy with elbow arthroscopic assistance for radial neck fracture reduction and fixation with a 2.4-mm 30° arthroscope [26].

Melchioni et al. in 2021 evaluated 26 patients treated by elbow arthroscopic debridement for post-traumatic elbow stiffness, posterior impingement and osteochondritis dissecans. The authors conclude that elbow arthroscopy performed by an expert surgeon in the paediatric and adolescent population is a safe procedure and allows to return to sports at previous levels [27].

Intra-articular group with abnormal joint anatomy, such as malunion and non-union, is treated by arthroscopy or open surgery. More in details, arthroscopic joint reshape is the choice for low grade of deformities when patients complain elbow stiffness, for example, coronoid fossa arthroplasty in malunion due to extension type of supracondylar fractures or radial head reshaping for dysmorphic radial head fracture sequelae.

In case of elbow stiffness associated with snapping of the medial border of triceps, posterolateral rotatory instability (PLRI) and tardy ulnar nerve palsy in cubitus varus deformities, open surgery with planned osteotomy is performed to correct the axis of distal humerus in the three dimensions (Fig. 8.13).

In 2022, Li et al., compared the result of conventional osteotomy with the three-dimensional (3D)-printed model and template guide osteotomy using the same surgical technique in 40 consecutive patients with cubitus varus deformity were included. The authors concluded the conventional osteotomy and 3D-printed model and osteotomy template techniques both met the treatment requirements of cubitus varus deformity. The 3D-printed template technique showed better osteotomy accuracy, but no significant advantage regarding the functional and cosmetic results than conventional osteotomy [28].

- **Capsular category** is linked to post-traumatic elbow stiffness. The initial insult causes intra-articular effusion or hemarthrosis. This causes the elbow to assume an antalgic position of flexion and co-contraction of the flexor and extensor muscle groups. Capsular thickening and contracture are the expression of complex interaction between myofibroblasts and mast

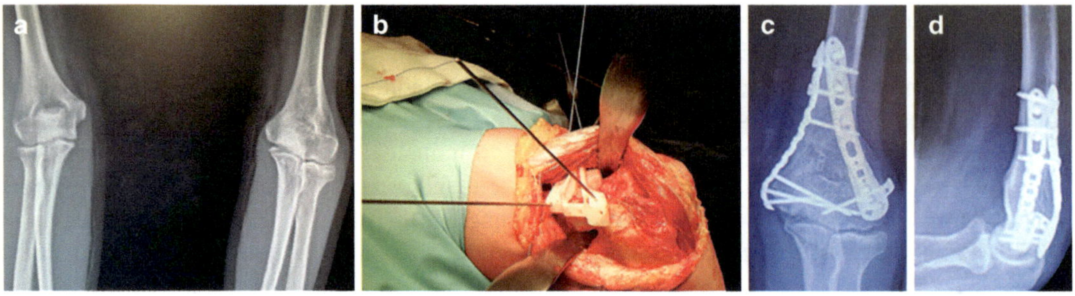

Fig. 8.13 Planned osteotomy for a varus deformity. (**a**) Preoperative both elbows X-rays; (**b**) intra-operative osteotomy with custom-made surgical cutting mask; (**c, d**) AP and LL post-operative X-rays

cells. Capsular contractures are also common with the intra-articular pathologies. Arthroscopic contracture release in capsular contracture can be challenging because the space between the articular surface and the overlying neurovascular structures is decreased, making them more vulnerable to iatrogenic injury. Arthroscopic and open contracture release can be associated technique in case of removal of hardware.

- **Extra-articular** pathologies such as HO, ulnar nerve neuropathy and muscle/tendon contractures are usually treated by an open procedure with resection or release of the offending structures.

The role of elbow contracture release in the very young population is unclear, with existing studies reporting conflicting results. Open surgical release is considered by some authors to be less predictable owing to conflicting reports of their efficacy [23, 29]. Stan et al., in a series of 37 patients, evaluate the efficacy of operative treatment for elbow contractures in patients younger than 21 years. Only 54% of children had an improvement of greater than 20°, and only 46% had a functional arc of motion (>100°). The authors demonstrated that in patients who had an intra-articular fracture or a complex fracture-dislocation, the outcomes of open arthrolysis are unpredictable both in terms or full range of motion (ROM) recovering and ROM improvement. In conclusion, the paediatric population is different in their response to the same operative techniques used similarly in the adult population.

Ek et al. reported the outcomes of 32 patients younger than 18 years old who underwent open elbow contracture release [30]. The mean time from the index injury to contracture release was 16.3 months. The authors report a total arc of motion improved from 69° to 123° ($p < 0.0001$). The function arc was >100° in 28 patients (88%), and 29 patients (91%) achieved >20° of improvement in their arc. Their results demonstrate significant improvements in range of motion that are maintained over time.

8.15.2 Technical Note from Authors

There are few surgical steps that could determine good outcomes in post-traumatic elbow arthrofibrosis.

- The first step is addressing the ulnar nerve. The risk of development of delayed onset ulnar neuropathy is strictly associated with elbow pain and stiffness. The ulnar nerve is at high risk of dysfunction after elbow arthrolysis for elongation and increased intraneural pressure, especially when considerable flexion is obtained [31]. Routine transposition is not performed by authors. At the end of surgery, the nerve is tested in maximum elbow flexion to check for any instability. In case of nerve luxation or subluxation, the nerve is anteriorly transposed in subcutaneous tissue.
- In post-traumatic elbow stiffness in presence of elbow hardware care must be taken to avoid manipulation of the elbow after hardware removal to avoid the possibility of an intraop-

erative fracture through the stress-risers left by screw holes. Anterior and posterior arthrolysis is the first step, and then the elbow motion is retested with gentle manipulation to check for ROM improvement. The implants removal is the final step of surgery. Removing hardware last, once motion has been regained, helps decrease the risk of intraoperative iatrogenic fractures. Intra-articular hardware prominence is an exception to this suggested progression.
- Soft tissue swelling control. Accurate haemostasis minimizes post-operative bleeding, and as consequences the intra-articular scar formation. It allows a faster range of motion with the reduction in soft tissue complications. Immediate post operative sling in extension at 'statue of liberty' is applied to maintain the upper arm elevate in the first night after surgery to drain oedema, arthroscopic saline solution and residual hematoma.

There are few reports in literature about the administration of steroid after elbow surgery to control swelling and pain, none for children [31].

Intravenous administration of tranexamic acid decreased the post-operative drainage volume and the total estimated blood loss and alleviated the elbow pain with motion during early post-operative days in patients undergoing open elbow arthrolysis [32]. There articles report safety of tranexamic acid in paediatric population in control perioperative blood loss [33–35]

- Pain control after arthrolysis for stiff elbow is crucial, mainly to allow early mobilization and maintain the arc of movement gained with surgery. A valid solution in post-operative pain control measures are catheters for the continuous administration of anaesthetic in the brachial plexus that have been seen to be very effective in the first 24–48 post-operative hours. The advantages of this approach versus isolated plexus block are a longer duration of block, reduction of the post-operative pain levels, lesser opioid consumption, and increased patient satisfaction. In our clinic, in adolescent and children, peripheral block is performed after general anaesthesia under ultrasound control. Only in adolescent and compliant patients we routinely use the catheters for the continuous administration of anaesthetic.
- Routinely reports with photos and chart degree the arc of elbow movement pre and post operatively. This will help patients, patient's parents and physiotherapist in post-operative rehabilitation to maintain the gained degree of movement.

References

1. Morrey BF, Askew LJ, Chao EY. A biomechanical study of normal functional elbow motion. J Bone Joint Surg Am. 1981;63(6):872–7.
2. Valone LC, Waites C, Tartarilla AB, Whited A, Sugimoto D, Bae DS, Bauer AS. Functional elbow range of motion in children and adolescents. J Pediatr Orthop. 2020;40(6):304–9. https://doi.org/10.1097/BPO.0000000000001467.
3. Mennen U, van Heest A, Ezaki MB, Tonkin M, Gericke G. Arthrogryposis multiplex congenita. J Hand Surg Br. 2005;30(5):468–74. https://doi.org/10.1016/j.jhsb.2005.06.004.
4. Lattanza L, Piper SL. Elbow stiffness in children and adolescents. In: Morrey's the elbow and its disorders. Elsevier; 2018. p. 349–55. https://doi.org/10.1016/B978-0-323-34169-1.00034-6.
5. Henrikson B. Supracondylar fracture of the humerus in children. A late review of end-results with special reference to the cause of deformity, disability and complications. Acta Chir Scand Suppl. 1966;369:1–72.
6. Hart ES, Turner A, Albright M, Grottkau BE. Common pediatric elbow fractures. Orthop Nurs. 2011;30(1):11–7; quiz 18–9. https://doi.org/10.1097/NOR.0b013e31820574c6.
7. Hyvönen H, Korhonen L, Hannonen J, et al. Recent trends in children's elbow dislocation with or without a concomitant fracture. BMC Musculoskelet Disord. 2019;20:294. https://doi.org/10.1186/s12891-019-2651-8.
8. Kluger G, Kochs A, Holthausen H. Heterotopic ossification in childhood and adolescence. J Child Neurol. 2000;15(6):406–13. https://doi.org/10.1177/088307380001500610.
9. Chen S, Yu S, Yan H, Cai J, Ouyang Y, Ruan H, Fan C. The time point in surgical excision of heterotopic ossification of post-traumatic stiff elbow: recommendation for early excision followed by early exercise. J Shoulder Elbow Surg. 2015;24(8):1165–71. https://doi.org/10.1016/j.jse.2015.05.044.
10. Lahoti O, Akilapa O. Not Kidding! Sequelae of elbow trauma in children. J Clin Orthop Trauma. 2021;20:101471. https://doi.org/10.1016/j.jcot.2021.06.001. Erratum in: J Clin Orthop Trauma. 2021 Jul 30;20:101540.

11. Patwardhan S, Omkaram S. Trash lesions around the elbow: a review of approach to diagnosis and management. Indian J Orthop. 2021;55(3):539–48. https://doi.org/10.1007/s43465-020-00333-x.
12. Gibson DA, Urs ND. Arthrogryposis multiplex congenita. J Bone Joint Surg Br. 1970;52(3):483–93.
13. Van Heest A, Waters PM, Simmons BP. Surgical treatment of arthrogryposis of the elbow. J Hand Surg Am. 1998;23(6):1063–70. https://doi.org/10.1016/S0363-5023(98)80017-8.
14. Tunçbilek E, Alanay Y. Congenital contractural arachnodactyly (Beals syndrome). Orphanet J Rare Dis. 2006;1(1):20. https://doi.org/10.1186/1750-1172-1-20.
15. Robertson S. FLNB disorders. 2008. In: Adam MP, Everman DB, Mirzaa GM, et al., editors. GeneReviews®. Seattle, WA: University of Washington, Seattle; 1993–2023.
16. Gharbaoui I, Kania K, Cole P. Spastic paralysis of the elbow and forearm. Semin Plast Surg. 2016;30(1):39–44. https://doi.org/10.1055/s-0035-1571255.
17. Kheder A, Nair KP. Spasticity: pathophysiology, evaluation and management. Pract Neurol. 2012;12(5):289–98. https://doi.org/10.1136/practneurol-2011-000155.
18. Claessen FM, Louwerens JK, Doornberg JN, van Dijk CN, Eygendaal D, van den Bekerom MP. Panner's disease: literature review and treatment recommendations. J Child Orthop. 2015;9(1):9–17. https://doi.org/10.1007/s11832-015-0635-2.
19. Chavda S, Abeid KA, Alhajri KK, Hasan NHA. Osteochondrosis of humeral capitellum, diagnosis and treatment—a case report. J Orthop Case Rep. 2021;11(7):74–7. https://doi.org/10.13107/jocr.2021.v11.i07.2324.
20. Macken AA, van Bergen CJA, Eygendaal D, The B. Diagnosis and treatment of osteochondritis dissecans of the elbow. Orthop Trauma. 2020;34(4):213–8. https://doi.org/10.1016/j.mporth.2020.05.004.
21. Bain G, Eygendaal D, van Riet RP, editors. Surgical techniques for trauma and sports related injuries of the elbow. Springer; 2020. https://doi.org/10.1007/978-3-662-58931-1.
22. Marinelli A, Bain GI. The stiff elbow: classification and treatment algorithm. ISAKOS Newslett. 2018;2:18–21.
23. Rane AA, Garcia BN, Wang AA. Closed manipulation under anesthesia for pediatric post-traumatic elbow arthrofibrosis. J Shoulder Elbow Surg. 2020;29(2):340–6. https://doi.org/10.1016/j.jse.2019.10.004.
24. Pavone V, Testa G, Restivo DA, Cannavò L, Condorelli G, Portinaro NM, Sessa G. Botulinum toxin treatment for limb spasticity in childhood cerebral palsy. Front Pharmacol. 2016;19(7):29. https://doi.org/10.3389/fphar.2016.00029.
25. Gouveia K, Zhang K, Kay J, Memon M, Simunovic N, Garrigues GE, Pollock JW, Ayeni OR. The use of elbow arthroscopy for management of the pediatric elbow: a systematic review of indications and outcomes. Arthroscopy. 2021;37(6):1958–1970.e1. https://doi.org/10.1016/j.arthro.2021.01.047.
26. Colozza A, Padovani S, Caruso G, Cavaciocchi M, Massari L. Arthroscopically-assisted reduction and pinning of a radial neck fracture in a child: a case report and review of the literature. J Med Case Rep. 2020;14(1):78. https://doi.org/10.1186/s13256-020-02390-0.
27. Micheloni GM, Tarallo L, Negri A, et al. Pediatric elbow arthroscopy: clinical outcomes and complications after long-term follow-up. J Orthop Traumatol. 2021;22:55. https://doi.org/10.1186/s10195-021-00619-2.
28. Li J, Wang J, Rai S, Ze R, Hong P, Wang S, Tang X. 3D-printed model and osteotomy template technique compared with conventional closing-wedge osteotomy in cubitus varus deformity. Sci Rep. 2022;12(1):6762. https://doi.org/10.1038/s41598-022-10732-9.
29. Stans AA, Maritz NGJ, O'Driscoll SW, Morrey BF. Operative treatment of elbow contracture in patients twenty-one years of age or younger. J Bone Joint Surg. 2002;84(3):382–7.
30. Ek ET, Paul SK, Hotchkiss RN. Outcomes after operative treatment of elbow contractures in the pediatric and adolescent population. J Shoulder Elbow Surg. 2016;25(12):2066–70. https://doi.org/10.1016/j.jse.2016.09.008.
31. Blonna D, Huffmann GR, O'Driscoll SW. Delayed-onset ulnar neuritis after release of elbow contractures: clinical presentation, pathological findings, and treatment. Am J Sports Med. 2014;42(9):2113–21. https://doi.org/10.1177/0363546514540448.
32. Cui H, Yu S, Ruan J, Sun Z, Li J, Chen S, Fan C. Intravenous tranexamic acid reduce postoperative drainage and pain after open elbow arthrolysis: a randomized controlled trial. J Shoulder Elbow Surg. 2021;30(8):1725–32. https://doi.org/10.1016/j.jse.2021.04.031.
33. Desai MJ, Matson AP, Ruch DS, Leversedge FJ, Aldridge JM 3rd, Richard MJ. Perioperative glucocorticoid administration improves elbow motion in terrible triad injuries. J Hand Surg Am. 2017;42(1):41–6. https://doi.org/10.1016/j.jhsa.2016.11.011.
34. Goobie SM, Faraoni D. Tranexamic acid and perioperative bleeding in children: what do we still need to know? Curr Opin Anaesthesiol. 2019;32(3):343–52. https://doi.org/10.1097/ACO.0000000000000728.
35. Ivasyk I, Chatterjee A, Jordan C, et al. Evaluation of the safety of tranexamic acid use in pediatric patients undergoing spinal fusion surgery: a retrospective comparative cohort study. BMC Musculoskelet Disord. 2022;23:651. https://doi.org/10.1186/s12891-022-05604-2.

Elbow Stiffness in Systemic Diseases

9

Valeria Vismara, Simone Cassin, and Paolo Angelo Arrigoni

Elbow stiffness is defined as the loss of movement greater than 30° in extension and loss of flexion of less than 120° [1]. A 50% reduction in elbow motion can reduce upper extremity function by 80%. It is the result of morphological and structural alterations of the bone and soft tissues, which may or may not follow a traumatic event. Trauma, burns, fractures, and pathologies of the nervous system are among the most common causes, together with rigidity occurring after surgical interventions [2].

Traumatic causes include [3] fractures, dislocations, soft tissue crush or burns, and head injury. Atraumatic causes include [2]:

- Osteoarthritis
- Inflammatory arthritis
- Rheumatoid arthritis
- Ankylosing spondylitis
- Psoriatic arthropathy
- Gout
- Enteropathic arthritis
- JIA
- Post-septic arthritis
- Hemophilia
- Congenital deformities
- Arthrogryposis
- Pterygium syndrome
- Congenital radial head dislocation

Elbow mobility depends on bone and soft tissue health. In case of trauma or pathology, their anatomy could be altered resulting in mechanical block and articular stiffness. Soft tissue thickening and heterotopic ossifications are common in response to traumatic events. Heterotopic ossification occurs in up to 3% of cases of simple dislocations and in up to 20% of fracture-dislocations. These percentages increase if elbow injury is associated with primary head injury, reaching values ranging from 79% to 86%. Predisposing factors to post-traumatic elbow stiffness are found in patient and fracture characteristics (comminuted fractures, exposed fractures, high energy trauma, infections, fragment devascularization, osteochondral defects, metabolic and cellular abnormalities) and in fracture treatment (incorrect osteosynthesis, soft tissue interposition, early mobilization). Moreover, intra- and extra-articular consolidation defects of elbow fractures can lead to stiffness and rigidity.

The three main elbow stiffness classification systems are those of Kay, Morrey, and Vidal. The first one is based on the structure that blocks movement and it consists of five types [4]:

V. Vismara · S. Cassin
Scuola di Specializzazione Ortopedia e Traumatologia, Università degli studi di Milano, Milan, Italy

P. A. Arrigoni (✉)
Clinica Ortopedica, Azienda Socio Sanitaria Territoriale Centro Specialistico Ortopedico Traumatologico Gaetano Pini-CTO, Milan, Italy

L. Pederzini et al. (eds.), *Stiffness of the Elbow, Wrist and Related Pathologies*,
https://doi.org/10.1007/978-3-031-81381-8_9

- Type I: Soft tissue contracture
- Type II: Soft tissue contracture with ossification
- Type III: Non-displaced articular fracture with soft tissue contracture
- Type IV: Displaced intra-articular fracture with soft tissue contracture
- Type V: Post-traumatic bony bars

The second one [5] is based on stiffness' etiology and anatomic location; it classifies the rigidity in:

- Extrinsic, caused by extra-articular causes including capsular, collateral ligament and muscle contractures, heterotopic ossifications, and extra-articular malunions
- Intrinsic, due to intra-articular adhesions, loose bodies, osteophyte formation or malalignment of the articular surface
- Mixed, in case of extrinsic contractures developing because of intrinsic pathology

The third one is based on the degree of severity of rigidity; it classifies the stiffness in four levels of severity:

- Very severe stiffness: ROM 180–150°
- Severe stiffness: ROM 150–120°
- Moderate stiffness: ROM 120–90
- Slight stiffness: ROM beyond 90°

However, it is important to highlight that stiffness should be evaluated not only in absolute terms but also relatively to the occupational and social life of the patient [6].

Recently, the Liverpool Elbow Score was validated too for assessing elbow stiffness severity [7].

Careful anamnesis and physical examination, together with radio-diagnostic imaging, help the physician towards the right diagnosis of the condition. Antero-posterior (AP) and latero-lateral (LL) projections X-rays allow identification of bony components and eventually of heterotopic ossifications which may limit the range of motion (ROM). While computed tomography (CT) scan with three-dimensional (3D) reconstruction may be helpful especially in identification of big osteophytes and irregular articular surface, magnetic resonance imaging (MRI) should be used when the physician suspects avascular necrosis or in case of post-traumatic elbow stiffness.

Surgical approach to these conditions should be taken into consideration only after failure of conservative treatment and in case of great functional compromise. Moreover, surgery should be delayed until inflammatory signs are no longer present. Only in the case of loose bodies or bony fragments found within the articular surface, surgery should be performed in a timely manner.

9.1 Intrinsic Causes

9.1.1 Osteoarthritis (OA)

Primary elbow osteoarthritis is a quite rare condition, affecting only 1–2% of the general population. It is often asymptomatic, being the elbow a non-weight bearing joint. When symptomatic, pain is the dominant presenting symptom followed by loss of range of motion (ROM), to which the elbow joint is prone.

Middle-aged men engaged in activities that subject the elbow to high force loads (e.g., heavy-machine operators, weightlifters, and professional overhead athletes) are at increased risk of developing elbow osteoarthritis. Indeed, in these subjects the elbow joint, in particular the ulna-humeral joint, is subject to forces which range from two to six times the body weight. Many other factors seem to increase the risk, such as ethnicity, genetics, ageing, bone mineral density, joint loading and malalignment and obesity.

Secondary elbow osteoarthritis is a much more common condition, which can arise following trauma, osteochondritis dissecans, synovial chondromatosis, and valgus extension overload syndrome [8].

Primary OA, differently from osteoarthritis in other joints, is mainly characterized by osteophyte formation, capsular contracture, and loose bodies, rather than loss of joint space. Initially, the main complaints are pain and movement restriction due to impingement of osteophytes at the extremes of the ROM. The lateral aspect of the elbow, the radio-humeral joint, is the first to be hit by articular degeneration. A posteromedial cartilage defect is often found and corresponds to a matched defect at the posterior part of the crest separating the trochlea from the capitellum. In contrast, the ulna-humeral articulation does not show this pattern of degeneration. This may be due to the fact that eccentric load contraction occurs at the center of the joint, destroying articular cartilage at the ulnar edge of the radial head and the corresponding crest. In secondary OA, misdiagnosed coronoid fractures, osteonecrosis, or repetitive hyperextension in the setting of medial laxity lead to osteophyte and loose bodies formation [9].

Reduction in the arc of motion is a common clinical finding in these patients, with an average 30° flexion contracture. These findings are also associated with ulnar neuropathy in almost 30–55% cases. To differentiate between primary and secondary OA, anamnesis and physical examination are keys. Pain at the end of arc of motion is suggestive of osteophyte impingement, whereas pain at the mid arc of motion suggests the presence of an osteochondral defect. Ulnar neuropathy signs should always be evaluated as well as the presence of prior surgery. In the latter case, infection should always be kept in mind as a cause of pain.

Synovial fluid aspirate may help in the diagnosis of this condition, together with a complete blood cell count, polymerase chain reaction (PCR), and erythrocyte sedimentation rate (ESR).

X-ray in two perpendicular projections, AP and LL, usually reveals anterior and medial osteophytes involving the coronoid process and a posteromedial osteophyte on the olecranon process. Radiographic changes are often present at the radio-capitellar joint, with preservation of the radio-capitellar and ulno-capitellar joints spaces. This finding is important to differentiate primary OA from inflammatory arthritis, which is characterized by narrowing of the joint spaces. Loose bodies, which usually present in the posterior compartment and proximal radio-ulnar joint, are often difficult to see with X-rays. For a better evaluation, CT scan or MRI is needed (Fig. 9.1).

Conservative treatment in these patients consists in rest, anti-inflammatory medications, and long-term modification of activity. Intra-articular steroid injects are not effective in the long term.

Operative treatment is often the real solution for these patients. There are many procedures available, both open and arthroscopic, to mitigate pain and improve range of motion, ranging from joint debridement, osteophyte excision to contracture release. When the disease is advanced and is characterized by joint space narrowing, interposition, or replacement arthroplasty may be the only solution. The best treatment option involves capsular release and removal of impingement osteophytes. Arthroplasty should be reserved for older, sedentary patients or for those in which all other treatments have failed [8]. When considering operative treatment, the patients must be informed of the need of early, controlled activity to restore a functional ROM after surgery, to regain as much as possible the arc of movement, which, despite optimal procedures, may not return to the native status.

9.1.2 Inflammatory Arthritis

Rheumatoid arthritis (RA) is the most common inflammatory arthritis affecting the elbow, followed by ankylosing spondylitis, psoriatic arthropathy and gout. Each condition is characterized by different and specific manifestations. Many other seronegative disorders, such as enteropathic arthritis, juvenile idiopathic arthritis (JIA), reactive arthritis, and systemic lupus erythematosus (SLE) disease may be associated with elbow stiffness, due to their inflammatory arthritis component. While synovitis is the hallmark of RA, enthesitis is the hallmark of seronegative arthritis. Independently of the underlying pathology, these patients are extremely fragile and require an extended team approach [10].

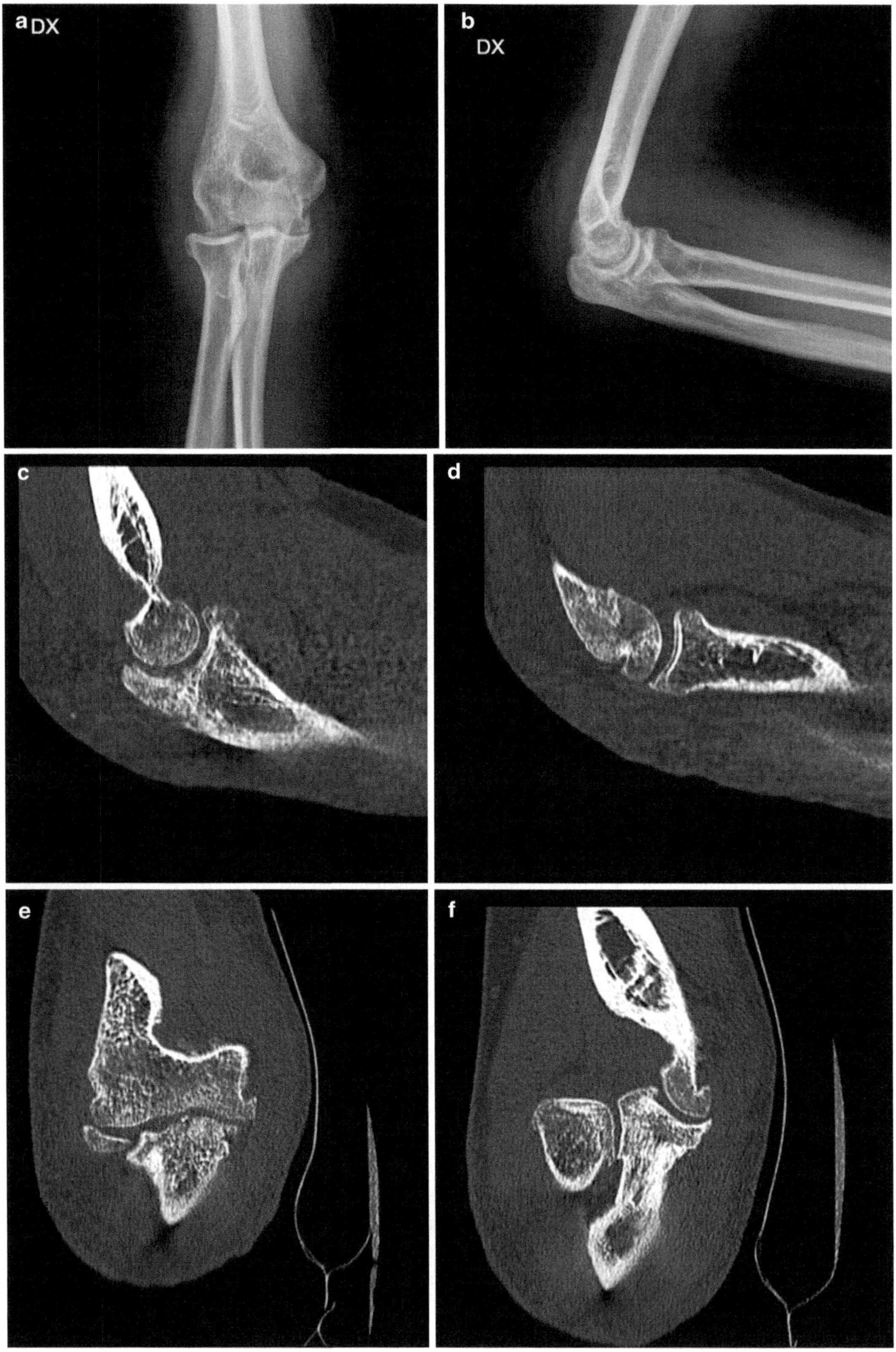

Fig. 9.1 Elbow AP (**a**) and LL (**b**) X-rays showing osteoarthritis features, like osteophytes formation, without extensive loss of joint space. CT scan images (**c–f**) in sagittal and coronal plane further show osteophytes present at both the radio-humeral and ulno-humeral interface

9.1.3 Rheumatoid Arthritis (RA)

Elbow stiffness affects 20–50% of patients with rheumatoid arthritis. Being RA is polyarticular symmetrical disease, elbow alone is involved in just 5% of cases. Its involvement is more frequently associated with the contralateral elbow, the adjacent shoulder (80% of cases), or the adjacent wrist (90%) [10].

RA starts from the synovium and then expands to the articular surfaces. As disease progresses, functional deterioration of the elbow joint occurs. Rheumatoid pannus, a typical feature of advanced disease, behaves as an erosive mass leading to progressive destruction of ligaments and bones, thereby causing joint instability, poor joint mechanics, and malalignment. Arthropathy is the last stage of disease. Therefore, by treating synovitis, either pharmacologically or surgically, physician can delay or prevent secondary joint damage [8].

Four RA types can be distinguished according to the type of damage that affects the elbow joint:

1. Classic soft tissue type: Characterized by synovial hypertrophy, increased joint laxity, malalignment, Z deformities, and instability
2. Osteoarthritic type: Characterized by stiff, hypertrophic joints, and preserved alignment
3. Nodular type: Characterized by subcutaneous nodules, which are partial sparing of tendons and bones
4. Mutilans type: Characterized by bone loss, joint destruction, and shortening

While X-ray and CT scan give the physician an idea of the degree of damage and ultrasound (US) is useful for evaluating enthesitis, the best imaging tool is MRI since it is superior in detecting inflammation at the bony attachment of tendons. Radiographic images are evaluated for joint space narrowing, osteophytes, heterotopic bone, bone quality, and deformities (Fig. 9.2). No radiographic classification exists. Extension and location of bony involvement in patients with heterotopic ossifications can be assessed through CT. Ligamentous integrity could be checked through MRI (Fig. 9.3). Finally, electrodiagnostic studies could be performed in case of nerve involvement [8].

Treatment in patients affected by RA is multidisciplinary and should be focused on pain relief rather than improvement in ROM. Involvement of adjacent joints and related disabilities should always be kept in mind in planning and deliver-

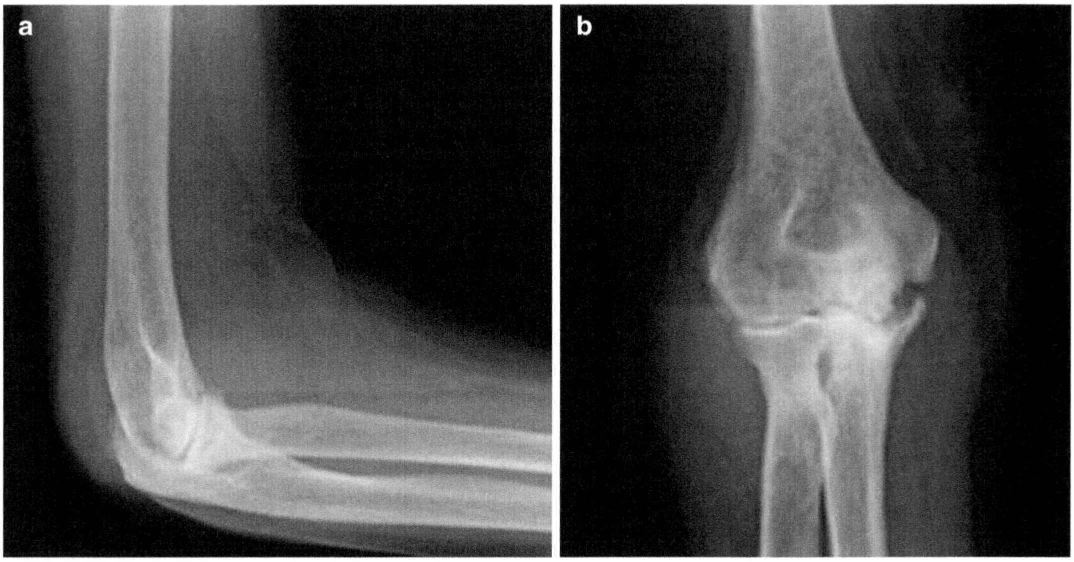

Fig. 9.2 X-rays of RA elbow (**a**) LL view and (**b**) AP view showing joint space narrowing and osteophytes formation

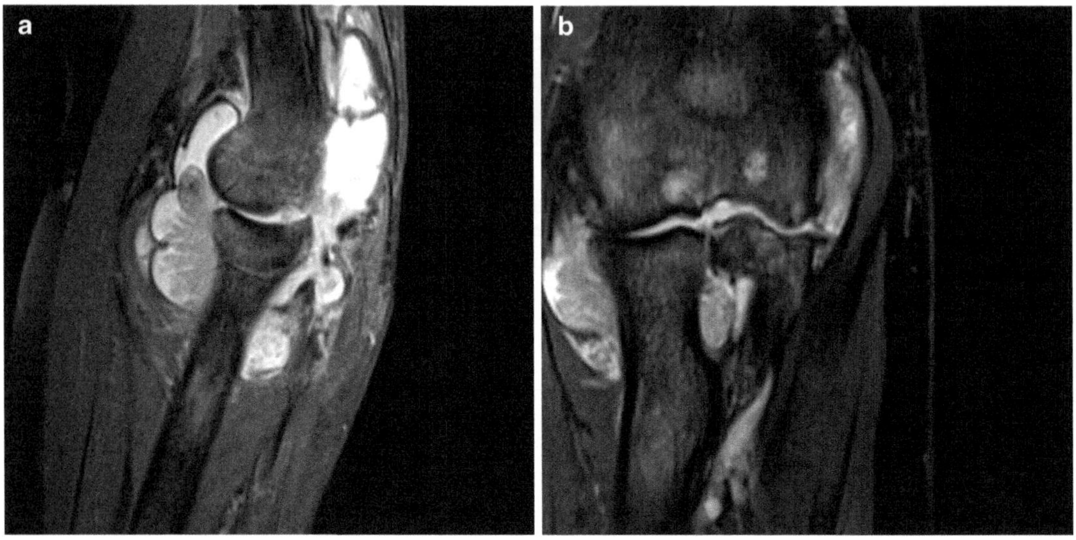

Fig. 9.3 MRI of RA elbow (**a**) sagittal view and (**b**) coronal view showing important synovitis and inflammation, loss of joint space and osteophytes formation

ing a comprehensive treatment. Moreover, prolonged synovitis and use of corticosteroids are involved too in the decision-making of the management plan. Anyhow, range of flexion should be restored as much as possible so to allow patients to perform activities of daily living, such as washing their face and feeding themselves.

With improvement in pharmacological approaches to this condition, the number of patients requiring surgery is decreasing. Anyway, when surgery is needed, biologic agents should be withheld for at least twice their half-lives before and after surgery to decrease the risk of peri-operative infection, whereas MTX can be continued, since no side effects have been witnessed.

Open or arthroscopic synovectomy has shown satisfactory results both in early and advanced phases of the disease. It remains controversial if ulnar nerve should be left in situ or transposed. The ulnar nerve can suffer either pre-operatively due to fixed flexion contracture, but also intra-operatively or post-operatively due to soft tissue fibrosis [8].

Capitellectomy can be performed when the proximal radio-ulnar joint is affected. This procedure increases only ROM without impacting on painful symptomatology. For this reason, it is often associated with open or arthroscopic synovectomy, yielding overall good clinical results. In case of severe, erosive, rheumatoid elbow, non-responding to pharmacological treatment, elbow arthroplasty is a valid option. Elbow arthrodesis, instead, should be taken into consideration only in case of chronic infections, failed arthroplasty, or severe bone loss. Luckily, the number of patients requiring total elbow replacement is decreasing due to better medical management. Linked total elbow replacement is the preferred choice, since it does not require a competent soft tissue envelope and it provides a painless yet functional elbow.

Complications in total elbow arthroplasty exist and are usually related to wound healing problems, infections, and periprosthetic fractures (due to the osteopenic and fragile bone of RA patients). Unfortunately, risk of infection in RA patients remains high, up to 6%, and consequences may be devastating, from clinical worsening to high mortality rate (2.7–18% according to literature). Interpositional arthroplasty has a limited role in these patients. Indeed, it provides good pain relief, but bony destruction often keeps progressing, making a future elbow arthroplasty revision much more difficult to perform.

Rheumatoid nodules are often found at the elbow joint. They are often signs of systemic disease and should be excised. Rheumatoid bursitis, which often involves the olecranon bursa, should be treated with aspiration and steroid injections.

9.1.4 Psoriatic Arthritis (PsA)

About 25% of patients with psoriasis develop psoriatic arthritis. Enthesitis, dactylitis, and presence of skin plaques are hallmarks of this disease. Indeed, skin involvement is present in most patients. PsA is most of the times a polyarticular symmetric condition; however, monoarticular, oligoarticular, or rheumatoid-like pattern of disease also exists. Synovitis is considered secondary to extra-capsular disease. Common features of PsA are preserved bone stock, paramarginal erosions, osteolysis, periostitis, and periarticular new bone. Enthesitis at the elbow joint is common. Surgeons should be careful and decide upon operative treatment when skin disease is stable or in remission. Moreover, surgery can lead to the development of psoriatic plaques in unaffected skin due to the Koebner phenomenon could lead to the development of psoriatic plaques in unaffected skin [10, 11].

9.1.5 Gout

Gout at the elbow joint can present either as olecranon bursitis, more typically, or as a painful and destructive mono-arthropathy. In the latter case, differential diagnosis with septic arthritis is mandatory, though early joint aspiration. Uric acid crystals are the hallmarks of gout and lead to easy identification of the condition. Recent researches [12] showed that hyperuricemia is a risk factor for poor performance and post-operative pain and stiffness in patients undergone elbow arthrolysis.

9.1.6 Systemic Lupus Erythematous (SLE)

SLE is a chronic autoimmune disease which affects peripheral joints, in particular the hands and feet. Articular involvement, even if common, is often transient and reversible, deforming and non-erosive (which helps with the differential diagnosis with RA). Jaccoud arthropathy, instead, has features in between SLE and RA, being an erosive symmetrical polyarthritis, with SLE like features. For this reason, it has also been addressed as Rhupus syndrome.

9.1.7 Septic Arthritis

Septic elbow arthritis is a rare but serious and dangerous condition, which can affect both children and adults and can lead to the development of fulminant sepsis leading to high mortality rates. Infections can occur either through the hematogenous route, by continuous spreading or by direct inoculation after elbow trauma. Open and arthroscopic elbow surgery puts patients at higher risk, together with concomitant disease, immunocompromised state, and advanced age. Prompt treatment and proper antibiotic therapy are essential for these patients. Stiffness, along with pain, edema, and erythema are classical signs which should alert the physician. Diagnosis is based on clinical symptoms and confirmed by laboratory findings. ESR, C-reactive protein (CRP), and white blood cell (WBC) counts are sensible, but not specific markers. Synovial fluid markers have a much better sensitivity for infection, especially WBC count. CT and MRI are the best imaging techniques to highlight bone and soft tissue infections. X-rays and US are readily available tools and are useful for early identification of soft tissue effusion and osteomyelitis but have low sensitivity. MRI is especially indicated when osteomyelitis is suspected.

Treatment of these patients relies on surgery, antibiotics, and elbow immobilization. Surgery should not be delayed in case MRI is not readily accessible. The lateral approach to the elbow joint allows direct control of the joint after debridement and synovial excision. Copious irrigation is key for the management of this condition. Arthroscopic drainage has shown promising results, especially when promptly carried out (within 2 days) and in the absence of prior elbow complaints [13].

Cultures should be made intra-operatively for pathogen identification. The most reported pathogen is *Staphylococcus aureus*, even though Gram-negative bacteria have also been isolated. Moreover, *methicillin-resistant Staphylococcus aureus* (MRSA) incidence is increasing.

Empirical antibiotic therapy, with anti-staphylococcal agents, should be started as soon as possible, after surgery, and tailored later based on the pathogen identified and antibiogram sensitivity. Antibiotic treatment should be continued until normalization of biological inflammatory markers and clinical evaluation, usually up to 6 to 12 weeks (about 3 months). The elbow joint should not be kept in cast for too long to avoid post-operative elbow stiffness and to rapidly improve ROM.

Functional outcome after a well-performed treatment is satisfactory. Stiffness is the most common reported complication due to the expanded fibrosis of the synovial membrane and capsular joint. Rehabilitation and physiotherapy are mandatory and should be started early on. Luckily, joint destruction occurs only in case of delayed and inadequate treatment of the infection. In children, growth plates are rarely affected, thereby growth disturbances and malalignment are rare, in contrast to osteomyelitis [14].

9.1.8 Hemophilia

Hemophilia is an X-linked condition characterized by deficiency or functional defect of coagulation factors VIII or IX, resulting in an increased bleeding tendency. Recurrent intra-articular bleeding is a hallmark of severe hemophilia. The elbow joint is the second most common site of arthropathy in hemophiliac patients, after the knee joint. Anyhow, it is still not yet known how many episodes of intra-articular bleeding are required to start an irreversible damage to the articular cartilage. Bleeding into the joint leads on one hand to hemosiderin accumulation within synovial macrophages, causing hypertrophic synovitis, and on the other hand, it directly affects cartilage metabolism, favoring cartilage destruction. Stiffness of the elbow joint is the direct consequence of chronic hypertrophic synovitis, where the synovium is replaced by dense scar tissue, resulting in severe contracture of the joint. Moreover, the abnormal synovium can act like an AV fistula, producing excessive blood supply to the epiphyseal plates of children, resulting in angular deformities [15].

Radiological assessment can guide the physician to identify the severity of the condition. Different classifications of hemophiliac arthropathy have been proposed. Patterson et al. classify the conditions based on eight radiological parameters: osteoporosis, hypertrophy of the end plate, loss of joint space, irregular subchondral surface, subchondral cysts, erosion of the joint surfaces, and deformity of the joint. Moreover, three different radiological patterns have been described:

1. Predominantly medial component with humeral-ulnar involvement
2. Characterized by medial spur formation, joint narrowing, and subperiosteal new bone formation
3. Predominantly lateral component with radial head enlargement and subperiosteal new bone formation of the lateral supracondylar ridge of the humerus
4. Medial and lateral component with generalized osteophytes, reduction in joint space, and subchondral cysts

In the first group, ulnar nerve involvement is more common; in the second group posterolateral joint pain and stiffness are the most common clinical findings, whereas in the third group stiffness was the main finding.

Medical treatment requires correction of the defect by replacement through factor concentrates, plasma and platelets. When hemophiliac arthropathy develops, treatment goals are symptoms alleviation, prevention of articular destruction, and ROM preservation. In acute setting, anti-inflammatory drugs and factor replacement is key. In case of tense and painful hemarthrosis, arthrocentesis could be useful under factor replacement cover. Synoviorthesis, meaning the injection within the joint of pharmacological agents, (radioactive gold, yttrium-90, phosphorus-32 rifampin, osmic acid, and hyaluronic acid) prevents the onset of arthropathy by decreasing the frequency and recurrence of intra-articular bleeding. This procedure should be considered after a 3-month period in which factor replacement and physiotherapy do not control synovitis.

When conservative treatment fails, many surgical options exist, from synovectomy to resection of the radial head, excision arthroplasty, arthrodesis, interposition arthroplasty, and total elbow replacement.

9.2 Extrinsic Causes

9.2.1 Heterotopic Ossifications

Heterotopic ossifications are the most common extrinsic cause of elbow contracture, leading to elbow stiffness and eventually complete bony ankylosis. They are associated with direct trauma, central nervous system trauma and thermal burns. They are usually a result of local or systemic insult, which lead to the deposition of mature lamellar bone into extraosseous soft tissue. Small heterotopic elbow ossifications can follow a self-limited course, without long-term symptoms or impairment; on the contrary, extensive ossifications may lead to clinically important contractures and ankylosis. In the latter case, surgery can be an option to relieve patient's symptomatology.

Conservative treatment consists of physical therapy, anti-inflammatory medications and manipulation under anesthesia. Nonsteroidal anti-inflammatory drugs (NSAIDs), such as indomethacin, could be used as prophylactic to prevent heterotopic ossifications by inhibiting the osteogenic differentiation of progenitor cells. These measures, however, have limited effects.

Surgical treatments include contracture release, excision of formations, radiation therapy, and botulinum toxin injections [16, 17].

9.2.2 Post-burn Contractures

Thermal injuries to both superficial and deep tissues are often associated with the development of post-burn contractures. Upper limbs more commonly develop post-burn contractures. The shoulder is the most involved joint followed by the elbow. These contractures usually result in structural deformities, joint movement restriction and thereby in disability. When the elbow joint is affected, heterotopic ossifications often worsen the clinical picture of these patients. Unfortunately, non-operative treatment does not seem to be enough to allow these patients to recover a satisfactory ROM, especially in the acute setting. Instead, surgery, aimed at releasing and excising all the pathologic anatomical structures limiting elbow motion, can result in substantial improvement in elbow movement and return to daily life activities. Recurrence of contracture has been shown to be associated with long-standing contracture, flame burn, and incomplete contracture release. Peri-operative radiation therapy may be useful to decrease the risk of HO recurrence and thereby post-operative elbow stiffness and pain [18–20].

References

1. Søjbjerg JO. The stiff elbow. Acta Orthop Scand. 1996;67(6):626–31. https://doi.org/10.3109/17453679608997771.
2. Nandi S, Maschke S, Evans PJ, Lawton JN. The stiff elbow. Hand (N Y). 2009;4(4):368–79. https://doi.org/10.1007/s11552-009-9181-z.
3. Evans PJ, Nandi S, Maschke S, Hoyen HA, Lawton JN. Prevention and treatment of elbow stiffness. J Hand Surg Am. 2009;34(4):769–78. https://doi.org/10.1016/j.jhsa.2009.02.020.
4. Kay NR. Arthrolysis of the post-traumatic stiff elbow. In: Stanley D, Kay N ed. Surgery of the elbow. London: Arnold, 1998:228-234.
5. Morrey BF. The posttraumatic stiff elbow. Clin Orthop. 2005;431:26–35.
6. Pizzetti M, Fredella D, Erriquez A. Post-traumatic elbow stiffness. Curr Concepts Orthop Surg. 1991;2:195–9. https://doi.org/10.1007/978-3-7091-4127-4_23.
7. Sun Z, Fan C. Validation of the Liverpool Elbow Score for evaluation of elbow stiffness. BMC Musculoskelet

Disord. 2018;19(1):302. https://doi.org/10.1186/s12891-018-2226-0.

8. Gallo RA, Payatakes A, Sotereanos DG. Surgical options for the arthritic elbow. J Hand Surg Am. 2008;33(5):746–59. https://doi.org/10.1016/j.jhsa.2007.12.022.
9. Gramstad GD, Galatz LM. Management of elbow osteoarthritis. J Bone Joint Surg Am. 2006;88(2):421–30. https://doi.org/10.2106/JBJS.E.00568.
10. Dott C, Chin K, Compson J. Inflammatory arthritis and the elbow surgeon. J Clin Orthop Trauma. 2021;20:101492. https://doi.org/10.1016/j.jcot.2021.101492.
11. Conaghan PG, Coates LC. Improving recognition of psoriatic arthritis. Practitioner. 2009;253(1724):15–8.
12. Xiong H, Sun Z, Chen S, Liu W, Peng S, Wang W, Fan C. Effect of hyperuricemia on functional outcomes and complications in patients with elbow stiffness after open arthrolysis combined with hinged external fixation: a retrospective study. J Shoulder Elb Surg. 2020;29(7):1387–93. https://doi.org/10.1016/j.jse.2020.02.021.
13. Van den Ende KI, Steinmann SP. Arthroscopic treatment of septic arthritis of the elbow. J Shoulder Elb Surg. 2012;21(8):1001–5. https://doi.org/10.1016/j.jse.2011.07.019.
14. Kaziz H, Triki MA, Mouelhi T, Bouattour K, Naouar N, Ben Ayeche ML. Septic elbow arthritis in children: epidemiology and outcome. Arch Pediatr. 2019;26(1):38–43. https://doi.org/10.1016/j.arcped.2018.11.001.
15. Utukuri MM, Goddard NJ. Haemophilic arthropathy of the elbow. Haemophilia. 2005;11(6):565–70. https://doi.org/10.1111/j.1365-2516.2005.01146.x.
16. Salazar D, Golz A, Israel H, Marra G. Heterotopic ossification of the elbow treated with surgical resection: risk factors, bony ankylosis, and complications. Clin Orthop Relat Res. 2014;472(7):2269–75. https://doi.org/10.1007/s11999-014-3591-0.
17. Freibott CE, Bäcker HC, Shoap SC, Tedesco LJ, Galle SE, Rosenwasser MP. Treatment methods for post-traumatic elbow stiffness caused by heterotopic ossification. J Shoulder Elb Surg. 2020;29(7):1380–6. https://doi.org/10.1016/j.jse.2020.02.026.
18. Manske MC, Hanel DP. Postburn contractures of the elbow and heterotopic ossification. Hand Clin. 2017;33(2):375–88. https://doi.org/10.1016/j.hcl.2016.12.014.
19. Maender C, Sahajpal D, Wright TW. Treatment of heterotopic ossification of the elbow following burn injury: recommendations for surgical excision and perioperative prophylaxis using radiation therapy. J Shoulder Elb Surg. 2010;19(8):1269–75. https://doi.org/10.1016/j.jse.2010.05.029.
20. Balumuka DD, Galiwango GW, Alenyo R. Recurrence of post burn contractures of the elbow and shoulder joints: experience from a Ugandan hospital. BMC Surg. 2015;9(15):103. https://doi.org/10.1186/s12893-015-0089-y.

Part II

Elbow: Pre-operative Planning

Elbow Stiffness: Preoperative Planning (Considerations on Soft Tissues and Bone)

10

Giuseppe Giannicola, Sebastien Prigent, Andrea Amura, and Pasquale Sessa

10.1 Introduction

The surgical treatment of the stiff elbow is a challenging condition that may lead to unsatisfactory clinical results and complications, even when performed by expert elbow surgeons. For this reason, accurate pre-operative planning may be considered more important for this condition than for other types of elbow surgery. In order to properly address the causes of elbow stiffness, a systematic examination of the elbow is mandatory: this allows the surgeon to evaluate the components (soft tissues, bone, or both) that are potentially responsible for the stiffness. This evaluation should always be conducted by considering general factors such as age, functional demands, comorbidities, expectations, and the time of onset of stiffness. A proper imaging study protocol, alongside an accurate clinical evaluation, is the starting point for the surgical planning: a varying combination of different imaging techniques allows a comprehensive understanding of the pathology.

G. Giannicola (✉) · S. Prigent · A. Amura
Department of Anatomical, Histological, Forensic Medicine and Orthopedics Sciences, "Sapienza" University of Rome–Policlinico Umberto I, Rome, Italy

P. Sessa
Department of Orthopedics and Traumatology, Azienda Ospedaliera San Camillo-Forlanini, Rome, Italy

In this chapter, for the sake of clarity, an introductory section on imaging techniques is followed by a separate discussion of bone and soft tissue disorders that may contribute to elbow stiffness. It should be borne in mind that soft tissue and bone disorders are generally not isolated: these two conditions are often encountered in a varying combination in clinical practice. In most cases of elbow stiffness, a custom surgical strategy is required.

10.2 General Considerations

10.2.1 Patient History

The first step in the treatment of elbow stiffness consists in collecting data on the patients' personal medical history. It is essential to distinguish between congenital or acquired causes of elbow stiffness since the treatment strategies may be different.

Congenital causes of elbow stiffness are less frequent and generally encompass a wide spectrum of malformations of the distal humerus or proximal radius and ulna (or both), either as isolated entities or in association with specific syndromes caused by genetic disorders [1]. In the latter case, the concomitant involvement of nervous or vascular structures is frequent and should be considered in the pre-operative planning. Acquired causes of elbow stiffness are instead

L. Pederzini et al. (eds.), *Stiffness of the Elbow, Wrist and Related Pathologies*,
https://doi.org/10.1007/978-3-031-81381-8_10

generally related to a previous traumatic event (post-traumatic elbow stiffness) or degenerative and inflammatory diseases.

When dealing with patients with post-traumatic stiffness, the following points should be addressed.

1. **The initial trauma:** It is important to collect all the data available on the initial elbow injury, including initial imaging (X-rays, computed tomography (CT), and magnetic resonance imaging (MRI)). The classification of the original injury pattern allows the surgeon to better understand which elbow structures were originally involved and what role they play in the current stiffness: a simple elbow dislocation that evolves into stiffness is substantially different from a fracture-dislocation of the elbow in which bony structures were initially involved.
2. **The initial medical or surgical treatment or non-treatment:** Although untreated elbow injuries are typical of third-world countries, the rare cases in which they are still encountered in developed countries are observed mainly in rural areas or in elderly patients seeking medical advice a long time after the injury. Since these conditions were not diagnosed in the acute setting and were left untreated, a thorough imaging and clinical examination should be performed in the chronic setting. Untreated fractures with malunion or nonunion are the most common conditions: the distal humerus, the proximal radius or proximal ulna, or a combination of these, might be involved.

   When considering an injury that was initially treated conservatively, it is important to ascertain whether a cast or splint immobilization was used and, if so, for how long. In patients treated with splints, it is useful to find out whether range of motion (ROM) was allowed from the beginning or only in the final phase of treatment; other important aspects that must be investigated are whether the patient received any physical therapy and, if so, the type and duration of physical therapy. Excessively long immobilization (>3 weeks) or aggressive physical therapy might be a cause of post-traumatic elbow stiffness.

   In patients who have already undergone previous surgical treatments, several points should be considered. The time elapsed from trauma to surgery is a key point as treatments in the subacute or chronic setting yield a higher risk of complications (such as heterotopic ossifications) and unsatisfactory results. The surgical report should be carefully examined to understand what surgical approach was performed, the type of fixation devices or arthroplasty that were implanted (Fig. 10.1), how the soft tissues (ligaments and capsule) were managed, and whether the ulnar nerve was isolated or transposed. The surgeon should investigate complications that might have occurred during the postoperative period, such as delayed wound healing or infection, persistent postoperative fever, prolonged use of antibiotics, and history of delayed union or nonunion that might have extended the duration of immobilization.
3. **Time since the onset of stiffness:** The timing of the patient's presentation is a pivotal point in the choice of treatment in elbow stiffness. According to the current literature [2], no surgery is required in most cases of extrinsic stiffness before 6–12 months have elapsed since the original trauma or treatment because physical therapy with dedicated protocols and skilled physical therapists may still be able to play a role up to then. In such patients, it is important to monitor improvements in elbow ROM at 45- to 60-day intervals. In our opinion, when a correct rehabilitation protocol is being applied, the lack of significant improvements in a 2-month interval may represent a turning point in the treatment strategy regardless of the time elapsed since the initial injury.

   In case of stiffness dating from a long time before, such as in the sequelae of a pediatric injury, particular attention should be paid to the evaluation of the secondary anatomical degenerative modifications, including dysmorphisms of the radial head, trochlear notch, and distal humerus. In such patients, it is very important

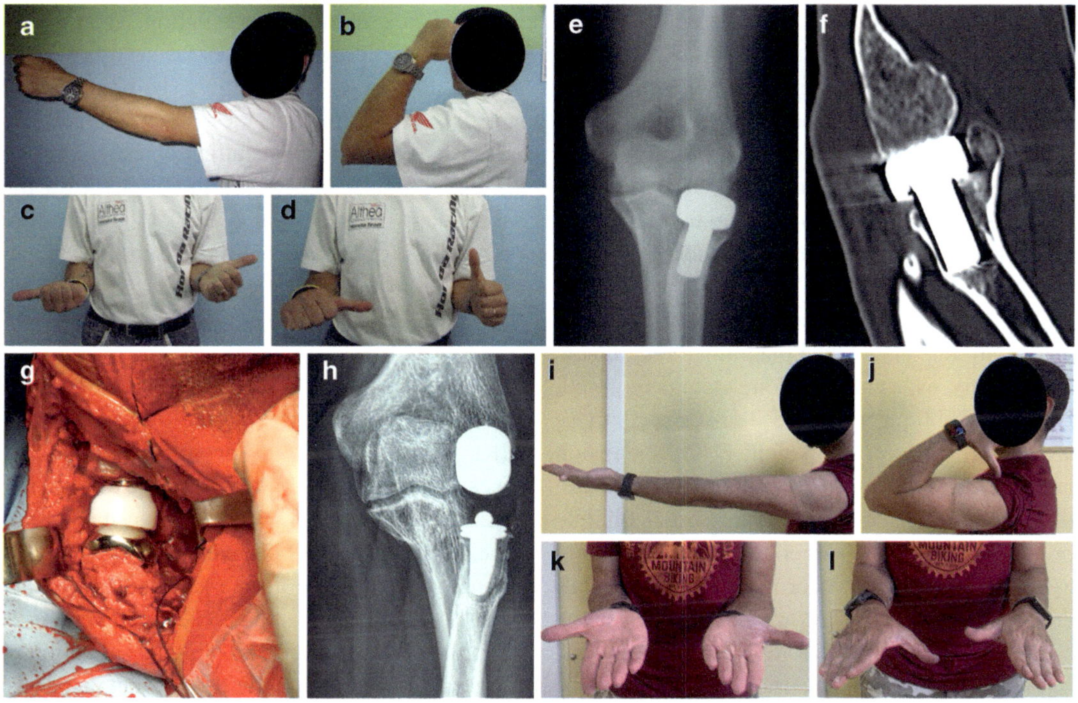

Fig. 10.1 Clinical case of a patient affected by elbow stiffness and pain, previously treated for a fracture of the radial head. A monobloc loose-fit radial head arthroplasty was implanted. Preoperative range of motion in extension (**a**), flexion (**b**), supination (**c**), and pronation (**d**). Preoperative X-rays (**e**) showing overstuffing of the radial head prosthesis: the height of the implant exceeds that of the radial notch, and a lateral widening of the joint space is visible in the ulno-humeral joint. CT scan (**f**) demonstrating overstuffing of the radial head prosthesis and degeneration of the articular surface of the humeral capitellum. An open-release procedure and a radio-capitellar arthroplasty were performed (**g**). Postoperative X-rays show the restoration of radial length and joint alignment (**h**). Clinical results in extension (**i**), flexion (**j**), supination (**k**) and pronation (**l**)

to properly assess the muscular and tendinous structures separately from the bony structures, since any fibrosis makes the surgical results very unpredictable, as has been observed in the sequelae of stiffness due to obstetric paralysis [3]. In cases of stiffness secondary to intra-articular malunions, the time interval between trauma and surgery significantly affects the possibility of performing a corrective osteotomy. In chronic instabilities, degenerative changes in the articular surface require prosthetic replacement after 6–9 months [4]. In patients affected by inflammatory diseases, it is fundamental to consult a rheumatologist to understand when the specific medical therapy is no longer able to control the disease, particularly with regard to pain relief and the progression of articular surface degeneration.

10.3 Imaging

As in all elbow disorders, an in-depth imaging study is required to correctly identify the type of stiffness.

10.3.1 X-Rays

Plain X-rays of the elbow are the typical initial evaluation tool. Conventional anteroposterior (AP) and lateral views of the elbow should be performed; in case of severe lack of extension, a double AP of the elbow should be performed: one perpendicular to the distal humerus (to assess distal humerus morphology) and one perpendicular to the forearm (to visualize the joint lines and evaluate congruency). If such views are not possible due to severe flexion contracture, a CT examination is required. In rotational stiffness, the AP view in full pronation, full supination, and neutral rotation should be obtained to evaluate the radial head morphology. The lateral view of the elbow should be performed at 90° to the distal humerus; this view is fundamental to rule out joint incongruency such as that observed in posterolateral instability and radial drift; moreover, proper distal bowing of the humerus can be evaluated with this view when planning a total elbow arthroplasty, especially if a long stem is required. Additional oblique views (45°) can be used: these are performed with the patient in full extension and forearm rotation in pronation (medial side) or supination (lateral side). The medial oblique projection allows the surgeon to more accurately assess the trochlea and coronoid profile; the lateral oblique projection allows a better view of the radio-capitellar joint. These additional oblique X-ray projections are now used less following the introduction of high-resolution computed tomography (CT).

10.3.2 CT

The CT scan is the most efficient and accurate technique for surgical planning, with its superiority over plain X-rays in identifying causes of elbow stiffness being widely recognized [5, 6]. CT scans should be performed with a maximum 0.6 mm slice thickness and with 2D and 3D reconstructions. Osteophytes, heterotopic ossifications (HO), dystrophic calcifications, articular bone erosion, subchondral cysts, free intra-articular osteochondral bodies, and loose fragments can easily be assessed by performing a CT scan. A CT scan with contrast enhancement or CT angiography can be used, respectively, in infections and as a means of evaluating the relationships with vascular structures, and thus choose the safest surgical approach.

CT scans are also required to assess articular nonunions and bone deformities such as malunions of the intra- or extra-articular portions of the distal humerus and proximal radius and ulna: the relative deformity axes can be drawn and computed by rendering simulation. When osteotomies are needed in cases of complex malunions, the CT examination of the contralateral side is required to plan the osteotomy, particularly when custom-made cutting jigs are required. CT arthrography is believed to be useful for the assessment of non-ossified intra-articular loose bodies and for the evaluation of capsular retraction and thickening [7].

10.3.3 MRI

MRI generally plays a secondary role in the assessment of elbow stiffness [8]. Soft-tissue assessment, especially in cases of capsular and/or ligament thickening, can reveal a low signal intensity (e.g., in both T1- and T2-weighted images). Intra-articular adherences can be seen as tissue bands connecting the joint capsule to osseous structures if enough fluid is present inside the joint. Fibrotic changes of the fat pads can be seen in non-fat saturated T1-weighted sequences. MRI is also useful if synovitis, ligament and tendon injuries, or neuropathies are associated with stiffness [9]. Benign or malignant soft tissue tumors can be evaluated through an MRI with or without contrast enhancement [10]. In patients with synovial chondromatosis or other forms of aggressive synovitis, the MRI might play a role alongside PET. An MRI with contrast enhancement may be performed in patients with suspect elbow joint infection or when a close relationship of vascular and neural structures with bony spurs or ossification needs to be investigated.

10.3.4 Scintigraphy

The scintigraphy with marked autologous leucocytes is indicated to rule out infections, especially in unclear cases or in subclinical presentations, and when metal devices have been previously implanted (plates, arthroplasties). As the results of this examination may be affected by other types of inflammatory conditions, the scintigraphy should be performed after a reasonable time interval from any other surgical procedure (at least 6 months). The three-phase bone scintigraphy with technetium may be useful to evaluate osseointegration and the loosening of arthroplasty components.

10.4 Patient Considerations

10.4.1 The Patient's Expectations

The patient's hand dominance, work activities, recreational vocations and, above all, expectations should be carefully and extensively discussed when considering surgical treatment for elbow stiffness. Most minor limitations in ROM may be irrelevant or have an acceptable impact on daily living activities; on the other hand, in certain patients with specific requirements, even small articular restrictions may be of paramount importance: this is the case, for example, for soldiers and police officers who require complete elbow extension to be able to use firearms. Some athletes also need a complete ROM to perform sport-specific activities. It should be remembered that rotational stiffness with lack of supination is tolerated to a far lesser extent than loss of pronation since compensatory movements of the shoulder are ineffective in the former. The patient's expectations in terms of pain resolution are even more closely related to final satisfaction and quality of life [11]. Since elbow surgery for the treatment of stiffness does not come without complications and the results might be uncertain in some cases, indications should be accurately tailored according to the patient's real needs and expectations. It is necessary to explain to patients that the surgical procedure may not fully match their expectations.

10.4.2 Skin

The physical examination of a patient affected by elbow stiffness starts with the observation of the skin layer. Scars from previous surgical interventions should be noted (site, length, trophism). Surgical incisions should be planned according to the quality of the skin, the local blood supply, and the previous surgical scars. Potential avascular flaps deriving from poorly planned surgical incisions should be avoided, considering the very thin soft-tissue layer that surrounds the joint.

The presence of fistulae or local signs of past or current infection should be ruled out. Indeed, subclinical presentations of articular infection may be the cause of elbow pain and stiffness: for this reason, laboratory examinations and appropriate imaging (CT, MRI, bone scintigraphy with autologous marked leucocytes) should be performed to rule out infection, as should a consultation with an infectious diseases physician if a substantial suspicion exists. In cases of strong clinical suspicion in which a conclusive diagnosis is difficult to obtain, an articular biopsy should be planned before more invasive surgical approaches are performed.

Skin burns and consequent contractures are one of the most evident causes of elbow stiffness: the number, location, and extension of skin contractures should be noted. A consultation with a plastic surgeon is mandatory to define the most appropriate surgical strategy, which may involve skin flaps or other reconstructive techniques to avoid skin damage during surgical manipulation of the elbow and to guarantee adequate soft-tissue coverage at the end of the procedure.

10.4.3 Elbow Range of Motion

A clinical examination of the elbow should be conducted in order to define the planes and the severity of stiffness. Elbow stiffness may involve the flexion-extension arc, the pronation-supination axis, or both (combined elbow stiffness). Both values should be measured and reported in the patient's clinical data. Moreover, they should be used as a basis for a thorough discussion with the patient on their expectations following surgery, in particular with regard to the degree of elbow motion that may be obtained with the surgical procedure. In cases of combined involvement, the severity of stiffness on the two motion planes may differ: in such circumstances, the surgeon should discuss the possibility of addressing the stiffness on either just one or both planes, depending on the patient's individual requirements. A comparison with the non-involved side in each patient may prove useful to evaluate what the normal ROM is, since variability in maximum flexion and extension has been reported in different individuals: it ranges from −30° to 10° for extension and 130° to 160° for flexion, and depends above all on age and sex; similarly, significant differences may be found between individuals in the rotatory plane of the forearm [12, 13]. Minor stiffness patterns may not benefit from surgical interventions since elbow stiffness is expected to relapse by a certain degree after the surgical procedure. During the physical examination, the presence or absence of a firm mechanical stop at terminal degrees of motion should be noted: patients with elastic tissues might still benefit from physical therapy. Crepitus during the arc of motion may point to the presence of arthritis, synovitis, nonunion, or fracture.

10.4.4 Neurological Examination

A thorough and accurate neurological examination is mandatory in order to exclude both sensory and motor neurological defects of the ulnar, median, or radial nerves. Ulnar neuropathy is often associated with elbow trauma, degenerative diseases, and surgical procedures [14].

The position of the ulnar nerve should always be determined (in situ vs. transposed) in patients that have undergone previous surgical procedures in order to plan the correct approach. If a neurolysis or an anterior transposition has previously been performed, signs and symptoms of ulnar neuritis should be ruled out or noted, if present. It should be borne in mind that perineural scars that limit nerve gliding or stretching may cause the onset of neurological symptoms when procedures aimed at increasing elbow range of motion are performed: the release of the ulnar nerve should be considered a routine procedure in elbow stiffness treatment, with some authors advocating a routine prophylactic transposition of the ulnar nerve, even in mild forms of elbow stiffness characterized by a limitation only in the final degrees of extension [14, 15]. The median and radial nerves are less commonly involved in the pathoanatomy of elbow stiffness and are not routinely addressed; however, if symptoms are present, neurolysis should also be performed [14]. In particular, the relationships between the radial and median nerves and large ossifications should be carefully evaluated.

Appropriate clinical tests for both sensory and motor functions should be performed. Diagnostic tests such as electroneuromyography, nerve conduction studies, or static and dynamic ultrasonography should be considered in order to objectively quantify the potential deficits and to avoid legal claims [16]. Moreover, the neurological examination should always be integrated with diagnostic imaging (CT or MRI with contrast enhancement, dynamic ultrasonography): fibrous scars, compressions from improperly applied hardware or osteophytes and HO, as well as the location of the nerves in case of local anatomy deformities are of utmost importance when planning surgical debridement. A careful examination is also indispensable to be able to plan and obtain the surgical instruments needed to decompress neurological structures that are circumferentially surrounded by HO.

10.5 Bone Considerations

10.5.1 Malunion

Malunions of the proximal ulna, proximal radius, or distal humerus are all possible causes of elbow stiffness due to mechanical limitations in ROM. Surgical technical errors or lack of accuracy in the reduction of fractures are the main reasons for malunions.

10.5.1.1 Proximal Ulna Malunions

The normal anatomy of the proximal ulna features a dorsal bow (proximal ulna dorsal angulation, PUDA) ranging from 0° to 14° [17, 18], with the apex being located on average 47 mm distal to the tip of the olecranon. The PUDA, which has been observed in 96% of the population, is symmetrical. According to several authors, it plays a substantial role in ulnar malunions [17, 19–21] and, consequently, in radial head subluxations resulting from proximal ulnar malunion greater than 5° [19]. The proximal ulnar varus angle (on average 8° [17]) should also be taken into account when evaluating the sequelae of previous ulnar fractures.

An accurate evaluation of both standard X-rays, including those from the uninvolved side, and of CT examinations allows the surgeon to detect malunions of the proximal ulna and to plan adequate corrective osteotomies. Corrective osteotomies should address the deformity in all the planes involved: the basic rules for planning an ulnar osteotomy refer to the identification of the anatomical axes in the bone segment, defined as the line located at the center of the medullary canal, which is in turn defined by its inner borders. In case of deformity, the intersection of the axes defines the CORA (center of rotation of angulation), which is where an osteotomy should be performed. Closure or opening wedge osteotomies depend on the specific deformity pattern to be addressed. Rotational abnormalities on the axial plane and length defects or elongations should also be addressed. When the possibility of using bone grafts is being evaluated and an autologous graft is being considered, an accessory surgical field exposing the iliac crest or other bone donor sites should be prepared. Although the use of allografts avoids donor site morbidity, a lower osteoinductive and osteogenetic potential is to be expected if they are used.

The close relationship between the proximal ulna and radius must be underlined: sagittal malunions of the ulna with significant angulation, especially if combined with annular ligament insufficiency, are responsible for radial head subluxation and proximal radio-ulnar joint maltracking, as reported by Sandman et al. [19], with consequent elbow ROM limitation. Similarly, coronal plane deformities (varus or valgus) are related to rotational stiffness [22]. In particular, Snow et al. reported that varus deformities of the ulna mainly cause a loss of pronation whereas valgus deformities mainly cause a loss of supination.

10.5.1.2 Distal Humerus Malunions

Distal humerus malunions account for the 30% of all complications in the treatment of distal humerus fractures, especially when conservative management is adopted (Fig. 10.2).

The complex anatomy of this humeral portion is the main reason for the difficulties encountered in fracture reduction and proper fixation: it should be borne in mind that the distal humerus features several specific angles on the sagittal, coronal and axial planes: the main angles are (1) a mean 30°-40° of anterior angulation of the distal epiphysis in relation to the humeral shaft axis; (2) a mean "carrying angle" of 4°–7° on the coronal plane and (3) a mean 5°–7° of internal rotation of the articular spool in relation to the humeral shaft. These "normal values" should be restored when addressing distal humeral fractures.

Malunions may also affect the intra-articular portion of the humerus, resulting in improper tracking between the trochlea and the capitellum and the greater sigmoid notch and/or the radial head.

Intra-articular malunion of the distal humeral epiphysis with secondary deformity may be responsible for elbow pain, stiffness, ulnar nerve symptoms, and post-traumatic osteoarthritis due to joint maltracking [23]. Corrective osteotomies for intra-articular malunions should be considered in the case of preserved joint surfaces (Figs. 10.3, 10.4, and 10.5), while they are contraindicated in cases of articular loss or severe joint degeneration; in the latter cases, prosthetic replacement is necessary. As for all deformities, a CT scan with 3D reconstructions is mandatory to properly understand the deformity and plan the osteotomy with the correct degree of angular or rotational correction. General rules for deformity assessment, as previously reported, should be followed. Nowadays preformed cutting guides, based on CT reconstructions of the deformity, can easily be obtained and greatly improve the accuracy of correction; computer simulations of deformity correction may also prove useful as a means of assessing whether the planned osteotomy correction is appropriate.

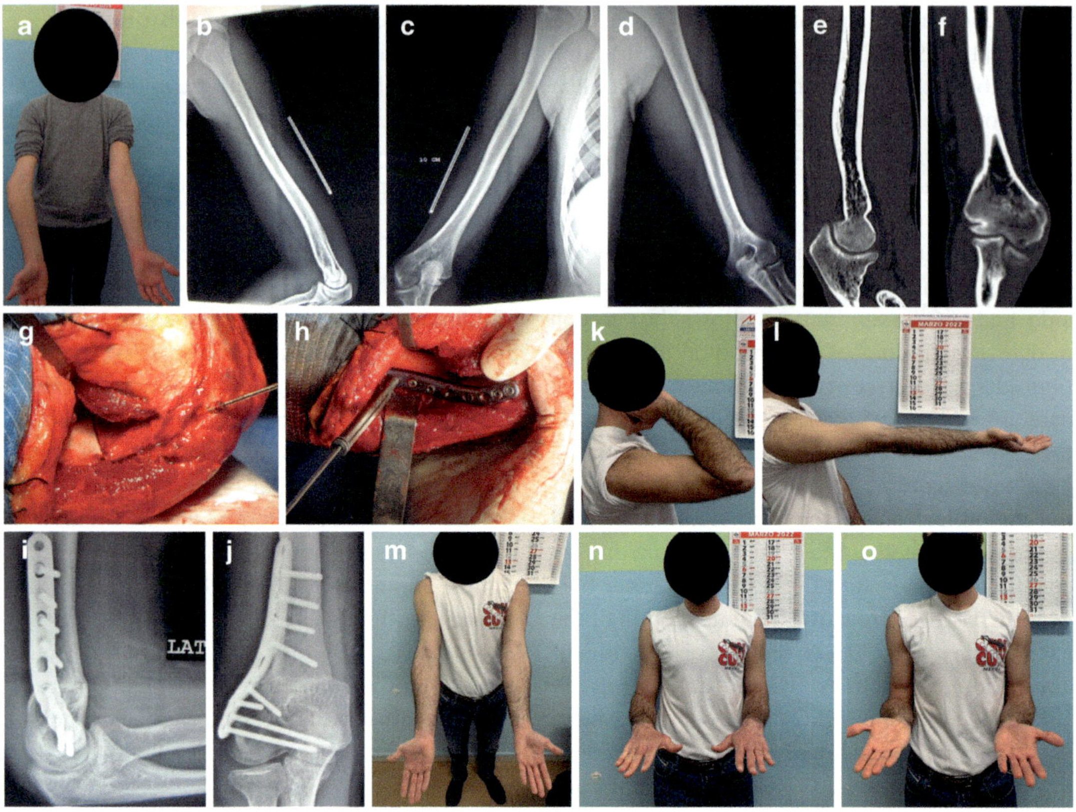

Fig. 10.2 Young patient with elbow stiffness and pain caused by severe post-traumatic varus deformity (**a**). Preoperative X-rays were performed with a metal landmark that allows to make measurements to accurately plan the corrective osteotomy (**b, c**). X-rays of the contralateral side are required to calculate the native axes of the patient's elbow (**d**). The CT scan allows to better investigate the deformity, to assess the degree of joint surfaces degeneration and investigate other possible causes of stiffness (**e, f**). The correction of the deformity was performed through a lateral wedge osteotomy of the humeral metaphysis (**g**). Fixation with a precontoured lateral locking plate (**h**). Postoperative X-rays (**i, l**) and clinical results (**k–o**) after 6 years

10.5.1.3 Proximal Radius Malunions

The proximal radius may, owing to its intrinsic anatomical variability [24], be prone to malunions, especially when fixation is performed with anatomical pre-contoured plates that do not match the patient's individual anatomy. A deformity of the radial head may cause rotational stiffness and pain (Fig. 10.6). Intra-articular or extra-articular osteotomies can be planned by using 3D reconstructions and patient-tailored preformed cut jigs; alternatively, an RHA can be performed if technically feasible and if radial drift is absent. If an RHA is not possible, the only alternative solution might be the excision of the radial head, which must be preceded by an accurate evaluation of the longitudinal stability of the forearm.

10.5.2 Nonunion

Nonunions of the distal humerus, proximal ulna, or radius can cause or be associated with elbow stiffness (Fig. 10.7). Nonunions can be located at an extra-articular or intra-articular site and may determine stiffness when associated with significant deformity or joint incongruency due to the same mechanisms as those described above for malunions. The type of nonunion (atrophic, hypertrophic, oligotrophic), the presence of active infec-

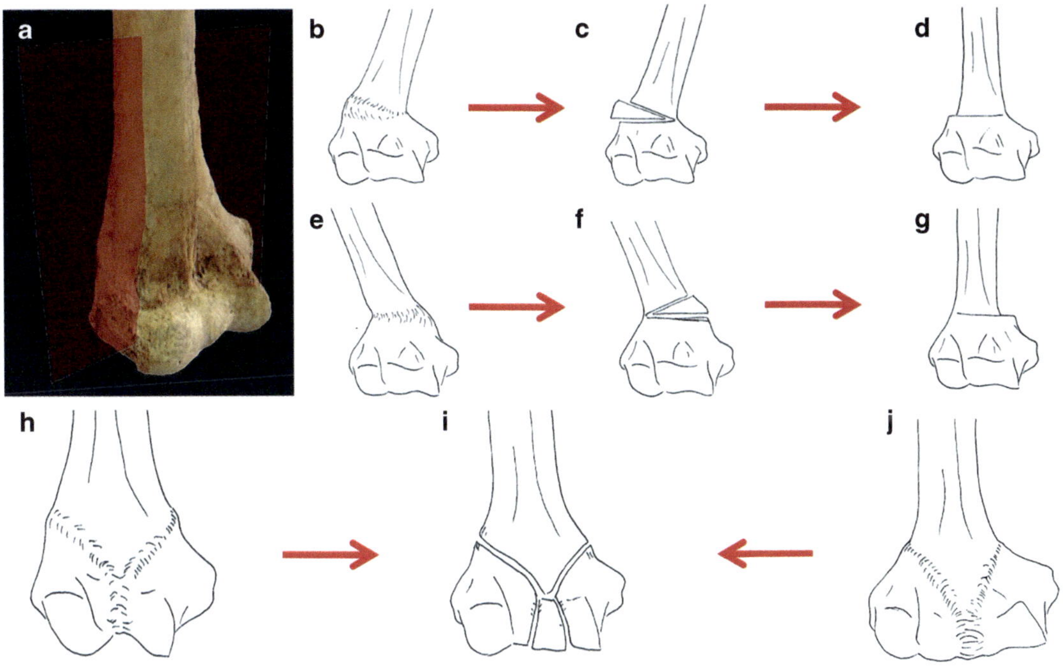

Fig. 10.3 Preoperative planning of corrective osteotomies for humeral deformities affecting the coronal plane (**a**). For extra-articular deformities in varus (**b**) or valgus (**e**) a metaphyseal lateral (**c**) or medial (**f**) subtraction wedge osteotomy should be performed to obtain the humeral axis restoration (**d, g**). For intra-articular malunions with inferior (**h**) or superior (**j**) tilt an addition or subtraction osteotomy (**i**) is required

tion (infected nonunion), fixation devices (hardware failure), or other possible causes should be accurately investigated. Appropriate surgical planning is based on an understanding of the biomechanics underlying the fracture nonunion and follows the same steps as normal nonunion treatment (X-ray, CT, samples to rule out infection, fixation revision, and grafting, if needed). Additional release to obtain a mobile elbow is performed according to the specific stiffness pattern.

10.5.3 Heterotopic Ossifications

Heterotopic ossifications around the elbow can be the consequence of elbow trauma, surgery, immobilization, or skin burns [25–28]. The reported incidence of HO after elbow injury varies greatly, ranging from 3% to 89% [29]; this variability may be explained both by the inappropriate use of the term and by the radiological interpretation of ectopic bone formation. The HO stage should be classified according to the Hastings and Graham classification, which is based on the presence of symptoms, the axes of motion involved, and the severity of stiffness [30]. When planning surgery in patients with HO, the following features should be carefully considered:

- **Location:** HO can be located anteriorly, posteriorly, or around the collateral ligaments (medial and lateral). The most common site for HO formation is the posterolateral aspect of the elbow. Several studies have pointed out that HO location is dependent on the initial injury pattern, since surgically treated distal humerus fractures tend to form around the medial collateral ligament (MCL) or along the torn soft tissues, whereas in proximal radius and ulna fractures, they tend to occur around the previous fracture site [26, 31]. The location of HO is of paramount importance when planning the surgical excision, as previously

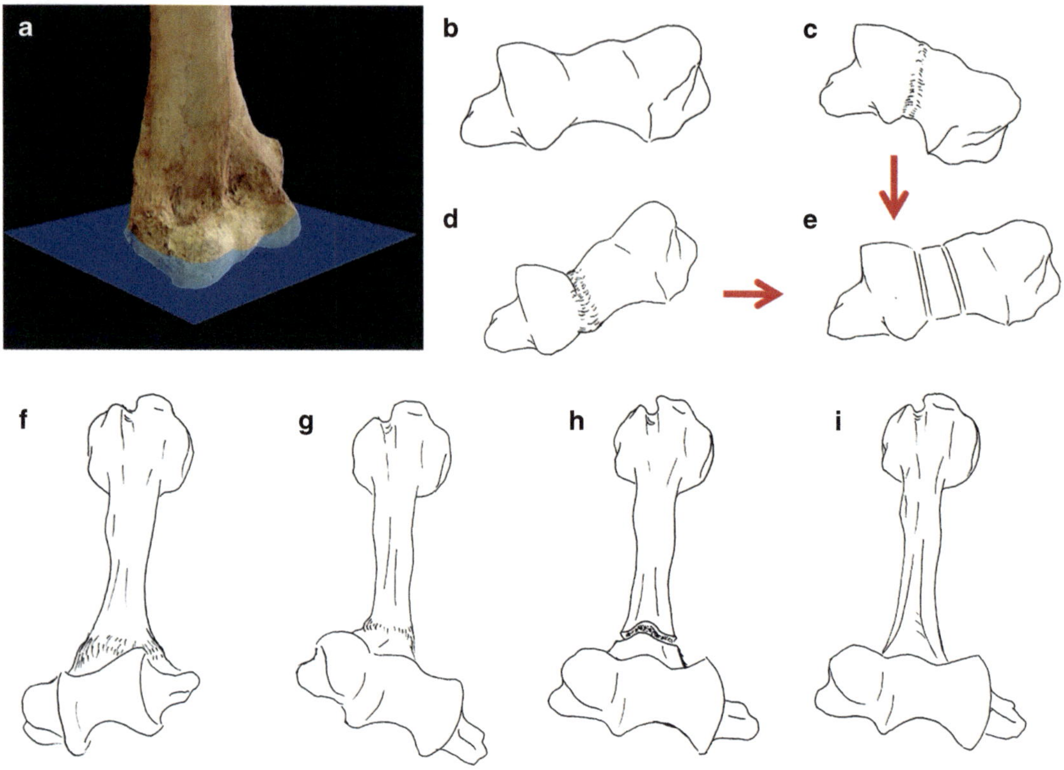

Fig. 10.4 Preoperative planning of corrective osteotomies for humeral deformities affecting the axial plane (**a**). Normal anatomy (**b**). For intra-articular malunions with posterior (**c**) or anterior (**d**) angulation, an addition osteotomy (**e**) is required. For extra-articular deformities in external (**f**) or internal (**g**) rotation a metaphyseal rotational osteotomy should be performed (**h**) to obtain the humeral axis restoration (**i**)

discussed, because of the possible proximity of the ossifications to neurovascular structures. Moreover, elbow instability may occur after HO removal when HO is located around the collateral ligaments; in such cases, the planning of a ligamentous reconstruction and/or external fixation after elbow contracture release is recommended. Another option in such cases is a two-staged procedure, as suggested by O'Driscoll: the first surgical procedure is aimed exclusively at intra-ligamentous HO removal, followed by a period of cast immobilization; after a minimum time of 3 months, circumferential release of the elbow is performed without reconstruction of the ligaments.

- **Relationship with surrounding structures:** a careful examination of the preoperative imaging, particularly of the elbow CT scan, is important to define whether any neurovascular structures are involved (Fig. 10.8). In case of vessel or nerve entrapment within the HO, the planning should involve a vascular surgery consultant or include neurosurgical advice to ensure that excision is performed without complications. In some cases, specific neurosurgical devices (for example, Kerrison forceps) may prove indispensable to perform neurolysis or vascular isolation. A safe zone of cleavage of the HO with the other soft tissue structures should be identified on imaging and evaluated with the help of consultants. The operation should also be thoroughly discussed with the patient since intraoperative lesions might determine permanent sequelae.
- **Timing:** The correct timing for HO excision is a matter of debate in the literature: some authors suggest that the procedure should be

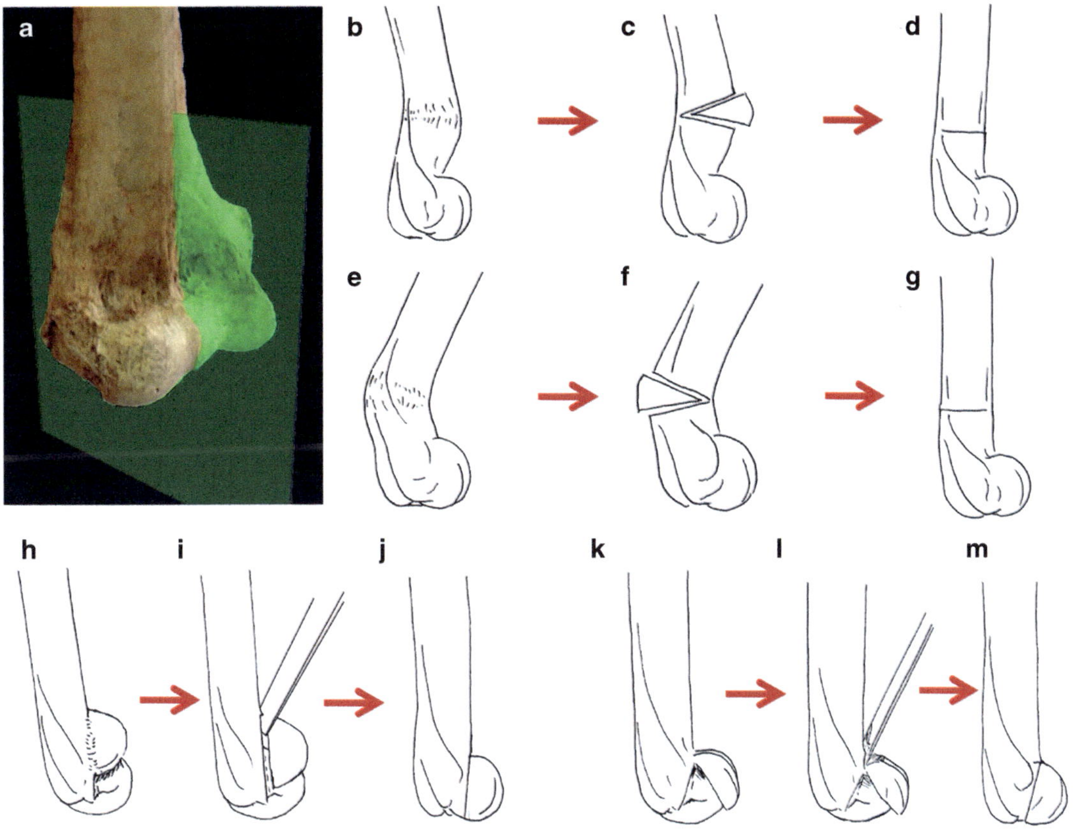

Fig. 10.5 Preoperative planning of corrective osteotomies for humeral deformities affecting the sagittal plane (**a**). For extra-articular deformities in recurvatum (**b**) or procurvatum (**e**) a metaphyseal anterior (**c**) or posterior (**f**) subtraction wedge osteotomy should be performed to obtain the humeral axis restoration (**d, g**). For intra-articular malunions with vertical translation (**h**) or flexion angulation (**k**) of the humeral capitellum intra-articular osteotomies (**i, l**) are required to restore the capitellum position (**j, m**)

delayed for at least 12 months following the original injury or surgical treatment in order to ensure that the condition of the HO is "mature," thereby preventing an acute relapse due to an ongoing, incomplete process. It is our opinion that HO should be treated when a well-defined trabecular pattern with smooth edges can be identified in the X-rays, regardless of the time that has elapsed.

10.5.4 Synostoses

Elbow synostoses mainly affect forearm rotation since it usually occurs as a bony union between the proximal radius and ulna. Elbow flexion may, however, also be affected when a bony bridge connects the distal humerus to the proximal radius or ulna. Apart from congenital causes, in which a distorted anatomy is to be expected as a consequence of abnormal bone growth, most cases result from post-traumatic conditions. Synostoses can be classified according to the Jupiter and Ring classification [32]. Proximal radioulnar synostoses can be classified according to the Viola and Hastings classification [33]. Plain X-rays of the forearm, elbow, and wrist and a CT scan of the forearm should be obtained in order to define the anatomy, location, and size of the synostosis. CT 3D reconstructions are very helpful as a means of characterizing synostosis and planning surgery (Fig. 10.9). Synostoses should not be surgically addressed before the maturation process is complete: this can be

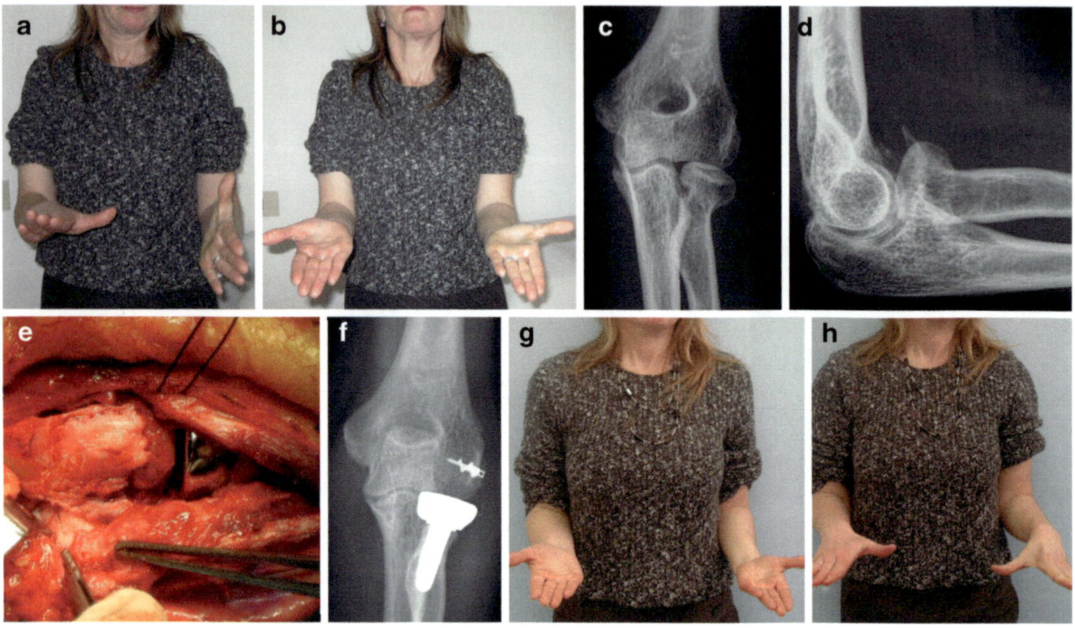

Fig. 10.6 Clinical case of a patient affected by post-traumatic rotational stiffness. The patient was previously conservatively treated for a radial head fracture. Preoperative ROM in pronation (**a**) and supination (**b**). Preoperative X-rays showing malunion of the radial head (**c, d**). An open elbow release and a radial head arthroplasty were performed, followed by the reconstruction of the lateral collateral ligament (**e**). Postoperative X-rays (**f**) and clinical results (**g, h**)

demonstrated by means of a serial radiological examination that points to a stable condition. Whether or not serum levels of alkaline phosphatase are useful for this purpose is debated [34, 35]. Delaying surgery by 1 to 2 years is currently believed to be the safest approach to ensure that synostoses do not recur as a result of an incomplete maturation process [36, 37]. Surgery should be customized according to the location and size of the synostosis, and strategies designed to prevent a recurrence should be adopted [38] (Fig. 10.10).

10.5.5 Prominent Hardware

The presence of prominent hardware in the articular surfaces deriving from previous surgical procedures may be the cause of elbow pain and stiffness (Fig. 10.11). The location and number of prominent hardware as well as the clinical signs and symptoms should be thoroughly investigated so as to allow their removal to be planned. The timing of the removal of any hardware must take into account previous fracture healing as well as the status of the articular cartilage since cartilage wear may have occurred. In general, the removal of prominent fixation devices should be planned as soon as possible to avoid further damage to the articular surfaces, especially in patients with intra-articular hardware. An accurate evaluation of the spatial relationship between prominent hardware and neurovascular structures should also be conducted. A standard diagnostic imaging evaluation with X-rays and CT scan is normally sufficient to identify and locate such devices.

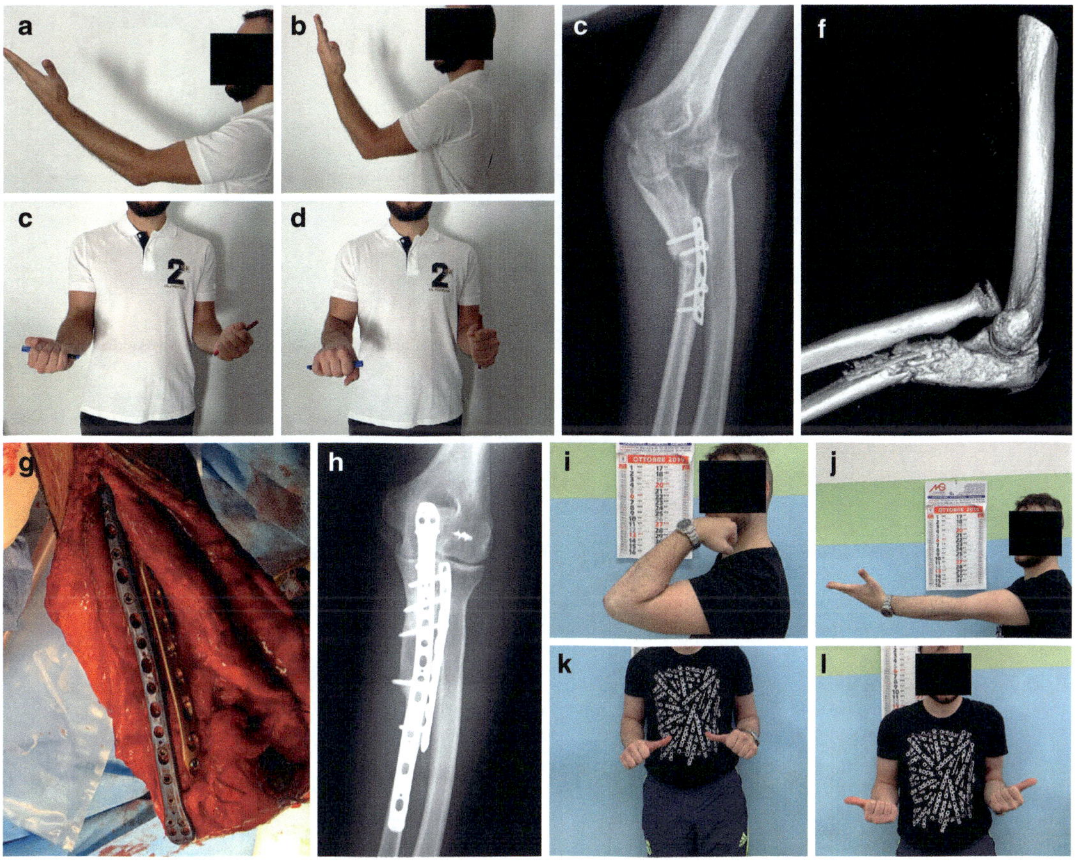

Fig. 10.7 Clinical case of a patient affected by nonunion of the ulnar diaphysis. The patient complained about pain and stiffness. (**a**) Preoperative ROM in extension, (**b**) flexion, (**c**) supination and (**d**) pronation. The patient had previously undergone multiple surgical procedures and the preoperative X-rays (**e**) and CT scan (**f**) showed a failed plate osteosynthesis of the ulnar fracture with the development of nonunion, severe deformity and radial head dislocation. A debridement of the nonunion site was performed to obtain the restoration of the ulnar axis, length and rotation, and the reduction of the radial head dislocation. Autologous bone grafting, double plate fixation, c elbow release and lateral collateral ligament reconstruction were also performed (**g**). Postoperative X-rays (**h**) and clinical results (**i–l**)

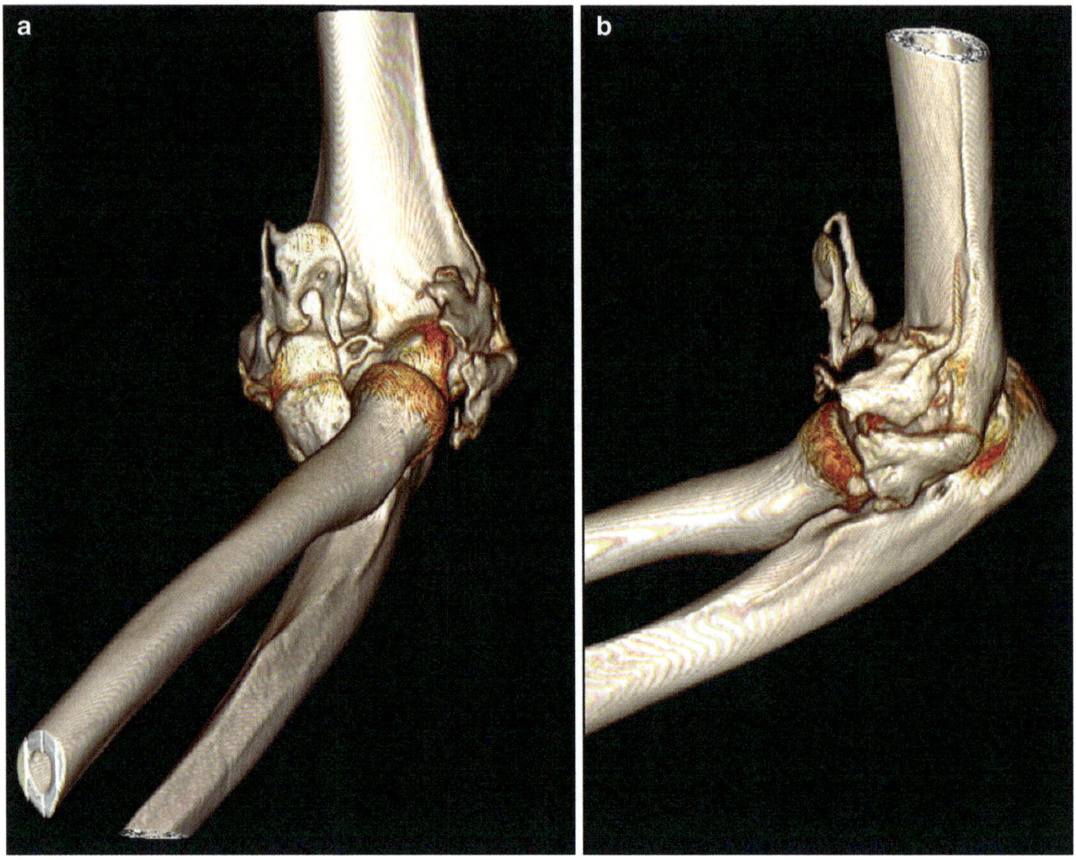

Fig. 10.8 Preoperative CT scan of a patient affected by symptomatic heterotopic ossifications (**a, b**) around the anterior capsule and the lateral collateral ligament. The execution of a CT scan is mandatory to plan this type of surgery and locate the exact position and morphology of the ossifications

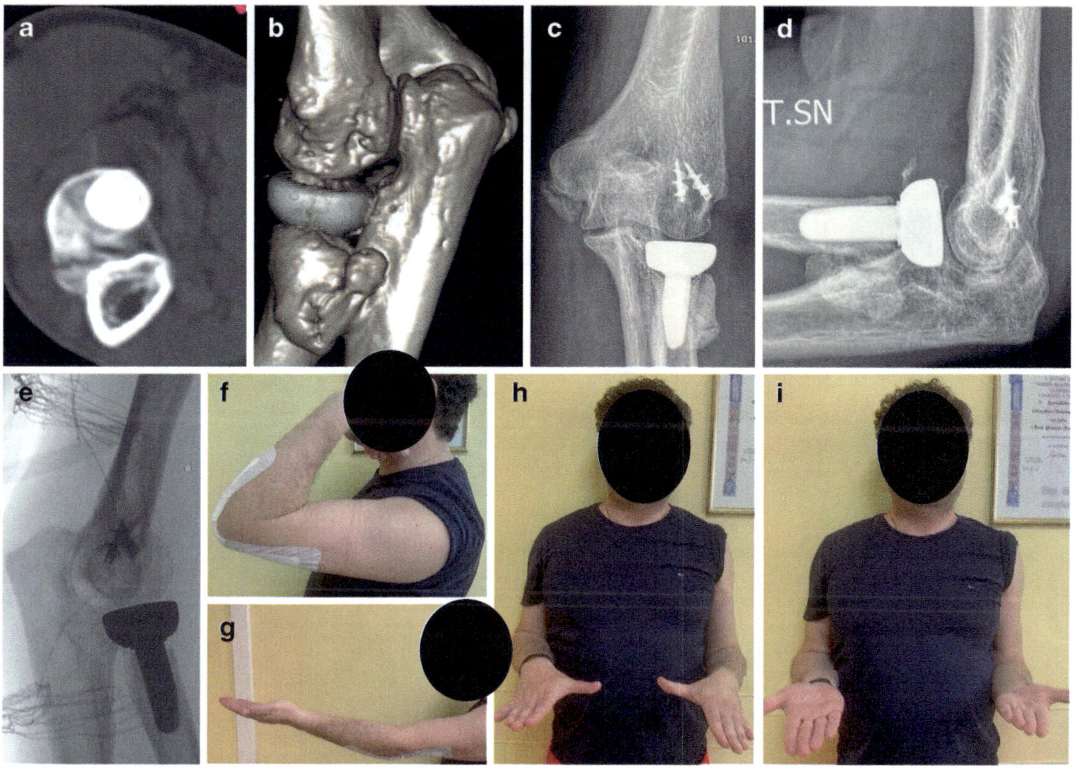

Fig. 10.9 Clinical case of a patient affected by post-traumatic rotational stiffness. The patient was previously surgically treated for a terrible triad of the elbow with the implant of an anatomical radial head arthroplasty, coronoid osteosuture and lateral collateral ligament reinsertion. Preoperative CT scan (**a, b**) and X-rays (**c, d**) showing a proximal radio-ulnar synostosis. An open pericapitellar release with excision of the synostosis was performed. Postoperative X-rays (**e**) and clinical results (**f–i**)

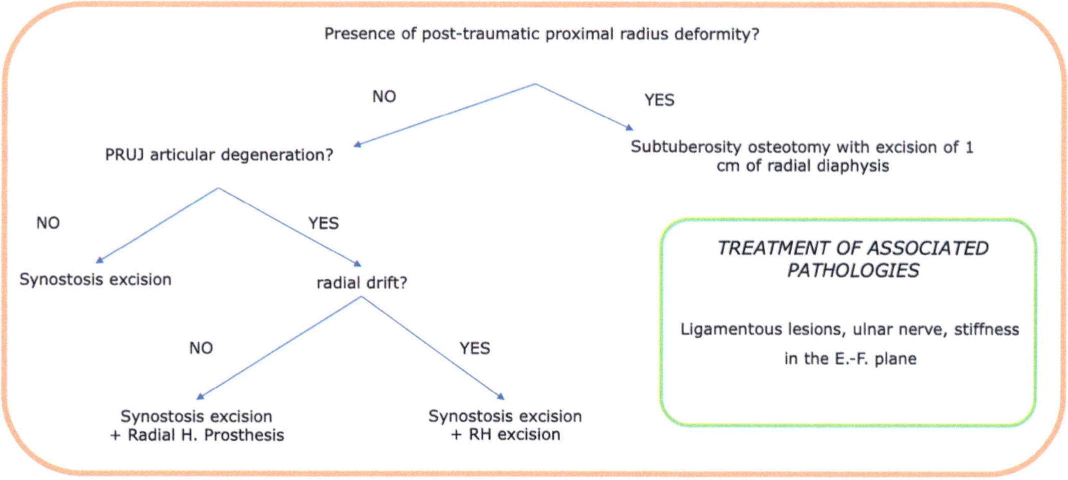

Fig. 10.10 Therapeutic algorithm for the treatment of post-traumatic proximal radioulnar synostoses

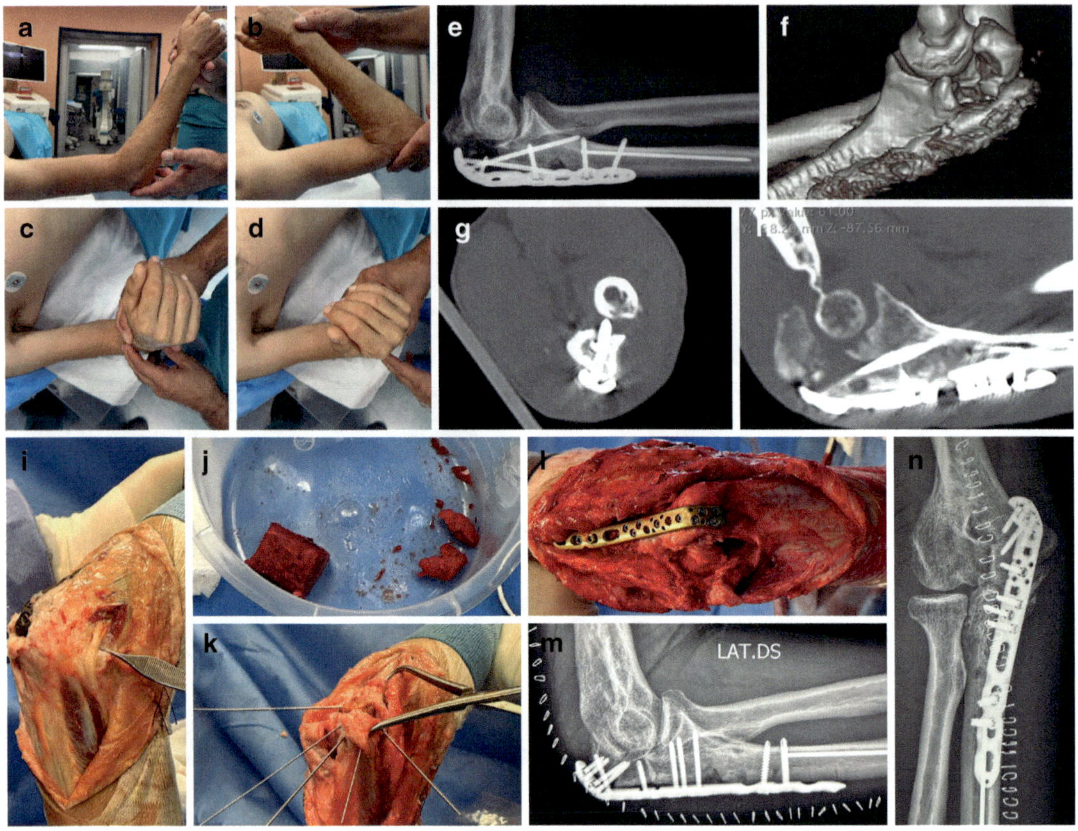

Fig. 10.11 Clinical case of a patient affected by elbow stiffness and nonunion of a surgically treated olecranon fracture associated with ulnar sensitive neuropathy. Preoperative ROM in extension (**a**), flexion (**b**), pronation (**c**), and supination (**d**). The preoperative X-rays (**e**) and CT scan (**f, h**) showed a failed plate fixation of the olecranon with secondary displacement of the proximal fragment with proximal migration and development of nonunion. The rotational stiffness is caused by a prominent screw in the radial notch that can be seen in the preoperative CT images (**g**). Removal of the plate, ulnar nerve transposition (**i**), and debridement of the nonunion site were performed to obtain the reduction of the olecranon fragment (**k**), followed by autologous bone grafting (**j**) and new plate fixation (**l**). The result is shown in the postoperative X-rays (**m, n**)

10.6 Soft Tissue Considerations

10.6.1 Medial and Lateral Collateral Ligaments

Medial and lateral collateral ligament complexes are fundamental structures for elbow stability and motion. When retracted or ossified, these complexes may become one of the causes of elbow stiffness. The MCL complex has an antero-inferior insertion on the medial epicondyle. Its three bundles exert varying degrees of tension along the elbow ROM and may affect motion in different ways when retracted or ossified. A retracted posterior bundle of the MCL is responsible for the lack of flexion in stiff elbows; its section is a routine part of the release surgical procedures since its contribution to stability is limited and no instability should be expected following its section [39–41]. On the other hand, the anterior bundle reaches its maximum tension in extension, and when retracted it may limit the last 30° of extension; however, to prevent the elbow from becoming unstable, only partial sections of the anterior bundle can be performed since it is the main constraint for valgus stability. The ulnar bundle of the LCL (LUCL) represents the main constraint for posterolateral stability, while the radial bundle (LRCL) and the annular ligament play a role in varus and PRUJ stability. The role of the LCL complex in the onset of elbow stiffness is not understood so well and has been discussed less in the literature. No standard procedures have been described for the lateral collateral ligament complex release, as most procedures on ligaments are performed on the medial side. Every effort should be made to preserve the LUCL or to reconstruct it using a graft in case of instability secondary to extensive elbow release. We believe that a more limited improvement in ROM that does not excessively damage the LCL complex and the anterior band of MCL is the best approach to adopt in the majority of such cases.

The square ligament (SL) of the elbow is a discrete ligamentous structure that joins the radial neck to the lower border of the lesser sigmoid notch and may be involved in elbow rotatory stiffness. It consists of three distinct bundles in 70% of cases and of a single bundle in 30% of cases [42]. The anterior bundle is tensioned in supination while the posterior bundle is tensioned in pronation. In maximal pronation and supination, all the bundles (when present) are equally tightened. The SL, when tightened, moves the radial head closer to the ulna and consistently contributes to forearm transverse and longitudinal stability [42]. However, no descriptions of standard SL release in elbow rotatory stiffness procedures are present in the literature, although they have been reported in several biomechanical studies [42] and performed in one early clinical series [43]. The interosseous membrane of the forearm (IOM) plays a role in forearm stability, load transfer, and the load-sharing mechanism between the radius and ulna. Ossification of the IOM is a known source of forearm rotational stiffness, with several techniques having been described for the removal of HO affecting this membrane; however, no studies have discussed the possibility of the release or controlled sectioning of the IOM to address rotatory stiffness.

Elbow stiffness may conceal subtle forms of elbow instability, the stiffness itself being a consequence of pain due to elbow instability. A preliminary evaluation of elbow stability is mandatory and dedicated clinical tests for both the medial and lateral side should be performed. The valgus stress and moving-milking valgus stress tests are used for the medial compartment; the drawer test, the tabletop relocation test, the pivot-shift test, and the varus stress test are used for the lateral side. When doubts persist or the clinical examination is not conclusive, an MRI of the elbow may help to identify collateral ligament abnormalities. Stress rays or a dynamic evaluation using fluoroscopy or sonography may also be indicated.

Ligament contractures or ossifications within the ligaments are issues that need to be addressed when treating elbow stiffness. A partial or total release of the MCL and LCL have been described in the literature [27, 39] as surgical steps associated with anterior and posterior capsulectomy that can be performed to regain both elbow flexion and extension. No standardized guidelines exist to define the extent to which ligaments should be released; however, partial ligament release is unlikely to cause elbow instability. Every effort should be made to preserve the anterior quarter of the MCL and the ulnar band of the LCL. In other words, the non-vital parts of the collateral ligaments can be released as a routine step, while complete detachment of the ligaments with subsequent reinsertion should be performed exclusively in refractory forms of stiffness when a partial release is not effective. In the case of ossified ligaments, since the removal of the ligament itself causes elbow instability, a ligamentous reconstruction procedure with grafts, with or without external fixation, should be performed.

10.7 Capsule

Anterior and posterior capsulectomy are routinely performed in surgical release procedures. Regardless of the surgical approach, the anterior and posterior thickened capsules preventing elbow extension and flexion, respectively, must be removed. Attention needs to be paid to avoid damaging the collateral ligaments and the radial nerve that lies anteriorly to the anterior capsule.

Capsulectomy can be performed via open release or arthroscopically.

References

1. Kozin SH. Congenital differences about the elbow. Hand Clin. 2009;25(2):277–91. https://doi.org/10.1016/j.hcl.2008.12.007.
2. Sun C, Zhou X, Yao C, Poonit K, Fan C, Yan H. The timing of open surgical release of post-traumatic elbow stiffness: a systematic review. Medicine (Baltimore). 2017;96(49):e9121. https://doi.org/10.1097/MD.0000000000009121.
3. Cao J, Stutz C, Beckwith T, Browning A, Mills J, Oishi SN. Elbow release and tricepsplasty in arthrogrypotic patients: a long-term follow-up study. J Hand Surg Am. 2020;45(6):549.e1–7. https://doi.org/10.1016/j.jhsa.2019.08.002.
4. Giannicola G, Sessa P, Calella P, Gumina S, Cinotti G. Chronic complex persistent elbow instability: a consecutive and prospective case series and review of recent literature. J Shoulder Elb Surg. 2020;29(4):e103–17. https://doi.org/10.1016/j.jse.2019.11.021.
5. Zubler V, Saupe N, Jost B, Pfirrmann CWA, Hodler J, Zanetti M. Elbow stiffness: effectiveness of conventional radiography and CT to explain osseous causes. AJR Am J Roentgenol. 2010;194:W515–20.
6. Lombard C, Teixeira P, Germain E, Dodin G, Louis M, Blum A, Gillet R. Elbow stiffness imaging: a practical diagnostic and pretherapeutic approach. J Clin Med. 2021;10(22):5348. https://doi.org/10.3390/jcm10225348.
7. Carlier Y, Lenoir H, Rouleau DM, Mansat P, Vidil A, Ferrand M, Bleton R, Herrisson O, Salabi V, Duparc F, et al. Arthroscopic debridement for osteoarthritis of the elbow: results and analysis of predictive factors. Orthop Traumatol Surg Res. 2019;105:S221–7.
8. Everding NG, Maschke SD, Hoyen HA, Evans PJ. Prevention and treatment of elbow stiffness: a 5-year update. J Hand Surg. 2013;38:2496–507.
9. Sun Z, Li J, Cui H, Ruan H, Wang W, Fan C. A new pathologic classification for elbow stiffness based on our experience in 216 patients. J Shoulder Elb Surg. 2020;29:e75–86.
10. Athlani L, Rouizi K, Granero J, Hossu G, Blum A, Dautel G, Gondim Teixeira PA. Assessment of scapholunate instability with dynamic computed tomography. J Hand Surg Eur Vol. 2020;45:375–82.
11. Giannicola G, Bullitta G, Sacchetti FM, Scacchi M, Polimanti D, Citoni G, Cinotti G. Change in quality of life and cost/utility analysis in open stage-related surgical treatment of elbow stiffness. Orthopedics. 2013 Jul;36(7):e923–30. https://doi.org/10.3928/01477447-20130624-24.
12. Morrey BF. Functional evaluation of the elbow. In: Morrey BF, Sanchez-Sotelo J, Morrey ME, editors. Morrey's the elbow and its disorders. 5th ed. Philadelphia: Elsevier; 2018. p. 66–74.
13. Soucie JM, Wang C, Forsyth A, Funk S, Denny M, Roach KE, Boone D, Hemophilia Treatment Center Network. Range of motion measurements: reference values and a database for comparison studies. Haemophilia. 2011;17:500–7. https://doi.org/10.1111/j.1365-2516.2010.02399.x.
14. Adolfsson L. Post traumatic stiff elbow. EFORT Open Rev. 2018;3(5):210–6. https://doi.org/10.1302/2058-5241.3.170062.
15. Shuai C, Hede Y, Shen L, et al. Is routine ulnar nerve transposition necessary in open release of stiff elbows? Our experience and a literature review. Int Orthop. 2014;38:2289–94.
16. Merolla G, Porcellini G, Bullita G, Giannicola G. Evaluation of UCL by ultrasound. In: Pederzini L, Eygendaal D, Denti M, editors. Elbow and sport. Heidelberg: Springer; 2016. p. 79–84. https://doi.org/10.1007/978-3-662-48742-6_15.
17. Beşer CG, Demiryürek D, Özsoy H, Erçakmak B, Hayran M, Kızılay O, et al. Redefining the proximal ulna anatomy. Surg Radiol Anat. 2014;36(10):1023–31. https://doi.org/10.1007/s00276-014-1340-4.
18. Rouleau DM, Faber KJ, Athwal GS. The proximal ulna dorsal angulation: a radiographic study. J Shoulder Elb Surg. 2010;19(1):26–30. https://doi.org/10.1016/j.jse.2009.07.005.
19. Sandman E, Canet F, Petit Y, Laflamme GY, Athwal GS, Rouleau DM. Radial head subluxation following malalignment of the proximal ulna: a biomechanical study. J Orthop Trauma. 2013;28(8):464–9. https://doi.org/10.1097/BOT.0000000000000058.
20. Baecher N, Edwards S. Olecranon fractures. J Hand Surg Am. 2013;38(3):593–604.
21. Edwards SG, Weber JP, Baecher NB. Proximal forearm fractures. Orthop Clin North Am. 2013;44(1):67–80. https://doi.org/10.1016/j.ocl.2012.09.001.
22. Snow BJ, Javidan P, Itamura JM, Lee TQ. The effects of varus or valgus malalignment of proximal ulnar fractures on forearm rotation. J Orthop Trauma. 2014;28(3):143–7. https://doi.org/10.1097/BOT.0b013e31829f5ebc.
23. Kinaci A, Buijze GA, Leeuwen DH, Jupiter JB, Marti RK, Kloen P. Corrective osteotomy for intraarticular distal humerus malunion. Arch Bone Jt Surg. 2016;4(2):161–5.
24. Giannicola G, Manauzzi E, Sacchetti FM, Greco A, Bullitta G, Vestri A, Cinotti G. Anatomical variations of the proximal radius and their effects on osteosynthesis. J Hand Surg Am. 2012;37(5):1015–23. https://doi.org/10.1016/j.jhsa.2012.02.005.
25. Pontell ME, Sparber LS, Chamberlain RS. Corrective and reconstructive surgery in patients with postburn heterotopic ossification and bony ankylosis: an evidence-based approach. J Burn Care Res. 2015;36:57–69.
26. Foruria AM, Augustin S, Morrey BF, Sanchez-Sotelo J. Heterotopic ossification after surgery for fractures

and fracture dislocations involving the proximal aspect of the radius or ulna. J Bone Joint Surg Am. 2013;95(10):e66.
27. Lindenhovius AL, Linzel DS, Doornberg JN, Ring DC, Jupiter JB. Comparison of elbow contracture release in elbows with and without heterotopic ossification restricting motion. J Shoulder Elb Surg. 2007;16(5):621–5.
28. Hong CC, Nashi N, Hey HW, Chee YH, Murphy D. Clinically relevant heterotopic ossification after elbow fracture surgery: a risk factors study. Orthop Traumatol Surg Res. 2015;101(2):209–13.
29. Wahl EP, Casey PM, Risoli T Jr, Green CL, Richard MJ, Ruch DS. Heterotopic ossification formation after farctures around the elbow. Eur J Orthop Surg Traumatol. 2021;31(6):1061–7. https://doi.org/10.1007/s00590-020-02855-4.
30. Hastings H 2nd, Graham TJ. The classification and treatment of heterotopic ossification about the elbow and forearm. Hand Clin. 1994;10(3):417–37.
31. Foruria AM, Lawrence TM, Augustin S, Morrey BF, Sanchez-Sotelo J. Heterotopic ossification after surgery for distal humeral fractures. Bone Joint J. 2014;96-B(12):1681–7.
32. Jupiter JB, Ring D. Operative treatment of post-traumatic proximal radioulnar synostosis. J Bone Joint Surg Am. 1998 Feb;80(2):248–57. https://doi.org/10.2106/00004623-199802000-00012.
33. Viola RW, Hastings H II. Treatment of ectopic ossification about the elbow. Clin Orthop Relat Res. 2000;370:65–86.
34. Garland DE, Hanscom DA, Keenan MA, Smith C, Moore T. Resection of heterotopic ossification in the adult with head trauma. J Bone Joint Surg Am. 1985;67(8):1261–9.
35. Tibone J, Sakimura I, Nickel VL, Hsu JD. Heterotopic ossification around the hip in spinal cord-injured patients: a long-term follow-up study. J Bone Joint Surg Am. 1978;60(6):769–75.
36. Failla JM, Amadio PC, Morrey BF. Post- traumatic proximal radio-ulnar synostosis: results of surgical treatment. J Bone Joint Surg Am. 1989;71(8):1208–13.
37. Vince KG, Miller JE. Cross-union complicating fracture of the forearm: part I. Adults. J Bone Joint Surg Am. 1987;69(5):640–53.
38. Giannicola G, Spinello P, Villani C, Cinotti G. Post-traumatic proximal radioulnar synostosis: results of surgical treatment and review of the literature. J Shoulder Elb Surg. 2020 Feb;29(2):329–39. https://doi.org/10.1016/j.jse.2019.07.026.
39. Wada T, Ishii S, Usui M, Miyano S. The medial approach for operative release of post-traumatic contracture of the elbow. J Bone Joint Surg Br. 2000;82-B:68–73.
40. Itoh Y, Saegusa K, Ishiguro T, Horiuchi Y, Sasaki T, Uchinishi K. Operation for the stiff elbow. Int Orthop. 1989;13:263–8.
41. Ruch DS, Shen J, Chloros GD, Krings E, Papadonikolakis A. Release of the medial collateral ligament to improve flexion in post-traumatic elbow stiffness. J Bone Joint Surg Br. 2008;90:614–8.
42. Otayek S, Ait Tayeb AEK, Assabah B, Viard B, Dayan R, Lazure T, Soubeyrand M. Squared ligament of the elbow: anatomy and contribution to forearm stability. Surg Radiol Anat. 2016 Mar;38(2):237–44. https://doi.org/10.1007/s00276-015-1539-z.
43. Bert JM, Linscheid RL, McElfresh EC. Rotatory contracture of the forearm. J Bone Joint Surg Am. 1980;62:1163–8.

Part III

Surgical Treatment of Degenerative Stiff Elbow

11 Surgical Treatment of Degenerative Stiff Elbow Open Management

Pierre Mansat

11.1 Introduction

Primary osteoarthritis of the elbow remains uncommon. It is most often secondary to overuse, traumatic history, lesions of osteochondritis dissecans, or synovial chondromatosis. Asymptomatic for a long time, the clinical presentation can be variable, resulting in a more or less painful loss of mobility more or less painful. The imaging assessment allows the evaluation of the osteo-cartilaginous lesions and specifies the position of osteophytes and foreign bodies. If initially medical treatment is the rule to decrease pain and keep a functional range of motion, in case of failure thea surgical treatment can be discussed. It consists of joint cleaning, with excision of the osteophytes and eventually capsule release. These can be performed arthroscopically or by an open procedure. In case of advanced alteration of the joint space, the choice is made between open arthrolysis with interposition or replacement with an elbow prosthesis.

11.2 Physiopathology

The elbow is considered a non-load-bearing joint. However, the resultant force generated in the humero-ulnar joint can thus reach one time body weight while carrying out daily activities [1]. Chadwick and Nicol [2] have shown that during the effort of lifting, mobilization, or weight lifting of 2 kg, this resultant could reach two times body weight. Whether the effort is repeated and sustained, this resultant can reach up to three times body weight [1]. Finally, dynamics charges when throwing or lifting weights generate high forces of more than six times body weight [3].

Primary osteoarthritis of the elbow seems to begin at the side of the joint, especially at the level of the radiohumeral joint. Goodfellow and Bullough [4] dissected 28 elbows between 18 and 88 years old at the time of their death and observed that the involvement of this joint increased with age. A posteromedial defect on

P. Mansat (✉)
Département d'Orthopédie-Traumatologie, Clinique Universitaire du Sport, Institut Recherche Riquet, Hôpital Pierre Paul RIQUET, CHU Purpan, Toulouse, France
e-mail: mansat.p@chu-toulouse.fr

L. Pederzini et al. (eds.), *Stiffness of the Elbow, Wrist and Related Pathologies*,
https://doi.org/10.1007/978-3-031-81381-8_11

the radial head was consistently found and corresponded to a mirror lesion at the posterior part of the crest separating the trochlea from the capitulum. Degenerative damage was not found in a similar way at the humero-ulnar joint. Murato [5] concluded that the osteoarthritis progressed from lateral to medial, due to excess stress at the central part of the joint destroying the cartilage in the ulnar part of the radial head, and the corresponding trochlear crest. Tsuge and Mizuseki [6] confirmed this hypothesis by showing that the impairment initially predominated over the radiohumeral joint before to extend to the humero-ulnar compartment. These osteo-cartilaginous modifications are associated with a thickening of the anterior and posterior joint capsule as shown by Suvarna et al. [7].

11.3 Epidemiology

Elbow osteoarthritis was recognized in the English literature only in 1955 during a study on British miners [8]. Since then, several reports have confirmed this entity [4, 9, 10], but the first description of both clinical and radiographic changes was published in Japan in the 1970s separately by Minami [11] and Kashiwagi [12]. Rostock, out of a population of 744 miners, found a 32.8% incidence of elbow osteoarthritis [13]. Conversely, Hunter found only a low incidence in heavy workers [14]. Later, Lawrence [8] showed that the miners using pneumatic jackhammers presented a higher incidence of elbow osteoarthritis than other workers (31% vs. 16%). Finally, Stanley [15] in a population of 1000 patients found a correlation between the type of activity and the incidence of osteoarthritis of the elbow. It therefore seems that strength activities are a decisive factor in the occurrence of this osteoarthritis, confirming the fundamental studies by Carter et al. [16].

The incidence of primary osteoarthritis of the elbow was evaluated at 1% to 2% of patients with elbow osteoarthritis [17]. Doherty and Preston reported an incidence of 7% in their practice of rheumatology, with frequent association with other articular locations, with 60% of cases a involvement of the metacarpophalangeal joint of the 2nd and 3rd rays of the hand titled the "Missouri metacarpal syndrome" [18]. Elbow osteoarthritis occurs mainly in men with a sex ratio of 4:1 [11, 12, 19–21]. The age of onset is around 50 [18], but some authors have observed surprising variations with extremes of 20 to 65 years [20, 21]. For nearly 60% of patients, a predisposing activity requiring repeated use of the limb in an upward position is highlighted. Stanley reported that 10% of 124 men who carried out manual strength activities presented with osteoarthritis of the elbow and none had less than 40 years [15]. The dominant side is interested in 80% to 90% of cases, with bilateral involvement varying from 25% to 60% of cases [18, 21].

11.4 Etiology

Trauma, osteochondritis dissecans, chondromatosis synovium, and the overuse of the elbow in extension-valgus have been associated with the occurrence of osteoarthritis of the elbow [22–27]. Although there does not appear to be a direct association between an episode of elbow dislocation and the subsequent occurrence of osteoarthritis, elbow dislocations with a fracture of the anteromedial facet of the coronoid appear to be more arthrogenic [28]. In the absence of diagnosis of this fracture and in the absence of reduction, osteoarthritis can develop rapidly. Radial head trauma in children can also lead to osteonecrosis, which can secondarily progress to osteoarthritis [27]. These traumatic events may have been forgotten in adulthood, leading misdiagnosis of primary osteoarthritis. Lesions of osteochondritis dissecans of the capitulum have an arthrogenic evolutionary potential. Two studies, one on 53 patients followed for 12 years, and the other of 31 patients followed for 23 years, have made it possible to know the natural history of osteochondritis dissecans of the capitulum and showed that, in 50% of cases, the patients continued to have symptoms during daily activities and that more than 50% had radiographic signs of osteoarthritis [22, 26, 29]. Overuse of the elbow in the extension valgus is a recognized cause of osteoarthritis in throwing athletes. Repetition constraints in hyperextension will induce the formation of osteophytes at the posteromedial part of the olecranon and at the medial part of the olecranon fossa with the formation of foreign bodies [23, 30].

11.5 Clinical Presentation

Loss of the last degrees of extension is the most common symptom, leading the patient to consult [12, 15, 31]. However, it is not uncommon for moderate pain to be associated. Stiffness is most often the dominant problem [18]. Pain occurs mainly at the end of extension in almost all patients, and at the end of flexion in half of the cases. More rarely, symptoms are present throughout along the arc of motion. An episode of painful locking can reflect the presence of loose bodies in the joint [12, 31, 32, 33]. The arc of motion is classically deficient by about 30° in extension, for a flexion reaching 120°. The arc of prono-supination is only rarely reduced [31, 34, 35].

Irritation of the ulnar nerve is noted in 26% to 55% of patients with elbow osteoarthritis [20, 31, 33, 35]. This impairment must be sought during the initial examination because it will influence the therapeutic decision, as well as the surgical technique. The interrogation makes it possible to determine the etiology of the osteoarthritis. The youngest patients often have a traumatic history [15]. The activity of the patient must be specified because it is not unusual that hard work is at the origin of this osteoarthritis. The intensity of the pain and the importance of the repercussion on function vary from patient to patient. The importance of the symptomatology, the localization of the pain, the mechanical symptoms, the presence of pain at rest or occurring at night, and the type of pain are important factors in clinical history. A joint effusion may also exist. This one is highlighted on palpation at the point of puncture located in the middle of the triangle represented by the lateral condyle, the radial head, and the tip of the olecranon. When examining joint mobility, it is important to note if pain is present only at the extremes of motion or if it is present throughout the arc of motion. Indeed, the conflict related to peripheral osteophytes is the origin of pain in forced extension or flexion, while chondral lesions are responsible for pain throughout along the arc of motion. A complete neurovascular examination should be part of the initial examination. It must look for suggestive clinical signs of compression of the ulnar nerve at the elbow which results by sensory disturbances in the fifth finger of the hand, and a positive Tinel's sign on percussion of the nerve in its gutter. Finally, a surgical history should always ask the question of a possible infection. In case of doubt, in addition to an inflammatory assessment, a bone scan and joint aspiration with microbiological examination can help make the diagnostic.

11.6 Radiographic Evaluation

Due to the low frequency of this pathology and its uncharacteristic presentation, synovial biopsies and arthroscopic explorations have been performed for diagnostic purposes [19, 36]. However, when one is familiar with this pathology, it is obvious that these examinations ultimately provide little additional diagnostic elements [14, 15]. X-ray examination is usually sufficient to make the diagnostic. Indeed, the images are characteristic. Dalal et al. [37] showed that in elbow osteoarthritis, osteophytes are present in more than 85% of cases, mainly around the olecranon (96% of cases), next to the coronoid (90% of cases) and radial head (86% of cases); narrowing of the humero-radial space is observed in 58% of cases, and the humero-ulnar joint in 16% of cases. The degenerative changes are therefore often more advanced in the lateral compartment [21, 31–33, 35]. Moreover, there exists frequent ossification and filling of olecranon and coronoid fossae [11] (Fig. 11.1). The preservation of humero-ulnar and humero-radial joint space is commonly observed even at an advanced stage of osteoarthritis. An important narrowing of the joint space without true osteophytes must rather make evoke an inflammatory rheumatism. Intra-articular foreign bodies may be difficult to visualize on standard X-rays and nearly 30% are not detected, especially in the posterior compartment and in the proximal radio-ulnar joint [36, 38]. More specific examinations, such as arthro-CT, make it possible to better evaluate osteophytes, locate any foreign bodies free in the joint, and assess the condition of the articular cartilage (Fig. 11.2). For Morrey [39], foreign bodies can be found in 50% of cases, frequency which also corresponds to the involvement of the radial head. A retro-olecranon view can be useful if there is ulnar nerve damage. More sophisticated examinations such as MRI are not useful in the diagnosis and evaluation of this pathology, except for synovial pathologies. At last, in the event of a clinical sign suggestive of damage to the nerve ulnar, an electromyographic assessment confirms this impairment, specifies the importance of compression, and gives a prognosis for recovery.

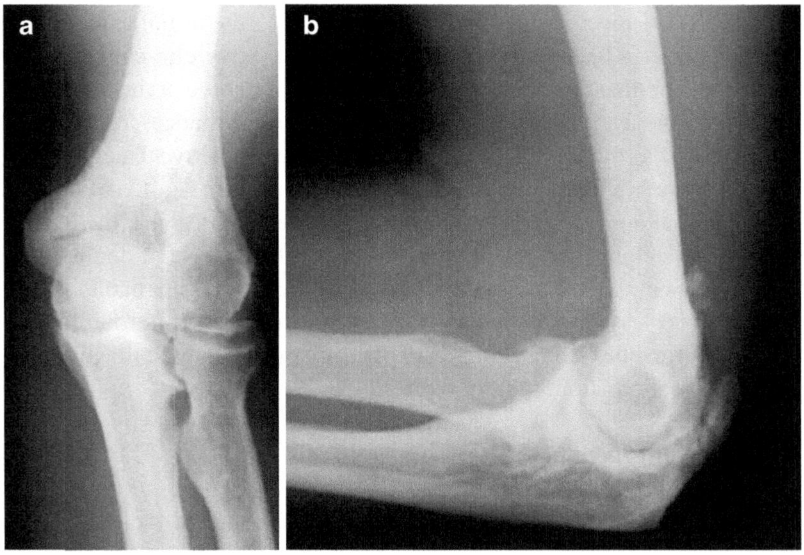

Fig. 11.1 Radiographic evaluation of a degenerative elbow: (**a**) A/P view; (**b**) Lateral view

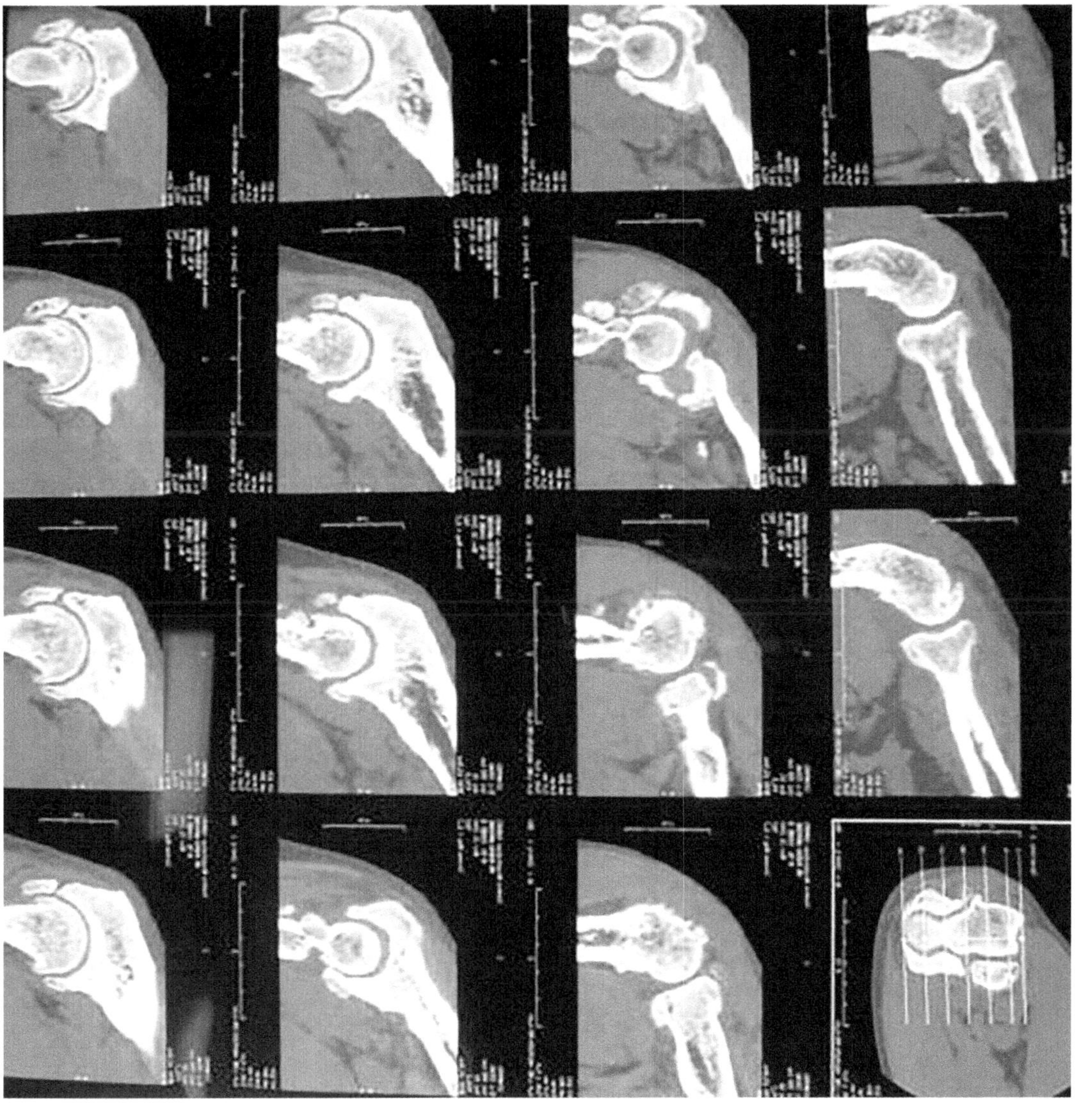

Fig. 11.2 CT-scan of a degenerative elbow

11.7 Treatment

11.7.1 Medical Treatment

Symptomatic treatment is the rule in the early stages because osteoarthritis of the elbow progresses slowly and is well tolerated for a long time. Rest, non-steroids anti-inflammatories drugs and the suppression of strength activities are the essential elements of this treatment. The realization of an intra-articular injection of corticosteroids can relieve the patient's pain transiently. However, these injections do not have a long-term effect and always have a risk of infectious complications. Visco-supplementation does not seem to have a place in the treatment of post-traumatic osteoarthritis of the elbow [40]. A specific rehabilitation program is not the rule for the conservative treatment of elbow osteoarthritis [18, 41]. However, prescription of a static splint is effective in stiffness and posttraumatic osteoarthritis of the elbow even if they are applied several months after the initial trauma [42].

11.7.2 Surgical Treatment

Several surgical options have been proposed to relieve patients' pain and improve their function. The choice depends on the main symptomatology and radiographic changes. Patients with limitation of range of motion of the elbow, with pain at the end of the arc of mobility, and joint space preservation can be treated successfully by joint debridement, excision of osteophytes, and capsular release [21, 31–33, 35, 43]. The patients having pain throughout the arc of motion associated with joint narrowing, and possibly a modification of the bone architecture, require techniques of resurfacing surgeries such as interposition-arthroplasty or total elbow prostheses [44–48].

11.7.2.1 Non-prosthetic Surgical Treatment

Joint Debridement and Humeroulnar Arthroplasty

Joint debridement, performing a capsulectomy and resection of osteophytes, a procedure called humero-ulnar arthroplasty, is indicated when the loss of motion is the predominant symptom. The ideal candidate for this intervention is the young and active subject or patient with mechanical symptoms, pain at the end of the arc of motion and moderate stiffness having withstood non-surgical conservative treatment [31, 33, 35].

The Outerbridge procedure, popularized by Kashiwagi [12], was intended to remove foreign bodies and osteophytes via a posterior approach associated with a fenestration of the olecranon fossa. This allows access to the anterior compartment and coronoid osteophytes. The use of a trephine to create this fenestration makes it possible to eliminate the debris generated by a cutter by carrying out clean resection [49] (Fig. 11.3).

However, the column procedure through lateral approaches allows better access to the anterior compartment for the realization of capsular release, removal of loose bodies, and resection of humeroradial osteophytes [31, 43, 50]. The column procedure allows as well the approach of the posterior compartment by lifting the triceps from the lateral column. Sometimes a second approach may be necessary to release the medial side of the joint [33, 35]. Finally, for some authors, a simple posterior skin incision allows, in performing two large lateral and medial subcutaneous flaps, the approach of both elbow sides [21, 31, 32]. The ulnar nerve can thus be, if necessary, released or transposed anteriorly.

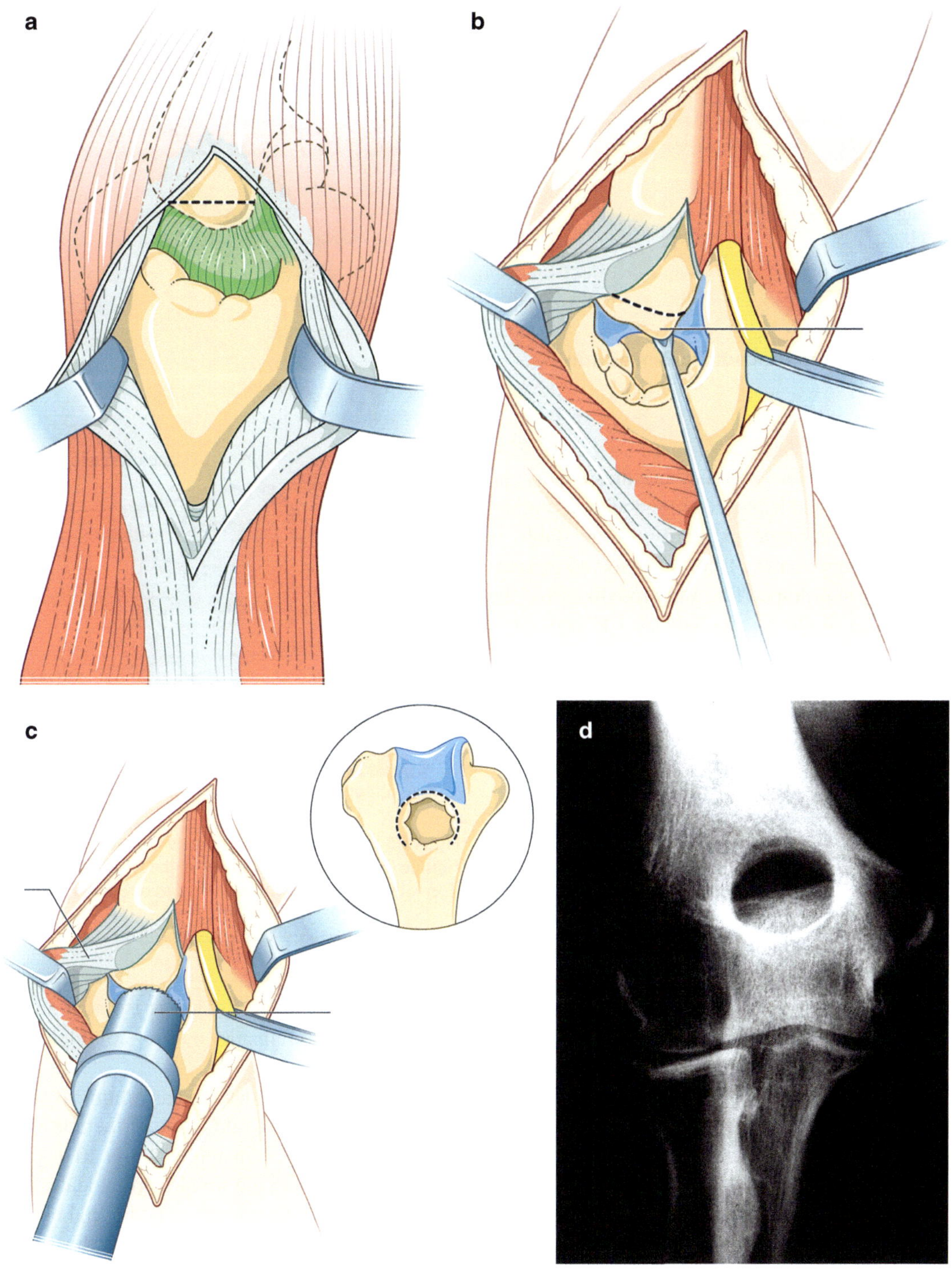

Fig. 11.3 Ulno-humeral arthroplasty: (**a**) posterior incision through the triceps; (**b**) resection of olecranon osteophytes; (**c**) fenestration of the olecranon fossa with a trephine; (**d**) radiographic results. (From: Mansat P. Arthrose du coude. EMC (Elsevier Masson SAS, Paris), Appareil locomoteur, 14-361-A-10, 2007)

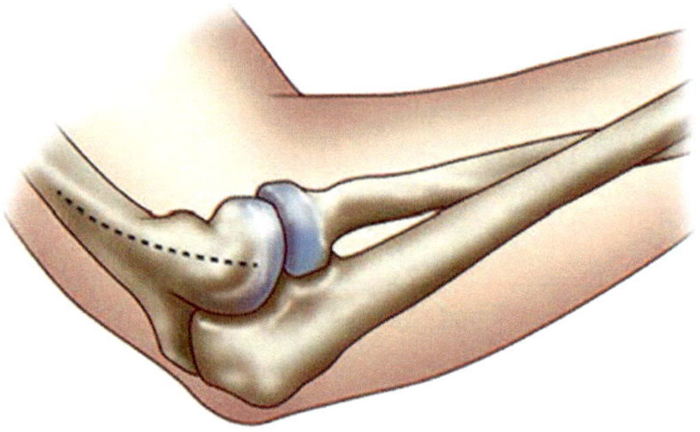

Fig. 11.4 Column procedure: lateral incision (Reproduced from S. Antuña, R. Barco (eds.), Essentials In Elbow Surgery, https://doi.org/10.1007/978-1-4471-4625-4_6, © Springer-Verlag London 2014)

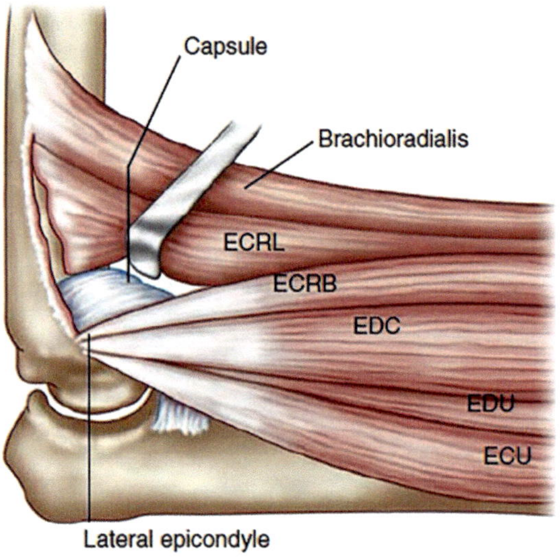

Fig. 11.5 Column procedure: exposition of the anterior capsule through a window between the ECRL and ECRB. (Reproduced from S. Antuña, R. Barco (eds.), Essentials In Elbow Surgery, https://doi.org/10.1007/978-1-4471-4625-4_6, © Springer-Verlag London 2014)

Lateral Column Procedure: Procedural Steps [51]

Positioning and Exposure

Either general or regional anesthesia may be used. The patient is placed supine with a sandbag under the ipsilateral extremity, or the table is tilted 10 degrees away from the involved extremity. The arm is draped free and brought across the chest. The proximal one-half of a Kocher incision, which extends 3 to 5 cm proximal to and 3 cm distal to the epicondyle, is used if there is no previous incision and if there are no symptoms related to the ulnar nerve (Fig. 11.4).

Exposing the Anterior Capsule

In order to release the anterior aspect of the capsule with minimum disruption of normal tissue, the fleshy origin of the extensor carpi radialis longus (ECRL) and the distal fibers of the brachioradialis are identified. Release of the origin of the ECRL and the distal fibers of the brachioradialis from the humerus using a cutting cautery provide direct access to the superolateral aspect of the capsule (Fig. 11.5). The brachialis is swept from the anterior aspect of the capsule with a periosteal elevator.

The capsule is entered at the anterior radiohumeral joint, and an assessment of the thickness of the capsule is noted. A retractor with a blade–shaft angle of 130 degrees protects the brachialis, the radial and median nerve, and the brachial artery. The anterior aspect of the capsule is grasped and excised as far medially as possible (Fig. 11.6). The most medial aspect of the capsule can sometimes be difficult to visualize but can be palpated. This is isolated and is incised from the inside out to complete the release.

The elbow is extended, and any remnant adhesion is gently lysed. At this time, if there is a full extension or if the extension is within 10 degrees of normal and there are no radiographically evident spurs on the olecranon, no additional release is needed. The capsule is left open, and the wound is closed.

Exposing the Posterior Capsule

If flexion is limited, if extension is not complete, or if posterior impingement pain is present, the

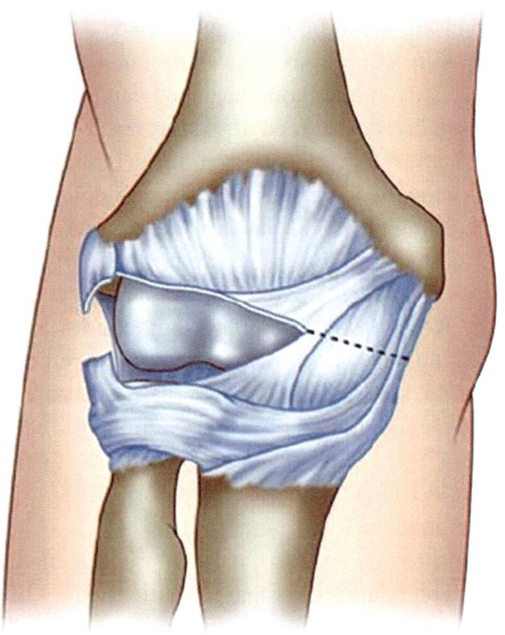

Fig. 11.6 Column procedure: excision of the anterior capsule. (Reproduced from S. Antuña, R. Barco (eds.), Essentials In Elbow Surgery, https://doi.org/10.1007/978-1-4471-4625-4_6, © Springer-Verlag London 2014)

posterior column is exposed. The triceps is elevated from the posterior aspect of the humerus along with the humeral attachment of the anconeus. The posterior aspect of the capsule is released, and the olecranon fossa is cleaned of soft tissue. The tip of the olecranon is removed with an osteotome if there are osteophytes. A high-speed burr can be useful to remove anterior and/or posterior humeral osteophytes. The amount of flexion and extension of the elbow is assessed. Typically, full extension is readily attained. If there are at least 130 degrees of flexion, nothing more needs to be done posteriorly. If flexion is limited, the coronoid is inspected and any osteophytes are removed.

If any of the concerns with the ulnar nerve are present, the ulnar nerve is inspected. It is decompressed or translocated. If simply decompressed, the stability of the nerve in the cubital tunnel is assessed through the full arc of flexion and extension.

Medial Column Procedure: Procedural Steps [52]

If a medial approach is chosen, the same steps are described on the medial side.

Approach

The skin incision may be a posterior skin incision or a midline medial one. The key to this exposure is the identification of the medial supracondylar ridge of the humerus. At this level, the surgeon can locate the medial intermuscular septum, the origin of the flexor–pronator muscle mass, and the ulnar nerve.

Exposing the Ulnar Nerve and the Medial Fascia

Once the medial intermuscular septum is identified, the medial antebrachial cutaneous nerve is identified, traced distally, and protected. If previously anterior transposition was performed, the ulnar nerve should be fully identified and mobilized before proceeding.

Exposing the Anterior Capsule for Excision and Incision

The septum is excised from the insertion on the supracondylar ridge to the proximal extent of the wound, usually about 5 to 8 cm. Many of the veins and perforating arteries at the most distal portion of the septum require cauterization. Once the septum has been excised, the flexor–pronator muscle mass should be divided parallel to the fibers, leaving roughly a 1.5-cm span of flexor carpi ulnaris tendon attached to the epicondyle.

The surgeon then returns the supracondylar ridge and begins elevating the anterior muscle with a Cobb elevator. Subperiosteally, the anterior structures of the distal humeral region proximal to the capsule are elevated to allow the placement of a wide Bennett retractor. As the elevator moves from medial to lateral, the handle of the elevator is lifted carefully, keeping the blade of the elevator along the surface of the bone (Fig. 11.7).

Once the Bennett retractor is in place and the medial portion of the flexor–pronator has been incised, the plane between muscle and capsule

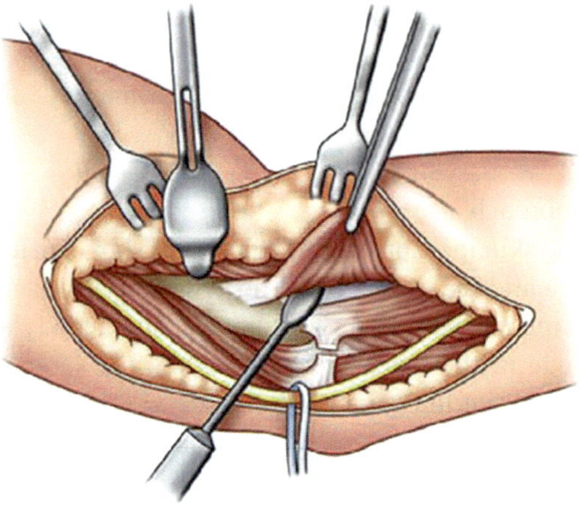

Fig. 11.7 Exposition of the anterior capsule through a medial approach after elevation of the anterior muscles. (Reproduced from S. Antuña, R. Barco (eds.), Essentials In Elbow Surgery, https://doi.org/10.1007/978-1-4471-4625-4_6, © Springer-Verlag London 2014)

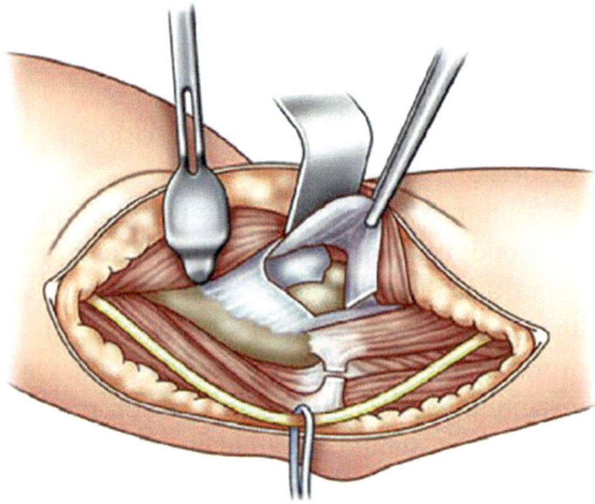

Fig. 11.8 Excision of the anterior capsule through a medial approach. (Reproduced from S. Antuña, R. Barco (eds.), Essentials In Elbow Surgery, https://doi.org/10.1007/978-1-4471-4625-4_6, © Springer-Verlag London 2014)

should be carefully elevated. As this plane is developed, the brachialis muscle is encountered from the underside. This muscle should be kept anterior and elevated from the capsule and anterior surface of the distal humerus.

The anterior capsule should be excised (Fig. 11.8) to the extent that it is practical and safe. It is helpful first to incise the capsule from the medial to the lateral aspect along the anterior surface of the joint. Once this edge of the capsule is incised, it can be lifted and excised as far distally as is safe. From this vantage, and after capsule excision, the radial head and capitellum can be visualized and freed of scar, as needed.

In cases of primary osteoarthritis of the elbow, removing the large spur from the coronoid is crucial. Using the Cobb elevator, the brachialis muscle can be elevated anteriorly for 2 cm from the coronoid process. With the elevator held in position, protecting the brachialis but anterior to the coronoid, the large osteophyte can be removed with an osteotome. The brachialis insertion is well distal to the tip of the coronoid.

Exposing and Excising the Posterior Capsule and Bone Spurs

The posterior capsule of the joint is exposed. The supracondylar ridge is again identified (Fig. 11.9). Using the Cobb elevator, the triceps is elevated from the posterior distal surface of the humerus. The exposure should extend far enough proximal to permit the use of a Bennett retractor. The posterior capsule can be separated from the triceps as the elevator sweeps from proximal to distal. The posterior medial joint line should also be identified, as it is often involved by osteophytes or heterotopic bone. In contracture release and in primary osteoarthritis, the tip of the olecranon usually must be excised to achieve full extension. The posteromedial joint line is easily visualized, but the posterolateral side must also be carefully palpated to ensure clearance. In case of persistent of flexion deficit, release of the posterior band of the medial collateral ligament can give some more degrees of motion to achieve full flexion. Kamineni et al. demonstrated the need for economical resection of the slope medial aspect of the olecranon in osteoarthritis in throwing sportsmen, with excess resection of the posteromedial osteophyte being a source of instability for the elbow [53]. Several studies have made it possible to evaluate the results of humero-ulnar arthroplasty at medium and long-term follow-up [31, 33–35, 54]. Wada et al. [35] reported 85% satisfactory results on 33 elbows followed for an average of 121 months. Phillips in another study also found 85% satisfactory results according to the

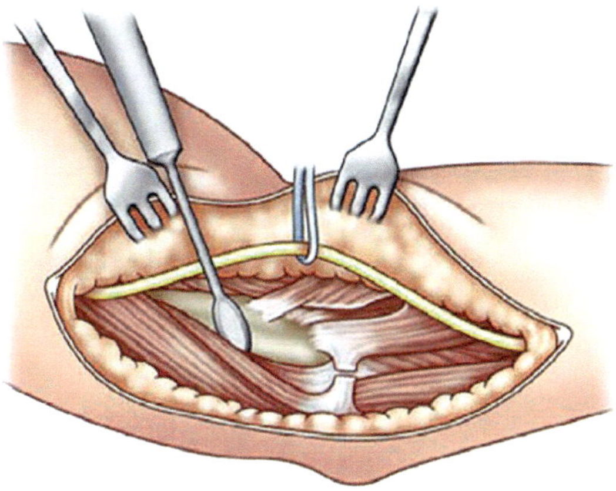

Fig. 11.9 Exposition and excision of the posterior capsule and spurs through a medial approach. (Reproduced from S. Antuña, R. Barco (eds.), Essentials In Elbow Surgery, https://doi.org/10.1007/978-1-4471-4625-4_6, © Springer-Verlag London 2014)

DASH score (Disability Arm Shoulder Hand score) and the MEPS (Mayo Elbow Performance Score) on 20 treated elbows [54]. Antuna et al. found 34 satisfactory results out of 46 at 18 months of follow-up [31]. The intervention usually allows the suppression of pain in most cases [31, 34, 35]. Wada et al. noted that 76% of patients who performed heavy work before the intervention were able to resume their activity [35]. Motion gains have been variable and less reproducible with a tendency to recurrence of stiffness and especially the loss of extension. Some advocate systematic anterior capsulectomy when there is a loss of extension greater than 20° or when the stiffness is the predominant symptom. Despite these clinical successes, radiographic signs of recurrence with filling of the fossae could be noted in 10 of the 20 operated elbows [54, 55]. It seems that this rate of recurrence increases with follow-up [31, 35]. However, there is no real radio-clinical correlation, the radiographic signs are not associated with recurrence of stiffness or the onset of pain. Forster et al. [32] defined the predictors of the Outerbridge-Kashiwagi procedure: the intensity of the preoperative pain, the existence of preoperative compression of the ulnar nerve, and a duration of evolution less than 2 years are good prognostic factors. The final result seems independent of the etiology (in particular trauma), and preoperative range of motion. Postoperative ulnar nerve damage is not uncommon [31, 34, 35]. Antuna et al. reported an incidence up to 28% after the performance of humero-ulnar arthroplasty, six patients requiring revision surgery for neurolysis [31]. These authors recommend carrying out an associated neurolysis with or without anterior transposition when there is a symptomatology preoperatively or when the flexion does not exceed 100°, and when we expect to recover 30° to 40° in this range of motion. Ulnar nerve involvement was noted in two patients who have benefited from manipulation of the elbow under anesthesia for stiffness that recurred 8 weeks after surgical release. Manipulation under anesthesia is therefore not recommended in case of recurrence of stiffness if the patient has not previously benefited from an anterior transposition of the ulnar nerve [31]. The use of adjustable static splint is recommended by some [55]. The concept is based on the postural elongation of the capsule allowing gain of motion.

Extensive Arthrolysis with Tissue Interposition

When joint damage is extensive, with destruction of the cartilage, a simple release with joint debridement is no longer sufficient. In young subjects, tissue interposition may be the indication of choice, with elbow prostheses being reserved for older patients. The technique consists of an extensive lateral approach to achieve a reshaping of the articular surface, an excision of the various osteophytes, and a joint resurfacing by tissue interposition on the humeral side only, or on both articular sides. The interposing tissue can be skin, fascia lata, or Achilles tendon allografts [44, 46, 56]. The collateral ligament is repaired and the elbow is protected by an articulated external fixator for 45 days (Fig. 11.10). This technique allows more often to obtain an elbow with a functional range of motion with limited pain level. However, the main complication is represented by instability and lack of strength. This technique must therefore be compared with other therapeutic options before being offered to the patient. Cheng [44] reviewed 13

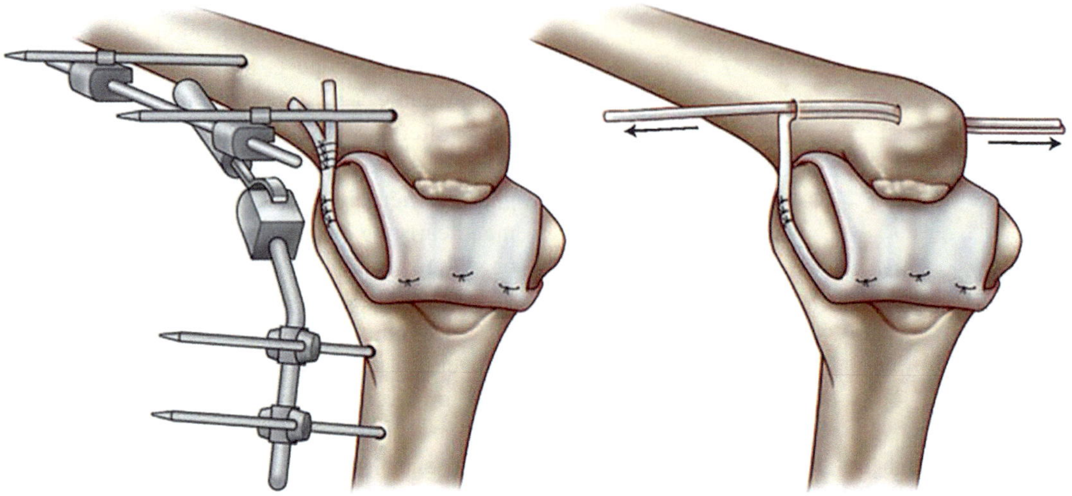

Fig. 11.10 Interposition arthroplasty with Achilles tendon interposition and external fixator. (Reproduced from S. Antuña, R. Barco (eds.), Essentials In Elbow Surgery, https://doi.org/10.1007/978-1-4471-4625-4_6, © Springer-Verlag London 2014)

patients with 63 months of follow-up; indolence was obtained in 69% of cases, with 62% satisfactory results. Eight complications were to be deplored, including four neurological impairments. The determining prognostic factor was the preoperative instability. Indeed, unstable elbows preoperatively often remained unstable postoperatively.

Radiocapitellar Hemiarthroplasty

Radiocapitellar arthritis can result from trauma or primary degenerative arthritis. In cases of previous excision of the radial head and with the increasing use of metallic radial head prostheses, radiocapitellar arthritis can be expected to be seen more frequently. Kachoeei et al. [57] reported the results in 19 cases of metallic capitellar resurfacing arthroplasty combined with metal backed, polyethylene radial head arthroplasty (i.e., radiocapitellar hemiarthroplasty). Range of motion, pain, and functional scores improved significantly from the preoperative to the final follow-up visit. According to the Mayo Elbow Performance Index outcome scores, they reported 9 excellent, 5 good, 3 fair, 0 poor, and 2 missing data. There was no pain in 11 patients, mild pain in 5, and moderate pain in 3. Radiographic assessment showed no significant progress in ulnohumeral arthritis, although 3 elbows showed osteoarthritis progression to a higher grade. There were no major complications, including infection, revision, disassembly of the components, or conversion to total elbow arthroplasty. Survival of the radio-capitellar arthroplasty was 100% (Fig. 11.11).

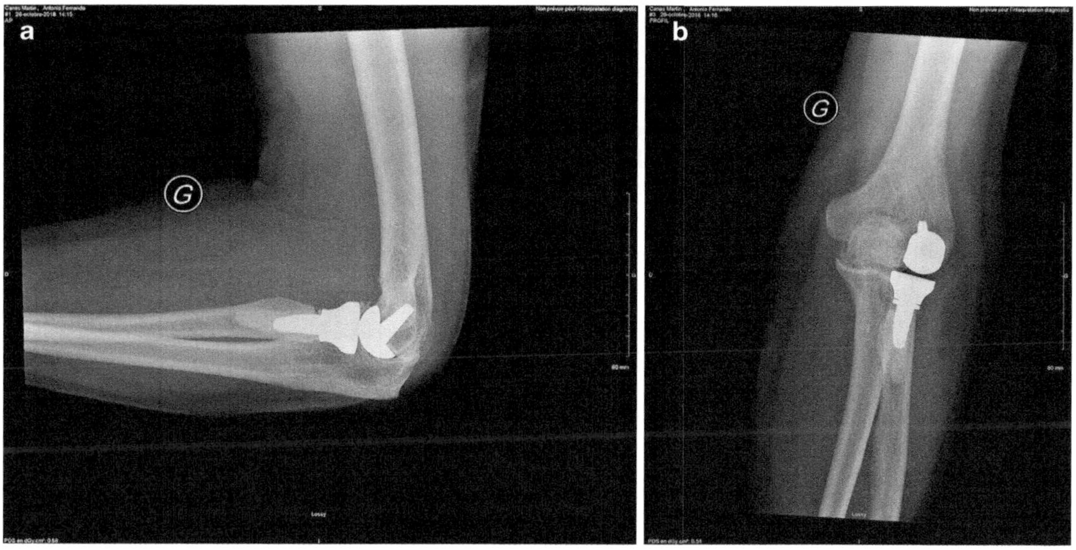

Fig. 11.11 Radiocapitellar hemiarthroplasty: (**a**) A/P view; (**b**) lateral view

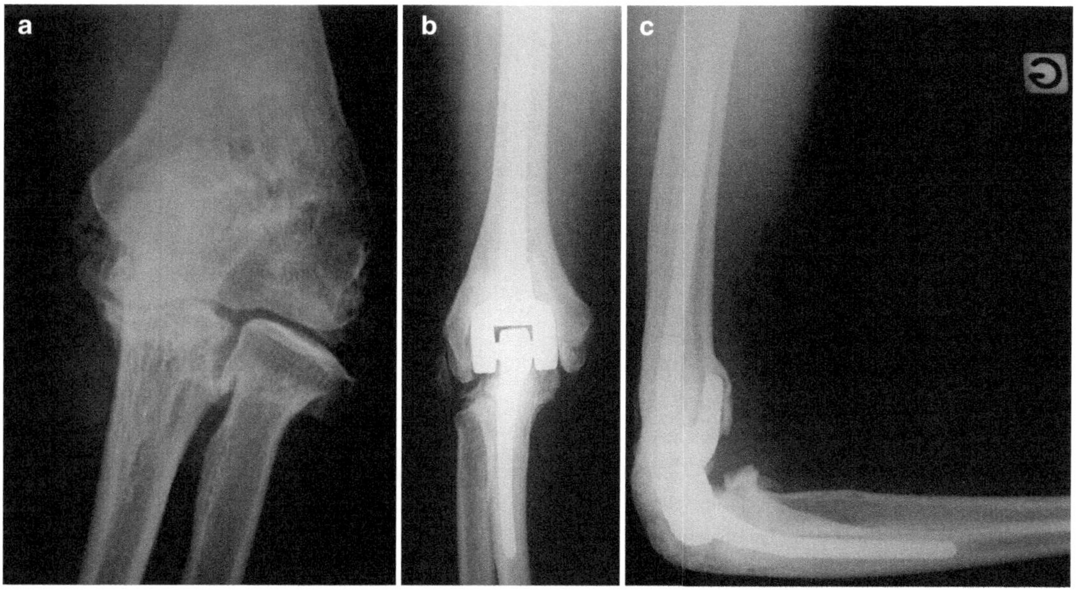

Fig. 11.12 Advanced elbow arthritis (**a**) treated with a total elbow arthroplasty (**b, c**)

Total Elbow Prostheses

The indication of total elbow prosthesis for primary osteoarthritis is uncommon. Indeed, osteoarthritis mainly affects the young and active patients with high demand. These patients are not ideal candidates for replacement arthroplasty because of the problem of longevity of the implants. However, improvements in implant designs have improved their long-term survival. Classically, the prostheses are indicated in patients over 70 with low-level activity and pain on mobilization of the elbow throughout the arc of motion, when the other therapeutic options cannot be realized (Fig. 11.12).

Most studies have included in their series of prostheses, only a few cases of primary osteoarthritis (5 out of 725). Only three studies [45, 47, 48] report a total of 34 elbows with primary osteoarthritis, treated with total elbow prosthesis (Fig. 11.6). The complications observed in these three studies were essentially of a mechanical nature with fracture of the implant, osteolysis and loosening of the prosthesis, and elbow instability. We must therefore be particularly careful before proposing this therapeutic option. In the presence of significant stiffness, the resurfacing implants are likely to be unstable given the extensive arthrolysis required for recovery joint amplitudes. The longevity of the implants therefore depends on the patient, their activity, and the surgical technique.

11.8 Indications

Treatment for elbow osteoarthritis depends on the age of the patient, his degree of activity, and the importance of the joint lesions. When it comes to peripheral osteoarthritis, often by overuse, with pain appearing only in extreme flexion and extension positions, after the failure of conservative treatment, joint cleaning with resection of osteophytes, removal of articular foreign bodies and anterior and posterior capsulectomy is the treatment of choice. Depending on the experience of the surgeon, and the importance of bone changes, procedures can be performed arthroscopically or by the column procedure. When osteoarthritis is global, with pain throughout the arc of motion, tissue interposition can be proposed in the young subject, while an elbow prosthesis can be discussed in the older subject.

References

1. An KN, Morrey BF. Biomechanics of the elbow. In: Morrey BF, editor. The elbow and its disorders. 3rd ed. WB Saunder; 2000. p. 43–60.
2. Chadwick EK, Nicol AC. Elbow and wrist joint contact forces during occupational pick and place activities. J Biomech. 2000;33:591–600.
3. Goldberg VM, Figgie HE 3rd, Inglis AE, Figgie MP. Total elbow arthroplasty. J Bone Joint Surg Am. 1988;70:778–83.
4. Goodfellow JW, Bullough PG. The pattern of ageing of the articular cartilage of the elbow joint. J Bone Joint Surg Br. 1967;49:175–81.
5. Murato H, Ikuta Y, Murakami T. Anatomic investigation of the elbow joint with specific reference to aging of the articular cartilage. J Shoulder Elbow Surg. 1993;2:175–81.
6. Tsuge K, Mizuseki T. Debridement arthroplasty for advanced primary osteoarthritis of the elbow. Results of a new technique used for 29 elbows. J Bone Joint Surg Br. 1994;76:641–6.
7. Suvarna SK, Stanley D. The histologic changes of the olecranon fossa membrane in primary osteoarthritis of the elbow. J Shoulder Elbow Surg. 2004;13:555–7.
8. Lawrence JS. Rheumatism in coal miners. III. Occupational factors. Br J Ind Med. 1955;12:249–61.
9. Mintz G, Fraga A. Severe osteoarthritis of the elbow in foundry workers. Arch Environ Health. 1973;27:78–80.
10. Ortner DJ. Description and classification of degenerative bone changes in the distal joint surface of the humerus. Am J Phys Anthrop. 1968;28:139.
11. Minami NM. Roentgenological studies of osteoarthritis of the elbow joint. Jpn Orthop Assoc. 1977;51:1223–36.
12. Kashiwagi D. Intra-articular changes of the osteoarthritic elbow, especially about the fossa olecrani. Jpn Orthop Assoc. 1978;52:1367–82.
13. Rostock P. Gelenkschaden durch arbeiten mit presluftwerkzeugen und andere schwere. Roperliche Arbeit Medizinische Klinik. 1936;11:341–3.
14. Hunter D, McLaughlin A, Perry K. Clinical effects of the use of pneumatic tools. Br J Indust Med. 1945;2:10–6.
15. Stanley D. Prevalence and etiology of symptomatic elbow osteoarthritis. J Shoulder Elbow Surg. 1994;3:386–9.
16. Carter DR, Beaupré GS, Wong M, Smith RL, Andriacchi TP, Schurman DJ. The mechanobiology of articular cartilage development and degeneration. Clin Orthop. 2004;427S:69–77.
17. Huskisson EC, Dieppe PA, Tucker AK, Cannell LB. Another look at osteoarthritis. Ann Rheum Dis. 1979;38:423.
18. Doherty M, Preston B. Primary osteoarthritis of the elbow. Ann Rheum Dis. 1989;48:743–7.
19. Doherty M, Watt I, Dieppe PA. Influence of primary generalized osteoarthritis on development of secondary osteoarthritis. Lancet. 1983;2:8.
20. Minami M, Kato S, Kashiwagi D. Outerbridge-Kashiwagi's method for arthroplasty of osteoarthritis of the elbow: 44 elbows followed for 8–16 years. J Orthop Sci. 1996;1:11.
21. Morrey BF. Primary arthritis of the elbow treated by ulno-humeral arthroplasty. J Bone Joint Surg Br. 1992;74:409–13.

22. Bauer M, Jonsson K, Josefsson PO, Linden B. Osteochondritis dissecans of the elbow. A long-term follow-up study. Clin Orthop. 1992;284:156–60.
23. Bennett JB, Green MS, Tullos HS. Surgical management of chronic medial elbow instability. Clin Orthop. 1992;278:62–8.
24. Mueller T, Barthel T, Cramer A, Werner A, Gohlke F. Primary synovial chondromatosis of the elbow. J Shoulder Elbow Surg. 2000;9:319–22.
25. Schmitt H, Hansmann HJ, Brocai DR, Loew M. Long-term changes of the throwing arm of former elite javelin throwers. Int J Sports Med. 2001;22:275–9.
26. Takahara M, Ogino T, Sasaki I, Kato H, Minami A, Kaneda K. Long-term outcome of osteochondritis dissecans of the humeral capitellum. Clin Orthop. 1999;363:108–15.
27. Young S, Letts M, Jarvis J. Avascular necrosis of the radial head in children. J Pediatr Orthop. 2000;20:15–8.
28. Sanchez-Sotelo J, O'Driscoll SW, Morrey BF. Medial oblique compression fracture of the coronoid process of the ulna. J Shoulder Elbow Surg. 2005;14:60–4.
29. Klekamp J, Green NE, Mencio GA. Osteochondritis dissecans as a cause of developmental dislocation of the radial head. Clin Orthop. 1997;338:36–41.
30. Wilson FD, Andrews JR, Blackburn TA, McCluskey G. Valgus extension overload in the pitching elbow. Am J Sports Med. 1983;11:83–8.
31. Antuna SA, Morrey BF, Adams RA, O'Driscoll SW. Ulnohumeral arthroplasty for primary degenerative arthritis of the elbow: long-term outcome and complications. J Bone Joint Surg Am. 2002;84:2168–73.
32. Forster MC, Clark DI, Lunn PG. Elbow osteoarthritis: prognostic indicators in ulnohumeral debridement—the Outerbridge-Kashiwagi procedure. J Shoulder Elbow Surg. 2001;10:557–60.
33. Oka Y. Debidement arthroplasty for osteoarthritis of the elbow: 50 patients followed mean 5 years. Acta Orthop Scand. 2000;71:185–90.
34. Oka Y, Ohta K, Saitoh I. Debridement arthroplasty for osteoarthritis of the elbow. Clin Orthop. 1998;351:127–34.
35. Wada T, Isogai S, Ishii S, Yamashita T. Debridement arthroplasty for primary osteoarthritis of the elbow. J Bone Joint Surg Am. 2004;86:233–41.
36. O'Driscoll SW, Morrey BF. Arthroscopy of the elbow. Diagnostic and therapeutic benefits and hazards. J Bone Joint Surg Am. 1992;74:84–94.
37. Dalal S, Bull M, Stanley D. Radiographic changes at the elbow in primary osteoarthritis: a comparison with normal aging of the elbow joint. J Shoulder Elbow Surg. 2007;16(3):358–61.
38. Ward WG, Belhobek GH, Anderson TE. Arthroscopic elbow findings: correlation with preoperative radiographic studies. Arthroscopy. 1992;8:498–502.
39. Morrey BF. Primary degenerative arthritis of the elbow: ulnohumeral arthroplasty. In: Morrey BF, editor. The elbow and its disorders. 3rd ed. WB Saunder; 2000. p. 799–808.
40. Van Brakel RW, Eygendaal D. Intra-articular injection of hyaluronic acid is not effective for the treatment of post-traumatic osteoarthritis of the elbow. Arthroscopy. 2006;22:1199–203.
41. Gramstad GD, Galatz LM. Management of elbow osteoarthritis. J Bone Joint Surg Am. 2006;88:421–30.
42. Doorberg JN, Ring D, Jupiter JB. Static progressive splinting for posttraumatic elbow stiffness. J Orthop Trauma. 2006;20:400–4.
43. Mansat P, Morrey BF. The column procedure: a limited lateral approach for extrinsic contracture of the elbow. J Bone Joint Surg Am. 1998;80:1603–15.
44. Cheng SL, Morrey BF. Treatment of the mobile, painful arthritic elbow by distraction interposition arthroplasty. J Bone Joint Surg Br. 2000;82:233–8.
45. Espag MP, Back DL, Clark DI, Lunn PG. Early results of the Souter-Strathclyde unlinked total elbow arthroplasty in patients with osteoarthritis. J Bone Joint Surg Br. 2003;85:351–3.
46. Hausman MR, Birnbaum PS. Interposition elbow arthroplasty. Technol Hand Upper Extr Surg. 2004;8:181–8.
47. Kozak K, Adams RA, Morrey BF. Total elbow arthroplasty in primary degenerative osteoarthritis of the elbow. J Arthroplasty. 1998;13:837–42.
48. Schoch BS, Werthel JD, Sánchez-Sotelo J, Morrey BF, Morrey M. Total elbow arthroplasty for primary osteoarthritis. J Shoulder Elbow Surg. 2017;26(8):1355–9. https://doi.org/10.1016/j.jse.2017.04.003.
49. Morrey BF. Post-traumatic contracture of the elbow. Operative treatment, including distraction arthroplasty. J Bone Joint Surg Am. 1990;72:601–18.
50. Mansat P, Morrey BF. Extrinsic contracture: lateral and medial column procedures. In: Morrey BF, editor. The elbow and its disorders. 4th ed. Saunders/Elsevier; 2009. p. 487–98.
51. Morrey B, Mansat P. Capsular release for flexion contracture: the column procedure. In: Morrey BF, editor. Master techniques in orthopaedic surgery. 3rd ed. Wolters Kluwer; 2015. p. 243–51.
52. Mansat P, André A, Bonnevialle N. Extrinsic contracture release: medial "over the top" approach. In: Wiesel S, editor. Operative techniques in orthopaedic surgery, vol. 3. Wolters Kluwer/Lippincott Williams & Wilkins; 2010. p. 3413–9.
53. Kamineni S, ElAttrache NS, O'Driscoll SW, Ahmad CS, Hirohara H, Neale PG, An KN, Morrey BF. Medial collateral ligament strain with partial posteromedial olecranon resection. A biomechanical study. J Bone Joint Surg Am. 2004;86:2424–30.
54. Phillips NJ, Ali A, Stanley D. Treatment of primary degenerative arthritis of the elbow by ulnohumeral arthroplasty: a long-term follow-up. J Bone Joint Surg Br. 2003;85:347–50.
55. Morrey BF. Splints and bracing at the elbow. In: Morrey BF, editor. The elbow and its disorders. 3rd ed. WB Saunder Company; 2000. p. 150–4.
56. Larson AN, Morrey BF. Interposition arthroplasty with an Achilles tendon allograft as a sal-

vage procedure for the elbow. J Bone Joint Surg Am. 2008;90(12):2714–23. https://doi.org/10.2106/JBJS.G.00768.

57. Kachooei AR, Heesakkers NAM, Heijink A, The B, Eygendaal D. Radiocapitellar prosthetic arthroplasty: short-term to midterm results of 19 elbows. J Shoulder Elbow Surg. 2018;27(4):726–32. https://doi.org/10.1016/j.jse.2017.12.013.

Arthroscopic Management of Stiff Elbow

12

G. Cataldo, A. F. Cheli, G. Caldarera, L. Pederzini, and A. Celli

12.1 Introduction

Elbow osteoarthritis is a degenerative condition that affects about 2% of the population. It can be classified into primary and secondary. The primary form, sometimes idiopathic, is most frequently observed in individuals who participate in competitive sports or repetitive manual labour. It is most commonly observed in the dominant arm and in the male sex. Risk factors include genetic predisposition, osteoarticular malalignment, aging, recurrent microtrauma, excessive loading, laxity and dysplasia. Secondary arthrosis most commonly arises from post-traumatic injuries such as fracture–luxations resulting in ossification disorders. In a minority of cases, it is related to other causes such as rheumatoid arthritis, haemophilia, osteochondritis dissecans and osteochondromatosis.

Despite the aforementioned partition, typical radiological and clinical findings, as well as treatment options do not present relevant differences in the two groups.

Although initial treatment is usually nonsurgical, OA often progresses and has historically been managed with an open surgery approach. In recent years, however, there has been increasing use of arthroscopy, which in selected cases has shown comparable or better results than similar open procedures.

Unlike other joints, such as the hip and knee, the clinical presentation of osteoarthritis of the elbow revolves around the presence of osteophytes, capsule retraction and the formation of loose bodies, rather than a narrowing of the joint space [1]. The osteophytes responsible for the typical symptomatology of osteoarthritis, as described in the study by YW Lim et al. [2], is mainly located in the ulnohumeral joint (with the highest percentage in the anterocoronoid region, 95%), followed by the anterior (23%) and posterior (27%) humeroradialis compartments; these data challenge the conventional belief (supported by previous studies on cadaveric elbow specimens whose joints were not necessarily symptomatic [3]) that elbow arthritis progresses from the radiohumeral joint to the ulnohumeral joint.

12.2 Biomechanics

The elbow muscles can generate high joint reactive forces during loading, while the contact zone is relatively small: due to this condition, the force developed on the articular surface during elbow

G. Cataldo · A. F. Cheli · G. Caldarera
Orthopaedic Unit, New Civil Sassuolo Hospital, Modena, Italy

L. Pederzini (✉)
Department of Orthopedics, Hesperia Hospital, Modena, Italy

A. Celli
Orthopaedic Unit, Hesperia Hospital, Modena, Italy

L. Pederzini et al. (eds.), *Stiffness of the Elbow, Wrist and Related Pathologies*,
https://doi.org/10.1007/978-3-031-81381-8_12

movement is relatively high, especially during axial loading. Repeated excessive loading leads to cartilage fragmentation, with subsequent production of intra-articular loose bodies and the formation of osteophytes [4].

When the elbow is flexed, the forearm axis changes from valgus to varus; simultaneously, the varus-valgus laxity of this particular joint allows the radial head to rise relative to the capitellum when applying varus pressure. Therefore, when the elbow reaches its functional position (which is flexion more often than extension), the radial head rises and 93% of the axial force is conveyed to the ulna [5]; the medial ulnohumeral compartment (where osteophytes usually occur first) is then subjected to greater mechanical stress. While this is more likely to occur in OA secondary to prolonged hard work or sport, the lateral portion of ulnohumeral joint is rarely affected in primary OA: the bony architecture of this articular structure has a high degree of congruity, which preserves the articular cartilage until the final stage of OA [6].

The presence of peripheral osteophytes is clinically manifested by pain and stiffness. Pain is reported from the early stages of the disease, especially during terminal flexion–extension movements; it is caused by the impingement of the osteophytes on the coronoid and olecranon fossae. Stiffness is the result of osteophyte growth into a space-occupying lesion, leading to secondary capsular contracture.

Secondary OA can also result from direct cartilage damage, fractures malunions or persistent elbow instability, which causes biomechanical changes with increasing cartilage loss. Repetitive hyperextension of the lateral elbow in overhead throwing athletes can cause laxity of the medial elbow, resulting in typical posteromedial osteophytes and loose bodies: the humeroradial compartment shows early radiographic degeneration because it is exposed to maximum load.

Degeneration is mainly localised near the posteromedial radial head and the crest separating the trochlea from the capitellum. The posteromedial ulnohumeral joint is often subsequently affected.

12.3 Pathoanatomy

Inflammatory mechanism is involved in primary OA of the elbow. Joint damage can be triggered by a variety of factors or conditions, such as ageing, obesity and genetic predisposition, leading to a vicious cycle of chronic local inflammation that progressively leads to OA. The inflammatory mediators involved include cytokines (such as TNF-α, IL1-β, IL-6), growth factors, chemokines, prostaglandins, leukotrienes and adipokines. If the inflammatory cascade is not contained, it can lead to chondrocyte hypertrophy, apoptosis, loss of intra-articular homeostasis and ultimately clinical OA.

12.4 Physical Examination

Typical symptoms of elbow OA are joint stiffness and pain with maximal flexion and extension; pain manifests strongly on maximal extension and is related to the conflict created by the presence of osteophytes, mainly in the fossa of the olecranon; the pain involves the entire range of motion only in more advanced forms.

Rest pain is rare and often due to the inflammatory state.

In advanced stages, crepitus and joint locking may also be present. Symptomatic ulnar neuropathy can be reported in 26–55% of patients [1].

Clinical examination should always include assessment of 'articular range of movement and stability, as well as the presence of joint block and crackling sensation.

12.5 Imaging

Radiographs are usually sufficient for the diagnosis of elbow OA. According to Dalal [7], the most important radiological aspects are a well-preserved humeroulnar joint line, intra-articular loose bodies and osteophytes, especially in the anterior coronoid surface and the medial compartment of the humeroulnar joint [2]. Joint space narrowing may not be relevant or indicative of the diagnosis or severity of OA, even in the later stages of the disease. Loose bodies are absent on plain radiographs in 30% of cases, especially when located in the posterior elbow and proximal radio-ulnar joints. The absence of gross osteophytes and the presence of joint narrowing suggest inflammatory arthritis.

CT scans and 3-dimensional reconstructions are highly recommended for surgical planning and are useful in diffuse degenerative disease or difficult post-traumatic deformity.

12.6 Classifications

The main radiological classifications for elbow OA are those proposed by Broberg and Morrey (BM) and Hastings and Rettig (HR). The BM system is usually used for post-traumatic OA; it is based on osteophyte formation and joint space narrowing and can be summarised as follows: grade 1: mild joint space narrowing with minimal osteophyte formation; grade 2: moderate joint space narrowing with moderate osteophyte formation; grade 3: severe degenerative change with severe joint destruction. The HR system is used for primary OA and is based on the presence of subluxation and involvement of the radiocapitellar joint: Class I: degeneration of the margins of the ulnotrochlear joint with the presence of coronoid and olecranon spurs; absence of degenerative changes within the radiocapitellar joint; Class II: Class I with mild narrowing of the joint space within the radiocapitellar joint without subluxation of the radial head; Class III: Class II with radiocapitellar subluxation.

Both of these systems have shown good reliability in grading the severity of elbow OA; however, no substantial superiority of one system over the other has been demonstrated [8].

Another reliable system is the Hastings and Graham (HG) classification [9], which classifies OA according to its functional impact on elbow ROM. Class I of the HG system indicates the presence of H.O. without limitation; class II subdivides according to functional limitation of the elbow (IIA, limited flexion–extension; IIB, limited pronation-supination; II C, limitation in both planes); class III represents radiographic and functional ankylosis (IIIA, ankylosis in flexion–extension; III B, ankylosis in pronation-supination; III C, ankylosis in both planes).

12.7 Conservative Treatment

In the early stages of the pathology, symptoms are treated with non-steroidal anti-inflammatory drugs (NSAIDs), immobilisation with braces, injections (glucocorticoids or viscosupplementation) and physiotherapy. The rehabilitation process aims to restore and maintain the range of motion (ROM) of the elbow, increase stability and protect the joint from any mechanical stress during daily activities. For athletes, treatment options also include physiotherapy, strengthening of the flexor and pronator muscles and platelet-rich plasma (PRP) injections.

12.8 Surgical Options

In the advanced stages of the disease, when pain and joint stiffness do not respond to conservative treatment, there is an indication for surgical treatment.

Surgical options can be divided into two main categories: arthroscopic, usually used in early stages of OA and in younger patients, and open.

Overall, the treatment options are as follows:

1. Arthroscopic capsular release/loose bodies and osteophytes removal
2. Open capsular release
3. Debridement of the arthroplasty
4. Arthroplasty with distraction interposition
5. Replacement arthroplasty

A more complete description of these options and their indications is presented in Table 12.1.

Table 12.1 The OA process produces an **elbow stiffness** with variable presentation. The aim of the table is to subdivide this process into main patterns and to summarise their principal treatment options

Elbow stiffness	Main injury	Associated lesions	Functional limitations	Treatment options
Grade 1	Contracture of soft tissue	– Capsular/ ligaments contracture – Tendon/muscle contraction	Flexion: – Posterior capsule – Posterior band of LCM Extension: – Anterior capsule – Anterior band of LCM Flexion–extension: – Anterior and posterior capsule – LCL, posterior band of LCM	**Rehabilitation program** **Surgical release:** – Arthroscopic – Open limited approach
Grade 2	*HO*: – Limited areas (medial, lateral, anterior or posterior) – Myositis ossificans – Bone bridge – Ankylosis	Contracture of soft tissue	According to HG classification IIA: limited Flexion–extension IIB: limited Pronation–supination IIC: limited on Both planes III: Ankylosis	**Arthroscopic surgery:** – Class II with minor HO **Open surgery:** – Limited approach (class II): HO excision – Extensile approach (class III): bone bridge excision
Grade 3	Limited cartilage damage: – Less than 50% of articular surface – Articular marginal bone deformity – Osteophytes Extensive cartilage damage: – More than 50% of articular surface – Major bone deformity – Instability	– Contracture of soft tissue – HO	Severe functional impairment	**Limited cartilage damage:** Limited debridement: – Arthroscopic – Kashiwagi's procedure Extensile debridement: – Tsuge's procedure **Extensive cartilage damage:** – Interposition arthroplasty – Replacement arthroplasty

12.9 Arthroscopic Capsular Release

Arthroscopic treatment is used in cases of mild to moderate elbow osteoarthritis with pain at the maximum range of motion and stiffness caused by loose bodies, osteophytes and capsule retraction.

The main indications are the removal of loose bodies (following trauma, OCD or synovial chondromatosis), removal of symptomatic osteophytes in the early stages of OA, and stiffness as the main symptom in non-traumatic conditions (e.g. inflammatory disease, synovitis or loose bodies) or post-traumatic conditions.

Contraindications include severe joint deformity, advanced arthritis, previous elbow surgery that may complicate arthroscopy, and uncertain anatomy or possible ulnar nerve instability [10]. In addition, arthroscopic debridement appears to be less successful than open surgery when the flexion–extension arc is less than 90° [11].

Several predictive factors regarding the outcome of arthroscopic debridement for elbow OA have been described in the literature. Men tend to show greater improvements in pain reduction and strength gain than women. Manual workers report greater improvements in functional scores, pain and strength. On the other hand, occupational injury/illness status correlates with poorer satisfaction and outcomes.

12.10 Operative Technique

After appropriate induction of endotracheal general anaesthesia and placement of a perineural catheter for post-operative pain management—the anaesthetic is injected at the end of surgery after assessment of nerve integrity—the patient is placed in the prone position on the operating table. The shoulder is abducted to 90° and the arm is flexed to 90°, supported by a frame parallel to the operating table. It is essential that the surgeon assesses the ROM and stability of the elbow before starting.

A non-sterile tourniquet is applied to the upper arm outside the operating field and inflated to 250 mmHg.

After preparing a sterile field, all bony landmarks and arthroscopic portals (posterior, superior anteromedial and superior anterolateral) are marked with a marker.

After locating the soft spot, an 18-gauge needle is inserted in the centre of the triangular area bounded by the lateral epicondyle, radial head and olecranon—and approximately 20–30 mL of sterile saline is insufflated to distend the joint space.

Insufflation expands the joint capsule and safely moves the neurovascular structures to a more anterior position. The joint is inflated by a pump at 35–50 mmHg throughout the procedure. Three posterior and two anterior portals are used throughout.

We start the procedure by creating a posterolateral portal.

The second portal is created 1.5 cm proximal to the previous one. The use of these portals ensures that the joint field can be observed and posterior pathologies can be treated with special instruments. After a complete posterior view of the proximal radio-ulnar joint, the surgeon creates the final posterior portal corresponding to the olecranon fossa, adjacent to the medial edge of the triceps, 2–3 cm proximal to the tip of the olecranon. This allows complete debridement of the olecranon fossa and its lateral surface (Fig. 12.1a).

The arthroscope position is then changed to the straight posterior portal and the posterior compartment is once again explored.

The size and location of the osteophytes are the key indicators to determine the best medial approach, with care taken to preserve the ulnar nerve. If they are small, they are removed arthroscopically, protecting the ulnar nerve, using a retractor inserted through an accessory subcutaneous portal posterior to the nerve. If they are large, it is advisable to resect them through a small arthrotomy in the final stage of the technique to avoid extravasation of fluid during arthroscopy.

In stiff elbows, ulnar neurolysis is highly recommended before the medial approach: in this situation, the nerve may be overstretched during intraoperative flexion–extension and during the following physiotherapy. The superior anteromedial portal (2 cm anterior and 2 cm distal to the medial epicondyle) is then created to examine the anterior compartment; the medial antebrachial cutaneous nerve may be injured during the procedure. The antero-lateral portal is then created using an inside–out technique: a Wissinger rod is inserted 3 cm proximally and 2 cm anteriorly to the lateral epicondyle and a plastic cannula is inserted through the rod, which is then removed; care must be taken due to the proximity of the radial nerve, the posterior antebrachial cutaneous nerve and the posterior interosseous nerve; the inside–out technique reduces the risk of nerve damage [10]. The cannula is required for shaver insertion and subsequent anterior debridement; these portals allow visualisation of the anterior trochlea, capitellum, coronoid process and fossa, radiocapitellar and ulnohumeral joints.

Anterior capsulectomy may be necessary, especially in secondary post-traumatic OA characterised by the presence of a thick capsule. Anterior capsulectomy is performed with basket forceps 1 cm proximal to the apex of the coronoid, first from lateral to medial and then in the

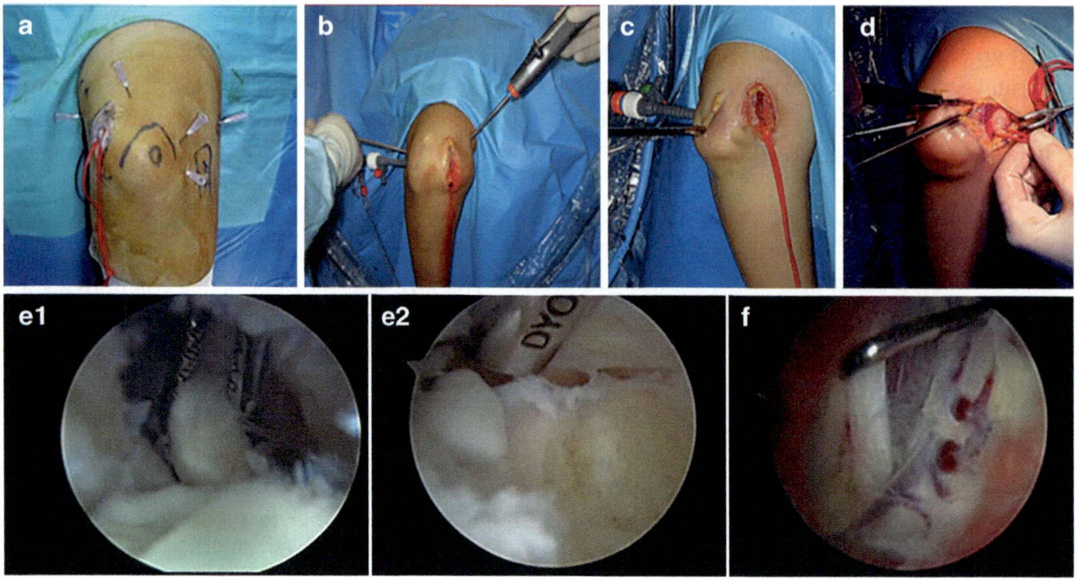

Fig. 12.1 Elbow arthroscopy is a suitable option for stiff elbow with mild OA and minor H.O. (**a**) five portals are commonly used (three posterior and two anterior); (**b**) ulnar nerve assessment if mandatory before surgery: if any neuropathy sign is present or in case of a limited preoperative flexion (under 100°), ulnar nerve release is highly recommended. This also helps to protect the nerve and work safely in the posteromedial compartment; (**c**) intra-articular loose bodies can be removed with forceps; (**d**) olecranon spurs can be removed and olecranon fossa can be re-shaped with a shaver or burr; (**e**) after complete and careful anterolateral capsulectomy the posterior interosseous nerve can be seen (**e1**, **e2**, **f**)

opposite direction; this procedure can also be performed with radiofrequency. After the anterior capsulectomy, the branch of the radial nerve can be observed: this is important in the treatment of radial head problems in order to avoid neurological complications.

At the end of the technique, one or two drains are placed, the portals are sutured and the elbow is immobilised in a splint in various positions depending on the preoperative ROM limitation, usually in extension [1, 12].

12.10.1 Management of Nerves

According to Wada, 25–50% of patients with elbow OA have evidence of ulnar neuropathy [8].

It is necessary to perform ulnar neurolysis prior to arthroscopy in the following cases.

1. Preoperative flexion of less than 100°
2. Post-traumatic OA or previous surgery
3. Patient with preoperative ulnar nerve symptoms

To avoid injury to the posterior interosseous nerve, it is advisable to use an inside–out technique with an anterior superior lateral portal. When inserting the trocar through the hypertrophied capsule and osteophytes, the surgeon must be aware of the risk of injury. Sometimes, in severe disease, it may be necessary to create a dissection plane between the brachialis muscle and the capsule and then proceed with capsular excision [12].

12.10.2 Radial Head Resection

The main indication for this procedure is a limitation in pronation-supination motion at the end of arthroscopy. Resection may result in loss of strength recovery by the patient [13] or overloading of the ulnohumeral compartment, leading to valgus malalignment and ulnar nerve symptoms. Radial head resection can be partial or complete and is usually performed from the posterior to the anterior compartment.

The current literature is still conflicting about its effectiveness [14–18].

12.10.3 Extra-articular Posterior Band of the Medial Collateral Ligament (MCL)

Once all osteophytes have been removed, persistent stiffness in flexion can be treated by transecting the posterior ligament of the MCL with a scalpel blade from the humeral surface (more specifically, at the base of the ulnar groove). A mini-open approach is required. The true benefit of this procedure in terms of the ultimate restoration of elbow motion is still controversial [19].

12.10.4 Humeral Fenestration

The aim of this procedure is to access the coronoid process and anterior compartment from a posterior approach via a transtricipital portal and a small incision across the base of the olecranon fossa. The main advantage is a lower risk of neurovascular injury from the posterior approach than from the anterior approach. The olecranon incision is made with a motorised burr. The exposure of the anterior chamber remains limited compared to a proper anterior approach [13].

12.10.5 Capsulectomy

Capsulectomy as an optional procedure for stiffer elbows with OA can provide a significant improvement in ROM [20]. It also appears to provide better analgesic control in the postoperative period (probably related to partial denervation of the sensory branches of the radial, ulnar and median nerves) and to prevent recurrence (sometimes the healing process on the capsule after simple capsulotomy can lead to loss of ROM).

The patient's expectations of the operation should also be taken into account: if the main problem has been identified as conflict pain, a thorough removal of osteophytes may be appropriate. Capsulectomy is more likely to be indicated in post-traumatic OA, where the increased activity of fibromyoblasts on the capsule increases the risk of capsule contraction [21].

The technique has been described in detail by O'Driscoll [22]. He recommends starting arthroscopy in the posterior compartment before the anterior compartment; each step has been divided into four steps (entering the compartment and creating a view, creating a working space, removing the bone and finally capsulotomy). The authors suggest proximal humeral release and synovectomy prior to capsulotomy. Removing the capsule with a razor and dividing the remaining lateral capsule with scissors seems to improve the results of the procedure [23].

It should be performed by experienced surgeons as a potential risk of neurovascular damage has been described [13].

12.10.6 Microfractures and Chondroplasty

During osteophyte removal, it is possible to locate a limited area characterised by severe chondral damage and bone exposure: in this scenario, microfractures are advocated as a possible treatment [4].

12.11 Postoperative Rehabilitation and Return to Sport After Arthroscopic Procedure

In peri-operative period, the patient is given tranexamic acid and cortisone.

On the first day after surgery, rehabilitation begins with a slow continuous passive motion (CPM) machine through the full range of motion, four times a day for 40 min. From the second day, self-mobilisation for 30 min four times a day is added to the protocol. On the third day, the catheter is removed. On the fourth day, the drains are also removed. From the fifth day, if there is adequate pain control, the patient is discharged with a rehabilitation programme of 20 days combined with indomethacin for 6 weeks.

The splint is usually kept for 15–20 days. The first follow-up visit is scheduled after 1 week and then after 1 month. Physiotherapy is continued for 3–5 months.

The return to sport interval for throwing athletes with OA after arthroscopic surgery was estimated by Jhan S.W. et al. to be 2 ± 1.5 months for training activities and 4.5 ± 1.5 months for return to competition [24].

12.12 Outcomes

Arthroscopic treatment can significantly improve elbow ROM, strength, functional scores and pain by removing osteophytes or mobile bodies in the joint. Improvement stabilises at an average of 6 months after surgery. Men and manual workers showed better results, as did those in the early stages of OA. A preoperative ROM of less than 90° is associated with poorer outcomes [23]. Complications such as local and superficial infection near the portals, subsequent mild elbow contracture (less than 20°), formation of heterotopic ossifications (obesity seems to be a risk factor) and deep infection have been described. Nerve damage is the most worrying complication of arthroscopic treatment, especially in post-traumatic or previous surgery cases: ulnar nerve lesions are the most common, but radial nerve branches and medial antebrachial cutaneous nerves can also be affected [1]. In limited ROM (usually when flexion is less than 100°), ulnar nerve isolation is recommended before arthroscopy.

12.13 Conclusion

In conclusion, it can be helpful to summarise the most common indications and relative contraindications for elbow arthroscopy in the setting of a stiff elbow.

12.13.1 Indications

- Mild or moderate ROM deficits
- Post-traumatic *(better results even in 'serius' stiffness but higher complication rate)*
- X-ray: bone spurs and loose bodies with preserved joint congruence

12.13.2 Relative Contraindications

- Heterotopic ossification
- Hardware in situ
- Muscle contractures
- Extra-articular fibrosis
- Rotational deficit (pronosupination)
- Severe chondral lesions/severe OA
- Anatomical variations due to previous surgery
- Patients >60 years old (worst results)
- Interval from disease onset >7 years (better results if <1 year)

References

1. Pederzini LA, Nicoletta F, Tosi M, Prandini M, Tripoli E, Cossio A. Elbow arthroscopy in stiff elbow. Knee Surg Sports Traumatol Arthrosc. 2014;22:467–73.
2. Lim YW, van Riet RP, Mittal R, Bain GI. Pattern of osteophyte distribution in primary osteoarthritis of the elbow. J Shoulder Elbow Surg. 2008;17:963–6.
3. Goodfellow JW, Bullough PG. The pattern of aging of the articular cartilage of the elbow joint. J Bone Joint Surg Br. 1967;49:175–81.
4. Kroonen LT, Piper SL, Ghatan AC. Arthroscopic management of elbow osteoarthritis. J Hand Surg Am. 2017;42:640–50.
5. Carlier Y, Desmoineaux P, Lenoir H, Vidil A, French Arthroscopic Society. Prospective comparative analysis of arthroscopic debridement for primary and post-traumatic elbow osteoarthritis. Orthop Traumatol Surg Res. 2019;105:S217–20.
6. Wysocki RW, Cohen MS. Primary osteoarthritis and posttraumatic arthritis of the elbow. Hand Clin. 2011;27(2):131–7.
7. Dalal S, Bull M, Stanley D. Radiographic changes at the elbow in primary osteoarthritis: a comparison with normal aging of the elbow joint. J Shoulder Elbow Surg. 2007;16:358–61.
8. Amini MH, Sykes JB, Olson ST, Smith RA, Mauck BM, Azar FM, Throckmorton TW. Reliability testing

of two classification systems for osteoarthritis and post-traumatic arthritis of the elbow. J Shoulder Elbow Surg. 2015;24(3):353–7.
9. Hastings H 2nd, Graham TJ. The classification and treatment of heterotopic ossification about the elbow and forearm. Hand Clin. 1994;10(3):417–37.
10. Hy C, Eygendaal D, The B. Elbow arthroscopy—indications and technique. J Clin Orthop Trauma. 2021;21(19):147–53.
11. Lim TK, Koh KH, Lee HI, Shim JW, Park MJ. Arthroscopic débridement for primary osteoarthritis of the elbow: analysis of preoperative factors affecting outcome. J Shoulder Elbow Surg. 2014;23:1381–7.
12. Pederzini LA, Di Palma F. Arthroscopic capsular release and debridement of elbow osteoarthritis: how I do it! In: Surgical techniques for trauma and sports related injuries of the elbow. Springer Nature; 2019. p. 759.
13. Desmoineaux P, Carlier Y, Mansat P, Bleton R, Rouleau DM, Duparc F, French Arthroscopic Society. Arthroscopic treatment of elbow osteoarthritis. Orthop Traumatol Surg Res. 2019;105:S235–40.
14. Kelly EW, Bryce R, Coghlan J, Bell S. Arthroscopic debridement without radial head excision of the osteoarthritic elbow. Arthroscopy. 2007;23:151–6.
15. Sochacki KR, Jack RA, Hirase T, McCulloch PC, Lintner DM, Liberman SR, Harris JD. Arthroscopic debridement for primary degenerative osteoarthritis of the elbow leads to significant improvement in range of motion and clinical outcomes: a systematic review. Arthroscopy. 2017;33:2255–62.
16. Galle SE, Beck JD, Burchette RJ, Harness NG. Outcomes of elbow arthroscopic osteocapsular arthroplasty. J Hand Surg Am. 2016;41:184–91.
17. Savoie FH, Nunley PD, Field LD. Arthroscopic management of the arthritic elbow: indications, technique, and results. J Shoulder Elbow Surg. 1999;8:214–9.
18. McLaughlin RE, Savoie FH, Field LD, Ramsey JR. Arthroscopic treatment of the arthritic elbow due to primary radiocapitellar arthritis. Arthroscopy. 2006;22:63–9.
19. Kim SJ, Kim JW, Lee SH, Choi JW. Retrospective comparative analysis of elbow arthroscopy used to treat primary osteoarthritis with and without release of the posterior band of the medial collateral ligament. Arthroscopy. 2017;33:1506–11.
20. Isa AD, Athwal GS, King GJW, MacDermid JC, Faber KJ. Arthroscopic debridement for primary elbow osteoarthritis with and without capsulectomy: a comparative cohort study. Shoulder Elbow. 2018;10:223–31.
21. Hildebrand KA, Zhang M, van Snellenberg W, King GJW, Hart DA. Myofibroblast numbers are elevated in human elbow capsules after trauma. Clin Orthop Relat Res. 2004;419:189–97.
22. O'Driscoll SW, Blonna D. Osteocapsular arthroplasty of the elbow: surgical technique. JBJS Essent Surg Tech. 2014;3:e15.
23. Carlier Y, Lenoir H, Rouleau DM, et al. Arthroscopic debridement for osteoarthritis of the elbow: results and analysis of predictive factors. Orthop Traumatol Surg Res. 2019;105:S221–7.
24. Jhan SW, Chou WY, Wu KT, Wang CJ, Yang YJ, Ko JY. Outcomes and factors of elbow arthroscopy upon returning to sports for throwing athletes with osteoarthritis. J Orthop Surg Res. 2018;13(1):280.

Part IV

Surgical Treatment of Post Traumatic Stiff Elbow

13 Open Management of the Post-traumatic Stiff Elbow

Adam C. Watts and Matthew N. O. Mathieson

13.1 Introduction

Open arthrolysis can be used to try to improve range of movement in patients developing impaired function due to elbow stiffness after trauma. The decision whether to use arthroscopic or open techniques will depend on the cause of stiffness, the experience of the treating surgeon and the wishes of the patient.

The three articulations of the elbow joint permit movement of the forearm and positioning of the hand in space. The elbow and forearm joints should be considered as a functional unit responsible for elbow flexion and extension and forearm pronation and supination, which enables us to manipulate our environment with such dexterity. The functional range of motion (ROM) of the elbow has been described by Morrey as 100° of flexion-extension, from 30° to 130° and 100° pronation-supination, from 50° supination to 50° pronation [1]. Sardelli et al. re-evaluated the functional arc of the elbow joint for modern daily activities and found that a greater range of motion is required for contemporary tasks [2].

A. C. Watts (✉)
Edge Hill University, Ormskirk, Lancashire, UK
e-mail: adam.watts@elbowdoc.co.uk

M. N. O. Mathieson
East Cheshire NHS Trust, Macclesfield, UK

13.2 Classification of Elbow Stiffness

The causes of elbow stiffness are classified according to either the structures involved or the location of the pathology.

13.2.1 Kay Classification

The classification system described by Kay is based on the causative structural components: type 1 (purely soft-tissue contracture), type 2 (soft-tissue contracture with ossification), type 3 (undisplaced articular fracture with soft-tissue contracture), type 4 (displaced intra-articular fracture with soft-tissue contracture) and type 5 (post-traumatic bony bars) [3].

13.2.2 Morrey Classification

The classification system described by Morrey is based on the anatomical location and the aetiological cause of the joint contracture, further divided into three categories: intrinsic, extrinsic and combined.

L. Pederzini et al. (eds.), *Stiffness of the Elbow, Wrist and Related Pathologies*,
https://doi.org/10.1007/978-3-031-81381-8_13

Intrinsic contractures are defined as lesions involving the articular surfaces, such as articular deformity, intra-articular adhesions, impinging osteophytes, loose bodies, fibrosis impinging on the olecranon or coronoid fossa and iatrogenic causes such as intra-articular metalwork [4, 5]. Extrinsic contractures are defined as lesions involving the surrounding soft-tissues which do not involve the articular surfaces such as skin and subcutaneous tissue, the joint capsule, collateral ligament contracture, muscular contractures and heterotopic ossification [4, 5]. Capsular contracture often occurs in association with intrinsic causes of elbow stiffness and mixed causes, intrinsic and extrinsic, are common. It is important when viewing imaging to consider hidden causes of elbow stiffness including low grade infection, instability, adhesions and neurogenic causes.

13.3 Post-traumatic Elbow Stiffness

The incidence of elbow stiffness following trauma has been reported to be between 3% and 20%. More recent studies, using Morrey's definition of functional stiffness, estimate the frequency to be between 8.4% and 12% [6, 7]. Estimates will depend on the timing of evaluation, as range of movement can continue to improve up to 9 months following injury. Stiffness in flexion-extension is reported to be more common than loss of pronation-supination [7]. Stiffness may be perceived differently depending on the individual's experience and it is important to consider the activities of daily living for that individual. Most can compensate for loss of up to 30° extension through small alterations in body positioning relative to the object; however, reduction in flexion proves more problematic as it is not possible to compensate for the lost movement when bending the elbow to reach the mouth, and a loss of flexion results in a greater loss of 'reach' in the sagittal plane compared to the equivalent number of degrees loss of extension (Fig. 13.1) [8].

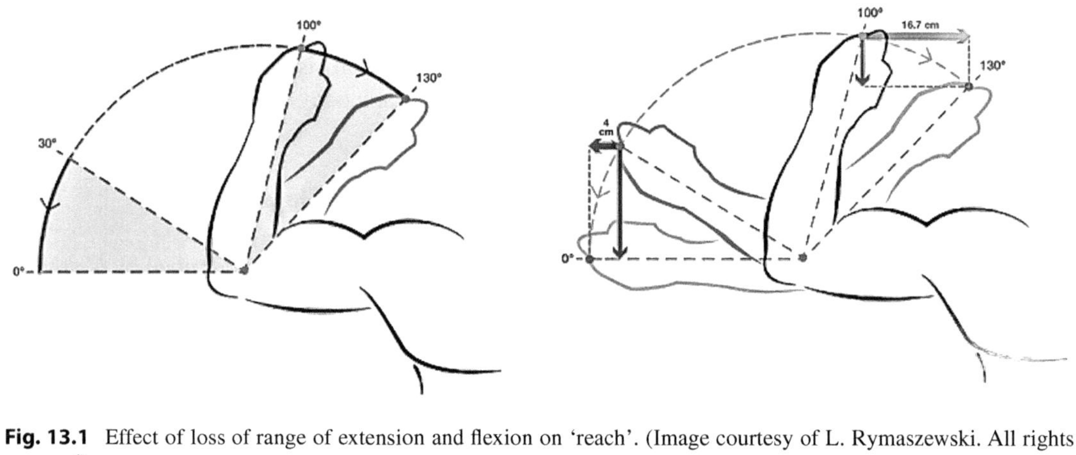

Fig. 13.1 Effect of loss of range of extension and flexion on 'reach'. (Image courtesy of L. Rymaszewski. All rights reserved)

13.4 Aetiology and Pathophysiology of the Post-traumatic Stiff Elbow

There are a number of causes of post-traumatic stiffness of the elbow. The elbow is thought to be prone to stiffness due to the complexity of the articulation, the congruity of the articular surfaces and poor proprioception of the elbow joint that inhibits recovery. It has been postulated that the degree of post-traumatic stiffness experienced is correlated with the severity of injury to the elbow [9, 10].

13.4.1 Soft-Tissue Contracture

Contractures of the soft-tissue surrounding the joint, particularly the capsule, can physically restrict elbow motion after traumatic injury leading to stiffness [11, 12]. Primarily comprised of collagen fibres and fibroblasts, the normal elbow capsule has a well organised, thin and compliant structure [13]. A number of different processes have been implicated in the process of capsular contracture. In the post-traumatic stiff elbow the capsule has been found to exhibit hypertrophy, reduced compliance and disorganised collagen. There is evidence of inflammatory cytokine activation, increased numbers of myofibroblasts and the presence of lymphocytic infiltration [12, 13]. Myofibroblasts are also thought to be activated through the mast cell-neuropeptide fibrosis axis: substance P and calcitonin-G-related peptide-mediated mast cell degranulation leading to myofibroblast activation in response to injury and pain [14]. A correlation has been reported between the proportion of myofibroblasts and the loss of elbow range of movement [14, 15]. Capsular contraction is also a key feature of arthrofibrosis, an inflammatory mechanism triggered by traumatic injury and mediated by pro-inflammatory cytokines [15]. The thickened and stiff joint capsule acts like a tie bar, restricting range of movement. The formation of a 'false capsule' along the margins of the trochlea articular cartilage may also restrict movement preventing the olecranon from gliding into the olecranon fossa in extension.

13.4.2 Heterotopic Ossification

Heterotrophic ossification (HO) is the inappropriate formation of lamellar bone within non-skeletal soft-tissue structures [11, 16, 17]. Heterotopic bone is histologically indistinguishable from native bone, and is formed through osteoid production and mineralisation via the differentiation of mesenchymal stromal cells into osteoblasts. HO can be benign, having no effect or limb function or pain, or can lead to variable restriction of range of movement depending on the extent of the new bone formation and the location. HO forming in the ligament can be very restrictive and is challenging to treat without disruption to the stabilising structures. At the elbow the classification described by Hastings and Graham is used; class I is HO without restriction of range of movement, Class II is HO causing a restriction of range of movement (IIA flexion/extension, IIB pronosupination, IIC restriction in both movements) and Class III is ankylosis of the joint by HO (Fig. 13.2) [18].

The overall risk of HO formation after trauma to the elbow is estimated to be 10% [19]. Several risk factors for HO formation around the elbow exist, the most important of which are traumatic

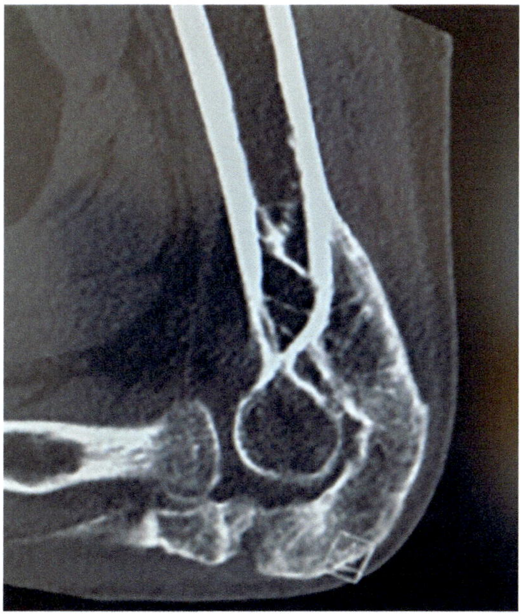

Fig. 13.2 Posterior post-traumatic heterotopic ossification causing ankylosis of the ulnohumeral joint

brain injury, burns, instability and delays to surgery [20, 21]. There is also a correlation between severity of traumatic injury and incidence and severity of HO. Prophylaxis, chemical or radiological, has not been shown to be any benefit in the prevention of HO after trauma [22]. Indeed, radiotherapy has been shown to cause harm due to unacceptable rates of non-union [23].

13.4.3 Fracture, Malunion and Non-union

Elbow stiffness may also be a result of the loss of normal anatomical and osseous geometry secondary to fracture malunion or non-union. Extra-articular fractures of the distal humerus may result in reduced elbow flexion through the loss of anterior translation of the articular surface, or through callus filling the olecranon or coronoid fossa. Intra-articular malunions, of the distal humerus, radial head or coronoid may lead to incongruity, mechanical blocks and instability. A painful non-union may result in elbow stiffness, with much of the elbow movement seen at the non-union rather than the joint itself. Intra-articular penetration of screws from osteosynthesis is not unusual following elbow trauma due to the complexity of the articulation, fracture patterns and variable anatomy (Fig. 13.3).

13.4.4 Joint Arthrosis

Arthrosis is a common sequela of elbow trauma and can be responsible for stiffness of the joint, either from pain inhibition or secondary features of arthrosis such as marginal osteophyte formation. While it can be radiographically classified into four distinct grades, detailing varying involvements of osteophyte formation and joint degeneration, the relationship between these findings and impairment are unclear (Fig. 13.4) [12, 24].

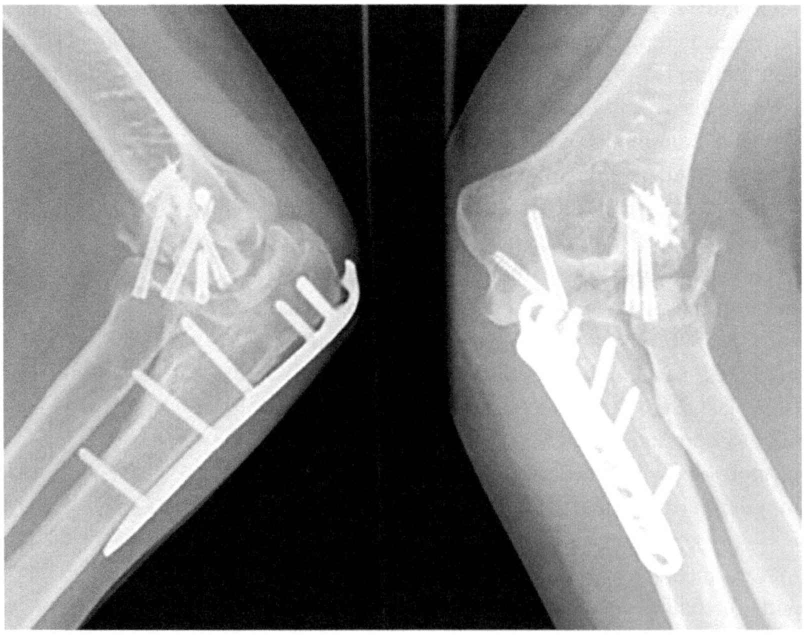

Fig. 13.3 Joint stiffness due to joint penetration by screws

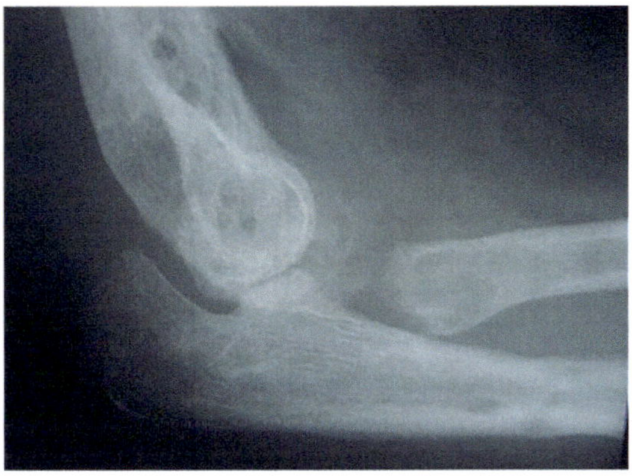

Fig. 13.4 Joint stiffness secondary to instability and post-traumatic arthrosis

13.5 Clinical Evaluation and Diagnosis of Post-traumatic Stiff Elbow

13.5.1 Clinical Evaluation

The clinician should undertake an assessment of the nature and energy of the elbow trauma, duration and progression of stiffness, pain inducing activities, symptoms indicative of ulnar neuropathy and locking or mechanical symptoms [8]. The elbow is commonly stiff following trauma and range of movement slowly improves over weeks to months but may reach a plateau. Progressive loss of elbow range of movement may indicate stiffness secondary to instability or neurogenic causes. Increasing pain may be an indicator of infection or arthrosis. Physical examination should include an assessment of the skin condition and soft-tissue envelope, measurement of elbow and forearm range of movement with a goniometer, stress testing for elbow stability and a comprehensive neurological assessment with specific focus on the ulnar nerve. The examination should include an assessment of the joints above and below the elbow with consideration of the influence of the kinetic chain.

Further investigations, following patient consultation, should be organised to enhance diagnostic certainty. Anteroposterior, lateral and, if necessary, radiocapitellar oblique radiographs should be obtained to provide a clear clinical picture, while concurrently allowing the clinician to identify potential causes or influential factors of the elbow stiffness. Computed tomography (CT) scan can provide useful information about the congruity of the joint surfaces, joint penetration by hardware and the location or extent of heterotopic ossification. Plain magnetic resonance imaging (MRI), MR arthrography or CT arthrography can be used to investigate for instability. Where infection is suspected blood tests should be undertaken to look for raised inflammatory markers and MRI or SPECT CT scans may influence clinician decision making (Fig. 13.5) [11].

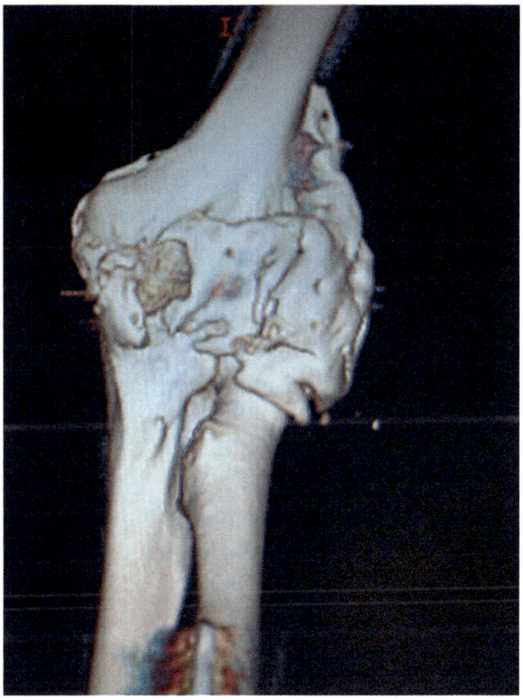

Fig. 13.5 3D CT scan of heterotopic ossification

13.6 Non-operative Management Options for the Treatment of Post-traumatic Stiff Elbow

The aims of treatment in the stiff elbow are to improve pain, range of movement and stability of the elbow to improve arm function. Achieving these goals requires the consideration of all available clinical information and interventional modalities to produce a patient-specific plan with joint decision making with the patient.

Consideration should be given to the utility of non-operative interventions particularly within the first 6 months after trauma in the absence of clear mechanical causes. The principle of non-operative management is to gradually achieve favourable increases in ROM while minimising inflammation [25]. Non-operative modalities include splinting, serial casting, continuous passive movement, occupational and physical therapy, and manipulation [26].

13.6.1 Static Progressive and Dynamic Splinting

Splinting is a conservative technique that harnesses both elastic and plastic forces to reduce contractures of the elbow's viscoelastic connective tissue [27]. It is split into two distinct categories: static progressive and dynamic. Static progressive splinting involves the stepwise progression of a constant force based on the creep loading principle [12, 27]. While the force applied is constant, it is not consistent—as tissues stretch, the force decreases over time until the next progression of force is applied [12]. Dynamic splinting, based on the stress relaxation principle, involves the application of a force, variable over time, to provide a consistent stretch on the tissues [12, 27]. There is no significant difference in outcomes comparing static progressive and dynamic splinting based on randomised controlled trials and a systematic review of the literature [28, 29]. There is also no evidence that splinting of any kind alters the natural history of post-traumatic elbow stiffness. Therefore, clinical decision-making regarding splinting modality should be guided by centre expertise, preference and patient factors.

13.6.2 Serial Casting

Zander and Healy have reported the use of serial casting in three patients with post-traumatic stiffness with average flexion contractures of 44° reduced to 11°, with results maintained over an average of 26 months [30]. More evidence is required to recommend this modality which is quite cumbersome for the patient.

13.6.3 Manipulation Under Anaesthesia

Manipulation under anaesthesia (MUA) remains a controversial procedure. There have been reports of good outcomes following MUA, although these studies focus on patients who have previously had surgery for elbow contractures, and therefore may not be accurately extrapolated to the population with primary post-traumatic stiffness [9, 12, 31, 32]. While MUA may be performed in the absence of fracture, or with radiographical evidence of osseous healing of a previous fracture, the procedure is not without risk [9, 27]. Reported adverse sequelae include transient ulnar neuropathies, periarticular fracture and formation or exacerbation of heterotrophic ossification [9, 25, 31]. There is insufficient evidence to recommend it as a treatment modality.

13.6.4 Physiotherapy

Initially, physiotherapy may focus on controlling inflammation, oedema and pain by cooling, compressing and elevating the joint [15]. Early mobilisation and graduated active-assisted stretch exercises are crucial for reducing the contractive effects of immobilisation on the soft and osteochondral tissues [15, 27, 33].

As described by Wolff and Hotchkiss, the supine overhead position provides maximised joint stabilisation for optimal early post-operative mobilisation of the elbow [27, 34]. This position reduces gravitational posterior vector forces at the elbow joint whilst also allowing the triceps to act as an elbow stabiliser resulting in minimised ulnohumeral distraction during exercise and allowing for isometric healing of the lateral collateral ligament [34–36]. The two exercises to be performed in the supine overhead position are active-assisted forearm pronation-supination and active-assisted elbow flexion-extension [34, 36]. Exercises are gradually progressed in ROM and reduced in assistance as tolerated with consideration of a protective ROM defined by surgery or injury [27]. As joint stability is achieved and scar tissue matures, the goals and techniques of physiotherapy shift on an individual patient basis [34]. Close monitoring and input from the surgeon, physiotherapist and patient are required to programme strengthening, endurance and functional exercises appropriate for the patient [34].

Passive mobilisations and stretching of the elbow joint have been discouraged because of concern that aggressive manipulation results in further trauma to the elbow through damage to the brachialis muscle and joint capsule [11, 27].

13.7 Open Management

Should more conservative measures be contraindicated or fail to provide desirable results, operative interventions may be considered to achieve the goals of treatment. Common surgical interventions include open arthrolysis or arthroscopic arthrolysis to improve range of movement. Relative contra-indications to arthrolysis include pain through movement, unless caused by misplaced metalwork and significant rest pain with evidence of joint degeneration where interposition arthroplasty or total elbow arthroplasty might be considered when infection has been excluded [11, 12].

Open arthrolysis is well suited for extra-articular pathologies, cases with concomitant rotational impairments, long-standing severe flexion contractures and those where previous surgeries which have distorted local anatomy [37]. It is also valuable in cases where arthroscopic approaches are contraindicated, where localisation of the ulna nerve proves difficult, where there is CT evidence of damage to brachialis placing the median nerve at risk or where the removal of hardware is required to improve function and ease symptoms [37, 38]. Good hand function is important and patients with lack of elbow function due to neurological injury may not benefit from surgical intervention [8].

Several techniques for open arthrolysis of the post-traumatic stiff elbow exist. The techniques can be considered as posterior, lateral, medial, anterior or combined approaches. Anterior approaches are not used in the author's practice due to the problem of persistent stiffness and risk of neurovascular injury [39].

The posterior Outerbridge–Kashiwagi (O–K) procedure is largely used for treatment of elbow osteoarthrosis but has been reported for the treatment of post-traumatic stiffness [38, 40]. It has largely been superseded by arthroscopic techniques or the column procedure. The author's preferred technique is a combination of column approaches, tailored to the pathology [4, 41–43].

13.7.1 Lateral Column Approach

Described by Morrey and associates, a lateral approach, termed as the 'lateral column procedure', has achieved good results and is considered highly versatile [26, 37, 44]. Anterior and posterior capsules can be released, impingement lesions and metalwork can be removed from the lateral elbow, but access to the medial side of the elbow is limited. A medial column approach will provide good access to the ulna nerve and medial structures, and the anterior and posterior capsule can be released, but the radiocapitellar joint cannot be accessed. Combining these approaches with a posterior midline triceps split, where required, will give good access to all necessary pathology. A decision whether to undertake the surgery through a posterior midline incision or separate medial and lateral approaches is determined by any previous surgical approach to the elbow, by the likelihood of the need for future surgery such as a total elbow replacement and by the preference of the surgeon and patient. The over-arching principle employed by the author is to minimise the raising of skin flaps as much as possible.

Under general anaesthesia, the patient is positioned supine with a sandbag laid underneath the ipsilateral shoulder and the arm, freely draped, brought across the thorax [4, 5]. Alternatively, the patient can be placed in the lateral decubitus position with the elbow draped over a bolster. The proximal one-half of a Kocher incision is made in the absence of a previous incision or ulnar neuropathy [4]. Symptomatic ulnar neuropathy may be explored through a midline posterior incision, allowing for decompression as required [4].

After identifying the origin of the extensor carpi radialis longus and the distal fibres of the brachioradialis, they are released from the humerus to provide access to the superolateral aspect of the capsule. At the radiohumeral joint, the capsule is entered anteriorly and the capsule thickness and orientation should be identified [4, 45]. Using a periosteal elevator, the brachialis should be swept from the anterior aspect of the capsule [4, 45]. The use of an angled retractor placed anteriorly provides protection for the brachialis, radial nerve, median nerve and brachial artery [4, 45, 46]. Subsequently, the anterior capsule is grasped, with the lateral half excised to at least the level of the coronoid and the medial half excised as far as safely visualised or palpated to complete the release [4, 45, 46].

The extension of the elbow should now be assessed [4, 45]. Should it fall within 5° of normal and there is an absence of an olecranon spur on radiographic assessment, the release is complete, the capsule should be left open and the wound should be closed [4, 45].

If the preceding criteria have not been met, further release of the posterior aspect of the capsule may be required [4, 45]. The triceps can be lifted from the posterior aspect of the humerus, gaining access to the posterior aspect of the capsule for release and the olecranon fossa to be cleaned of soft-tissue [4, 45]. The tip of the olecranon may also be excised should there be osteophytes visible [4]. ROM should be assessed once more, with reduced flexion below 130° being an indication for the inspection of the coronoid and removal of any osteophytes present (Fig. 13.6) [4].

Positive outcomes for the lateral column approach are widely reported. Post-operative improvements of the flexion-extension arc range from 35° to 50°, restoration of a functional arc has been reported in up to 30% of patients, and satisfactory results have been achieved in the majority of cases [4, 45, 47–50]. Morrey et al. reported an average increase in Mayo Elbow Performance Score of 19/100 points and Gunlach and Eygendaal an average increase in Elbow Function Assessment of 17/100 points [4, 47, 48]. Satisfaction with the outcome of surgery has been reported to be high [50].

In clinical practice since 1989, the lateral column procedure has been adopted widely [4, 37]. While there are many advantages to this approach, such as the versatility, speed, preservation of the lateral collateral ligament and stability of the elbow, disadvantages do exist [31, 37, 44, 51].

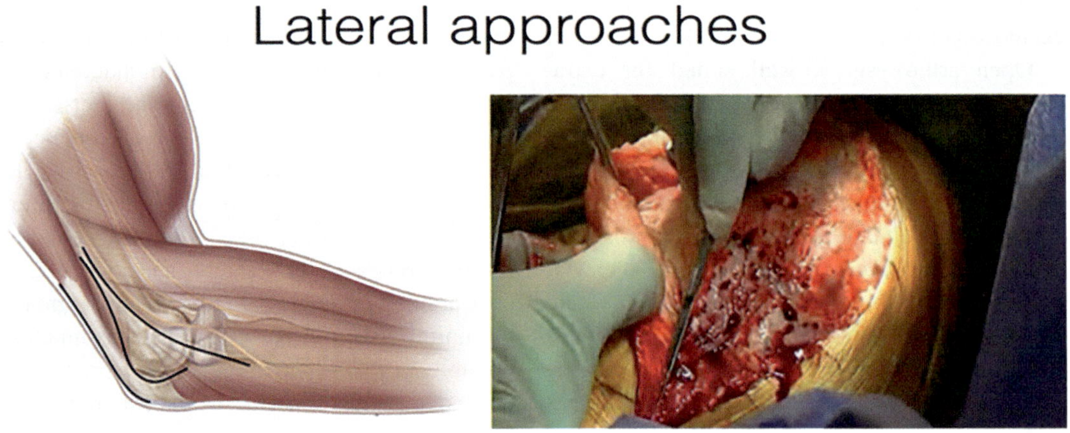

Fig. 13.6 Lateral approaches to the elbow

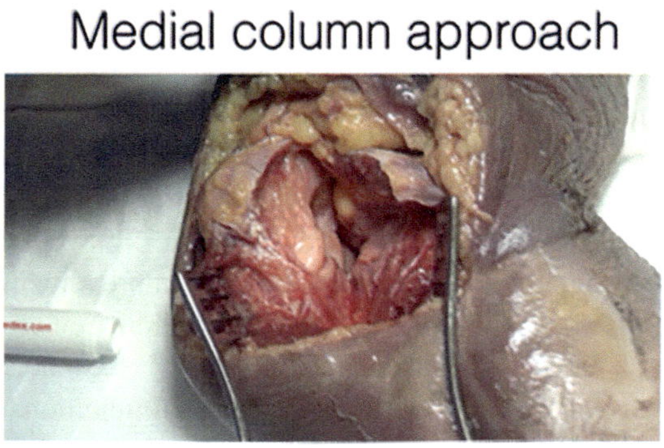

Fig. 13.7 Medial column approach

The approach does not provide adequate access to structures other than the radiohumeral joint, and therefore may not be the most suitable technique in the presence of extensive medial heterotopic ossification [44, 52]. In the presence of heterotopic ossification affecting the medial aspect of the radial head, the approach does not offer adequate visualisation of the radial nerve [9]. Should ulnar nerve dysfunction require surgical exploration, a medial approach is preferable to that of the lateral approach (Fig. 13.7) [52].

13.7.2 Outerbridge–Kashiwagi Procedure

Primarily for the treatment of mild–moderate arthritis of the elbow, the O–K procedure is a safe and effective procedure for patients suffering from post-traumatic contracture [38, 53]. Described by Kashiwagi in 1978, the O–K procedure consists of a posterior transhumeral osseous approach, providing access for the removal of osteophytes and loose bodies in the olecranon fossa, through splitting of the triceps, and the anterior compartment of the elbow and coronoid process, through the fenestration of the olecranon fossa membrane [54, 55].

A modified approach to the O–K procedure, as described by Morrey, is commonly used [56]. After a brachial plexus block is established, under general anaesthesia the patient is positioned supine with a sandbag laid underneath the ipsilateral scapula. A tourniquet can be applied to the arm, with the arm subsequently being draped freely and brought across the thorax [56]. To optimise elbow access, the patient is rotated 35° [56]. Alternatively, the patient can be placed in the lateral decubitus position with the arm over a bolster. A straight incision over the posterior aspect of the joint exposes the triceps fascia, where the triceps is subsequently split down the midline to provide access to the supracondylar bony columns [56]. If the ulnar nerve requires exploration or decompression, the medial margin and attachment of the triceps tendon are elevated to provide adequate access [56]. The medial quarter of the triceps attachment is now released, allowing for an osteotomy of the olecranon tip and removal of loose bodies from the olecranon fossa [56]. Directed slightly proximally, a trephine, of a slightly larger diameter than the original olecranon fossa, is used to core out and excise all osteophytes present and a ring of bone from both the olecranon and coronoid fossae to provide a clean opening through to the anterior aspect of the joint [56]. The elbow is flexed to bring the coronoid process into view through the hole excised by the trephine [56]. The anterior osteophyte of the coronoid is removed through the use of a curved 7 mm osteotome, obvious loose bodies are removed, and the anterior capsule is palpated for any remaining loose bodies [56]. Bone wax is applied to any exposed bone surfaces, a Gelfoam sponge is placed into the defect, drains are laid and the wound is closed [56].

The O–K procedure is not widely reported in the literature for the treatment of post-traumatic stiffness. One study, conducted by Brewley et al., reports results gained from a series of patients with post-traumatic sequelae [38]. The results of this study were encouraging, showing an average improvement in the flexion-extension arc of 54° alongside a mean MEPS improvement from 52 to 84 points [38].

Whilst the O–K procedure is safe and effective for the treatment of patients suffering from post-traumatic contracture, the disadvantage for this approach is that it does not allow access to the radiohumeral joint [53, 57].

13.7.3 Open Arthrolysis and Mechanical Distraction

In 1975, Volkov and Oganesian published a study detailing the use of external hinged distraction devices in the treatment of elbow contractures [58]. External hinged distraction devices use intraosseous pins and adjustable attachments to accurately align the joint surfaces, relieve static and dynamic loads and maintain a predetermined clearance between the articular surfaces throughout the full ROM [58]. The underlying theory behind the use of such devices is to permit the correct distribution of forces across articular surfaces and allow the development of a more anatomical shape to newly fashioned articular surfaces, post-open arthrolysis, through the use of an external artificial joint [58]. Since this initial study, the design of external hinged distraction devices has been continually refined and developed [59].

Contemporary approaches to open arthrolysis with the use of mechanical distraction have been described in the literature. Such approaches may be performed under general anaesthetic or with a brachial plexus block [59–61]. All operations are performed with the patient positioned supine and may be performed both with and without the use of tourniquet [59–61]. The procedure starts with the in-situ decompression of the ulnar nerve via a medial incision, where the decompressed nerve is reassessed throughout the procedure as appropriate [59–61]. Once the removal of impinging osteophytes or heterotopic bone is complete, often through medial, lateral or combination approaches, the application of the hinged fixator device starts [59–61]. The desired axis of rotation is identified through radiographic imaging and the use of K-wires [59–62]. With the K-wire situated over the desired axis of rotation, it now acts as a locus for the external hinged device to be accurately aligned and fixed [59–62]. Distraction is applied intra-operatively, and radiographically assessed for symmetrical average distraction, of at least double the physiological joint space as reported by Mader and Pennig, before the final fixation of the apparatus [59].

Medium term follow-up outcomes show satisfactory results for open arthrolysis with the use of an external hinged distraction device [60, 61]. Comparison of absolute ROM improvements between individual studies is difficult due to differing devices and surgical techniques; however, outcome score trends show positive improvement [60, 61]. The use of external fixation devices introduces additional complications, the most commonly reported being pin-related infections, although there were no serious reported infections [60, 61]. Determining the clinical effectiveness of external hinged distraction devices from these studies proves difficult due to inconsistent techniques and device, follow-up periods and outcome measures.

13.8 Post-operative Management After Open Management

Early mobilisation, often started on the first day post-operatively, helps to preserve ROM gained through the procedure to achieve a satisfactory result for the patient [63]. Good control of post-operative pain is important to encourage compliance with physiotherapy regimes. Various post-operative rehabilitation modalities have been documented and it is important that there is good communication between the surgical and physiotherapy team. It is equally important to communicate with the patient that the elbow will lose range of movement initially after open arthrolysis but that it will regain movement close to what is achieved on the operating table with improvements seen beyond 3 months after surgery [64].

13.8.1 Continuous Passive Motion

Continuous passive motion (CPM) is the sinusoidal oscillation of intra-articular pressure, produced by continuous passive movement of the joint through an external device [65]. CPM is advocated to be initiated in the early post-traumatic stages of joint injury with the aim of maintaining satisfactory articulation, reducing soft-tissue oedema and aiding in the clearance of joint hemarthrosis [65–67]. CPM has poor evidence demonstrating effectiveness, with some studies highlighting significantly raised treatment costs and procedural risks, such as bleeding, swelling and ulnar nerve irritation [11, 27, 67]. CPM may have advantages, however, in demonstrating to the patient in the early post-operative phase that their elbow can move through a good range, as it is likely that there will be some stiffening due to post-operative swelling, before gradually range of movement improves.

13.8.2 Splinting

Splinting has been used for 3–4 months post-operatively adjusted for the individual patient [63]. There is no significant difference in outcomes comparing static progressive and dynamic splinting based on randomised controlled trials and a systematic review of the literature, therefore clinical decision-making regarding splinting modality should be guided by centre expertise, preference and patient factors [28, 29].

13.8.3 Physiotherapy

Physiotherapy enhances post-operative rehabilitation; however, exercises must be appropriate for the stage of recovery. An example of a progressive physiotherapy programme has been described by Sun et al., gradually increasing in intensity and exercise complexity through the stages of recovery [60]. Early physiotherapy input and continued education and support seem important for achieving satisfactory outcomes; however, exact exercises and regimens are not strictly agreed upon throughout the literature [68]. A valuable resource for physiotherapy in the management of elbow stiffness from Val Jones, Specialist Elbow Physiotherapy Practitioner can be found on the British Elbow and Shoulder Society Website (https://bess.ac.uk/exercises-for-elbow-stiffness/).

13.9 Complications of Open Management

Reported complications include failure to restore a functional range of movement, ongoing pain, haematoma, ulnar neuropathies, infection, heterotopic ossification and a decrease in the range of motion [4, 31, 44, 45, 57, 69–72]. Measures can be taken to reduce the frequency of complications.

Ulnar neuropathy is a common post-operative complication, attributable to several causative factors including iatrogenic injury, increased stretching of the nerve, increased intra-neural pressure and the swelling, thickening or scarification of the fibro-osseous tunnel in which the ulnar nerve resides [73–77]. Ulnar neuropathy may be transient, however, to avoid stretch and compression injury post-operatively, it has been suggested to consider concurrently decompress and/or anteriorly transpose the nerve—particularly if there is a pre-operative flexion contracture greater than 100° [9, 31, 38, 44]. Consideration of prophylactic ulnar nerve decompression when there is an anticipated increase of flexion post-operatively of more than 30°, has also been suggested to reduce the risk of acute ulnar nerve palsy [70]. For the treatment of delayed onset ulnar neuropathy, it has been suggested that the efficacy of limited ulnar nerve decompression is thought to equal that of transposition, while also associated with lower complication rates, provided that the decompression is of sufficient length, 7–8 cm [78]. Mini-decompression of the ulnar nerve is not considered as successful as transposition or in-situ ulnar nerve decompression [78].

Heterotopic ossification is a concern following open arthrolysis, particularly when excising HO from trauma [73]. Whilst chemical prophylaxis is not used routinely following elbow trauma or arthrolysis, there may be benefit in preventing recurrence of HO [79]. The O–K procedure involves the fenestration of the olecranon fossa via dental burr and the drilling of osteophytes creating bone dust, which itself has been suggested to increase the risk of heterotopic ossification through the seeding of bone into extra skeletal tissue [55, 69, 72]. Subsequent modifications to the technique by Morrey have reduced the production of bone dust through the use of a trephine [55, 69].

Careful haemostasis is required before wound closure to reduce the chances of haematoma formation and, while not routinely done, wound drainage can be considered in patients where the complexity of the operation is increased [4, 45]. In the author's experience performing the surgery without a tourniquet, with careful intra-operative haemostasis and administration of intravenous tranexamic acid prior to incision will avoid this complication in most cases.

Re-fracture through previous fracture lines or new fractures as a result of weakening of the bone to due fenestration have been highlighted as concerns of elbow arthrolysis. Re-fracture can be avoided by ensuring that full range of movement is restored on the operating table before osteosynthesis plates are removed from the bone. Care is taken never to undertake passive stretch of the elbow after metalwork has been removed and where this technique is used the forces are applied close to the elbow joint to minimise the lever-arm. Biomechanical studies have demonstrated that fenestration may reduce the strength of the columns of the distal humerus and a case report has documented a column fracture [80, 81].

Whilst open arthrolysis is generally a successful procedure, we must understand the limitations. A study by Bręborowicz et al. highlighted the reduced durability of intra-operative ROM compared to those at final follow-up [43]. Intra-operative ROM values for extension, flexion and arc of motion were significantly increased, gaining an average of 33°, 18° and 51° respectively compared to pre-operative measurements [43]. However, at final follow-up, significant deterioration of ROM was observed for extension and arc of motion, losing an average of 13° and 14° respectively [43]. Flexion does not seem to be significantly affected [43]. Reduced post-operative versus intra-operative values are thought to be secondary to scarring of the joint capsule post-surgical trauma [43]. The only exception to the observed decline in ROM was a group of younger patients, with a larger proportion of more severe contractures, who were observed to gain ROM over time [43]. However, across all patient groups, the authors suggest an expected post-operative arc of motion value of 86% of the intraoperative arc of motion [43].

Discussions surrounding risks, benefits and expectations are key to the informed consent of procedures. Taking an individualised approach to risk assessment and the prediction of surgical outcomes provides the patient with adequate information to make informed decisions and equips the practitioner with the tools to appropriately counsel the patient. The Shanghai Prediction Model for Elbow Stiffness provides insight into both risk factors, associated with poor clinical outcomes, and the value of predictive models patient counselling, consent and expectation management [82].

13.10 The Authors' Approach

Under general anaesthesia with upper limb block the patient is placed in a lateral decubitus position with the elbow resting over a padded bar. A tourniquet is not used with the aim of avoiding the risk of haematoma, compressive nerve lesions and reperfusion oedema that can lead to significant swelling. Haemostasis is achieved through the use of monopolar diathermy and intravenous tranexamic acid.

The surgical approach is tailored to the patient's needs and pathology. The most consistent approach is through separate lateral Kocher and medial post-epicondylar incisions taking care to leave a 10 cm skin bridge between the two. Care is taken to avoid raising large skin flaps that can compromise the soft-tissue envelope and allow more space for haematoma to form. Through a lateral column approach, down the lateral ridge of the humerus between the extensor and flexor compartments, the anterior and posterior capsules can be elevated. Care is taken proximally not to extend as far as the radial nerve. Distally the incision can be extended into a Kaplan, EDC splitting or modified Kocher approach as described by Bain et al. (2015) depending on what needs to be done around the radial head to restore forearm rotation. The coronoid process can be excised, the coronoid fossa deepened and the tip of the olecranon removed through this lateral column approach. HO can be excised anteriorly or posteriorly through this approach but if more work is required in the olecranon fossa or medial aspect of the elbow, alternative ligament sparing windows are used.

Through the posteromedial incision the ulnar nerve is released at least 7 cm above and below the medial epicondyle. If the nerve is then unstable, if there is any compressive lesion in the floor of the cubital tunnel or if the elbow flexion is to be increased by more than 30, the ulna nerve is anteriorly transposed into a subcutaneous pocket with excision of the medial intra-muscular septum. Any remaining anterior or posterior capsule can be released. The medial olecranon can be excised as required and metalwork removed from the medial column. If having undertaken these steps there is still restriction of elbow flexion, the posterior band of the MCL is released which will often restore this motion. Care is taken to preserve the lateral ulna collateral ligament and the anterior band of the medial ligament. If HO involving the MCL is restricting motion this is carefully excised through a flexor tendon split between flexor carpi ulnaris and palmaris longus. If additional work is required in the olecranon fossa to restore elbow extension a posterior triceps midline split can be performed through the posteromedial incision and a burr and osteotomes used to remove bone.

Wounds are closed in layers with continuous sutures and no drain is used. The surgical aim is to restore full range of movement on the operating table, accepting that the patient will lose about 15% of what has been achieved, whilst maintaining elbow stability. If the elbow is found to be unstable at the time of surgery ligamentoplasty is usually sufficient to ensure good approximation of the ulnohumeral joint through range of movement, and to maintain radiocapitellar contact. Excision of a malunited or arthritic radial head can improve range of movement or pain without producing ulnohumeral instability. In some cases, a loose, overstuffed or malaligned radial head prosthesis needs to be removed to restore motion. Post-operatively the patient is placed on to a continuous passive motion device for up to a week if tolerated and this is followed by active out-patient physiotherapy exercises.

13.11 Conclusion

Elbow stiffness is common after trauma. Much of it can be prevented through early mobilisation, and when identified early non-surgical measures may improve the outcome for the patient and avoid the need for surgical intervention. Where necessary open surgery can improve the range of movement of the elbow and limb function. Combined open approaches allow access around the elbow joint without disrupting stability. Fenestration is rarely required and may weaken the distal humerus.

13.12 Future Directions for Research in Post-traumatic Stiff Elbow

Further investigation is ongoing to better understand the causes of post-traumatic elbow stiffness and to find effective prevention strategies. Abdel et al. studied a rabbit model of joint contracture, showing peak myofibroblast proliferation during the early phase post-injury [83]. The study also revealed greater numbers of myofibroblasts present in the posterior capsule, where injury has been shown to cause severe and permanent contracture [83, 84]. The significance of these finding, should it translate to the pathophysiology of joint contracture in humans, pertains to the early administration of myofibroblast targeting pharmacological agents for prophylaxis against joint contracture [83]. There have been suggestions towards the link between myofibroblastogenesis and the COX-2 pathway, with preliminary studies showing reduced scar tissue formation and improved passive knee extension with the administration of Celecoxib, a NSAID and selective cyclooxygenase-2 inhibitor, in rabbit models [85, 86]. Similarly, other pharmacological therapies that target profibrotic pathways, such as mast cell stabilisers, may provide similar anti-arthrofibrotic effects in future clinical studies [87].

13.13 Key Takeaways from the Chapter

Prevent post-traumatic stiffness by allowing early active mobilisation.

Open arthrolysis is affective in the treatment of extrinsic and intrinsic post-traumatic stiffness.

Successful outcomes require a multi-disciplinary approach between surgeons, physiotherapists and pain teams.

References

1. Morrey BF, Askew LJ, Chao EY. A biomechanical study of normal functional elbow motion. JBJS. 1981;63(6):872–7.
2. Sardelli M, Tashjian RZ, MacWilliams BA. Functional elbow range of motion for contemporary tasks. JBJS. 2011;93(5):471–7.
3. Kay N. Arthrolysis of the post-traumatic stiff elbow. In: Stanley DKN, editor. Surgery of the elbow. London: Arnold; 1998. p. 228–34.
4. Mansat P, Morrey BF. The column procedure: a limited lateral approach for extrinsic contracture of the elbow. JBJS. 1998;80(11):1603.
5. Morrey BF. Post-traumatic contracture of the elbow. Operative treatment, including distraction arthroplasty. JBJS. 1990;72(4):601.
6. Wessel LE, Gu A, Richardson SS, Fufa DT, Osei DA. Elbow contracture following operative fixation of fractures about the elbow. JSES Open Access. 2019;3(4):261–5.
7. Myden C, Hildebrand K. Elbow joint contracture after traumatic injury. J Shoulder Elb Surg. 2011;20(1):39–44.
8. Murray O, Macdonald D, Nunn T, Mceachan J, Rymaszewski L. Management of the post-traumatic stiff elbow. Shoulder Elbow. 2012;4(1):38–45.
9. Evans PJ, Nandi S, Maschke S, Hoyen HA, Lawton JN. Prevention and treatment of elbow stiffness. J Hand Surg Am. 2009;34(4):769–78.
10. Sojbjerg JO. The stiff elbow: how I do it. Acta Orthop Scand. 1996;67(6):626–31.
11. Akhtar A, Hughes B, Watts AC. The post-traumatic stiff elbow: a review. J Clin Orthop Trauma. 2021;19:125–31.
12. Mellema JJ, Lindenhovius ALC, Jupiter JB. The posttraumatic stiff elbow: an update. Curr Rev Musculoskelet Med. 2016;9(2):190–8.
13. Cohen MS, Schimmel DR, Masuda K, Hastings H 2nd, Muehleman C. Structural and biochemical evaluation of the elbow capsule after trauma. J Shoulder Elb Surg. 2007;16(4):484–90.
14. Charalambous CP, Morrey BF. Posttraumatic elbow stiffness. JBJS. 2012;94(15):1428–37.
15. Zhang D, Nazarian A, Rodriguez EK. Post-traumatic elbow stiffness: pathogenesis and current treatments. Shoulder Elbow. 2020;12(1):38–45.
16. Vanderstraeten G. Heterotopic ossification: a review. J Rehabil Med. 2005;37(3):129–36.
17. Attum B, Obremskey W. Posttraumatic elbow stiffness: a critical analysis review. JBJS Rev. 2016;4(9):e1.
18. Hastings H, Graham TJ. The classification and treatment of heterotopic ossification about the elbow and forearm. Hand Clin. 1994;10(3):417–37.
19. Wiggers JK, Helmerhorst GT, Brouwer KM, Niekel MC, Nunez F, Ring D. Injury complexity factors predict heterotopic ossification restricting motion after elbow trauma. Clin Orthop Relat Res. 2014;472:2162–7.
20. Orzel JA, Rudd TG. Heterotopic bone formation: clinical, laboratory, and imaging correlation. J Nucl Med. 1985;26(2):125–32.
21. Hong C, Nashi N, Hey H, Chee Y, Murphy D. Clinically relevant heterotopic ossification after elbow fracture surgery: a risk factors study. Orthop Traumatol Surg Res. 2015;101(2):209–13.
22. Bochat K, Mattin AC, Ricciardo BJ. The efficacy of nonsteroidal anti-inflammatories in the prevention of heterotopic ossification following elbow trauma surgery. JSES Int. 2021;5(4):793–6.
23. Hamid N, Ashraf N, Bosse MJ, Connor PM, Kellam JF, Sims SH, et al. Radiation therapy for heterotopic ossification prophylaxis acutely after elbow trauma: a prospective randomized study. JBJS. 2010;92(11):2032–8.
24. Guitton TG, Zurakowski D, van Dijk NC, Ring D. Incidence and risk factors for the development of radiographic arthrosis after traumatic elbow injuries. J Hand Surg Am. 2010;35(12):1976–80.
25. King GJW, Faber KJ. Posttraumatic elbow stiffness. Orthop Clin N Am. 2000;31(1):129–43.
26. Nandi S, Maschke S, Evans PJ, Lawton JN. The stiff elbow. Hand. 2009;4(4):368–79.
27. Jones V. Conservative management of the post-traumatic stiff elbow: a physiotherapist's perspective. Shoulder Elbow. 2016;8(2):134–41.
28. Veltman ES, Doornberg JN, Eygendaal D, van den Bekerom MPJ. Static progressive versus dynamic splinting for posttraumatic elbow stiffness: a systematic review of 232 patients. Arch Orthop Trauma Surg. 2015;135(5):613–7.
29. Lindenhovius ALC, Doornberg JN, Brouwer KM, Jupiter JB, Mudgal CS, Ring D. A prospective randomized controlled trial of dynamic versus static progressive elbow splinting for posttraumatic elbow stiffness. JBJS. 2012;94(8):694.
30. Zander CL, Healy NL. Elbow flexion contractures treated with serial casts and conservative therapy. J Hand Surg Am. 1992;17(4):694–7.

31. Jupiter JB, O'Driscoll SW, Cohen MS. The assessment and management of the stiff elbow. Instr Course Lect. 2003;52:93–111.
32. Spitler CA, Doty DH, Johnson MD, Nowotarski PJ, Kiner DW, Swafford RE, et al. Manipulation under anesthesia as a treatment of posttraumatic elbow stiffness. J Orthop Trauma. 2018;32(8):e304.
33. Bruno RJ, Lee ML, Strauch RJ, Rosenwasser MP. Posttraumatic elbow stiffness: evaluation and management. J Am Acad Orthop Surg. 2002;10(2):106.
34. Wolff AL, Hotchkiss RN. Lateral elbow instability: nonoperative, operative, and postoperative management. J Hand Ther. 2006;19(2):238–44.
35. Lee AT, Schrumpf MA, Choi D, Meyers KN, Patel R, Wright TM, et al. The influence of gravity on the unstable elbow. J Shoulder Elb Surg. 2013;22(1):81–7.
36. Schreiber JJ, Paul S, Hotchkiss RN, Daluiski A. Conservative management of elbow dislocations with an overhead motion protocol. J Hand Surg Am. 2015;40(3):515–9.
37. Siemensma MF, Windt AE, Es EM, Colaris JW, Eygendaal D. Management of the stiff elbow: a literature review. EFORT Open Rev. 2023;8(5):351–60.
38. Brewley EE, Gorman RA, Christmas KN, Simon P, Chapel RJ, Mighell MA. Use of a modified Outerbridge-Kashiwagi procedure for the treatment of posttraumatic elbow sequelae. J Shoulder Elb Surg. 2019;28(7):1387–94.
39. Aldridge JM III, Atkins TA, Gunneson EE, Urbaniak JR. Anterior release of the elbow for extension loss. JBJS. 2004;86(9):1955–60.
40. Minami M, Kato S, Kashiwagi D. Outerbridge-Kashiwagi's method for arthroplasty of osteoarthritis of the elbow—44 elbows followed for 8–16 years. J Orthop Sci. 1996;1:11–5.
41. Shafi M, Hattori Y, Doi K. Surgical technique of debridement arthroplasty of the elbow through medial/trans-flexor approach. Tech Hand Up Extrem Surg. 2009;13(3):151–4.
42. Tosun B, Gundes H, Buluc L, Sarlak AY. The use of combined lateral and medial releases in the treatment of post-traumatic contracture of the elbow. Int Orthop. 2007;31:635–8.
43. Bręborowicz M, Lubiatowski P, Długosz J, Ogrodowicz P, Wojtaszek M, Lisiewicz E, et al. The outcome of open elbow arthrolysis: comparison of four different approaches based on one hundred cases. Int Orthop. 2014;38:561–7.
44. Lindenhovius AL, Jupiter JB. The posttraumatic stiff elbow: a review of the literature. J Hand Surg Am. 2007;32(10):1605–23.
45. Morrey BF. Surgical treatment of extraarticular elbow contracture. Clin Orthop Relat Res. 2000;370:57–64.
46. Cheung EV, Steinmann SP. Surgical approaches to the elbow. J Am Acad Orthop Surg. 2009;17(5):325–33.
47. Gundlach U, Eygendaal D. Surgical treatment of post-traumatic stiffness of the elbow: 2-year outcome in 21 patients after a column procedure. Acta Orthop. 2008;79(1):74–7.
48. Husband J, Hastings H 2nd. The lateral approach for operative release of post-traumatic contracture of the elbow. JBJS. 1990;72(9):1353–8.
49. Marti RK, Kerkhoffs GMMJ, Maas M, Blankevoort L. Progressive surgical release of a posttraumatic stiff elbow: technique and outcome after 2–18 years in 46 patients. Acta Orthop Scand. 2002;73(2):144–50.
50. Sharma S, Rymaszewski L. Open arthrolysis for post-traumatic stiffness of the elbow: results are durable over the medium term. J Bone Joint Surg Br Vol. 2007;89(6):778–81.
51. Podgórski AP, Kordasiewicz B, Pomianowski S. The column procedure preserves elbow stability on biomechanical testing. Int Orthop. 2020;44(5):911–8.
52. Keschner MT, Paksima N. The stiff elbow. Bull NYU Hosp Jt Dis. 2007;65(1):24.
53. Vingerhoeds B, Degreef I, De Smet L. Debridement arthroplasty for osteoarthritis of the elbow (Outerbridge-Kashiwagi procedure). Acta Orthop Belg. 2004;70:306–10.
54. Phillips N, Ali A, Stanley D. Treatment of primary degenerative arthritis of the elbow by ulnohumeral arthroplasty: a long-term follow-up. J Bone Joint Surg Br Vol. 2003;85(3):347–50.
55. Kim PD, Grafe MW, Rosenwasser MP. Elbow stiffness: etiology, treatment, and results. J Am Soc Surg Hand. 2005;5(4):209–16.
56. Morrey B. Primary degenerative arthritis of the elbow. Treatment by ulnohumeral arthroplasty. J Bone Joint Surg Br Vol. 1992;74-B(3):409–13.
57. Forster MC, Clark DI, Lunn PG. Elbow osteoarthritis: prognostic indicators in ulnohumeral debridement—the Outerbridge-Kashiwagi procedure. J Shoulder Elb Surg. 2001;10(6):557–60.
58. Volkov M, Oganesian O. Restoration of function in the knee and elbow with a hinge-distractor apparatus. JBJS. 1975;57(5):591–600.
59. Mader K, Pennig D. Post-traumatic elbow stiffness-arthrolysis and mechanical distraction. In: European surgical orthopaedics and traumatology. Springer; 2014. p. 1479–507.
60. Sun Z, Cui H, Ruan J, Li J, Wang W, Fan C. What range of motion and functional results can be expected after open arthrolysis with hinged external fixation for severe posttraumatic elbow stiffness? Clin Orthop Relat Res. 2019;477(10):2319–28.
61. Kulkarni GS, Kulkarni VS, Shyam AK, Kulkarni RM, Kulkarni MG, Nayak P. Management of severe extra-articular contracture of the elbow by open arthrolysis and a monolateral hinged external fixator. J Bone Joint Surg Br Vol. 2010;92-B(1):92–7.
62. Liu S, Fan C-Y, Ruan H-J, Li F-F, Tian J. Combination of arthrolysis by lateral and medial approaches and hinged external fixation in the treatment of stiff elbow. J Trauma Acute Care Surg. 2011;70(2):373–6.
63. Sun Z, Liu W, Li J, Fan C. Open elbow arthrolysis for post-traumatic elbow stiffness. Bone Joint Open. 2020;1(9):576–84.
64. Higgs ZC, Danks BA, Sibinski M, Rymaszewski LA. Outcomes of open arthrolysis of the elbow with-

out post-operative passive stretching. J Bone Joint Surg Br. 2012;94(3):348–52.
65. Giori NJ. Continuous passive motion (CPM): theory and principles of clinical application. J Rehabil Res Dev. 2000;37(2):179–88.
66. Masci G, Cazzato G, Milano G, Ciolli G, Malerba G, Perisano C, et al. The stiff elbow: current concepts. Orthop Rev (Pavia). 2020;12(Suppl 1):8661.
67. Adolfsson L. Post-traumatic stiff elbow. EFORT Open Rev. 2018;3(5):210–6.
68. Pettersen PM, Eriksson J, Bratberg H, Myrseth LE, Bjørnstad LG, Johansen M, et al. Increased ROM and high patient satisfaction after open arthrolysis: a follow-up-study of 43 patients with posttraumatic stiff elbows. BMC Musculoskelet Disord. 2016;17(1):74.
69. Allen DM, Devries JP, Nunley JA. Ulnohumeral arthroplasty. Iowa Orthop J. 2004;24:49.
70. Jeon I-H, Lee S-M, Kim P-T. Acute ulnar nerve palsy after Outerbridge-Kashiwagi procedure. J Hand Surg Eur Vol. 2007;32(5):596.
71. Cohen AP, Redden JF, Stanley D. Treatment of osteoarthritis of the elbow: a comparison of open and arthroscopic debridement. Arthroscopy. 2000;16(7):701–6.
72. Chandrasenan J, Dias R, Lunn PG. Heterotopic ossification after the Outerbridge-Kashiwagi procedure in the elbow. J Shoulder Elb Surg. 2008;17(3):e15–e7.
73. Cai J, Wang W, Yan H, Sun Y, Chen W, Chen S, et al. Complications of open elbow arthrolysis in post-traumatic elbow stiffness: a systematic review. PLoS One. 2015;10(9):e0138547.
74. Cohen M. Post-traumatic contracture of the elbow: operative release using a lateral collateral ligament sparing approach. J Bone Joint Surg Br Vol. 1998;80(5):805–12.
75. Darlis NA, Kaufmann RW, Sotereanos DG. Open surgical treatment of post-traumatic elbow contractures in adolescent patients. J Shoulder Elb Surg. 2006;15(6):709–15.
76. Lindenhovius AL, Doornberg JN, Ring D, Jupiter JB. Health status after open elbow contracture release. JBJS. 2010;92(12):2187–95.
77. Shin R, Ring D. The ulnar nerve in elbow trauma. JBJS. 2007;89(5):1108–16.
78. Blonna D, O'Driscoll SW. Delayed-onset ulnar neuritis after release of elbow contracture: preventive strategies derived from a study of 563 cases. Arthroscopy. 2014;30(8):947–56.
79. Sun Y, Cai J, Li F, Liu S, Ruan H, Fan C. The efficacy of celecoxib in preventing heterotopic ossification recurrence after open arthrolysis for post-traumatic elbow stiffness in adults. J Shoulder Elb Surg. 2015;24(11):1735–40.
80. Degreef I, Van Audekercke R, Boogmans T, De Smet L. A biomechanical study on fracture risks in ulnohumeral arthroplasty. Chir Main. 2011;30(3):183–7.
81. Hong C-K, Chou A, Su W-R, Li C-L. A rare case of supracondylar humerus fracture after the Outerbridge-Kashiwagi procedure: a case report. Formosan J Musculoskel Disord. 2018;9(3):121–4.
82. Liu W, Sun Z, Xiong H, Liu J, Lu J, Cai B, et al. Development and validation of a prognostic nomogram for open elbow arthrolysis. Bone Joint J. 2022;104-B(4):486–94.
83. Abdel MP, Morrey ME, Barlow JD, Kreofsky CR, An K-N, Steinmann SP, et al. Myofibroblast cells are preferentially expressed early in a rabbit model of joint contracture. J Orthop Res. 2012;30(5):713–9.
84. Nesterenko S, Morrey ME, Abdel MP, An K-N, Steinmann SP, Morrey BF, et al. New rabbit knee model of posttraumatic joint contracture: indirect capsular damage induces a severe contracture. J Orthop Res. 2009;27(8):1028–32.
85. Trousdale WH, Limberg AK, Reina N, Salib CG, Thaler R, Dudakovic A, et al. Intra-articular celecoxib improves knee extension regardless of surgical release in a rabbit model of arthrofibrosis. Bone Joint Res. 2022;11(1):32–9.
86. Salib CG, Reina N, Trousdale WH, Limberg AK, Tibbo ME, Jay AG, et al. Inhibition of COX-2 pathway as a potential prophylaxis against arthrofibrogenesis in a rabbit model of joint contracture. J Orthop Res. 2019;37(12):2609–20.
87. Tibbo ME, Limberg AK, Salib CG, Turner TW, McLaury AR, Jay AG, et al. Anti-fibrotic effects of the antihistamine ketotifen in a rabbit model of arthrofibrosis. Bone Joint Res. 2020;9(6):302–10.

Arthroscopic Management of Proximal Radioulnar Joint Stiffness

14

Deepak N. Bhatia and Gregory I. Bain

14.1 Introduction

The proximal radioulnar joint (PRUJ) contributes to rotational range of motion and stability of the elbow joint. PRUJ pathology is an uncommon cause of rotational stiffness and can sometimes result in severe functional disability. At the milder end of the spectrum, PRUJ lesions involve peri-radial soft tissue adhesions, either isolated or as a part of global elbow stiffness. However, occasionally, bony involvement can result in a mechanical impingement and restricted arc of pronation-supination movement. Arthroscopy of PRUJ is a minimally invasive technique for visualization and excision of the impinging bony lesions and is associated with good functional outcomes [1, 2].

14.2 Indications and Contraindications

PRUJ arthroscopy is indicated in post-traumatic rotational elbow stiffness that occurs as a result of bony overgrowth/impingement and/or soft-tissue adhesions between the radial head/neck and proximal ulna. Fracture malunions of the radial head can result in PRUJ articular incongruency and loss of rotational range arc. Additionally, chronic contractures or periarticular adhesions between the annular ligament or quadrate ligament, and radial head/neck region add to the pathology. Heterotopic ossification around the PRUJ may also contribute to the overall stiffness and must be excised during the procedure (Fig. 14.1).

D. N. Bhatia (✉)
SportsDocs®, Sir HN Reliance Foundation Hospital and Research Center, Bandra, Mumbai, India

G. I. Bain
Department of Orthopedic Surgery, Flinders University of South Australia and Flinders Medical Centre, Adelaide, Australia
e-mail: greg@gregbain.com.au

L. Pederzini et al. (eds.), *Stiffness of the Elbow, Wrist and Related Pathologies*,
https://doi.org/10.1007/978-3-031-81381-8_14

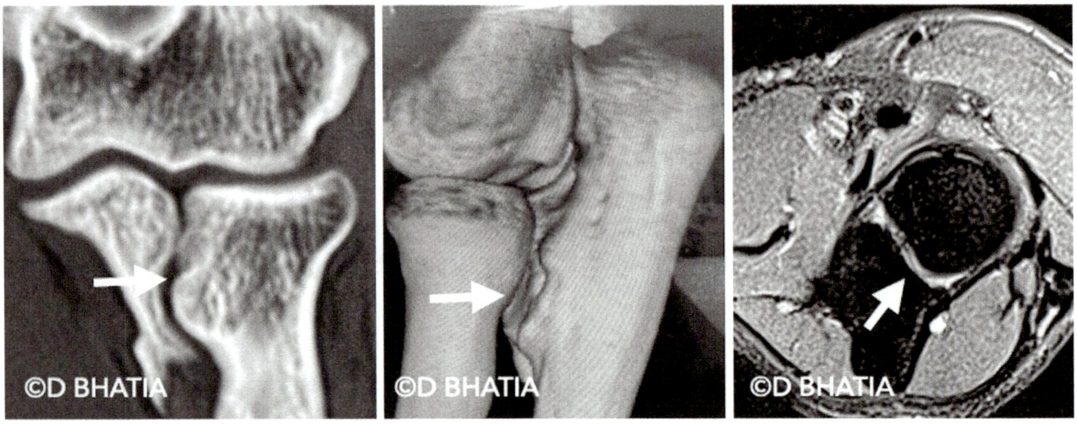

Fig. 14.1 Imaging of an elbow with severe rotational stiffness is shown. CT scans demonstrate an abnormal outgrowth from the radial head-neck junction (arrow, left image) and irregular outgrowths from the ulnar notch (arrow, middle image). The radial head is incongruent within the proximal radio-ulnar joint (arrow, right image) (copyright DN Bhatia)

Arthroscopic PRUJ debridement is contraindicated in radial head fracture malunions with severely deformed radial head anatomy, and these usually necessitate arthroscopic excision or recession procedures [3]. Other contraindications include congenital contractures, forearm deformities and advanced degenerative arthritis. Longstanding PRUJ stiffness is a relative contraindication; however, a release may be attempted in selected cases.

14.3 Surgical Technique

The surgery is performed with the patient in lateral decubitus position, and a tourniquet is used during the procedure. A 2.9 mm arthroscope (30° and 70° lens) and sheath (ConMed, Linvatec, Largo) are used, and gravity inflow is used to minimize fluid extravasation into the arm and forearm (Figs. 14.1, 14.2, 14.3, 14.4, and 14.5).

Portals: Four standard portals are used in the procedure:

- Proximal anteromedial (AM) and anterolateral portals (AL) are used for initial access to the radiocapitellar and lateral ulnotrochlear region and may be used as working portals for anterior PRUJ instrumentation.

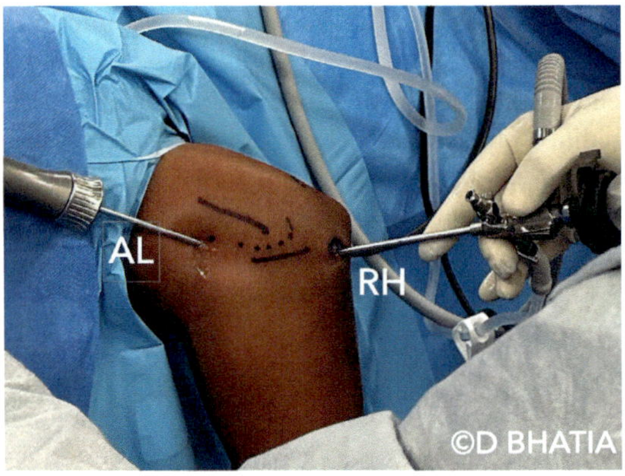

Fig. 14.2 A posterior 'radial head portal' (RH) is useful for visualization and working in combination with an anterolateral portal (AL). (Copyright DN Bhatia)

- The 'radial head portal' (RH) is used for visualization of PRUJ and may be used as an additional instrumentation portal [4] (Fig. 14.2).

PRUJ Access: PRUJ access is performed in three steps.

- **Annular ligament release:** Initial visualization of the PRUJ is performed via the standard AM portal. An AL portal is used for instrumentation and the thickened annular ligament is released from the anterior ulnar attachment.

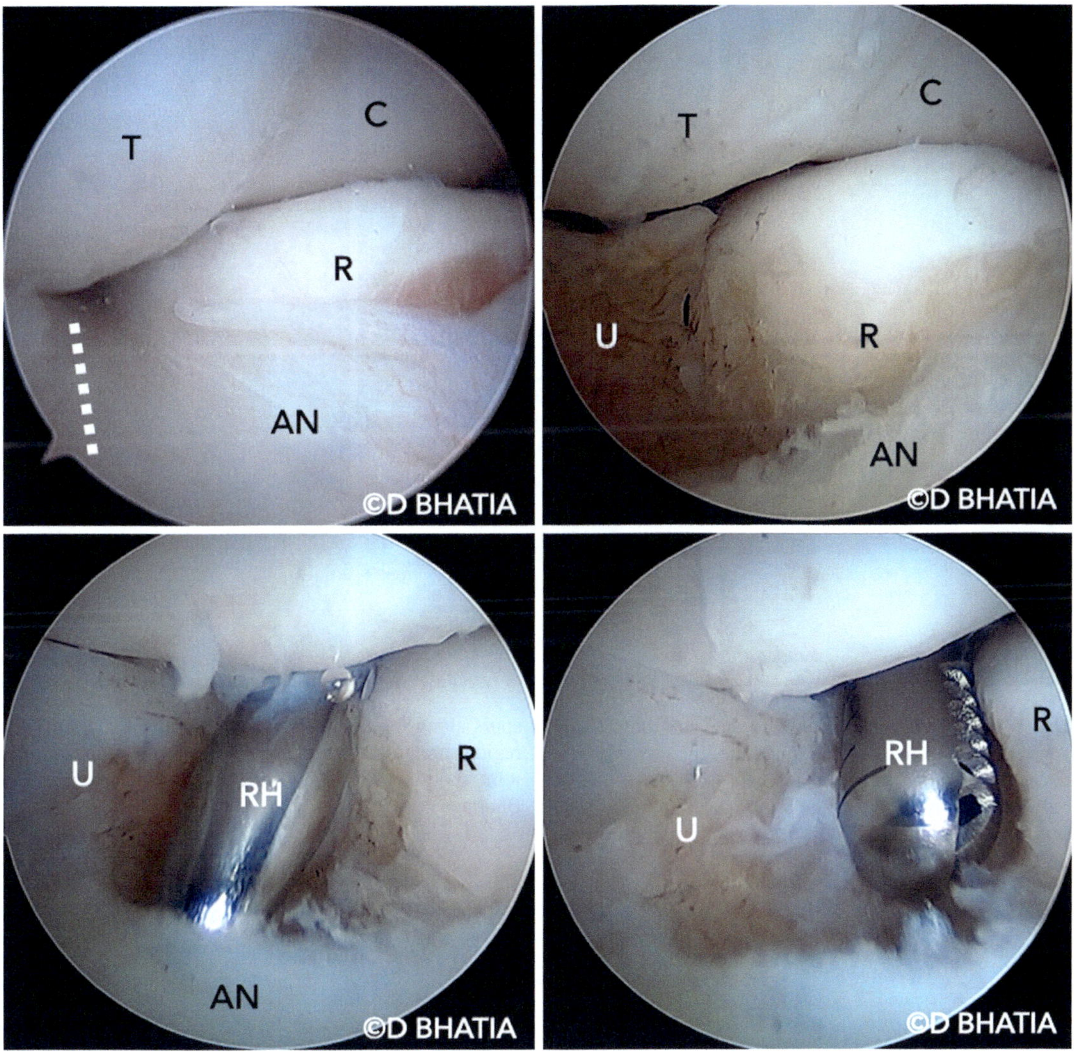

Fig. 14.3 Arthroscopic approach to proximal radio-ulnar joint (PRUJ) is shown. To gain access to PRUJ, the annular ligament (AN) is released anteriorly at its ulnar attachment (dotted line, top images). Next an obturator is passed from posterior to anterior via radial head portal (RH) and is directed between radial head (R) and ulnar notch (U). A shaver blade is passed via the same tract (RH) and the radial head is trimmed to create a working space. (*R* radial head, *C* capitellum, *T* trochlea). (Copyright DN Bhatia)

This release permits visualization of the entire PRUJ.

- **Radial head trimming:** A posterior RH portal is created, and a blunt obturator is passed into the PRUJ in a posterior to anterior direction. A 3.5 or 4 mm shaver blade is passed through this portal and initial resection/trimming of 2–3 mm of the ulnar aspect of radial head is performed to create space (Fig. 14.6).
- **Quadrate ligament release:** Next, the quadrate ligament is released along the anterior ulnar and entire radial attachments. This release provides further access to the impinging bone and contracted soft tissues inferior to the PRUJ.

Bone resection: Under AM portal visualization, an aggressive shaver blade is passed via RH portal. The ulnar aspect of radial head is

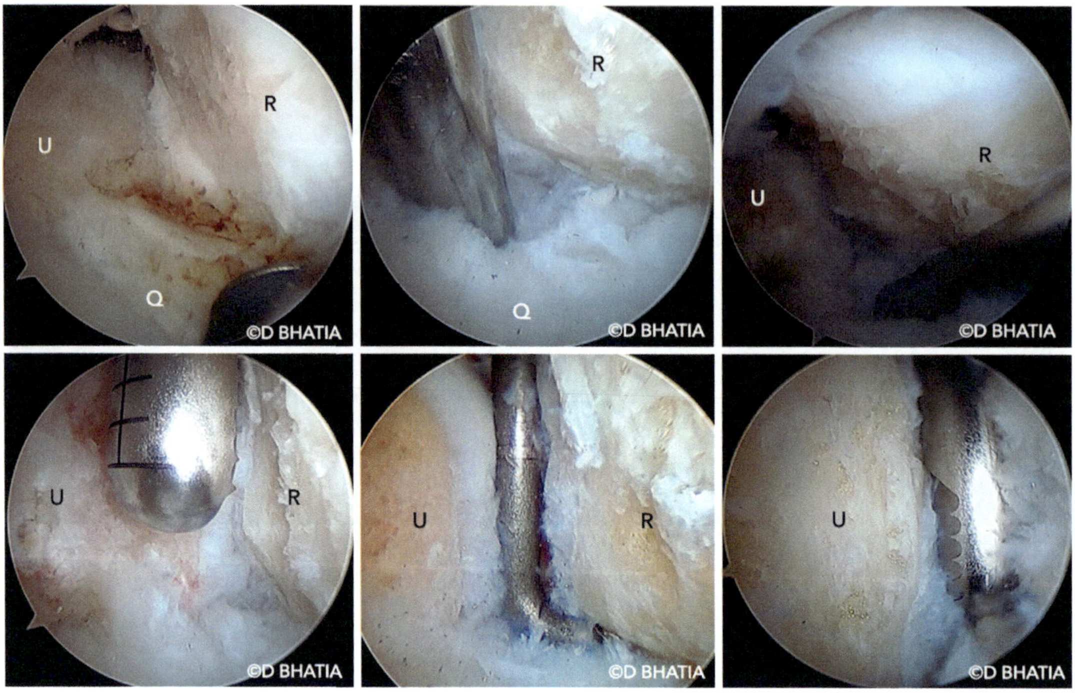

Fig. 14.4 Arthroscopic access to the sub-radial head zone is demonstrated. The quadrate ligament (Q) is released from its radial attachment (top left) and is retracted ulnarly to expose the region distal to radial head (top middle). The scarred soft tissues and impinging bone spurs along the radial (top right) and ulnar (bottom left) regions are burred for 1–2 cm distal to the radiocapitellar joint (bottom middle and left images). (Copyright DN Bhatia)

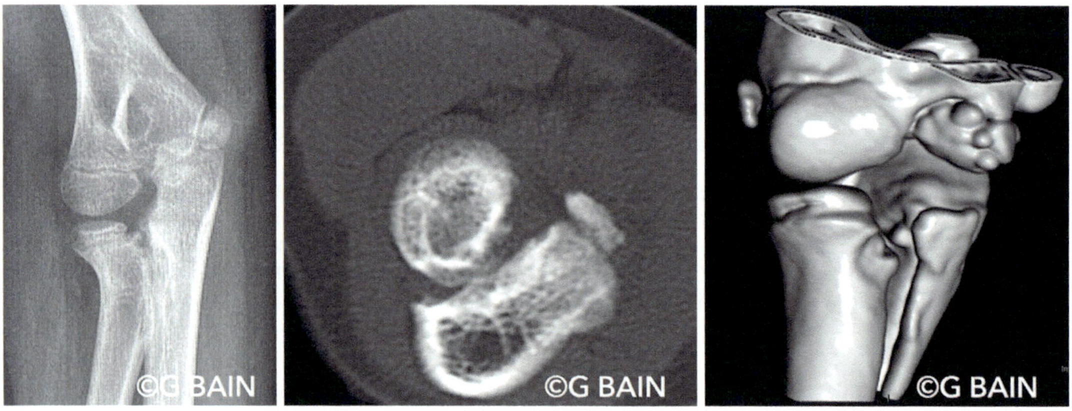

Fig. 14.5 Imaging of a patient with severe rotational restriction after a fall suffered 3 years ago. Radiographs and CT scan images show incongruence of the proximal radioulnar joint. (Copyright G Bain)

debrided; the forearm is rotated to identify impinging bone, and both radial head and radial aspect of ulna are debrided. The anterior aspect of radial head is difficult to reach via RH portal and is best approached via the AL portal. After initial debridement with a shaver, a burr is used to resect any remnant impinging bone. The visualization is changed to RH portal, and both AM and AL portals may be used to extend the debridement as required. Image

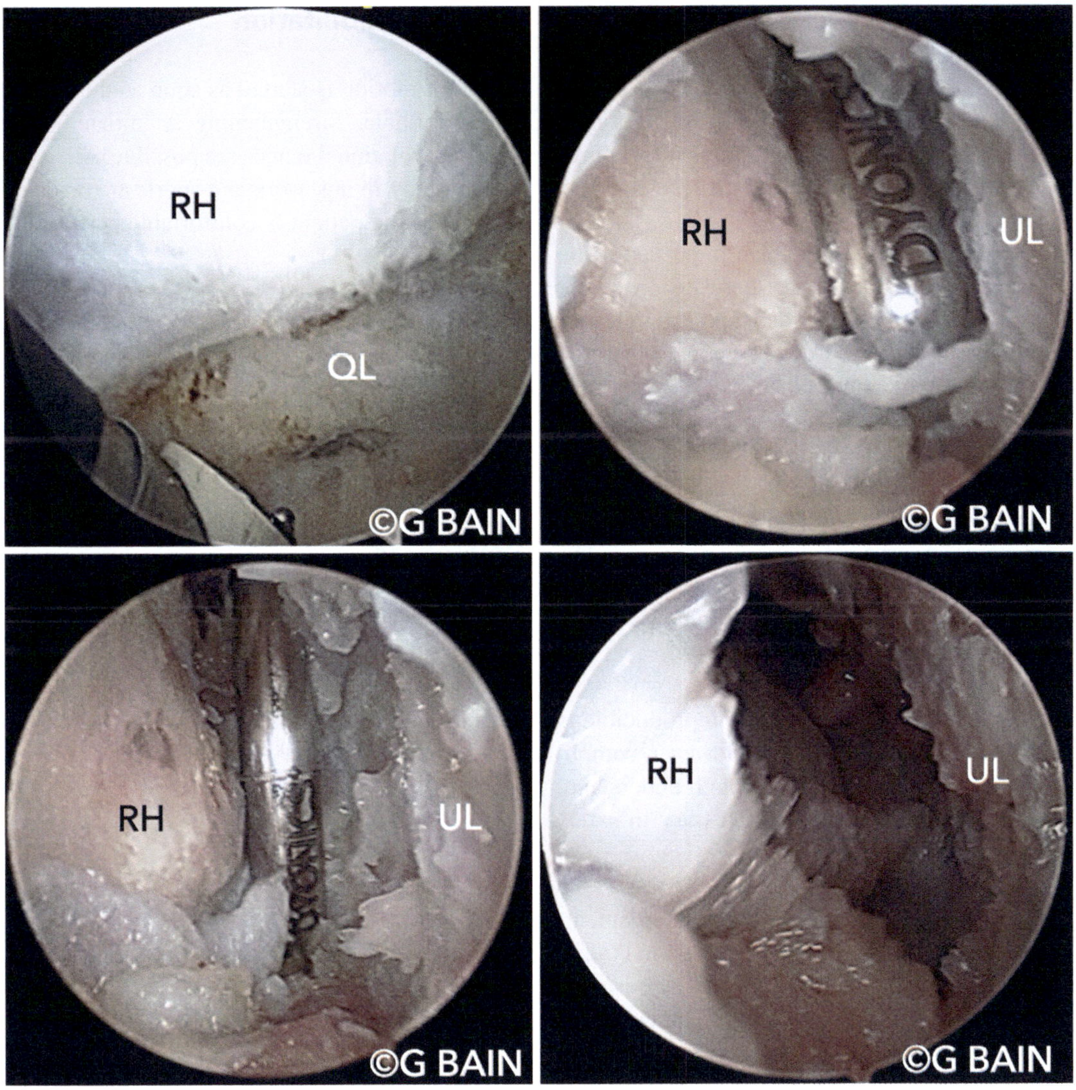

Fig. 14.6 Arthroscopic view of quadrate ligament (QL) release and debridement/burring of the radial (RH) and ulnar (UL) surfaces of the PRUJ (top images and bottom left image). Final view (bottom right) shows complete removal of the impinging spurs and irregular bone and complete rotational range was obtained. (Copyright G Bain)

guidance may be used to further guide the resection level.

Soft tissue resection: After releasing the annular and quadrate ligaments, the contracted and scarred soft tissue inferior to the PRUJ is identified. A probe is used to assess the extent of resection and the tissue is debrided using a shaver via RH portal. Forearm rotations are used throughout the procedure to guide resection.

A thorough lavage is given at the end of the procedure to remove any debris or bone fragments. The portals are closed and a compressive dressing is applied.

14.4 Tips and Tricks

- The RH portal provides excellent access for resection. Release of annular ligament prior to directing the obturator through RH portal allows clear visualization of the resection process [3, 4].
- The quadrate ligament is an important stabilizer of the PRUJ. Resection/excision of this ligament should be avoided, and a radial sided release is sufficient to gain access to the inferior impinging bone and soft tissues.
- The ulnar artery is in close proximity to the distal biceps tendon insertion on the radial tuberosity [5]. Neurovascular structures can be protected by restricting resection instruments to the area between the radius and ulna.

14.5 Complications

The technique has been safe and reproducible in the experience of both authors. However, complications are possible, and a thorough understanding of elbow arthroscopy is necessary to safely perform this procedure.

- Release of annular and quadrate ligaments may result in instability of the proximal radioulnar joint. This may be avoided by performing only a detachment of both ligaments from their bony insertions; this helps preserve ligament tissue and scarring in the region may help prevent instability.
- Initial trimming of the radial head may progress to painful restriction of rotational range; however, this has not been observed at follow-up assessments.
- The bony and soft tissue resection zone should not extend further distal to the radial neck region to avoid proximity to neurovascular structures.
- Further distal along the radial neck and proximal to the radial tuberosity, the transverse radio-ulnar ligament and oblique cord are at risk of iatrogenic damage [6, 7].

14.6 Rehabilitation

Range of motion is started as soon as the patient is comfortable. Strengthening is initiated once pain-free rotational ranges are possible. All activities of daily living, work and sports are resumed as soon as the patient is comfortable performing them.

Conflict of Interest The author(s) declare that they have no competing interests. All authors, their immediate family and any research foundation with which they are affiliated did not receive any financial payments or other benefits from any commercial entity related to the subject of this article.

References

1. Ek ET, Wang KK. Arthroscopic releases of the proximal radioulnar joint. In: Bhatia DN, Bain GI, Poehling GG, Graves BR, editors. Arthroscopy and endoscopy of the elbow, wrist and hand. Cham: Springer; 2022. https://doi.org/10.1007/978-3-030-79423-1_25.
2. Ek ET, Paul SK, Hotchkiss RN. Outcomes after operative treatment of elbow contractures in the pediatric and adolescent population. J Shoulder Elbow Surg. 2016;25(12):2066–70. https://doi.org/10.1016/j.jse.2016.09.008.
3. Bhatia DN. Arthroscopic resection of the radial head. In: Bain G, Eygendaal D, van Riet R, editors. Surgical techniques for trauma and sports related injuries of the elbow. Heidelberg: Springer, Berlin; 2020.
4. Bhatia DN. Arthroscopic radial head resection using the "radial head portal". In: Bhatia DN, Bain GI, Poehling GG, Graves BR, editors. Arthroscopy and endoscopy of the elbow, wrist and hand. Cham: Springer; 2022. https://doi.org/10.1007/978-3-030-79423-1_25.
5. Bhatia D, Naskar R, DeNiese P. Dynamic rotational alteration in positional relationship of neurovascular structures and distal biceps tendon insertion: a cadaveric study. J ISAKOS. 2019;4:296–301. https://doi.org/10.1136/jisakos-2019-000326.
6. Bhatia DN. Endoscopic anatomy of distal biceps tendon insertion and bicipitoradial bursa: a cadaveric study. J Shoulder Elbow Surg. 2021;30:1759–67. https://doi.org/10.1016/j.jse.2020.11.033.
7. Biewener A, Bischoff F, Rischke T, Tille E, Nimtschke U, Kasten P, Schaser KD, Nowotny J. Instability of the proximal radioulnar joint in Monteggia fractures-an experimental study. J Orthop Surg Res. 2019;14(1):392. https://doi.org/10.1186/s13018-019-1367-7.

15 Arthroscopic Management of the Stiff Elbow: Ankylosis and Arthrofibrosis

Tara Reza, Michael O'Brien, and Felix H. Savoie

15.1 Introduction

Arthroscopic treatment of elbow stiffness has evolved to become the mainstay of operative treatment of choice in many cases. Multiple pathologies lead to a stiff elbow that can be simplified into post-traumatic causes and arthritic causes. Arthritic elbow includes ulnohumeral, proximal radioulnar, and radiocapitellar joint deterioration. Post-traumatic stiff elbow includes capsular contracture, intra- and peri-articular adhesions, and arthrofibrosis. These contractures can happen after trauma, systemic disease, or surgery. This chapter will discuss elbow stiffness from its two sources: arthritic elbow and arthrofibrotic, often post-traumatic, stiff elbow. Though both causes lead to a stiff elbow, the etiology and management differ and will therefore be discussed in separate subsections.

15.2 What Is Elbow Stiffness?

Elbow stiffness has been defined as a loss of normal range of motion, leading to loss of flexion or the pronation/supination arc to <100°, which results in marked impairment of the ability to perform activities of daily living [1]. Arthrofibrosis of the elbow is a loss of both extension and flexion due to intrinsic and extrinsic abnormalities caused by dislocations, fractures, burns, head injury, arthritis conditions, or cerebral palsy [2–4]. Recently, elbow stiffness has been quantified as a loss of extension >30° and flexion of fewer than 120° [1]. While the definitions vary, a common motif is the functional loss of movement and ability to perform ADLs, which hinders recovery and rehab following trauma to the elbow [1]. The motion of the elbow is preserved with the tight congruence of articular surfaces, the posterior and anterior capsule, and the collateral ligaments; any alteration of these components can reduce the arc of motion of the elbow joint [5].

15.3 Pathology of Elbow Stiffness

Many factors lead to elbow stiffness, including soft tissue contractures, heterotopic bone formation as well as fracture nonunion or malunion, and arthrosis of the joint [1]. Arthrofibrosis is defined as loss of both flexion and extension of the elbow due to intrinsic and extrinsic abnormalities, as listed above [2, 6, 7]. Elbow stiffness can be classified as atraumatic or traumatic, as well as congenital or acquired, as outlined by Masci et al. [5]. Atraumatic causes include

T. Reza · M. O'Brien · F. H. Savoie (✉)
Department of Orthopaedic Surgery and Rehabilitation, Tulane University, New Orleans, LA, USA
e-mail: treza@tulane.edu; mobrien@tulane.edu; Fsavoie@tulane.edu

L. Pederzini et al. (eds.), *Stiffness of the Elbow, Wrist and Related Pathologies*,
https://doi.org/10.1007/978-3-031-81381-8_15

inflammatory arthritis (rheumatoid), post-septic arthritis, osteoarthritis, hemarthrosis, arthrogryposis, and congenital dislocation of the radial head [5, 8]. Fractures, burns, other trauma, and pathologies of the nervous system, such as cerebral palsy or brain injury are the most common etiologies of elbow stiffness [5, 8, 9].

15.4 The Nonarthritic Stiff Elbow

15.4.1 Pathology of Elbow Stiffness (Arthrofibrosis)

Contracture of the soft tissues physically restricts elbow motion, as the elbow capsule will thicken when traumatized [1]. The microbiology of capsule thickening is attributed to increased myofibroblasts and collagen crosslinks, as well as decreased water content and proteoglycan content [1, 10]. Though this physiologic response to trauma aids in wound healing and tissue repair, when overstimulated, the abundance of these components leads to contracture and scarring [1, 11]. The myofibroblasts are most prolific earlier after the traumatic event to the elbow [5, 12]. Hildebrand et al. found that post-traumatic pain and inflammation (substance P) induce mast cells mediated by neuropeptides which then stimulate myofibroblasts for fibrosis [13, 14]. The implication is that pain control may decrease fibrotic response post-traumatic, to reduce elbow stiffness [13]. Heterotopic ossification (HO) can lead to post-traumatic elbow stiffness, from the inappropriate formation of lamellar bone in non-skeletal tissue [1, 5]. HO mechanically blocks the elbow's normal range of motion. This physiologic block to joint movement is sometimes exacerbated by the creation of synostoses between the radius and ulna, hindering pronation and supination of the forearm [5, 15]. Risk factors for HO development include closed head injuries, burns, delay to surgery, as well as neurologic complications, though the most common is direct trauma [1] (Table 15.1). Often, surgical excision of HO has been delayed until it has clearly defined margins and smooth borders, to aid in locating it for excision [1]. Variations in fracture treatment affect post-traumatic elbow healing [5]. Alterations in joint anatomy following fractures of the distal humerus, for instance, can lead to elbow stiffness, obstructing the elbow's normal range of motion [1]. Fracture characteristics, such as whether it is comminuted, open, after high-energy trauma, de-vascularized, or followed by infection, can all predispose a post-traumatic elbow to stiffness [5]. Emphasis must be placed on achieving anatomic reduction for primary bone healing to restore the smooth articulation of the elbow joint [1]. Finally, joint arthrosis from trauma to the articular surface leads to osteophyte formation and degeneration, causing post-traumatic arthritis [1]. These osteophytes prevent a smooth range of motion at the articular surface [1].

Table 15.1 A listing of risk factors that lead to increased risk of formation of HO about elbow

Closed head injuries
Burns
Delay to surgery
Direct trauma (most common)

The ulnar nerve, in the setting of severe joint contractures, requires special attention. Ulnar nerve palsy can sometimes be prevented if there is a prophylactic ulnar nerve decompression [4, 16, 17] (Fig. 15.1).

Blonna and O'Driscoll completed a large retrospective study of elbow arthroscopy for elbow stiffness which found that ulnar nerve prophylactic decompression reduced the rate of ulnar nerve injury, delaying the onset of neuropathy [16, 18]. Indications for ulnar nerve exploration are listed in Table 15.2. Notably, preoperative arc of motion of 30° or less and/or lack of flexion past 90° increase the risk of delayed ulnar nerve palsy once motion is restored [2].

15.4.2 History of Arthroscopic Management of the Stiff Elbow

In the 1930s, Burman et al. performed a study using cadavers describing arthroscopy usage in elbows [2, 19]. Entering the 1980s, almost 50 years later, elbow arthroscopy finally caught

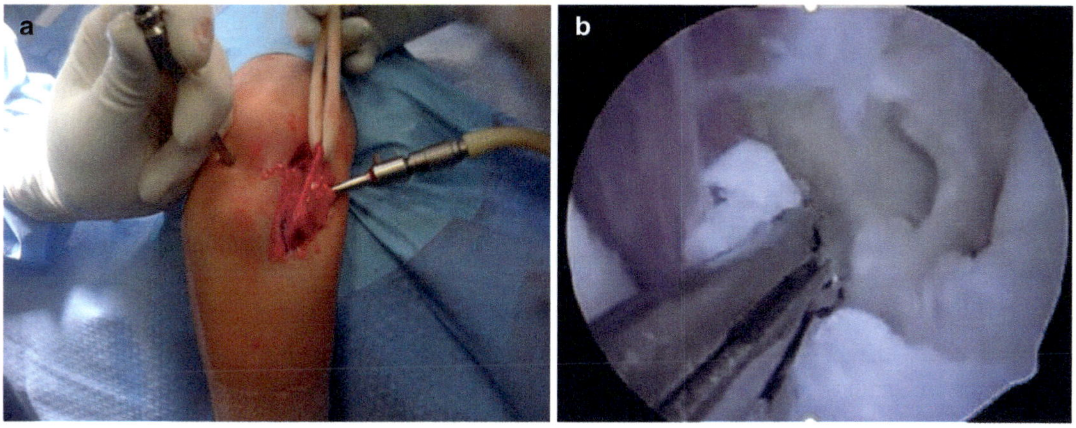

Fig. 15.1 (**a**) The ulnar nerve can be exposed and protected during arthroscopic ankylosis takedown as seen in this view with a Penrose drain holding the ulnar nerve away from the operating instruments. (**b**) Arthroscopic view of ulnar nerve decompression during arthroscopic ankylosis takedown

Table 15.2 Indications for ulnar nerve exploration

Preoperative ulnar nerve symptoms
Narrow cubital tunnel due to loose bodies/spurts
Previous ulnar nerve surgery
Preoperative arc of motion of 30° or less
Lack of flexion past 90°

up to knee and shoulder arthroscopy, as Poehling et al. and Andrews and Carson reported techniques of elbow arthroscopy, including different approaches from supine and prone positioning [20–22]. Poehling et al. specifically added the proximal medial portal from the prone position to the commonplace anteromedial and anterolateral portals, which were associated with injuries to the ulnar nerve [20, 23, 24]. This increased confidence in elbow arthroscopy, from an innovative approach to a safe procedure that would become more utilized and commonplace in the treatment of elbow stiffness [4, 20, 25, 26]. Andrews and Carson reported on elbow arthroscopy to remove loose bodies and debridement of synovectomy in rheumatic disease, debridement and lysis of adhesions in post-traumatic or atraumatic processes of the elbow, and debridement of osteochondritis dissecans of the radial head and capitellum [21]. In the 1990s, O'Driscoll, Morrey, Baker, and McGinty reported more studies on the use of arthroscopy of elbows, followed by specific treatment of elbow stiffness reported by Nowicki and Shall, Jones and Savoie, and Byrd [2, 27–31]. A common complication reported from these early studies was ulnar nerve neuropathy, which emphasized the need for consideration and safety during these procedures [8, 32].

15.4.3 Indications for Treatment

The primary indications for arthroscopic management of stiff elbow are pain and functional impairment refractory to non-operative management [2, 9, 33–36]. The American Academy of Orthopedic Surgeons defines a normal elbow range of motion from 0° to 146° of flexion [2, 34]. Motion less than the elbow's normal arc of motion in which activities of daily living are performed defines this functional impairment; while historically, Morrey et al. set the original definition of the elbow's functional arc of motion as 30–130° of flexion, 100° of flexion required for ADLs [34, 37, 38]. Painful elbow contractures <30° of extension or end extension <30° indicates arthroscopic management as well [34]. Another description is painful contracture of 30° or more that is functionally limiting and refractory to conservative treatment [39]. Elbow function is needed for basic every day motions, such as bringing the hand close to the face and reaching the hand out [16]. While there are some standard definitions of what is required for ADLs, certain activities may require more range of motion, such as personal hygiene, typing shoes, eating, and sporting activities [2]. For those who want a greater range of motion, such as athletes, the indications for arthroscopy treatment of stiff elbow extend to a larger range [6]. For manual workers and sportsmen, a slight decrease in range of motion with pain and hindrance of desired tasks are unacceptable to them, interfering with their livelihood [16, 38]. Specific age groups are more affected than others, such as active and young patients with increased functional demands [6, 8]. The indication for arthroscopy is, most importantly, the patient's decision, promoting shared decision-making with the physician [23]. Elbow stiffness of undetermined cause may also be an indication for arthroscopic diagnosis and further management [29].

15.4.4 Contraindications for Treatment

Mild and acute heterotopic ossification (HO) can be managed arthroscopically, while severe HO usually requires debridement with an open approach unless one is an expert arthroscopist [8]. Extensive contractures, extra-articular adhesions, and muscle contractures hinder successful arthroscopic treatment due to difficulties insufflating the joint, although Kamenini and Savoie have described an approach that begins extra-articularly to address these issues [4, 8]. Keener et al. report that loss of supination-pronation is a contraindication, and would be better addressed with an open approach, but McLaughlin and Savoie have described successful results in managing these issues [8, 40]. Submuscular ulnar nerve transposition is a relative contraindication as well, unless the course of the ulnar nerve can be determined by palpation, visual inspection, and ultrasound [8, 23]. Inexperience of the operative surgeon is an indirect contraindication, as close proximity of the neurovascular structures and a small working space makes arthroscopy of the elbow technically challenging [16, 33, 41]. As this procedure can prove extremely difficult, it should only be attempted by experienced arthroscopic surgeons [2]. Application of this procedure is limited by the extensive learning curve [33]. Baker et al. state that elbow arthroscopy is contraindicated when there is significant distortion of the joint, where safe entry of the arthroscope is inhibited by excess bony or soft tissue damage [29].

15.4.5 Anatomic Considerations

A stiff elbow is the result of changed anatomy within the elbow joint. There must be a thorough understanding of the pathogenesis, which comes from studying the altered anatomy; this is paramount to the surgeon [2]. A contracted joint does not behave normally, which leaves the neurovascular structures at risk as they cannot be safely displaced when the elbow is insufflated [2]. Three major structures are potentially associated with elbow stiffness, including ligaments, muscles, and the capsule [42, 43]. Arthroscopic capsulectomy is used for treating elbow stiffness, but may prove challenging if there are significant adhesions between the joint and the capsule, reducing the working space for arthroscopic exposure after insufflation [42, 44] (Fig. 15.2). Arthroscopy for elbow stiffness aims to remove fibrous tissue, resect osteophytes, release the capsule, and possibly excise the radial head [25].

Initial entrance into the elbow joint is guided by the often unaffected medial epicondyle and medial intramuscular septum [2]. To protect the median nerve and brachial artery from damage, the proximal anteromedial portal is placed more anteriorly, usually 2.5–3 cm anterior to the intermuscular septum, angling posterior to the brachialis muscle [2]. The posterior interosseous nerve can be affected by distal lateral elbow contracture or trauma due to the hypertrophy or adhesions that may bind the nerve [2]. While the proximal anteromedial portal should be used from an outside-in manner, the inside-out technique should be utilized for an anterior superior lateral portal to decrease the risk of injury to the posterior interosseous nerve [2]. A stiff elbow is contracted due to the hypertrophied injured soft tissue; this tissue can cause misdirection of the cannula through the skin and into the joint, neces-

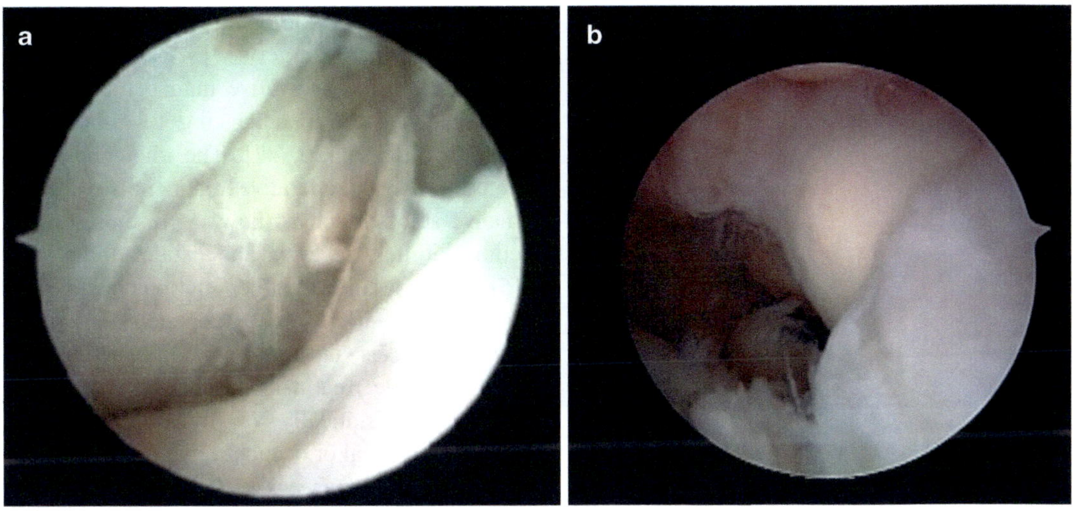

Fig. 15.2 Arthroscopic images found in a stiff elbow. (**a**) Adhesions and scarring in the capsule as evidenced in this anterior view. (**b**) Osteophytes and spurring present along medial gutter

sitating care during its placement into the joint [2]. In cases of severe contracture, developing a plane between the capsule and brachialis muscle safely allows the surgeon to incise and thus excise the capsule secondarily [2]. Retractors must be placed carefully to protect the brachialis muscle and the neurovascular structures in proximity during this approach [2]. An excessive olecranon deformity or hypertrophied adherent medial capsule can move the ulnar nerve, making the initial insertion into the posterior central portal into the olecranon fossa risky. When entering the olecranon fossa, it is important to enter centrally and not swerve medially to possibly injure the nearby neurovascular structures [2].

Prior to beginning the procedure, it is important to remember the relationship of the neurovascular structures to the capsule. From the anterior approach, the brachialis muscle lies between the anterior neurovascular structures, including the median nerve, radial nerve and brachial artery, and the capsule. Releasing and excising the capsule should be continued until the brachialis muscle fibers are visible, at which point the surgeon must stop [24]. The cutting blades and shavers are to be kept close to the humerus and avoid any anterior misstep so as to prevent injury of the neurovascular structures by brachialis muscle penetration [2]. A technique used to avoid these missteps is an additional anterior portal for protective retractors to hold the anterior neurovascular structures and brachialis muscle away from the operative field, decreasing the risk of complications [2, 45].

The radial nerve courses between the brachialis muscle and brachioradialis, at which point it divides into the posterior interosseous nerve and the superficial radial nerve at the level of the elbow joint. The posterior interosseous nerve then courses distal and lateral to the brachialis muscle, adjacent to the anterior aspect of the joint capsule in the distal half of the elbow joint. Hypertrophied joint capsule and scar tissue in this area may cling to the posterior interosseous nerve, putting it at risk of damage during the capsule's release. Prior to proceeding with the distal excision of the capsule, the nerve should be identified by the perineural fat and retracted [2]. Until the posterior interosseous nerve is identified, the excision of the capsule should remain close to the radial head [2]. Caution should also be exercised with the ulnar nerve, which should be identified posteriorly; excision should proceed below the nerve, while identifying and retracting it [2] (Fig. 15.3). If elbow flexion remains stiff after capsulectomy from a posterior approach, the posterior bundle of the medial collateral ligament may need to be released for improvement. This

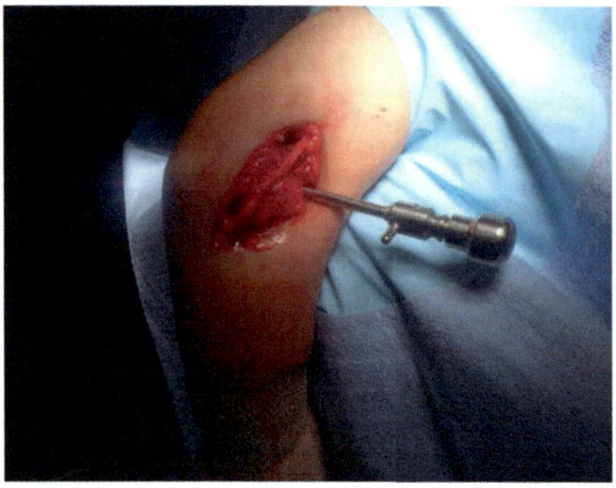

Fig. 15.3 Approach used to protect at-risk ulnar nerve

can decompress and protect the ulnar nerve simultaneously [42].

Elbow motion after trauma is affected by two muscles: brachialis for extension in the front and triceps for extension posteriorly; both muscles should be elevated off the humerus during arthroscopy for the stiff elbow. We routinely do this on all stiff elbows, and find it beneficial for successful results. When deciding between starting with an anterior or posterior approach, O'Driscoll et al. postulated that a posterior approach with work extending into the medial and lateral gutters will be challenging because of the soft tissue inflammation, while anterior compartment swelling can be controlled or maneuvered around with the use of retractors [46]. However, Savoie routinely prefers to begin anteriorly, feeling the anterior neurovascular structures are more at risk in extensive ankylosis takedown surgery and prefers to completely excise the anterior capsule and elevate the brachialis prior to moving to the posterior compartment (Fig. 15.4).

15.4.6 Non-operative Management

Stiffness following injury to a joint progresses in four stages: bleeding, edema, granulation tissue, and fibrosis [35]. Treatment options for elbow stiffness are divided into non-operative and operative management. Non-operative treatment is almost always attempted first, as patients should undergo a trial of non-operative therapy prior to consideration for surgery [2]. A course of 3 to 12 months of conservative management is recommended prior to advancing to arthroscopic surgical release [26, 47]. The choice between conservative and operative treatment is guided by many factors, such as how it presents, timing, comorbidities, severity, and patient compliance [5]. Non-operative treatment options include corticosteroid injections, non-steroidal anti-inflammatories, and activity modifications. Other non-operative treatment options include splinting, either statically or dynamically, serial casting, physical or occupational therapy, manipulation, continuous passive motion (CPM), and functional re-education [5]. Adjustable static splints provide a constant force at delineated intervals to exert stress and distraction to the elbow tissues, which reduces inflammation risk [5] (Fig. 15.5). According to Masci et al., dynamic splints are the most used device to treat elbow stiffness and are based on viscoelastic properties of the soft tissues around the joint to create a certain degree of deformation in response to a variable force [5]. However, we feel dynamic splinting often causes increased inflammation and pain, with negative results in most cases. Outcomes from non-operative treatment vary vastly from the return of range of motion or potentially losing some range of motion if the joint becomes increasingly inflamed. Manipulations for elbow stiffness have very mixed results and high complication rates and are not routinely recommended. Caution should be exercised in any non-operative therapy to prevent additional damage to the elbow capsule and increased arthrofibrosis [2].

15.4.7 Indications for Surgery

Operative management for elbow stiffness is primarily indicated by patients who fail conservative management techniques, as discussed above. Shared decision-making between the patient and the surgeon should be practiced, prior to further discussions of possible surgical management [2]. Prior to proceeding with surgical management,

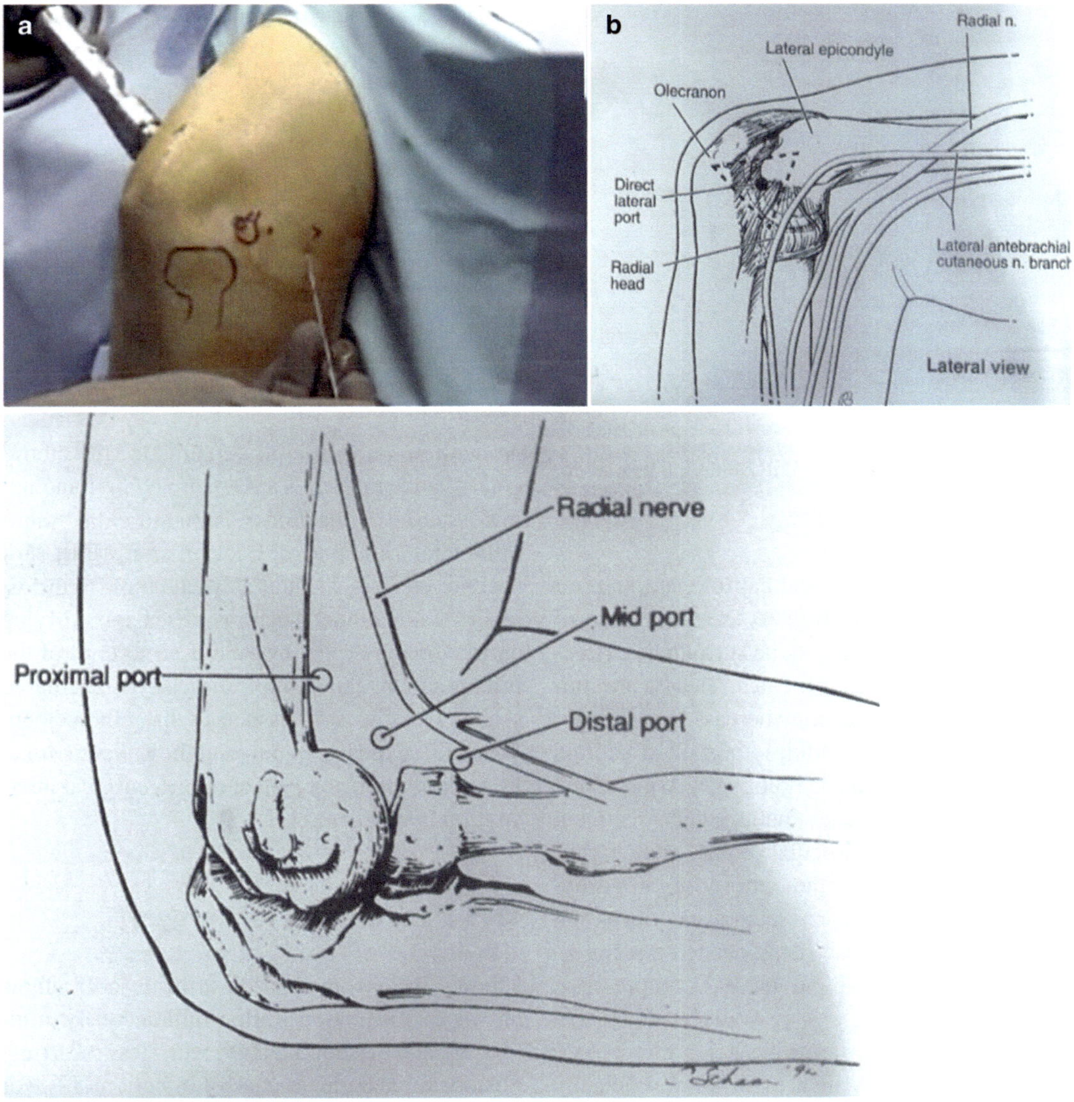

Fig. 15.4 Anterior portals utilized in arthrofibrosis takedown. (**a**) The proximal anterolateral portal. (**b**) The proximal anterolateral portal

the likely etiology of the condition, risks, benefits, expected results, and possible complications, such as the risk of ulnar nerve damage, should be evaluated and discussed between the surgeon and the patient [2].

Historically, elbow stiffness refractory to nonoperative management was addressed with open surgical approaches. However, advances in elbow arthroscopy beginning in the late 1980s with Jones and Savoie's report on successful management of arthrofibrosis as well as increased training in elbow arthroscopy have expanded the indications for arthroscopic treatment of elbow stiffness [32, 38, 48, 49]. Now, post-traumatic elbows can be successfully treated with arthroscopy. This procedure has the added benefit of using a minimally invasive approach that offers results comparable, if not better, than the open approach with fewer complications and faster readaptation and recovery [4, 15–17, 25, 48]. Open surgical release of elbow contracture increases soft tissue trauma from the capsule dis-

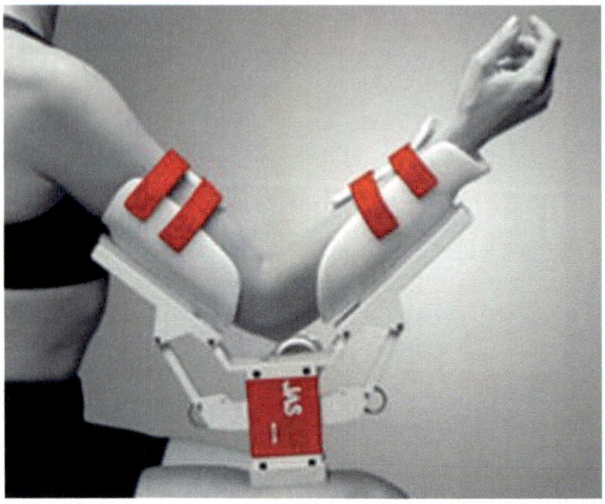

Fig. 15.5 Adjustable static and dynamic splints used for non-operative management

section, and scarring of the capsule and anterior structures, which can lead to the recurrence of contracture, and damage to the surrounding structures of the elbow [2, 16]. Open releases are limited by the approach, whereas arthroscopic management can use multiple portals to address the entire intrinsic joint pathology [2]. Arthroscopy permits diagnostic examination and treatment planning for intra-articular joint pathologies. Arthroscopy allows for the removal of intra-articular adhesions, capsular resection anteriorly and posteriorly, and release of associated scaring as well as metal removal and nerve decompression. Lubiatowski et al., as well as Kodde et al., recommend avoiding open arthrolysis for minor contractures and to only treat them arthroscopically to reduce the chance of worsening the contracture [16, 39]. Release of collateral ligaments, in addition to adhesions in the lateral and medial gutters, can be accomplished arthroscopically [2]. Overall, arthroscopic management of elbow stiffness is advantageous for improved visualization of the joint, smaller scars, reduced pain, faster rehabilitation, and shorter hospital stay [15, 47, 50] (Table 15.3). Outcomes following arthroscopic management of stiff elbow have proved favorable by many studies [8, 33, 36, 38, 51–57]. Of note, 2–3 weeks immediately following the surgery, some studies have reported a decrease in motion, that improves and surpasses original range of motion around 3 months [16, 47].

Table 15.3 Advantages of arthroscopic management of stiff elbow

Improved visualization of elbow joint
Smaller scars
Reduced pain
Faster rehabilitation
Shorter hospital stay

15.5 The Arthritic Elbow

15.5.1 Non-operative Management

As with non-arthritic post-traumatic stiff elbow, conservative measures are attempted first, including steroid injections, non-steroidal anti-inflammatories, and physical therapy [50]. For specific etiologies, such as rheumatoid arthritis, other medications, such as disease-modifying antirheumatic drugs, may be used to control the inflammation and reduce the risk of increased scarring of the soft tissues of the elbow joint. When these measures fail, and the patient's functional limitation and pain continue, surgical intervention is warranted [2].

15.5.2 Indications for Surgery

Elbow arthroscopy for the arthritic stiff elbow allows for evaluation while simultaneously minimizing soft-tissue damage with less scarring, postoperative pain, and risk of infection [58]. For the arthritic elbow, many factors should be considered to dictate the decision between arthroscopic management and total elbow arthroplasty. These factors include activity level, patient expectations, bone stock, age, and severity of the deformity [2]. Historically, an open approach was used, dating back to the Outerbridge–Kashiwagi procedure, which involves a triceps-splitting approach, debridement of the olecranon and a hole drilled between the coronoid fossa and olecranon. This would increase flexion and extension, and reduce impingement anteriorly and posteriorly [2]. Resection of the radial head improved function in inflammatory arthritis, such as in patients with rheumatoid arthritis (Fig. 15.6). The

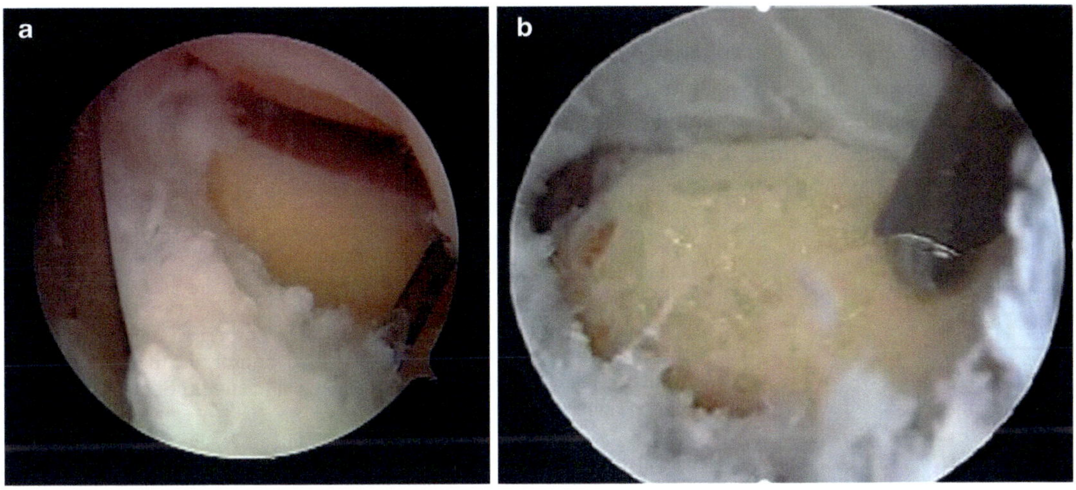

Fig. 15.6 Arthroscopic procedure when radial head excision is indicated and performed: (**a**) in this view from the medial portal significant radiocapitellar arthritis is visualized. (**b**) In the same view as "A" the radial head has been completely excised while preserving the annular ligament

same soft tissue principles apply when capsular contractures are accompanied by arthritis. However, the emphasis in an approach of a stiff arthritic elbow should focus more on intrinsic bony pathology [59]. Morrey modified the aforementioned approach by elevating, rather than splitting, the triceps, in an attempt to reduce intra-articular adhesions. Morrey's approach aided in the transposition of the ulnar nerve and increased range of motion [2]. Savoie et al. modified Morrey's approach, transitioning from open to arthroscopic treatment. Arthroscopic tools were used to fenestrate the coronoid and olecranon fossa, remove the radial head, if necessary, withdraw loose bodies and perform a synovectomy of the elbow capsule [53].

Technical pearls in managing the arthritic elbow include moving the medial proximal anterior portal about a cm more anterior to "get around" the anterior medial osteophytes, and allow better access to the coronoid osteophytes, deepening the radial fossa rather than excising the radial head, elevation of the triceps posteriorly and excision of the spur on the posterior capitellum. Preservation of the capsule is usually recommended if all spurs are excised completely, but one study found that preservation leads to worse outcomes, specifically decreased range of motion [60]. Many studies following the development of arthroscopic management of arthritic elbow showed positive outcomes, promoting the enduring success of this method for early, mid-, and late-stage arthritis, reducing the number of patients originally destined for complete elbow replacement [40, 52, 61, 62]. Kim et al. and Lubiatowski et al. found no difference in outcomes between patients with post-traumatic versus degenerative etiology [16, 33].

15.6 Conclusion

Due to advances in technology, the development of safe approaches, and increased arthroscopic training, arthroscopic management of elbow stiffness has become the treatment of choice in most cases. There are intrinsic and extrinsic etiologies that can lead to elbow stiffness, which must be considered when choosing operative management. Stiff elbow includes loss of motion due to post-traumatic capsular contractures, arthrofibrosis, and intra- and peri-articular adhesions, as well as arthritic elbow stiffness from joint deterioration. Indications for arthroscopic management are multifactorial and include the extent of elbow arc of motion loss, stiffness refractory to conservative management, pain, patient expectations for activities of daily living, and willingness to comply with post-operative therapy. A foundation of knowledge of the pathology and etiology of elbow stiffness, anatomical considerations for approaches, indications, and contraindications, with a patient-centered approach, will guide surgeons to positive outcomes following arthroscopic management of elbow stiffness.

References

1. Akhtar A, Hughes B, Watts AC. The post-traumatic stiff elbow: a review. J Clin Orthop Trauma. 2021;19:125–31.
2. Savoie FH, Field LD. Arthroscopic management of the stiff elbow. In: Morrey's the elbow and its disorders. Elsevier; 2009. p. 596–608.
3. Aldridge JM, Atkins TA, Gunneson EE, Urbaniak JR. Anterior release of the elbow for extension loss. J Bone Joint Surg Am. 2004;86(9):1955–60.
4. Willinger L, Siebenlist S, Lenich A, Liska F, Imhoff AB, Achtnich A. Arthroscopic arthrolysis provides good clinical outcome in post-traumatic and degenerative elbow stiffness. Knee Surg Sports Traumatol Arthrosc. 2018;26(1):312–7.
5. Masci G, Cazzato G, Milano G, Ciolli G, Malerba G, Perisano C, et al. The stiff elbow: current concepts. Orthop Rev (Pavia). 2020;12(Suppl 1):8661.
6. Schreiner AJ, Schweikardt N, Gühring D, Ahrend MD, Döbele S, Ahmad SS, et al. Arthroscopic arthrolysis leads to improved range of motion and health-related quality of life in post-traumatic elbow stiffness. J Shoulder Elb Surg. 2020;29(8):1538–47.
7. Zubler V, Saupe N, Jost B, Pfirrmann CW, Hodler J, Zanetti M. Elbow stiffness: effectiveness of conventional radiography and CT to explain osseous causes. AJR Am J Roentgenol. 2010;194(6):W515–20.
8. Keener JD, Galatz LM. Arthroscopic management of the stiff elbow. J Am Acad Orthop Surg. 2011;19(5):265–74.
9. Bruno RJ, Lee ML, Strauch RJ, Rosenwasser MP. Posttraumatic elbow stiffness: evaluation and management. J Am Acad Orthop Surg. 2002;10(2):106–16.
10. Biswas D, Wysocki RW, Cohen MS. Primary and posttraumatic arthritis of the elbow. Arthritis. 2013;2013:473259.
11. Cohen MS, Schimmel DR, Masuda K, Hastings H 2nd, Muehleman C. Structural and biochemical evaluation of the elbow capsule after trauma. J Shoulder Elb Surg. 2007;16(4):484–90.
12. Charalambous CP, Morrey BF. Posttraumatic elbow stiffness. J Bone Joint Surg Am. 2012;94(15):1428–37.
13. Hildebrand KA, Zhang M, Befus AD, Salo PT, Hart DA. A myofibroblast-mast cell-neuropeptide axis of fibrosis in post-traumatic joint contractures: an in vitro analysis of mechanistic components. J Orthop Res. 2014;32(10):1290–6.
14. Hildebrand KA. Posttraumatic elbow joint contractures: defining pathologic capsular mechanisms and potential future treatment paradigms. J Hand Surg Am. 2013;38(11):2227–33.
15. Karelson M, Launonen AP, Jokihaara J, Havulinna J, Mattila VM. Pain, function, and patient satisfaction after arthroscopic treatment of elbow in a retrospective series with minimum of 5-year follow-up. J Orthop Surg (Hong Kong). 2019;27(1):2309499019832808.
16. Lubiatowski P, Ślęzak M, Wałecka J, Bręborowicz M, Romanowski L. Prospective outcome assessment of arthroscopic arthrolysis for traumatic and degenerative elbow contracture. J Shoulder Elb Surg. 2018;27(9):e269–e78.
17. Rai S, Zhang Q, Tamang N, Jin S, Wang H, Meng C. Arthroscopic arthrolysis of posttraumatic and non-traumatic elbow stiffness offers comparable clinical outcomes. BMC Musculoskelet Disord. 2019;20(1):285.
18. Blonna D, Bellato E, Marini E, Scelsi M, Castoldi F. Arthroscopic treatment of stiff elbow. ISRN Surg. 2011;2011:378135.
19. Burman MS. Arthroscopy or the direct visualization of joints: an experimental cadaver study. Clin Orthop Relat Res. 1931;2001(390):5–9.
20. Poehling GG, Whipple TL, Sisco L, Goldman B. Elbow arthroscopy: a new technique. Arthroscopy. 1989;5(3):222–4.
21. Andrews JR, Carson WG. Arthroscopy of the elbow. Arthroscopy. 1985;1(2):97–107.
22. Everding NG, Maschke SD, Hoyen HA, Evans PJ. Prevention and treatment of elbow stiffness: a 5-year update. J Hand Surg Am. 2013;38(12):2496–507.
23. Savoie FH, O'Brien MJ, Field LD. Arthroscopy for arthritis of the elbow. Hand Clin. 2011;27(2):171–8, v–vi.
24. Thoreux P, Blondeau C, Durand S, Masquelet AC. Anatomical basis of arthroscopic capsulotomy for elbow stiffness. Surg Radiol Anat. 2006;28(4):409–15.
25. Temporin K, Shimada K, Oura K, Owaki H. Arthroscopic release for the severely stiff elbow. Musculoskelet Surg. 2020;104(1):81–6.
26. Wu X, Wang H, Meng C, Yang S, Duan D, Xu W, et al. Outcomes of arthroscopic arthrolysis for the post-traumatic elbow stiffness. Knee Surg Sports Traumatol Arthrosc. 2015;23(9):2715–20.
27. O'Driscoll SW, Morrey BF. Arthroscopy of the elbow. Diagnostic and therapeutic benefits and hazards. J Bone Joint Surg Am. 1992;74(1):84–94.
28. Morrey BF. Primary degenerative arthritis of the elbow. Treatment by ulnohumeral arthroplasty. J Bone Joint Surg Br. 1992;74(3):409–13.
29. Baker CL, Jones GL. Arthroscopy of the elbow. Am J Sports Med. 1999;27(2):251–64.
30. Nowicki KD, Shall LM. Arthroscopic release of a posttraumatic flexion contracture in the

elbow: a case report and review of the literature. Arthroscopy. 1992;8(4):544–7.
31. Byrd JW. Elbow arthroscopy for arthrofibrosis after type I radial head fractures. Arthroscopy. 1994;10(2):162–5.
32. Jones GS, Savoie FH. Arthroscopic capsular release of flexion contractures (arthrofibrosis) of the elbow. Arthroscopy. 1993;9(3):277–83.
33. Kim SJ, Moon HK, Chun YM, Chang JH. Arthroscopic treatment for limitation of motion of the elbow: the learning curve. Knee Surg Sports Traumatol Arthrosc. 2011;19(6):1013–8.
34. Vieira LA, Dal Molin FF, Visco A, Fernandes LF, Dos Santos MC, Cardozo Filho NS, et al. Arthroscopic treatment of elbow stiffness. Rev Bras Ortop. 2011;46(4):398–402.
35. Sanchez-Sotelo J. Arthroscopic management of elbow stiffness. J Exp Orthop. 2021;8(1):97.
36. Ball CM, Meunier M, Galatz LM, Calfee R, Yamaguchi K. Arthroscopic treatment of post-traumatic elbow contracture. J Shoulder Elb Surg. 2002;11(6):624–9.
37. Morrey BF, Askew LJ, Chao EY. A biomechanical study of normal functional elbow motion. J Bone Joint Surg Am. 1981;63(6):872–7.
38. Pederzini LA, Nicoletta F, Tosi M, Prandini M, Tripoli E, Cossio A. Elbow arthroscopy in stiff elbow. Knee Surg Sports Traumatol Arthrosc. 2014;22(2):467–73.
39. Kodde IF, van Rijn J, van den Bekerom MP, Eygendaal D. Surgical treatment of post-traumatic elbow stiffness: a systematic review. J Shoulder Elb Surg. 2013;22(4):574–80.
40. McLaughlin RE, Savoie FH, Field LD, Ramsey JR. Arthroscopic treatment of the arthritic elbow due to primary radiocapitellar arthritis. Arthroscopy. 2006;22(1):63–9.
41. Van Zeeland NL, Yamaguchi K. Arthroscopic capsular release of the elbow. J Shoulder Elb Surg. 2010;19(2 Suppl):13–9.
42. Dai J, Zhang G, Li S, Xu J, Lu J. Arthroscopic treatment of posttraumatic elbow stiffness due to soft tissue problems. Orthop Surg. 2020;12(5):1464–70.
43. Tucker K. Some aspects of post-traumatic elbow stiffness. Injury. 1978;9(3):216–20.
44. Nguyen D, Proper SI, MacDermid JC, King GJ, Faber KJ. Functional outcomes of arthroscopic capsular release of the elbow. Arthroscopy. 2006;22(8):842–9.
45. Aldridge JM, Katt B, Rizzo M, Beredjiklian P, Urbaniak JR. Anterior elbow release for post-traumatic flexion contractures in patients 21 years or younger. J Shoulder Elb Surg. 2020;29(7):1394–400.
46. Martinez-Catalan N, Sanchez-Sotelo J. Primary elbow osteoarthritis: evaluation and management. J Clin Orthop Trauma. 2021;19:67–74.
47. Cefo I, Eygendaal D. Arthroscopic arthrolysis for posttraumatic elbow stiffness. J Shoulder Elb Surg. 2011;20(3):434–9.
48. Sos C, Petit A, Brunet J, Rabarin F, Cast YS, Raimbeau G, et al. Comparison of results of arthroscopic arthrolysis between traumatic and degenerative elbow stiffness. Orthop Traumatol Surg Res. 2022;109:103436.
49. Geib TM, Savoie FH. Elbow arthroscopy for posttraumatic arthrosis. Instr Course Lect. 2009;58:473–80.
50. Poonit K, Zhou X, Zhao B, Sun C, Yao C, Zhang F, et al. Treatment of osteoarthritis of the elbow with open or arthroscopic debridement: a narrative review. BMC Musculoskelet Disord. 2018;19(1):394.
51. Degreef I, De Smet L. Elbow arthrolysis for traumatic arthrofibrosis: a shift towards minimally invasive surgery. Acta Orthop Belg. 2011;77(6):758–64.
52. Phillips BB, Strasburger S. Arthroscopic treatment of arthrofibrosis of the elbow joint. Arthroscopy. 1998;14(1):38–44.
53. Savoie FH, Nunley PD, Field LD. Arthroscopic management of the arthritic elbow: indications, technique, and results. J Shoulder Elb Surg. 1999;8(3):214–9.
54. Steinmann SP, King GJ, Savoie FH. Arthroscopic treatment of the arthritic elbow. Instr Course Lect. 2006;55:109–17.
55. Timmerman LA, Andrews JR. Arthroscopic treatment of posttraumatic elbow pain and stiffness. Am J Sports Med. 1994;22(2):230–5.
56. Somanchi BV, Funk L. Evaluation of functional outcome and patient satisfaction after arthroscopic elbow arthrolysis. Acta Orthop Belg. 2008;74(1):17–23.
57. Júnior JC, Zabeu JL, Junior IA, Mattos CA, Myrrha JP. Arthroscopic treatment of post-traumatic elbow stiffness. Rev Bras Ortop. 2012;47(3):325–9.
58. Sochacki KR, Jack RA, Hirase T, McCulloch PC, Lintner DM, Liberman SR, et al. Arthroscopic debridement for primary degenerative osteoarthritis of the elbow leads to significant improvement in range of motion and clinical outcomes: a systematic review. Arthroscopy. 2017;33(12):2255–62.
59. Peden JR, Savoie FH. Arthroscopy of the stiff elbow. Tech Orthop. 2006;21:331–9.
60. Lim TK, Koh KH, Lee HI, Shim JW, Park MJ. Arthroscopic débridement for primary osteoarthritis of the elbow: analysis of preoperative factors affecting outcome. J Shoulder Elb Surg. 2014;23(9):1381–7.
61. Cohen AP, Redden JF, Stanley D. Treatment of osteoarthritis of the elbow: a comparison of open and arthroscopic debridement. Arthroscopy. 2000;16(7):701–6.
62. Kwak JM, Sun Y, Kholinne E, Koh KH, Jeon IH. Surgical outcomes for post-traumatic stiffness after elbow fracture: comparison between open and arthroscopic procedures for intra- and extra-articular elbow fractures. J Shoulder Elb Surg. 2019;28(10):1998–2006.

Post-traumatic Elbow Stiffness: Complications and Treatments

16

Paweł Reichert, Maciej Kentel, Aleksandra Królikowska, and Robert Prill

16.1 Introduction

Painless movement in the elbow joint is extremely important for normal functioning because it allows people to move their hands in space. Elbow stiffness, a common condition associated with significant morbidity, is generally defined as elbow range of motion (ROM) <30–130° [1]. The resulting post-traumatic stiffness or fibrosis in the elbow joint limit functionally and negatively affects an individual's quality of life.

In a systematic review conducted by Cai on the complications of open elbow arthrolysis in post-traumatic elbow stiffness, nerve complications were observed in 8.6 ± 1.9% of cases, of which 18.6% required reoperation. Heterotopic ossification was observed in 5.6 ± 1.6% of cases, with 28.9% requiring revision surgery, and elbow instability was observed in 1.0 ± 0.7% of cases, with a reoperation rate of 25.0%. Infection was observed in 1.6 ± 0.9% of cases, with 53.8% requiring revision surgery, and pin-related complications were observed in 17.4 ± 8.0% of cases, with a reoperation rate of 13.3%. Other complications, including repeat elbow contracture, refracture, hematoma, synovitis, triceps avulsion, incomplete wound healing with a sinus, wound dehiscence and intra-articular bleeding, were observed in 5.7 ± 1.6% of cases, 63.0% of which required reoperation. The total complication rate was 24.3 ± 3.0%, and the reoperation rate was 34.0% [1].

Meanwhile, in a meta-analysis, Zhang reported a complication rate of open arthrolysis in elbow stiffness of approximately 10%. Common complications include superficial wound infections and nerve palsies [2]. Ulnar sensory neuropathy is the most common nerve complication after open arthrolysis, and approximately 25% of cases require operative decompression. Hematomas and seromas can occur

P. Reichert
Department of Orthopedics, Traumatology and Hand Surgery, Faculty of Medicine, Wroclaw Medical University, Wroclaw, Poland

Clinical Department of Orthopedics, Traumatology and Hand Surgery, Jan Mikulicz-Radecki University Hospital, Wroclaw, Poland
e-mail: pawel.reichert@umw.edu.pl

M. Kentel (✉)
eMKaMED Medical Center Traumotology and Ortopaedic Department, Wroclaw, Poland

A. Królikowska
Physiotherapy Research Laboratory, University Centre of Physiotherapy and Rehabilitation, Faculty of Physiotherapy, Wroclaw Medical University, Wroclaw, Poland
e-mail: aleksandra.krolikowska@umw.edu.pl

R. Prill
Center of Orthopaedics and Traumatology, University Hospital Brandenburg/Havel, Brandenburg Medical School Theodor Fontane, Brandenburg an der Havel, Germany

Faculty of Health Sciences Brandenburg, Brandenburg Medical School Theodor Fontane, Brandenburg an der Havel, Germany
e-mail: robert.prill@mhb-fontane.de

L. Pederzini et al. (eds.), *Stiffness of the Elbow, Wrist and Related Pathologies*,
https://doi.org/10.1007/978-3-031-81381-8_16

secondary to flap elevation in a vascular wound bed. Reflex sympathetic dystrophy has been reported after open arthrolysis in 1.5% of cases. Elbow instability is a rare but challenging complication of contracture release and is observed in 1.2% of cases.

Female Qian patients and patients with a lower preoperative range of motion are at greater risk of complications after open arthrolysis. Patients with a higher body mass index (BMI) experience more postoperative pain and less improvement in motion after open arthrolysis compared with patients of normal weight. In addition, patients with diabetes mellitus can expect less improvement in motion and poorer functional outcomes compared with normoglycemic patients.

According to Mittal, the increased immobilization time in conservatively treated patients may be a risk factor for elbow stiffness. Regarding the severity of elbow stiffness, 'multiple surgeries' may increase surgical treatment risks between mild/moderate and severe stiffness groups. Alcohol abuse may also have a negative effect on stiffness progression in patients after conservative therapy.

Elbow stiffness can be assessed and qualified according to two classifications.

Two Kay's classification is based on the offending structure:

- Type 1: soft tissue contracture
- Type 2: soft tissue contracture with ossification
- Type 3: nondisplaced articular fracture with soft tissue contracture
- Type 4: displaced articular fracture with soft tissue contracture
- Type 5: post-traumatic bony bars

Meanwhile, Morrey's classification is based on aetiology and location and classifies elbow stiffness as intrinsic, extrinsic and mixed.

Depending on the status of the ulnar nerve, the formation and localization of heterotopic ossification, the contracture severity, the appearance of the articular surface and the skill of the surgeon, open or arthroscopic arthrolysis can be useful [3]. The open procedure encompasses various approaches (lateral, medial, combined lateral and medial, posterior and anterior) [4]. As reported in the literature, there has been a tendency toward sufficient outcomes, especially in recent years. However, the occurrence of complications has not waned with time, which continues to vex specialists.

The first step in avoiding complications is prevention. Studies have frequently shown that the process of inflammation, as well as fibroblast and myofibroblast activation, starts soon after the initial injury. Consequently, to stave off elbow joint stiffness, it is important to initiate elbow motion immediately after injury or surgery. Early motion can consist of active exercise or continuous passive motion (CPM), with or without nerve blocks. Pain relief is vital after injury or surgery to start elbow movements [5]. Latterly, botulinum toxin A has been used intraoperatively after fracture fixation and after contracture release to prevent elbow stiffness in the postoperative period [6]. The prevention of myositis ossificans (MO) is based on three methods.

16.2 Nerve Complications

Nerve complications, defined as new-onset or intensification of nerve symptoms postoperatively, occur in 7–10% primary surgery and consist of ulnar, radial and median nerve symptoms and reflex sympathetic dystrophy. It was found that 14–19% of nerve complications involving the ulnar nerve required subsequent decompression surgery for the ulnar nerve, with or without transposition.

The associated clinical symptoms are caused by several factors. First, the procedure can cause iatrogenic injury to a nerve when the dissection is not done with great precision or is simply completed [7]. Second, an escalation in the length and intra-neural pressure of the ulnar nerve with a quick improvement ROM can contribute to neuropathy postoperatively [4, 8]. In addition, the normal fibro-osseous tunnel in which the ulnar nerve is located is susceptible to swelling, thickening and creating scar tissue after surgery [4, 9].

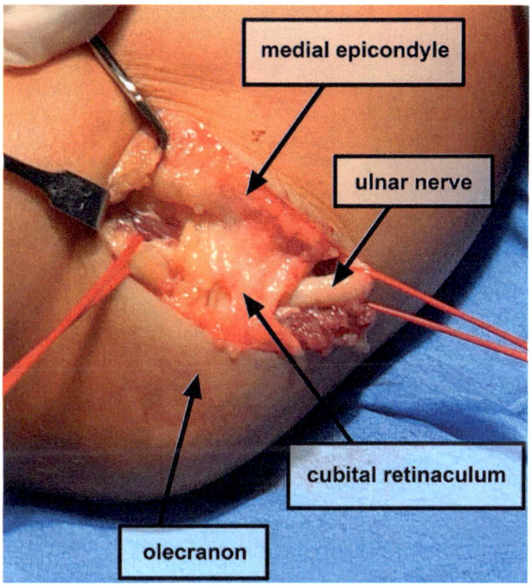

Fig. 16.1 Anatomical dissection in cubital tunnel—compression after elbow stiffness (Is that a screw or plate in the distal aspect of the ulnar N)

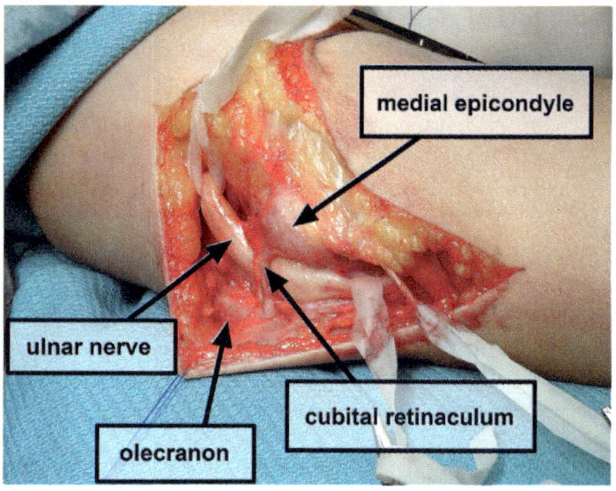

Fig. 16.2 Anatomical dissection in cubital tunnel—compression after elbow stiffness

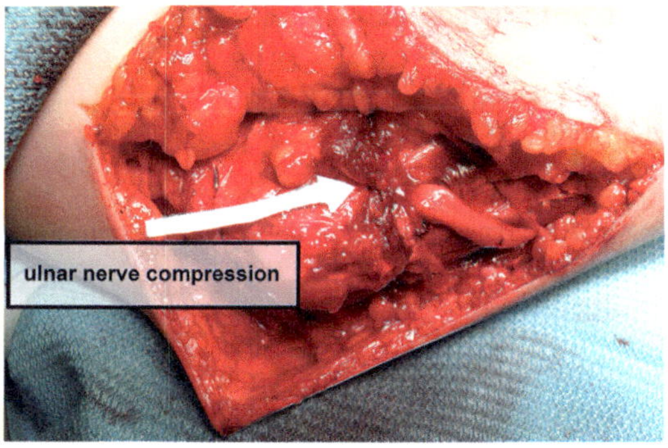

Fig. 16.3 Anatomical dissection in cubital tunnel—compression neuropathy (Is this a suture around the nerve)

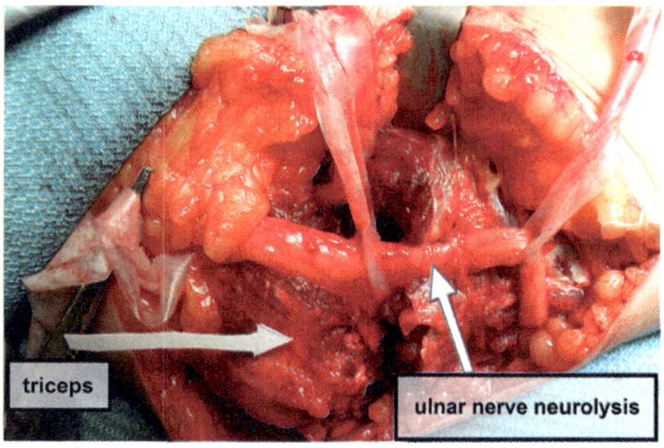

Fig. 16.4 Anatomical dissection in cubital tunnel—compression neuropathy

Because the ulnar nerve is highly vulnerable to pathologic changes in the area around the elbow and ulnar neuropathy is a strong predictor of improvement in health status after open or arthroscopic elbow arthrolysis [10], the application of an appropriate ulnar nerve intervention is crucial during arthrolysis (Figs. 16.1 and 16.2). The indications for ulnar nerve release include preoperative ulnar nerve symptoms [11–13], surgery using the medial approach [14–16], nerve entrapment at the time of the surgery [15, 16], severe flexion contracture [15, 16], large osteophytes or HO [17, 18], an inappropriate ulnar nerve bed [16, 17] and positive provocative tests for impingement of the ulnar nerve [18].

Routine ulnar nerve interventions may be a sensible approach during index elbow release to prevent ulnar nerve compression. The study suggested that routine decompression and subcutaneous anterior transposition are paramount to the prevention of nerve compression during the treatment of a stiff elbow. Some authors have suggested routine decompression of the ulnar nerve during arthroscopic release. Moreover, the decompression length of the ulnar nerve was shown to be crucial to the efficacy of prophylactic intervention, and a mini-decompression (4–6 cm) was less efficacious than a decompression of 7 cm or longer (Figs. 16.3 and 16.4). It has also been demonstrated that ulnar nerve

Table 16.1 Indications of release of the ulnar nerve with elbow surgery

– Clinical symptoms (paraesthesia in the ulnar nerve sensory distribution, point of tenderness and pain overlying the nerve at the medial aspect of the elbow, weakness affecting the ring or small finger, claw deformity, Wartenberg's sign) [1–3, 19, 20]
– Positive provocation tests (incl. Tinnel sign, Froment's test, elbow flexion test) [19]
– Patients with symptoms after conservative treatment failure [3]

Table 16.2 Based on the literature, we recommend a prophylactic ulnar nerve release in the following cases

– Asymptomatic, electrodiagnostically confirmed ulnar neuropathy [1]*
– Limitation of elbow extension of >60 degrees and flexion of <100 degrees [2, 19]
– Anticipated gains in ROM greater than 40 degrees [2]
– Those who undergo manipulation under anaesthesia in the early postoperative period to increase motion [2]
– Morphological changes of the ulnar nerve and surrounding tissues during surgery

*Conduction velocity <50 m/sec across elbow

decompression at a proper length reduced the incidence of ulnar nerve injury [17, 18]. However, studies evaluating the routine ulnar nerve electrodiagnostic tests of patients with elbow stiffness are still needed. We recommend electrodiagnostic testing for revision surgeries (Tables 16.1 and 16.2).

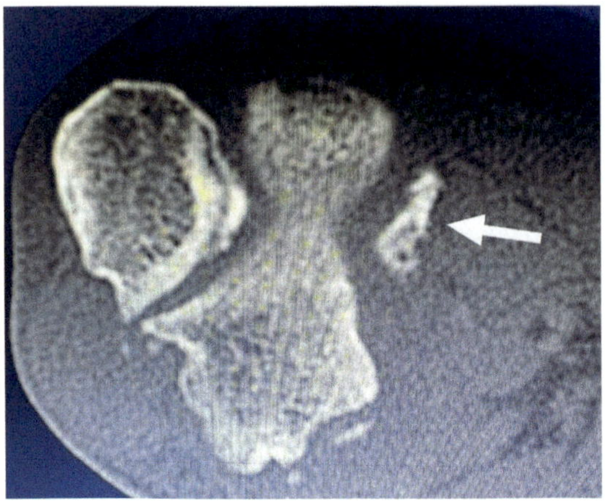

Fig. 16.5 Heterotopic ossification computed tomography (CT) coronal scan

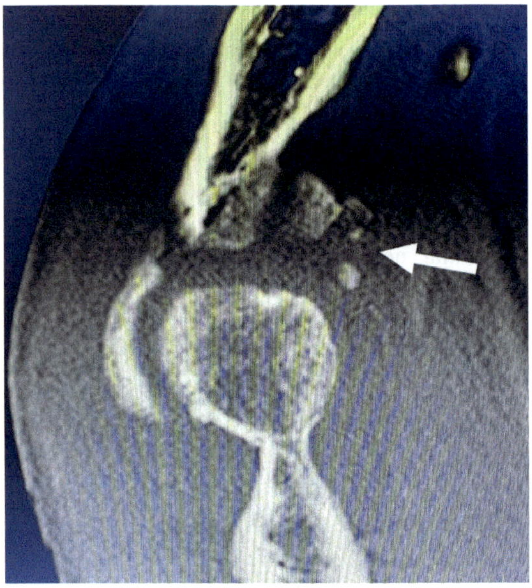

Fig. 16.6 Heterotopic ossification CT sagittal scan

16.3 Heterotopic Ossification (HO)

HO is observed in 6–9% cases including radiographic and clinical new-onset or recurrence [10, 13, 15]. Patients who do not regain a functional arc of motion due to postoperative HO are considered to have clinical new-onset or recurrence (Figs. 16.5 and 16.6).

HO is a major complication, and the way it arises remains unclear. Many studies have not reported the results of postoperative radiographic evaluation, and thus it is possible that the authors did not pay proper attention to the new-onset or recurrence of HO and that the actual incidence was much higher than expected [21]. HO of the elbow can present after direct trauma (fracture, dislocation or both), central nervous system injury or burn injury and can occur in patients with genetic diseases. Moreover, surgical dissection, possibly leading to soft-tissue insult, is related to HO. Clinical new-onset or recurrence of HO can lead to an inability to restore ROM, which is a possible indicator of adverse results in arthrolysis for stiff elbows caused by HO. In accordance with conclusions from elbow, acetabular and hip surgeries, a high body mass index (BMI), longer injury time and preoperative ROM are definitive risk factors in the development of HO [22]. These data may be consequential in determining the use of prophylactic interventions for patients with elbow stiffness. Although the preponderance of patients who had undergone these interventions reported having attained sufficient ROM with a low rate of recurrence in the selected studies, a small number of relative trials were conducted to evaluate the efficaciousness of these interventions for preventing the recurrence of HO after open elbow arthrolysis [23]. In extreme cases, including stiffness after distal humeral fracture, the final solution is elbow replacement (Figs. 16.7, 16.8, 16.9, and 16.10).

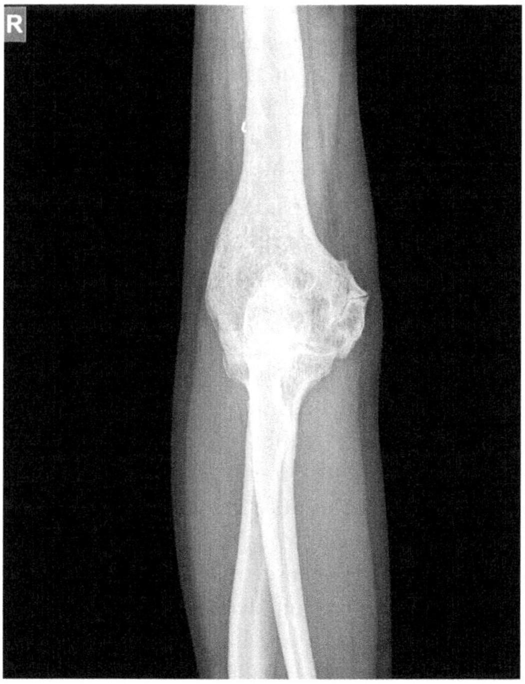

Fig. 16.7 Heterotopic ossification anteroposterior (AP) X-ray

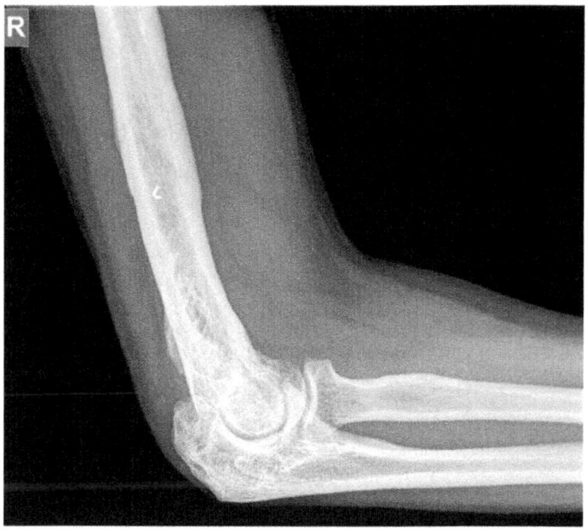

Fig. 16.8 Heterotopic ossification lateral X-ray

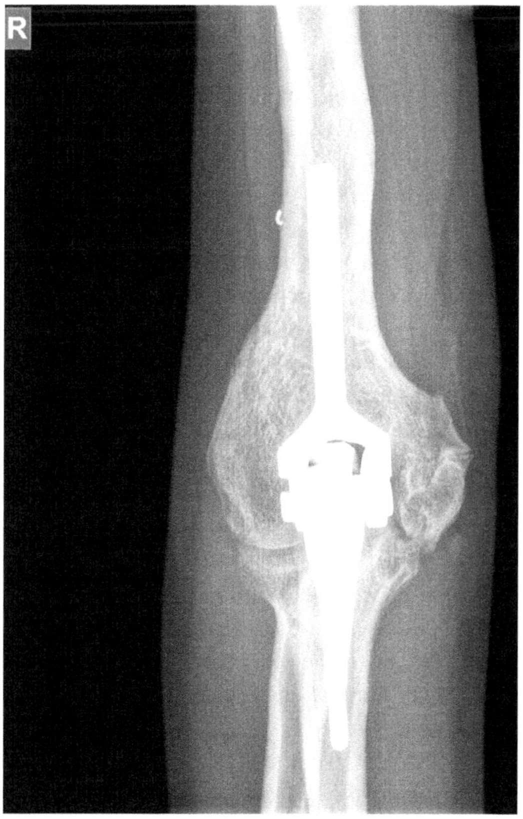

Fig. 16.9 Elbow replacement AP X-ray

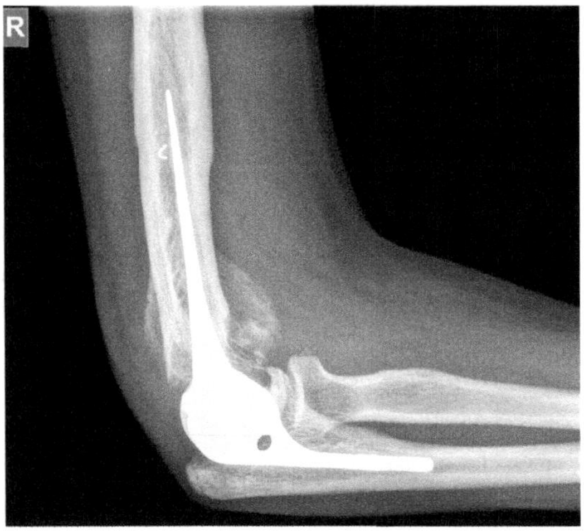

Fig. 16.10 Elbow replacement lateral X-ray

There are three methods for preventing HO:

1. Disrupting signal pathways—(prostaglandins) PGEs and bone morphogenetic proteins are required for the formation of ectopic bone. Non-steroidal anti-inflammatory drugs (NSAIDs) abate the formation of PGEs by inhibiting the cyclo-oxygenase enzyme. Drugs such as indomethacin, ibuprofen and naproxen are used to prevent myositis, particularly in the hip. Although their effects on the elbow are unclear, they are still being used.
2. Modifying the relevant progenitor cells in the target tissue—Stem cells are highly vulnerable to radiation, and irradiation prevents them from differentiating into osteoblasts. A 600–100 cGy dose of radiation is used to prevent HO.
3. Adapting the environment to be conducive to HO—Sodium etidronate inhibits angiogenesis, which is necessary for mineralization, that can prevent ossification. Radiation therapy can be used in concert with NSAIDs to prevent HO. That said, in the presence of a fracture, NSAIDs and irradiation must be used with caution, as they can result in non-union.

The use of NSAIDs is still controversial. In one study, the rate of HO after hip arthroscopy procedures approached 46% without prophylaxis, and the administration of NSAIDs decreased this to 4% [24]. A recent systematic review on HO after hip arthroscopy showed that all NSAIDs seem to be effective as HO prophylaxis [5]. Based on these findings and data from elbow contracture studies, we recommend the use of indomethacin (75 mg daily for 4 days) followed by naproxen (500 mg twice daily for 3 weeks) for patients with elbow contracture surgery with risk factors of HO and for all patients operated for recurrent HO [5, 6, 25]. Although forcible manipulation of stiff joints is believed to lead to increased HO, passive ROM exercises are effective and should be performed progressively with a low load and within tissue tolerance [25–27]. In a recently published systematic review, the use of radiotherapy (RT) only for elbow HO prevention was found to be more effective than the combination of radiotherapy (RT) with NSAIDs [4].

Conversely, in a meta-analysis, Henstenburg found no differences in demographic risk factors, HO occurrence, and ROM and MEPI scores between the use of NSAIDs and RT prophylaxis for HO of the elbow caused by trauma. Situational factors should be considered when selecting the proper prophylactic treatment strategy. Radiotherapy is needed to better delineate the clinical differences between different HO prophylaxis strategies.

Based on the literature, we recommend the use of HO prophylaxis in patients with increased BMI and those suffering from high-energy trauma, who are more likely to develop HO. Further, the use of radiation therapy to prevent HO of the elbow is supported by weak evidence [4, 25]. Because of lack of high-quality studies and the risk of adverse events, we do not recommend RT as a first-line intervention for the prevention of elbow HO [4]. In most studies, preoperative and postoperative radiotherapy were found to be equally efficient in the prevention of HO recurrence [4]. The most frequently used type of RT was a single dose of irradiation (7.0 Gy), and it has not been related to complications except in cases following osteosynthesis, in which concerns were raised regarding fracture union prevention by RT [4].

16.4 Myositis Ossificans (MO)

MO describes conditions involving heterotopic bone formation within soft tissues. It can be classified in two different groups: MO progressiva (genetic autosomal dominant rare disease) and MO traumatica (occurring after an injury) [7, 8]. Other terms used to describe ectopic bone formation in soft tissues are HO, paraosteoarthopathy and heterotopic calcification [9]. MO/HO refers to the formation of mature lamellar bone in soft tissue structures and not to the deposition of amorphous calcium salts in soft tissues. It is histologically identical to mature bone but is more metabolically active and lacks a true periosteal layer. It is formed by the stimulation of pluripotent stem cells, which produce osteoid and then mineralize. The risk factors for the development of MO are concomitant head injury, forceful and repeated manipulations, multiple surgical interventions within the first week of injury, thermal burns, longer time to surgery and a longer time to mobilization after surgery. Hastings and Graham presented the following classification of myositis around the elbow:

- Class I: does not cause functional limitation
- Class II: causes functional limitation
- Class IIA: flexion extension <100°
- Class IIB: supination–pronation <100°
- Class IIC: restriction of movements in both planes
- Class III: ankylosis in any plane
- Class IIIA: ankylosis in the flexion extension plane
- Class IIIB: ankylosis in the rotation plane
- Class IIIC: no motion in either direction

16.5 Infection

Infection instances, including arthroscopic or open elbow arthrolysis, occur in 1–2%. Treatment consists of intravenous or oral antibiotics as well as irrigation and debridement [28]. The severity of elbow stiffness, comparatively less active ROM, longer operation times, diabetes and increased prior operation times are potential risk factors for infection after open elbow arthrolysis. The use of the prophylactic method of intrawound application of vancomycin powder during open elbow arthrolysis was reported to significantly lessen the postoperative infection rate compared to the use of standard intravenous antibiotics after open elbow arthrolysis [29] Antibiotic prophylaxis achieved higher tissue antibiotic concentrations than those achieved with standard systemic antibiotics, which may reduce the risk of infection in elbow arthrolysis.

16.6 Compartment Syndrome

Acute compartment syndrome is a serious complication that results from high tissue fluid pressure in the closed osseofascial compartment, which leads to reduced capillary perfusion below the level necessary for tissue viability [11]. The most common causes are excessive bleeding, increased capillary permeability, burns, fractures and contusions [11]. Quick diagnosis and emergency treatment are essential, as the disease leads to irreversible necrotic changes in tissues after just 8 h [11]. Although very severe, it is not very common after elbow surgery. Intravia et al. found no compartment syndrome after 560 elbow arthroscopies [10].

16.7 Safe Tourniquet Usage

To avoid serious complications, we recommend the use of a tourniquet pressure of 250 mm Hg or less for fewer than 2 h [12].

16.8 Recurrent Stiffness

Repeat elbow contractures may occur for unknown or unreported reasons (excluding elbow contracture associated with HO mentioned in the studies). Unfortunately, in some cases it is a consequence of the first operation (arthroscopic or open), including synovitis, hematomas, triceps avulsion, incomplete wound healing, intra-articular bleeding or iatrogenic injuries, such as recurrent osteophytes, or refractures (intercondylar region of the distal humeral). Patients who fail to progress and experience medial elbow pain may have ulnar nerve entrapment. This needs to be assessed and decompressed if it is problematic.

16.9 Elbow Instability

Elbow instability is a common complication after complete arthrolysis for severe elbow stiffness. Instability can be identified and circumvented through a meticulous stress test for stability during surgery as well as the establishment of surgical techniques. The coronoid process is a critical stabilizer of the elbow, and it is crucial to avoid instability. The first step in assessing instability is to determine whether it is a bone or soft tissue problem. Fixation using a plate, screw, or anchor is necessary in the event of a loss of more than one-third of the articular surface. If primary fixation is not successful, reconstruction is required. The root causes of postoperative instability are initial injuries and iatrogenic violations of the collateral ligaments, which are essential to maintaining elbow stability [30, 31]. In general, during its release, the anterior band of the medial collateral ligament and the lateral collateral ligament should be preserved as the primary stabilizers of the elbow, according to early biomechanical and clinical studies [32–34].

In some cases, when the collateral ligaments are severely contracted or encased in HO, the ligaments may need to be released. Stability must be assessed intra-operatively. Ligament repair or reconstruction may be required to regain stability The transosseous suture and suture anchor repair techniques can be used to reattach the collateral ligaments and flexor–pronator and extensor tendons to the epicondyle and supracondylar ridge [35–37].

References

1. Andelman SM, Meier KM, Walsh AL, Kim JH, Hausman MR. Pediatric elbow arthroscopy: indications and safety. J Shoulder Elbow Surg. 2017;26(10):1862–6. https://doi.org/10.1016/j.jse.2017.07.005.
2. Andelman SM, Walsh AL, Sochol KM, Rubenstein WM, Hausman MR. Arthroscopic elbow contracture release in the pediatric patient. J Pediatr Orthop. 2018;38(9):e507–13. https://doi.org/10.1097/BPO.0000000000001216.
3. Attum B, Obremskey W. Posttraumatic elbow stiffness: a critical analysis review. JBJS Rev. 2016;4(9):e1. https://doi.org/10.2106/JBJS.RVW.15.00084.
4. Bachman DR, Fitzsimmons JS, O'Driscoll SW. Safety of arthroscopic versus open or combined heterotopic ossification removal around the elbow. Arthroscopy. 2020;36(2):422–30. https://doi.org/10.1016/j.arthro.2019.09.010.
5. Intravia J, Acevedo DC, Chung WJ, Mirzayan R. Complications of elbow arthroscopy in a community-based practice. Arthroscopy. 2020;36(5):1283–90. https://doi.org/10.1016/j.arthro.2019.11.108.
6. Jhan SW, Chou WY, Wu KT, Wang CJ, Yang YJ, Ko JY. Outcomes and factors of elbow arthroscopy upon returning to sports for throwing athletes with osteoarthritis. J Orthop Surg Res. 2018;13(1):280. https://doi.org/10.1186/s13018-018-0992-x.
7. Kim DS, Chung HJ, Yi CH, Kim SH. Comparison of the clinical outcomes of open surgery versus arthroscopic surgery for chronic refractory lateral epicondylitis of the elbow. Orthopedics. 2018;41(4):237–47. https://doi.org/10.3928/01477447-20180621-04.
8. Koh JL, Zwahlen BA, Altchek DW, Zimmerman TA. Arthroscopic treatment successfully treats posterior elbow impingement in an athletic population. Knee Surg Sports Traumatol Arthrosc. 2018;26(1):306–11. https://doi.org/10.1007/s00167-017-4563-1.
9. Kwak JM, Kholinne E, Sun Y, Lim S, Koh KH, Jeon IH. Clinical outcome of osteocapsular arthroplasty for primary osteoarthritis of the elbow: comparison of arthroscopic and open procedure. Arthroscopy. 2019;35(4):1083–9. https://doi.org/10.1016/j.arthro.2018.11.057.
10. Kwak JM, Kim H, Sun Y, Kholinne E, Koh KH, Jeon IH. Arthroscopic osteocapsular arthroplasty for advanced-stage primary osteoarthritis of the elbow using a computed tomography-based classification. J Shoulder Elbow Surg. 2020;29(5):989–95. https://doi.org/10.1016/j.jse.2019.09.036.

11. Kwak JM, Sun Y, Kholinne E, Koh KH, Jeon IH. Surgical outcomes for post-traumatic stiffness after elbow fracture: comparison between open and arthroscopic procedures for intra- and extra-articular elbow fractures. J Shoulder Elbow Surg. 2019;28(10):1998–2006. https://doi.org/10.1016/j.jse.2019.06.008.
12. Lanzerath F, Wegmann K, Hackl M, Uschok S, Ott N, Müller LP, Leschinger T. Surgical arthrolysis of the stiff elbow: a systematic review. Arch Orthop Trauma Surg. 2023;143(5):2383–93. https://doi.org/10.1007/s00402-022-04442-0.
13. Lubiatowski P, Ślęzak M, Wałecka J, Bręborowicz M, Romanowski L. Prospective outcome assessment of arthroscopic arthrolysis for traumatic and degenerative elbow contracture. J Shoulder Elbow Surg. 2018;27(9):e269–78. https://doi.org/10.1016/j.jse.2018.02.068.
14. Matsuura T, Iwame T, Suzue N, Kashiwaguchi S, Iwase T, Hamada D, Sairyo K. Long-term outcomes of arthroscopic debridement with or without drilling for osteochondritis dissecans of the capitellum in adolescent baseball players: a ≥10-year follow-up study. Arthroscopy. 2020;36(5):1273–80. https://doi.org/10.1016/j.arthro.2020.01.020.
15. Mellema JJ, Lindenhovius AL, Jupiter JB. The posttraumatic stiff elbow: an update. Curr Rev Musculoskelet Med. 2016;9(2):190–8. https://doi.org/10.1007/s12178-016-9336-9.
16. Mittal R. Posttraumatic stiff elbow. Indian J Orthop. 2017;51(1):4–13. https://doi.org/10.4103/0019-5413.197514.
17. Morrey BF, An KN. Articular and ligamentous contributions to the stability of the elbow joint. Am J Sports Med. 1983;11(5):315–9. https://doi.org/10.1177/036354658301100506.
18. Noticewala MS, Trofa DP, Vance DD, Jobin CM, Levine WN, Ahmad CS. Elbow arthroscopy: 30-day postoperative complication profile and associated risk factors. Arthroscopy. 2018;34(2):414–20. https://doi.org/10.1016/j.arthro.2017.08.286.
19. Ahmed AF, Alzobi OZ, Hantouly AT, Toubasi A, Farsakoury R, Alkhelaifi K, Zikria B. Complications of elbow arthroscopic surgery: a systematic review and meta-analysis. Orthop J Sports Med. 2022;10(11):23259671221137863. https://doi.org/10.1177/23259671221137863.
20. Arrigoni P, Cucchi D, D'Ambrosi R, Butt U, Safran MR, Denard P, Randelli P. Intra-articular findings in symptomatic minor instability of the lateral elbow (SMILE). Knee Surg Sports Traumatol Arthrosc. 2017;25(7):2255–63. https://doi.org/10.1007/s00167-017-4530-x.
21. Nowotny J, Löbstein S, Biewener A, Fitze G, Kasten P. Elbow arthroscopy in children and adolescents: analysis of outcome and complications. Eur J Med Res. 2018;23(1):42. https://doi.org/10.1186/s40001-018-0338-5.
22. Pederzini LA, Bartoli M, Cheli A, Nicoletta F, Severini G. Encouraging mid-term outcomes for arthroscopic autologous osteochondral transplant (OAT) in capitellum osteochondritis dissecans (OCD). Knee Surg Sports Traumatol Arthrosc. 2019;27(10):3291–6. https://doi.org/10.1007/s00167-019-05568-2.
23. Rai S, Zhang Q, Tamang N, Jin S, Wang H, Meng C. Arthroscopic arthrolysis of posttraumatic and non-traumatic elbow stiffness offers comparable clinical outcomes. BMC Musculoskelet Disord. 2019;20(1):285. https://doi.org/10.1186/s12891-019-2666-1.
24. Chen S, Yan H, Wang W, Zhang M, Hildebrand KA, Fan CY. Reconstruction of medial collateral ligament defects with a flexor-pronator fascia patch in complete open release of stiff elbows. J Shoulder Elbow Surg. 2017;26(1):133–9. https://doi.org/10.1016/j.jse.2016.09.030.
25. Carlier Y, Lenoir H, Rouleau DM, Mansat P, Vidil A, Ferrand M, Bleton R, Herrisson O, Salabi V, Duparc F, Kelberine F, Desmoineaux P, French Arthroscopic Society. Arthroscopic debridement for osteoarthritis of the elbow: results and analysis of predictive factors. Orthop Traumatol Surg Res. 2019;105(8S):S221–7. https://doi.org/10.1016/j.otsr.2019.09.002.
26. Jinnah AH, Luo TD, Wiesler ER, Li Z, Poehling GG, Tuohy CJ, Graves BR, Freehill MT, Papadonikolakis A. Peripheral nerve injury after elbow arthroscopy: an analysis of risk factors. Arthroscopy. 2018;34(5):1447–52. https://doi.org/10.1016/j.arthro.2017.12.004.
27. Karelson M, Launonen AP, Jokihaara J, Havulinna J, Mattila VM. Pain, function, and patient satisfaction after arthroscopic treatment of elbow in a retrospective series with minimum of 5-year follow-up. J Orthop Surg (Hong Kong). 2019;27(1):2309499019832808. https://doi.org/10.1177/2309499019832808.
28. Schreiner AJ, Schweikardt N, Gühring D, Ahrend MD, Döbele S, Ahmad SS, Baumann M, Hirschmann MT, Bozzi F, Ateschrang A. Arthroscopic arthrolysis leads to improved range of motion and health-related quality of life in post-traumatic elbow stiffness. J Shoulder Elbow Surg. 2020;29(8):1538–47. https://doi.org/10.1016/j.jse.2020.01.099.
29. Sun C, Zhou X, Yao C, Poonit K, Fan C, Yan H. The timing of open surgical release of post-traumatic elbow stiffness: a systematic review. Medicine (Baltimore). 2017;96(49):e9121. https://doi.org/10.1097/MD.0000000000009121.
30. Sun Z, Cui H, Ruan J, Li J, Wang W, Fan C. What range of motion and functional results can be expected after open arthrolysis with hinged external fixation for severe posttraumatic elbow stiffness? Clin Orthop Relat Res. 2019;477(10):2319–28. https://doi.org/10.1097/CORR.0000000000000726.
31. Sun Z, Li J, Cui H, Ruan H, Wang W, Fan C. A new pathologic classification for elbow stiffness based on our experience in 216 patients. J Shoulder Elbow

Surg. 2020;29(3):e75–86. https://doi.org/10.1016/j.jse.2019.08.001.
32. Temporin K, Shimada K, Oura K, Owaki H. Arthroscopic release for the severely stiff elbow. Musculoskelet Surg. 2020;104(1):81–6. https://doi.org/10.1007/s12306-019-00601-6.
33. Willinger L, Siebenlist S, Lenich A, Liska F, Imhoff AB, Achtnich A. Arthroscopic arthrolysis provides good clinical outcome in post-traumatic and degenerative elbow stiffness. Knee Surg Sports Traumatol Arthrosc. 2018;26(1):312–7. https://doi.org/10.1007/s00167-017-4630-7.
34. Xiong H, Sun Z, Chen S, Liu W, Peng S, Wang W, Fan C. Effect of hyperuricemia on functional outcomes and complications in patients with elbow stiffness after open arthrolysis combined with hinged external fixation: a retrospective study. J Shoulder Elbow Surg. 2020;29(7):1387–93. https://doi.org/10.1016/j.jse.2020.02.021.
35. Zheng W, Chen S, Song J, Liu J, Fan C. The influence of body mass index on outcome of open arthrolysis for post-traumatic elbow stiffness. J Shoulder Elbow Surg. 2017;26(5):809–14. https://doi.org/10.1016/j.jse.2016.12.065.
36. Zhou Y, Cai JY, Chen S, Liu S, Wang W, Fan CY. Application of distal radius-positioned hinged external fixator in complete open release for severe elbow stiffness. J Shoulder Elbow Surg. 2017;26(2):e44–51. https://doi.org/10.1016/j.jse.2016.09.019.
37. Zhu W, Wang W, Mao X, Chen Y. Arthroscopic management of elbow synovial chondromatosis. Medicine (Baltimore). 2018;97(40):e12402. https://doi.org/10.1097/MD.0000000000012402.

17 Hemi-Joint Replacement Arthroplasty in Stiff Elbow

Marinelli Alessandro, Buondonno Catello, Riva Marta, and Guerra Enrico

17.1 Introduction

Management of elbow stiffness caused by end-stage arthritis in young and/or active patients is challenging. In those patients, who suffer from intense pain and severe stiffness, when alternative procedures have failed or are not indicated, an elbow hemiarthroplasty (EHA) can be considered. Especially if the ulnar articular surface is still partially preserved, EHA can save the patients from the profound lifelong functional and activity restrictions required by a joint replacement with a total elbow arthroplasty (TEA) [1].

Elbow hemiarthroplasty (EHA) consists of a partial replacement of the elbow joint, involving only the humeral component. It is composed of three modular parts: (1) a humeral stem, that needs to be cemented; (2) an anatomical spool designed to replicate the distal humerus shape; (3) a cannulated pin, which is used to connect the spool to the stem (Fig. 17.1).

Over the last decade, EHA has become, especially in Europe, an attractive treatment option for not fixable distal humerus fractures in young and/or active patients. Other less common indications are malunions, nonunions, and avascular necrosis [2–6]. More rarely EHA has been also used to treat stiffness caused by post-traumatic or degenerative arthritis. The rationale of using EHA is to overcome the current limits of TEA. In particular, the advantages of EHA respect to TEA include preservation of ulnar and radial bone stock, decreased risk of component loosening, absence of polyethylene wear, and decreased surgical time.

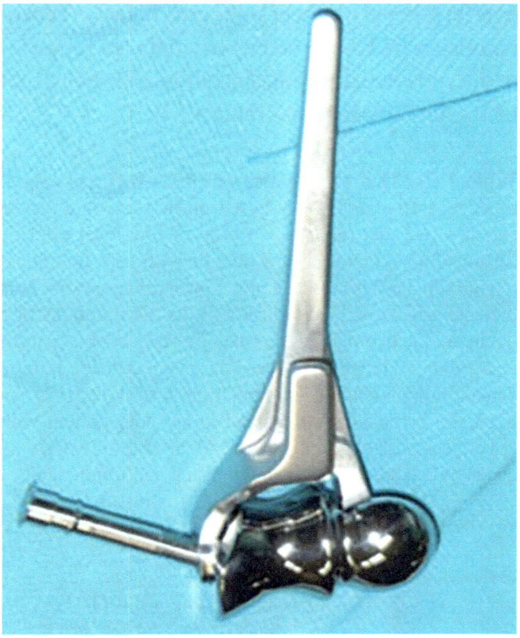

Fig. 17.1 EHA is composed by a flanged stem, an anatomical spool, and a cannulated pin that connect the previous two parts

M. Alessandro · B. Catello · R. Marta
G. Enrico (✉)
Shoulder and Elbow Department, IRCCS Rizzoli Orthopedic Institute, Bologna, Italy
e-mail: enrico.guerra@ior.it

L. Pederzini et al. (eds.), *Stiffness of the Elbow, Wrist and Related Pathologies*, https://doi.org/10.1007/978-3-031-81381-8_17

Compared to TEA the potential disadvantages of EHA are the risks of instability and, in particular in patients with a pre-existing post-traumatic or degenerative joint, of progressive joint osteoarthritis due to the direct contact of the metallic trochlea against the articular surfaces of the greater sigmoid notch and radial head.

However, in the existing literature there are limited data regarding indications and outcomes in the setting of stiffness and post-traumatic arthritis.

17.2 Indications

EHA can be considered an option in case of elbow stiffness only if there is a significant degenerative arthritis of a distal humeral surface, causing pain and stiffness, associated with an absent or mild ulnar degenerative changes. In all other cases, other treatments must be considered first. Activity modification, oral analgesics, and injections can be initially proposed to the patient to relieve symptoms. Surgical options can range from open or arthroscopic osteocapsular arthroplasty (capsular release and loose bodies/osteophytes removal) or interposition arthroplasty, elbow arthrodesis, or total joint replacement (Table 17.1).

Table 17.1 The management of elbow stiffness caused by degenerative arthritis is based on its stage and on the patient's age and requests. In case of low-level arthritis causing few symptoms in a patient with low functional requests, regardless the age, the conservative treatment is indicated. If a low-level arthritis limits the functions of a young and active patient, an open or arthroscopic arthroplasty can be indicated. In case of severe arthritis in high demanding patient an interposition arthroplasty or an EHA can be considered, instead in an older patient with lower requests, especially if the ulnar side is extremely degenerated, a total elbow prosthesis is more indicated

Arthritis	Demands	Treatment
↓	↓	Conservative treatment
↓	↑	Osteocapsular arthroplasty *(young and active patients)*
↑	↑	Interposition VS EHA
↑	↓	TEA *(old and low demanding patients)*

↑: High level, ↓: Low level

17.3 Contraindications

Absolute contraindications to EHA are represented by a local or systemic infection of the elbow. Because of unconstrained nature of the EHA implants, the joint stability relies on the congruence of their design with the radio-ulnar surfaces and on the integrity of the primary and secondary elbow stabilizers: medial and lateral columns with their corresponding collateral ligaments, radial head, olecranon, and coronoid.

Therefore, EHA is also contraindicated in case of lack of medial or lateral column, irreparable MCL or LCL lesions or radial head osteotomy, and coronoid or olecranon significant defect. In these cases, a linked TEA should be considered instead. Relative contraindications to EHA for a stiff elbow are a pre-existing degenerative ulnar osteoarthritis due to the risk of persistence or increase of the postoperative pain and stiffness. Contraindications to EHA include also patients affected by elbow stiffness that can be treated with more conservative and predictable treatments.

17.4 Preoperative Planning

Before considering performing an EHA, a careful and accurate planning is necessary.

Medical history: The presence of concomitant diseases, level of physical activity, and needs of the patient must be evaluated. Metal hypersensitivity and previous surgeries around the elbow must be investigated, asking for the attesting documents and surgical reports, if they are available.

Clinical evaluation: The elbow skin condition must be checked and the presence of previous scars or of an ongoing local infection must be ruled out. The neurovascular condition of the involved upper limb must be examined. The position of the ulnar nerve must be assessed, to evaluate if a previous transposition has been performed.

Imaging: Imaging evaluation must confirm a joint deformity not treatable with more conservative treatments. Orthogonal plain radiographs are almost always completed by a computer tomography (CT) with two-dimensional (2D) and three-dimensional (3D) reconstruction. Unfortunately, virtual planning software allowing to plan or navigate the surgery is not available for elbow replacement at the moment.

Instrumentation: The surgeon must ensure to have the necessary instrumentation to implant the humeral prosthesis and to repair the elbow stabilizers if they are injured. Latitude EV implant (Stryker) is the only hemiarthroplasty implant available on the market at the time of this writing (Fig. 17.2b).

It is an anatomic, modular, and cemented implant with an interchangeable spool for conversion to linked or unlinked TEA, without need for humeral exchange. The spool is cannulated, to allow ligament repair through the center of rotation of the implant.

In addition to the elbow replacement system provided by the company, other necessary instruments are as follows:

Tourniquet, bean bag if the lateral decubitus is decided, oscillating saw, high speed burr, low viscosity cement, cement restrictor and gun, C-arm machine for intraoperative fluoroscopy.

In case of previous osteosynthesis, a detailed list of the previously implanted hardware is needed to allow the surgeon to have the specific removal tools available. The previous operative report is useful to understand the triceps management formerly performed and to confirm the ulnar nerve position.

Informed consent: EHA is a complex operation. Because of the possible alternative treatments and complications, before performing EHA for a stiff elbow, an exhaustive informed consent is necessary. Providing to the patient a detailed information about his/her current elbow condition, the available solutions and informing about realistic expectations and possible complications of an elbow replacement foster trust in the patient–physician relationship and allows the patient to take part in the decision-making process.

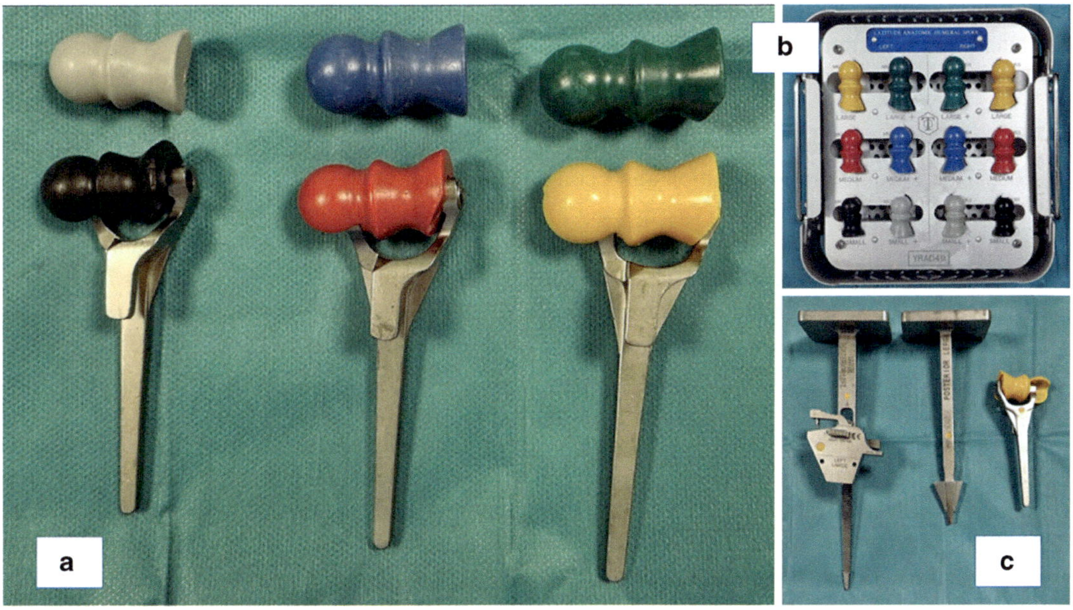

Fig. 17.2 Latitude EV Trial instrumentation. (**a**) Anatomic humeral stems are of three different sizes (small black, medium red, large yellow). (**b**) Anatomic spools are of six different sizes for right and six for left side (small black, small + gray, medium red, medium + blue, large yellow, large + green). (**c**) Humeral broaches and humeral cut guides are specific for each trial stem

17.4.1 Surgical Approach Decision

The strategic choice of the surgical exposure is certainly the first basic step to obtain good EHA implant and minimize complications.

EHA can be implanted using several approaches, each with its advantages and limits. Regardless of the selected approach, the insertion of the elbow prosthesis requires to manage the elbow extensor mechanism to expose the joint, to perform the distal humerus joint resection, to determine the correct size of the implant and the right direction of insertion and height of the prosthesis, and, lastly, to carefully reinsert the collateral ligaments. Whenever it's possible, preserving the triceps attachment reduces the risk of overstuffing and weakness of the extensor system, allowing an early active motion in the postoperative phase [7].

Based on the different triceps management, the most suggested approaches to implant an EHA in elbow stiffness are as follows:

- Olecranon osteotomy
- Triceps splitting
- Lateral para-olecranon approach [8]
- Tongue approach

The choice among these approaches should be based on the specific elbow situations and considering the surgeon preferences.

17.4.1.1 Olecranon Osteotomy

This approach allows the greatest joint exposure, but in case of an unexpected instability with the necessity to convert to a TEA, surgical difficulties grow much more. Moreover, this approach is associated with possible complications such as osteotomy delayed union, nonunion, malunion, prominent hardware, intra-articular adhesions, and arthritis. Moreover, the intact sigmoid notch is important to choose the correct size of the implant spool as well as the triceps tension is an important landmark to identify the correct length of the implant: all these reasons make the olecranon osteotomy not the ideal approach to perform an EHA.

17.4.1.2 Triceps Splitting

This approach consists in dissecting longitudinally the triceps, detaching its insertion on both sides of the olecranon. Using this approach, dislocating the elbow is necessary to release the collateral ligaments from the condyles. At the end of surgery, after having implanted the prosthesis, the ligaments must be sutured back to the bone and the two sides of this soft tissue "envelope" must be closed using side-to-side stiches. The triceps needs to be reattached to the olecranon as strongly as possible with multiple transosseous sutures. Shahane-Stanley [9] proposed a modification of this technique, performing the triceps split 75% laterally and 25% medially. The medial part is then detached subperiosteally and reflected medially as a single unit; the lateral part of the triceps with the anconeus and extensors is dissected according to the needs of the procedure being undertaken. Lately, Nestorson et al. [10] described in a small number of cases of EHA implantation, a modification of the original Campbell approach with a mid-line triceps split and detaching only the lateral half of the triceps, leaving the medial half inserted on the olecranon. Through this approach the joint can be dislocated and the humeral canal can be prepared. More recently Phadnis et al. [2] published a cases series where the triceps had been split in 1/3 lateral and 2/3 medial, with a second window performed on the medial border of the triceps to access the medial condyle and collateral ligament.

17.4.1.3 Lateral Para-olecranon Approach

The lateral para-olecranon approach exposes the ulno-humeral joint through medial and lateral arthrotomies, leaving the insertion of the central triceps tendon attached to the olecranon. The posterolateral arthrotomy is performed distally to the olecranon using the Boyd approach. Proximally the triceps tendon is split between the central tendinous attachment to the olecranon and its lateral expansion, and the lateral half of the triceps. The lateral part of the triceps, along with the anconeus, is retracted laterally as a single unit. On the medial side, the ulnar nerve is released and transposed, the triceps muscle is released from the medial intermuscular septum and dorsal aspect of the distal humerus. At the end of the surgery, the medial and lateral soft tissues are repaired back to the distal humerus, using the central hole of the implant spool. The triceps split is then closed. This approach allows an immediate elbow rehabilitation, without risk of triceps failure. This is our suggested approach to implant an EHA for elbow stiffness.

17.4.1.4 Tongue Approach

The triceps fascial tongue approach, originally described in 1940 by Van Gorder for T-type distal humeral fractures, has been recently reproposed as a possible approach for total elbow arthroplasty [11, 12]. Although to date the tongue approach has never been described to implant an EHA, it should be considered as a possible approach. O'Driscoll recently proposed a variant of the tongue approach, called Diamond pop-up exposure (personal communication) that, to provide adequate visualization of the articular surface, which has the peculiarity of dissecting collateral ligaments from the ulnar insertions and that can be considered as a possible approach to insert an EHA in a stiff and arthritic elbow.

17.5 Personal Experience

In our department, we have implanted 25 HEA in the last 15 years. Only in two cases was the indication for elbow stiffness associated with a significant arthritis: One case was a sequela of a shear fracture, and the second case was a patient affected by a genetic disease causing precocious polyarticular arthritis. All the two elbows have been revisioned at a mean of 7 years (1 case at 6 years and 1 case at 8 years). In both cases, EHA gave a pain relief and a range of motion (ROM) improvement for the first years (3 years for case 1, 2 years for case 2), with a subsequent progressive onset of pain and ROM decrease. All the two elbows have been later revisioned, converting the humeral implant in a total elbow arthroplasty, at a mean of 7 years (8 case 1, 6 case 2). The patient of case 2, considering the experience of the first treated elbow, requested directly a total elbow for the other stiff, arthritic and painful elbow, which became more symptomatic a few years after.

17.5.1 Case 1

A 54-year-old woman (school teacher) presented to our clinic with stiffness and pain at her left elbow 3 years after a shear fracture treated in another hospital with ORIF with Kirschner wires (K-wires) and resulted in malunion of the distal humerus (Figs. 17.3 and 17.4). The patient complained of an increasing left elbow pain with significant limitation during daily living activities. The ROM was 100–30° in flexion–extension with a full forearm rotation and without signs of ulnar nerve neuropathy.

Three years after the original trauma, an elbow hemiarthroplasty was performed using the olecranon osteotomy approach to properly expose the articular portion of the distal humerus. Soft tissue adhesions and heterotopic ossifications were removed. Two months after surgery the pain was greatly reduced and the ROM was 125–20° in flexion–extension with good radiographic result (Fig. 17.5a and b).

One year later a second surgery was performed to remove the olecranon screw. Starting from the 2-year follow-up the patient began to present a progressive pain, functional limitations, and ROM reduction. Conservative treatment was carried out until the pain and functional limitations worsened significantly. Clinical exams, labs, and X-rays did not show any sign of infection. At the 8-year follow-up (Fig. 17.6a and b), the ROM was 90–30° in flexion–extension (Fig. 17.7a and b), full pronosupination, and severe elbow pain. The patient underwent to a total elbow arthroplasty. At 6-year follow-up after TEA, the patient presents occasional moderate pain with a functional ROM (130–10°, full forearm rotation) and good radiographic result (Fig. 17.8a and b).

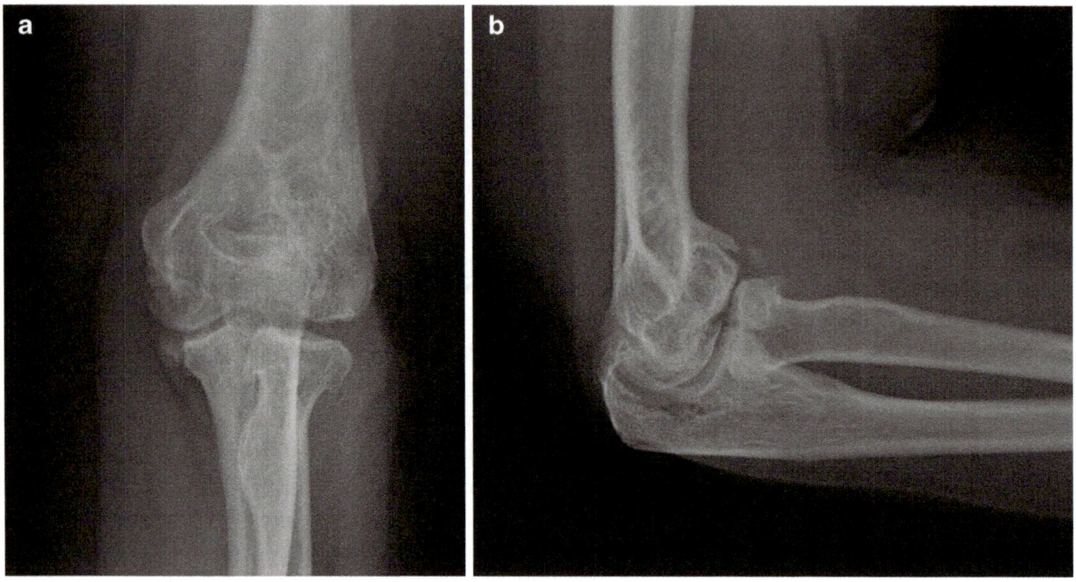

Fig. 17.3 (**a** and **b**) Anteroposterior (AP) and lateral X-rays showing malunion of the distal humerus as a result of a shear fracture (2A according to Dubberley classification) treated with K-wires that had been successively removed

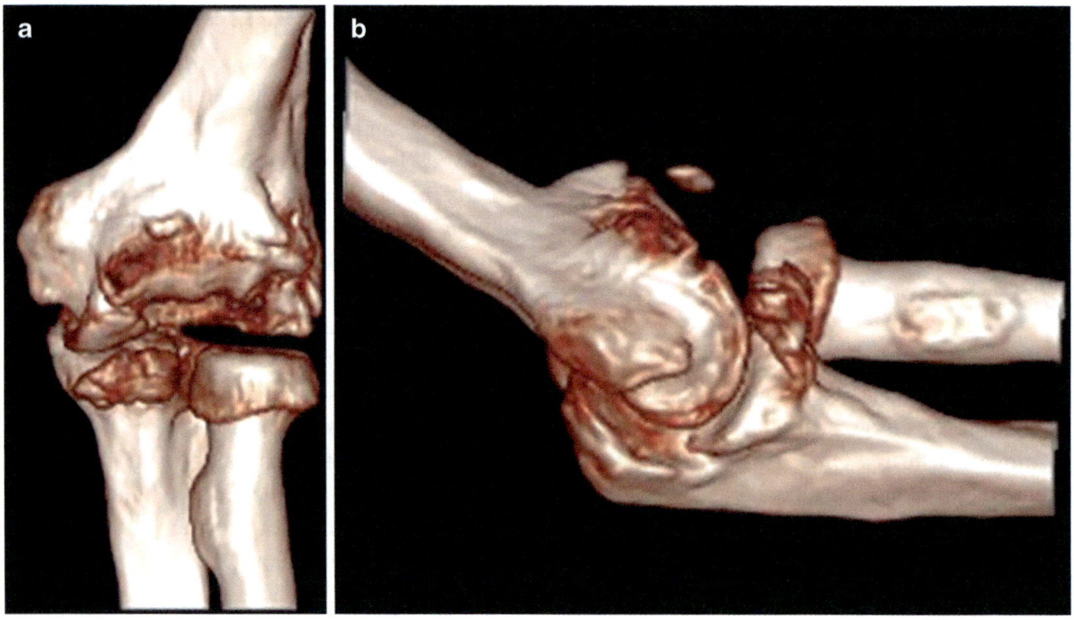

Fig. 17.4 (**a** and **b**) 3D-CT scan showing deformity and arthritis especially on the humeral articular surface

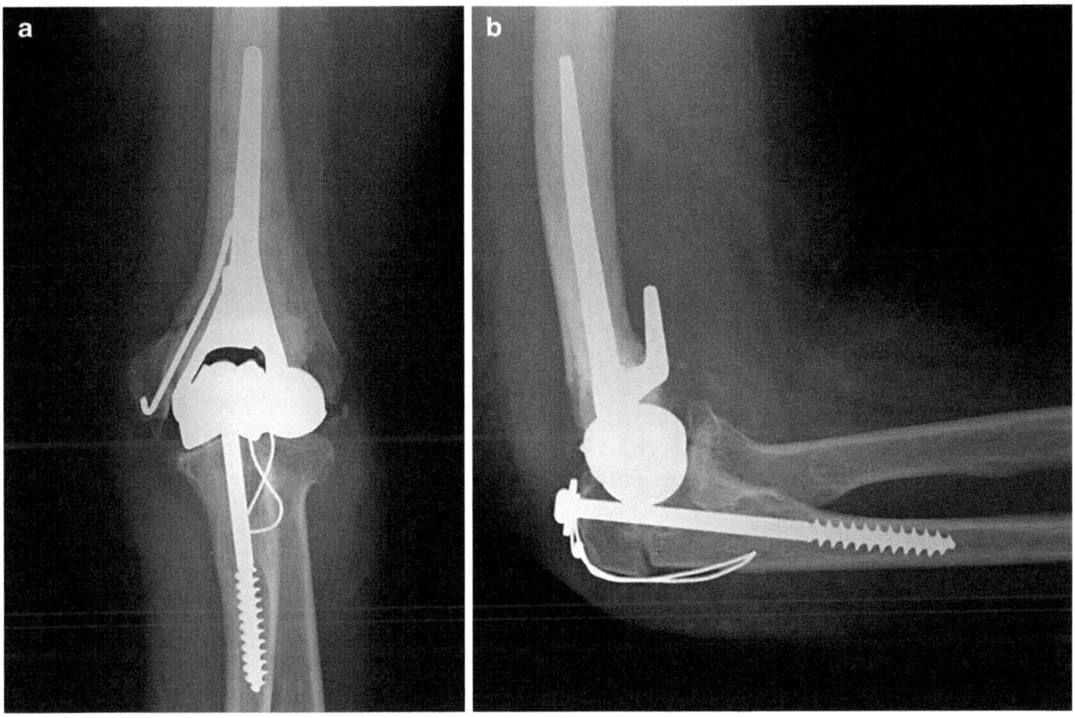

Fig. 17.5 (**a** and **b**) AP and lateral X-rays at 2-month follow-up. An olecranon osteotomy approach was used. A K-wire has been used to fix an undisplaced fracture of the medial column

17.5.2 Case 2

A 35-year-old woman affected from epiphyseal chondrodysplasia presented to our clinic with significant bilateral elbow pain and severe functional limitations, at the beginning more severe on the right side, with ROM restricted to 90–75° in flexion–extension and 20°-0–20° in forearm rotation. The preoperative CT scan showed severe hypertrophic arthritis of the right elbow (Fig. 17.7). Considering her young age and high functional requests, an hemiarthroplasty was considered as the most appropriate indication (Fig. 17.8).

In this case, a triceps splitting approach was performed in order to expose the joint (Fig. 17.9).

The patient came back to our clinic 6 years later with severe pain to the right elbow and ROM blocked at 80° of flexion–extension and 50°-0-10° in forearm rotation (Fig. 17.10). The patient asked for surgery and the hemiarthroplasty was converted to a total elbow prosthesis.

At 6-year follow-up of the total elbow arthroplasty (Fig. 17.11), the patient was pain free, with ROM of 130–80° in flexion–extension, 50° forearm rotation deficit. The prosthesis does not show any sign of radiographic loosening (Figs. 17.12 and 17.13).

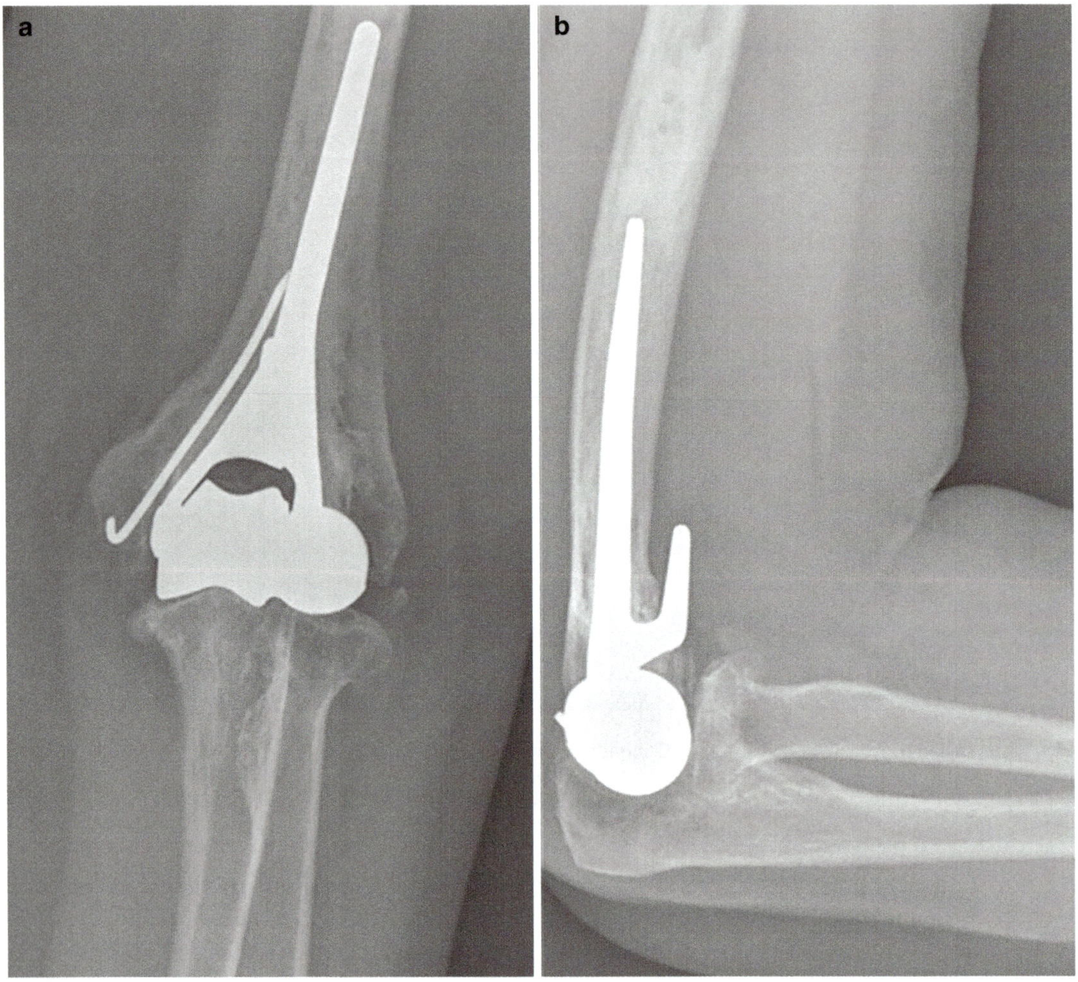

Fig. 17.6 (**a** and **b**) AP and lateral view at 8-year follow-up of left elbow hemiarthroplasty

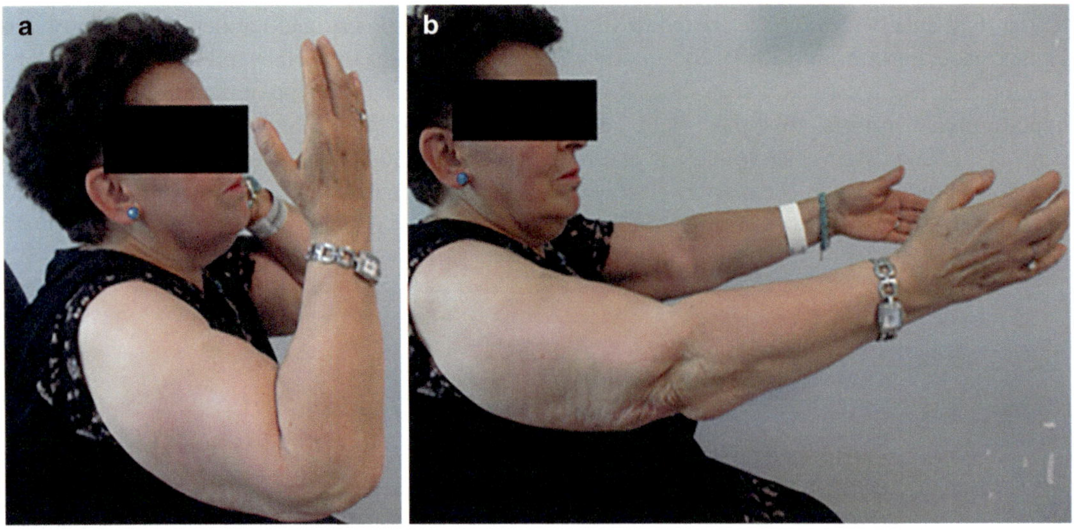

Fig. 17.7 (**a** and **b**) Eight-year follow-up of left elbow hemiarthroplasty: active ROM 90–30° with severe pain and functional limitation in daily living activities

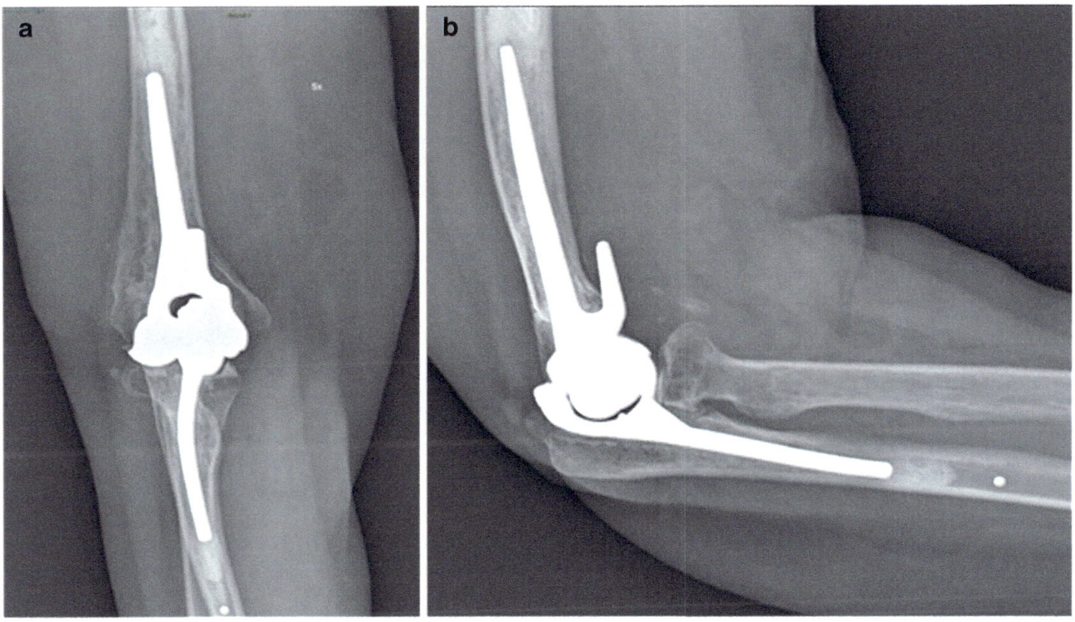

Fig. 17.8 (**a** and **b**) AP and lateral view at 6-year follow-up for a TEA

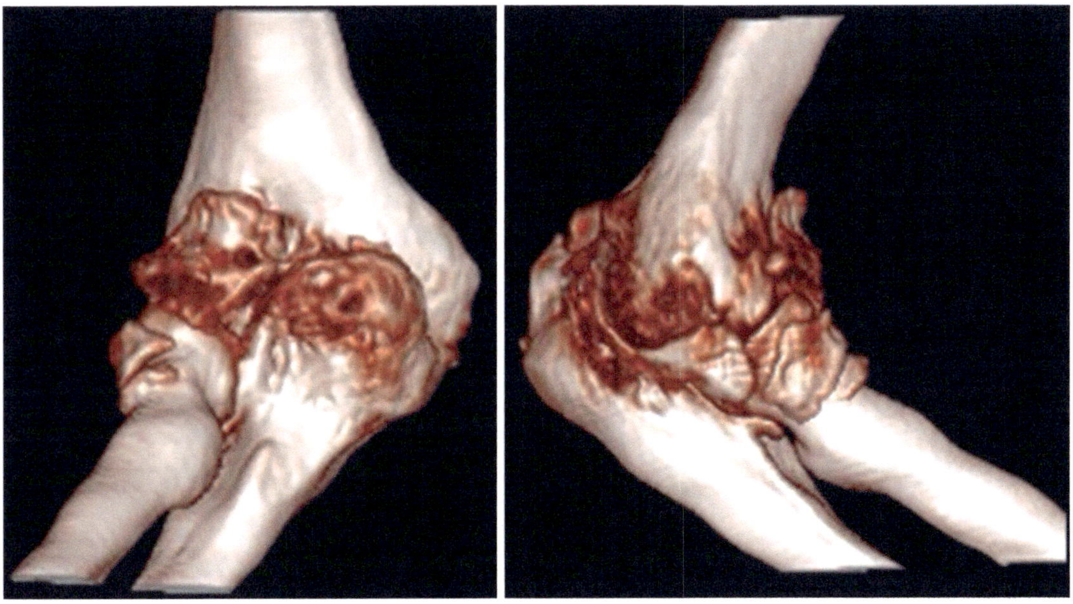

Fig. 17.9 Preoperative CT scan of the right elbow affected by an arthritic elbow joint of a 35-year-old woman

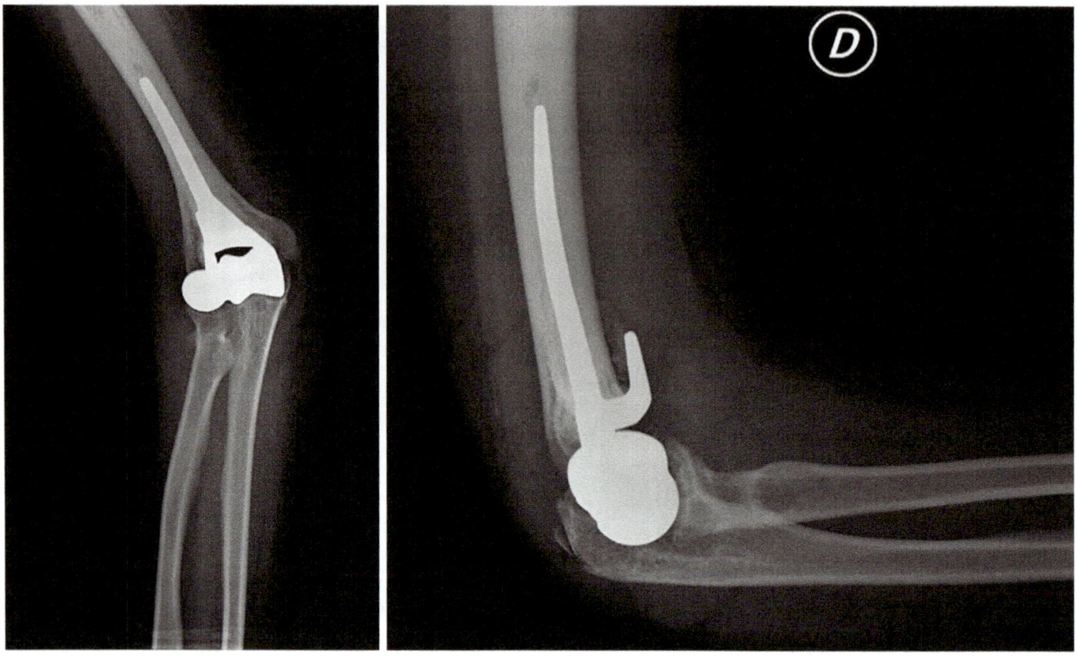

Fig. 17.10 X-rays showing the right elbow hemiarthroplasty at 2-year follow-up

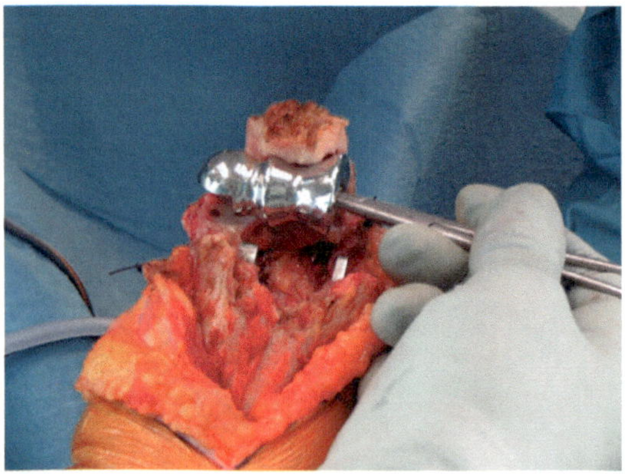

Fig. 17.11 Intraoperative elbow joint exposure

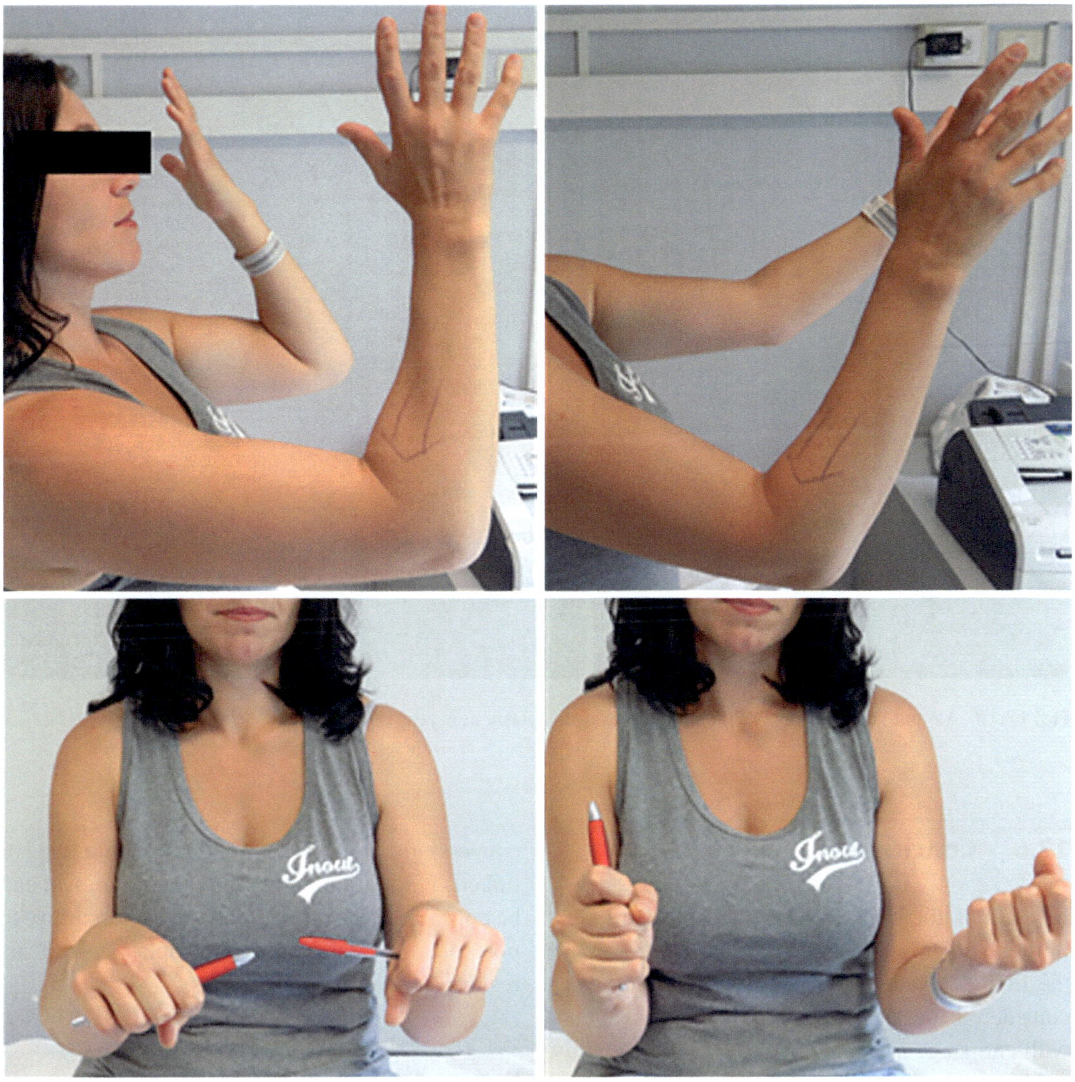

Fig. 17.12 Six-year follow-up of the right elbow hemiarthroplasty: the patient complained limited ROM and pain during daily living activities

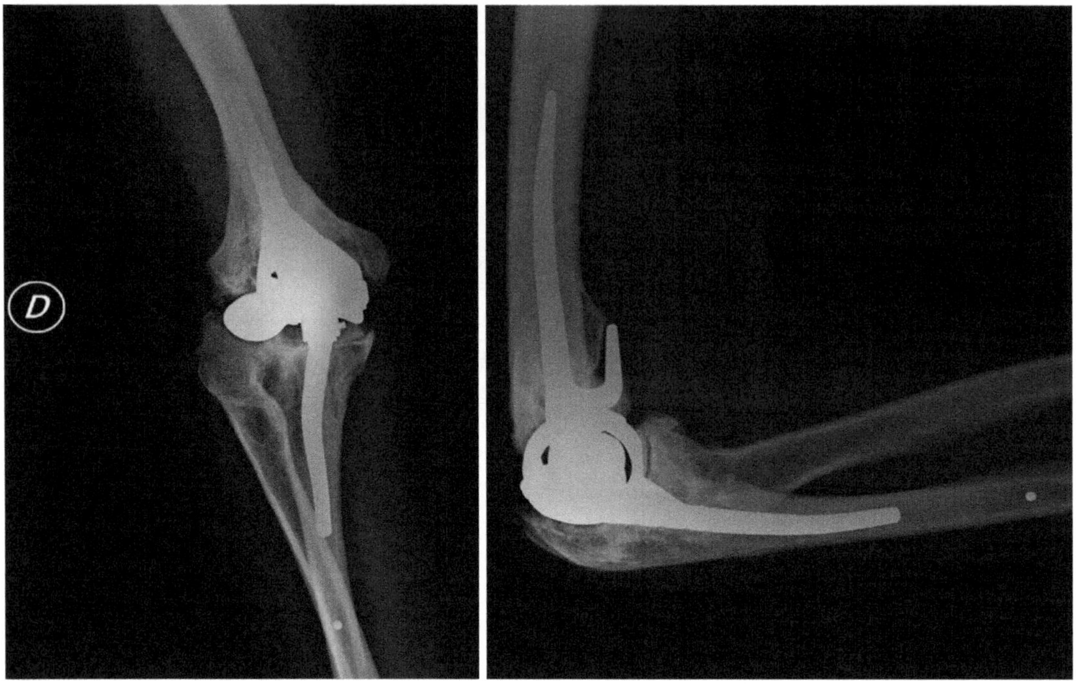

Fig. 17.13 AP and lateral X-rays of the total elbow arthroplasty at 6-year follow-up

17.6 Conclusion

Indications for EHA in elbow stiffness are very limited and only few cases have been reported in the literature until now. EHA can be cautiously considered for selected young or active patients with end-stage arthritis involving only or mainly the humeral surface, in whom alternative procedures have failed or cannot considered.

Based on our limited experience and on the literature available, after an EHA implant for elbow stiffness the ROM improvement is predictable only in the short term and it frequently worsens over time due to progressive increase of arthritis on the native proximal ulnar and radius surface. According to the literature, only about half of patients with surviving implants present a good to excellent MEPS at mid-term follow-up. Moreover, high rates of complications and revision surgery, included revision to TEA, can be expected already in the first years following surgery. However, the possibility of a subsequent conversion from EHA to TEA (unlinked or linked) without humeral component removal can be considered in selected patient a a possibility to postpone a total elbow arthroplasty with its resulting functional limitations.

References

1. Werthel JD, Schoch B, Adams J, Steinmann S. Outcomes after hemiarthroplasty of the elbow for the management of posttraumatic arthritis: minimum 2-year follow-up. J Am Acad Orthop Surg. 2019;27(19):727–35. https://doi.org/10.5435/JAAOS-D-18-00055.
2. Phadnis J, Watts AC, Bain GI. Elbow hemiarthroplasty for the management of distal humeral fractures: current technique, indications and results. Shoulder Elbow. 2016;8(3):171–83. https://doi.org/10.1177/1758573216640210. Epub 2016 Apr 21
3. Rotini R, Ricciarelli M, Guerra E, Marinelli A, Celli A. Elbow hemiarthroplasty in distal humeral fractures: Indication, surgical technique and results. Injury. 2020; https://doi.org/10.1016/j.injury.2020.11.020. S0020-1383(20)30946-3. Epub ahead of print

4. Celli A, Ricciarelli M, Guerra E, Bonucci P, Ritali A, Cavallo M, Rotini M, Rotini R. Elbow hemiarthroplasty for acute distal humeral fractures and their sequelae: medium- and long-term follow-up of 41 cases. J Shoulder Elb Surg. 2022;31(5):1015–25. https://doi.org/10.1016/j.jse.2021.12.030. Epub 2022 Jan 26
5. Parsons M, O'Brien RJ, Hughes JS. Elbow hemiarthroplasty for acute and salvage reconstruction of intra-articular distal humerus fractures. Tech Shoulder Elb Surg. 2005;6(2):87–97.
6. Jukes CP, Dirckx M, Phadnis J. Current concepts in distal humeral hemiarthroplasty. J Clin Orthop Trauma. 2021;19:224–30. https://doi.org/10.1016/j.jcot.2021.05.025.
7. Guerra, E., Zaccaro, R., Marinelli, A., Cavallo, M., Bettelli, G., Rotini, R. (2020). Chapter 5: Surgical approaches for elbow replacements. In: Castoldi, F., Giannicola, G., Rotini, R. (eds) Elbow arthroplasty: current techniques and complications. Cham: Springer pg 57–73.
8. Studer A, Athwal GS, JC MD, Faber KJ, King GJ. The lateral para-olecranon approach for total elbow arthroplasty. J Hand Surg Am. 2013;38(11):2219–2226.e3. https://doi.org/10.1016/j.jhsa.2013.07.029.
9. Shahane SA, Stanley D. A posterior approach to the elbow joint. J Bone Joint Surg Br. 1999;81(6):1020–2. https://doi.org/10.1302/0301-620x.81b6.9696.
10. Nestorson J, Ekholm C, Etzner M, Adolfsson L. Hemiarthroplasty for irreparable distal humeral fractures. Bone Joint J. 2015;97-B(10):1377–84. https://doi.org/10.1302/0301-620X.97B10.35421.
11. Marinello PG, Peers S, Styron J, Pervaiz K, Evans PJ. Triceps fascial tongue exposure for total elbow arthroplasty: surgical technique and case series. Tech Hand Up Extrem Surg. 2015;19(2):60–3.
12. Na KT, Song SW, Lee YM, Choi JH. Modified triceps fascial tongue approach for primary total elbow arthroplasty. J Shoulder Elb Surg. 2018;27:887–93. https://doi.org/10.1016/j.jse.2018.01.005.

Total Joint Replacement in Post-traumatic Elbow Stiffness

18

Andrea Celli, Cataldo Giacomo,
and Luigi Pederzini

18.1 Introduction

Elbow stiffness can involve severe limitations in upper limb use, thus hampering patients' activities of daily living. The condition can due to an articular deformity caused by degenerative changes. Primary degenerative arthrosis of the elbow is often ascribed to repeated microtrauma from work or sport activities. Demographic studies have demonstrated a different incidence of primary elbow arthritis in different populations, but it is unclear whether it stems from genetic or environmental factors. Men are much more affected than women (ca. 4: 1 ratio) [1, 2]. The age at presentation is about 50 years, although patients as young as 20 years and patients aged 65 years have also been described [1, 2]. The dominant limb is involved in 80–90% of patients whereas bilateral involvement is found in 25–60% [1, 2]. Post-traumatic arthritis (PTA) is more common than primary arthritis, being a sequela of complex elbow injuries such as dislocation, fracture–dislocation, and articular fracture. Patients with PTA are frequently young and active, often with high expectations and a desire to return to their previous level of activity. Pain is associated with joint stiffness and deformity. Patients present soft-tissue retraction, bone loss or deformity, and joint instability [3, 4].

18.2 Clinical and Radiological Evaluation

The clinical picture of PTA is highly variable both because of the variable pain intensity and because of the possible association with joint deformity, contractures, stiffness, bone loss, and instability due to the primary trauma (e.g., fracture of the humerus, radius or ulna, dislocation, ligament injuries) or of earlier treatments and procedures. The clinical evaluation considers not only range of motion (ROM) and pain but also instability, nerve deficiency, and soft-tissue injury. Computed tomography (CT) (Fig. 18.1a–f) and magnetic resonance imaging (MRI) are useful to define bone loss, articular cartilage lesions, size and shape of heterotopic ossification, presence of loose bodies, and capsule and ligament lesions [1–4].

A. Celli (✉)
Department of Orthopaedic and Traumatology Surgery, Shoulder and Elbow Unit, Hesperia Hospital, Modena, Italy

C. Giacomo
Department of Orthopaedic, Traumatology and Arthroscopic Surgeries, Nuovo Ospedale di Sassuolo, Modena, Italy

L. Pederzini
Department of Orthopedics, Hesperia Hospital, Modena, Italy

L. Pederzini et al. (eds.), *Stiffness of the Elbow, Wrist and Related Pathologies*,
https://doi.org/10.1007/978-3-031-81381-8_18

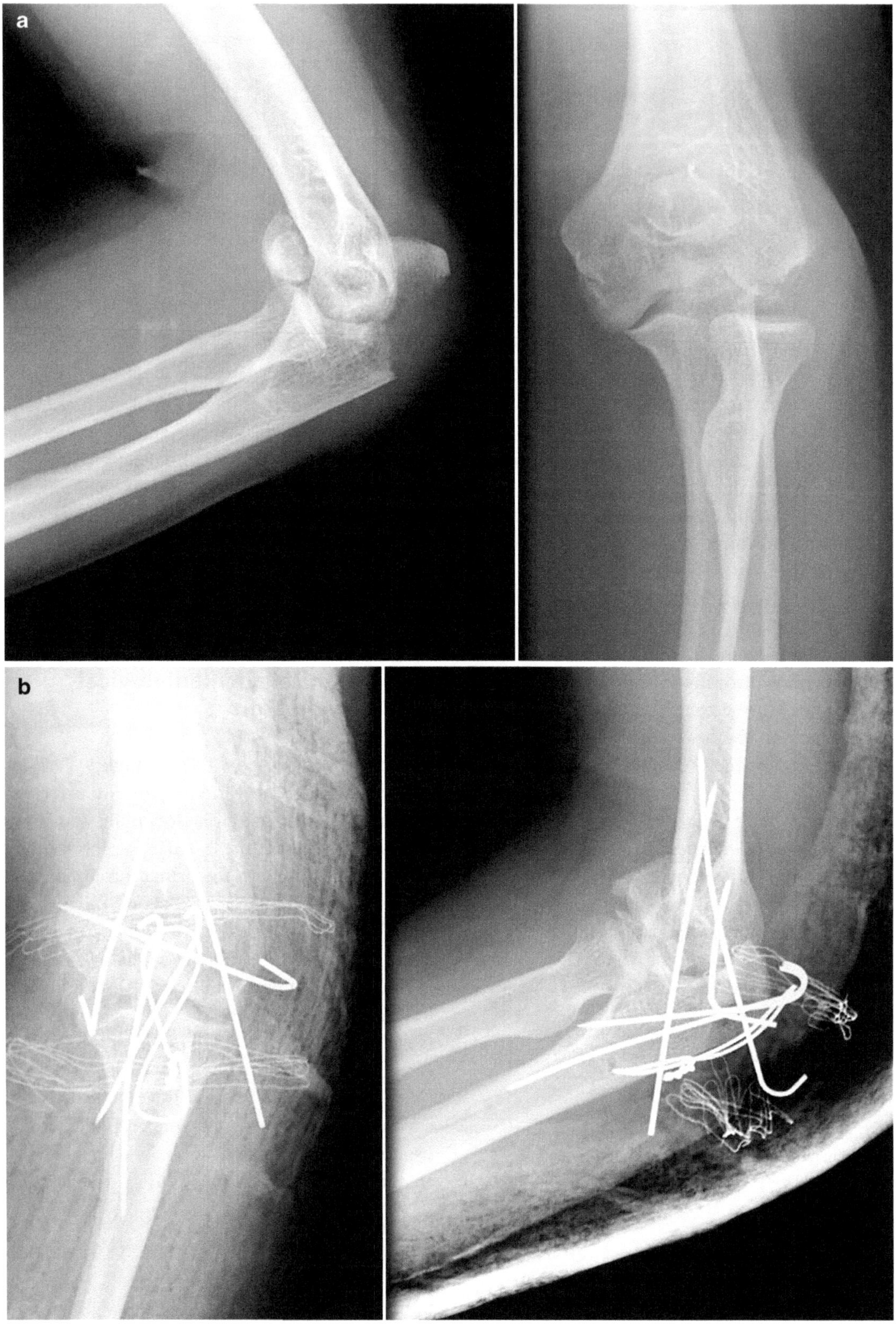
a
b

Fig. 18.1 (**a**–**f**) A 48-year-old female, sedentary, right hand dominant, left elbow, closed distal humeral, and olecranon articular fractures (**a**). Treated with open reduction and internal fixation using percutaneous Kirschner wires and olecranon cerclage (**b**). X-rays at 8 months (**c**). X-rays at 14 months, with severe pain and stiffness (**d**). CT scan with three-dimensional (3D) reconstructions (**e**, **f**) helps to define the extension of the articular damage in terms of joint deformity and loose of the articular congruency defining the possibility to recover motion and stability with or without an elbow replacement

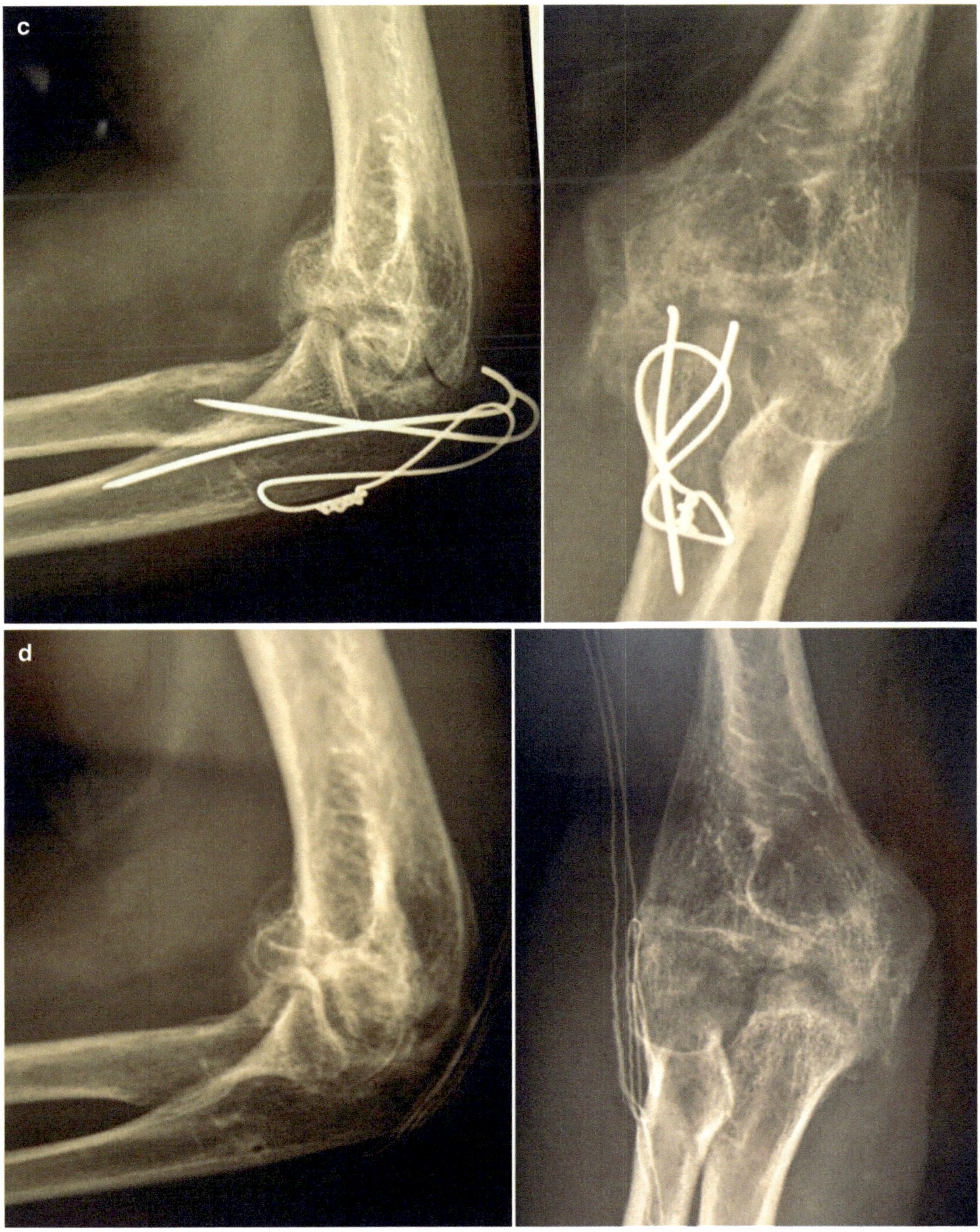

Fig. 18.1 (continued)

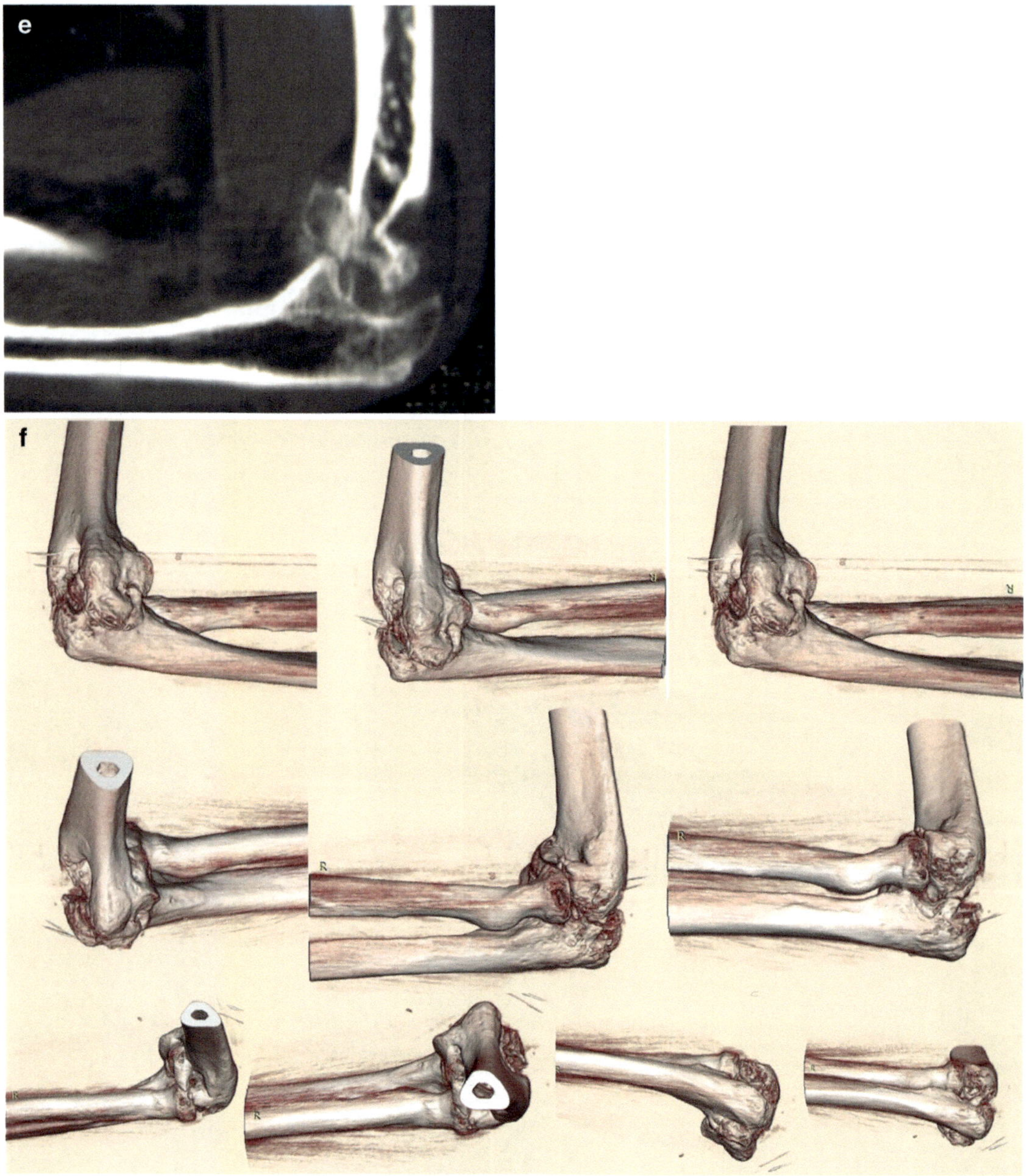

Fig. 18.1 (continued)

18.3 Indications for Total Elbow Replacement

Total elbow arthroplasty (TEA) is a salvage procedure for stiff elbow, because the prosthesis involves considerable limitations of elbow motion. TEA (linked or unlinked) may be considered in elderly and low-demand patients with an elbow contracture associated with severe arthritic changes of the joint surfaces [5–7], whereas in young patients it may be considered if no other treatment options are feasible [8]. A semiconstrained linked implant is recommended for patients with complete elbow ankylosis and stiffness [8]. In such situations, complete soft-tissue release, ulnar nerve transposition, and resection of joint surfaces and any impinging heterotopic bone are needed. The surgical technique depends on the implant being used, any prior incisions, and surgeon preference. In all cases, the ulnar nerve must be identified and released or transposed. Optimal biomechanical conditions include aggressive soft-tissue release and adequate bone resection [5–8].

18.4 Surgical Technique

Most surgical approaches used for TEA require mobilization of the elbow extensor mechanism. The ulnar nerve is routinely isolated and transposed anteriorly to a subcutaneous pocket. Although the authors' preferred triceps exposure is the anconeus-triceps lateral flap approach [9] (Fig. 18.2a, b), the triceps-reflecting Bryan-Morrey approach, [10] triceps splitting, and an extended lateral Kocher approach [11] are also useful techniques. Triceps-sparing approaches are desirable, although in some patients with post-traumatic conditions it is hampered by tendon retraction and scar tissue, which can limit the ROM in flexion [12]. Linked semiconstrained implants have an intrinsic stability provided by the hinge and do not require ligament repair or preserved epiphyseal bone. In contrast, unlinked prostheses are sometimes difficult to implant in patients with PTA, due to deformity of the humeral condyles and to collateral ligament deficiency. Bone loss is merely a relative contraindication. Post-traumatic instability is not incompatible with TEA, as it requires a semiconstrained implant. In fact, the condition is well managed with this device.

18.4.1 Surgical Steps

With the patient in supine decubitus, a posterior skin incision is made to gain medial and lateral exposure or to exploit a previous incision. The ulnar nerve is isolated and prepared for subsequent anterior transposition in a subcutaneous pocket at the end of the procedure. Selection of the triceps exposure technique is related to the soft-tissue retraction. Preservation of the olecranon insertion is desirable, but lengthening the triceps tendon is sometimes necessary to increase the ROM, particularly in flexion. In patients without triceps tendon retraction, we prefer the anconeus-triceps lateral flap approach [9] which allows sparing the medial portion of the tendon, reflecting its lateral portion in continuity with the anconeus muscle (Fig. 18.2a, b). In patients with extensile soft-tissue contractures, release of the common flexor and extensor muscles from the humeral insertion with the medial and lateral ligaments helps to improve the surgical exposure and the final ROM. The prosthetic components are inserted using the proper technique and low-viscosity cement. Resection of the osteophytes and of the tip of the coronoid process is necessary to avoid impingement with the anterior flange and between bone and the prosthetic components, which would cause considerable forces around the implant, particularly on the ulnar component. The radial head is preserved if there is no significant malalignment or impingement. To gain extension the humeral component may need to be seated up to 5 mm farther proximal than usual, to help release the anterior soft-tissue envelope in extension. Subcutaneous anterior transposition of the ulnar nerve must avoid secondary points of possible compression during motion. Drains are placed in the anterior compartment, in the posterior compartment, and in the subcutaneous space.

18.4.2 Postoperative Care

The arm is elevated with the elbow extended in a splint using cryotherapy for pain and edema control. The patient begins passive and active flexion–extension (motion is encouraged as tolerated and in relation to the swelling, pain and the triceps approach used). The patient is asked to avoid single-event lifting exceeding 5 kg and repetitive lifting exceeding 2.5 kg.

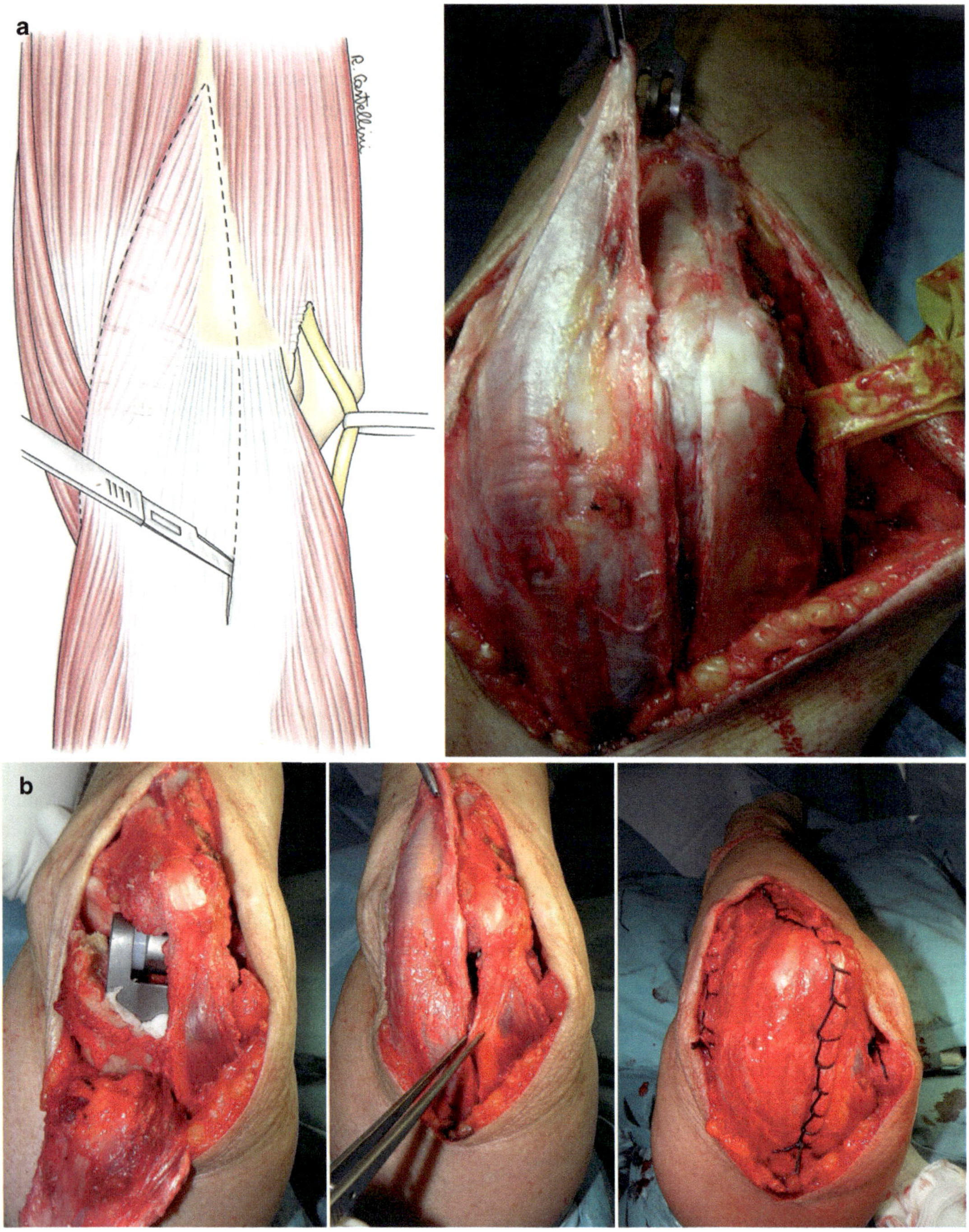

Fig. 18.2 (**a** and **b**) The anconeus-triceps lateral flap approach [9] allows to keep intact the medial part of tendon reflecting the lateral part in continuity with the anconeus muscle

18.5 Results

TEA is very attractive as it provides the best early functional results; however, it is associated with the risk of mechanical failure, especially in younger patients [13–17]. Schneeberger et al. [18] published the results of 41 patients with post-traumatic osteoarthritis who received the Coonrad-Morrey prosthesis. Their mean age at the time of surgery was 57 years (range, 32–82 years) and the mean follow-up was 5 years. The results were considered satisfactory in 83% of cases, with 73% of the patients reporting mild or no pain. However, there was a 27% complication rate, including five fractures of the ulnar component and two revisions due to polyethylene wear. The authors concluded that elbow arthroplasty should be relatively contraindicated in patients who are unable to comply with postoperative restrictions.

At the Mayo Clinic [19], 85 consecutive patients with PTA underwent semiconstrained TEA; 69 elbows with a retained primary prosthesis were followed up for a mean period of 9.1 years (range, 2–20.5). A total number of 16 primary arthroplasties (19%) failed due to isolated bushing wear, infection, component fracture, or component loosening; four showed radiographic signs of loosening; and three showed substantial radiographic wear. Forty-seven (68%) patients achieved good or excellent clinical results according to objective criteria and 74% of patients were subjectively satisfied with their outcome at the final follow-up visit.

An alternative strategy in younger patients is interposition arthroplasty as the primary procedure, although they need to be informed that pain relief with this option is not reliable [8].

18.5.1 Complications

Although complications are frequent in patients with post-traumatic conditions, careful preoperative planning and surgery execution improve function and relieve pain [20–23]. The main complications include periprosthetic loosening, mechanical failure, infection, triceps rupture, and nerve palsy [20].

18.6 Discussion

PTA is often disabling as it entails pain and loss of motion. Bone deficiency is common and a flail limb may result from fracture nonunion. Such circumstances represent a relative contraindication for TEA. In these cases, there is no reliable alternative treatment. Arthrodesis is not a good salvage procedure as the essential function of the elbow is to position the hand in space through joint flexion and extension (Fig. 18.3). Interposition arthroplasty, the common treatment for these patients, has unpredictable results with a risk of late deterioration (Fig. 18.4a, b). Although TEA remains the best treatment, especially in the older, low-demand age group (Fig. 18.5a–f), younger patients with PTA place excessive demands on the implant and experience a relatively high failure rate. Bushing wear and component loosening or fracture are seen more commonly in the intermediate and long term, whereas aseptic loosening is relatively uncommon. Strict limb use limitations are necessary to reduce the risk of complications; heavy work is not allowed and a lifting limit of 5 kg is recommended.

Elbow joint replacement has improved continuously over time. Widespread use of some designs has enabled identification of successful elements as well as opportunities for improvement. Current hot topics in elbow arthroplasty

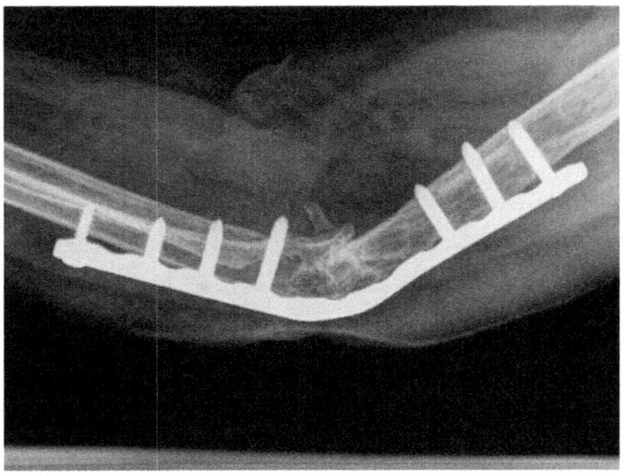

Fig. 18.3 Arthrodesis is not a good salvage procedure since the essential function of the elbow is to allow the hand to be placed in space

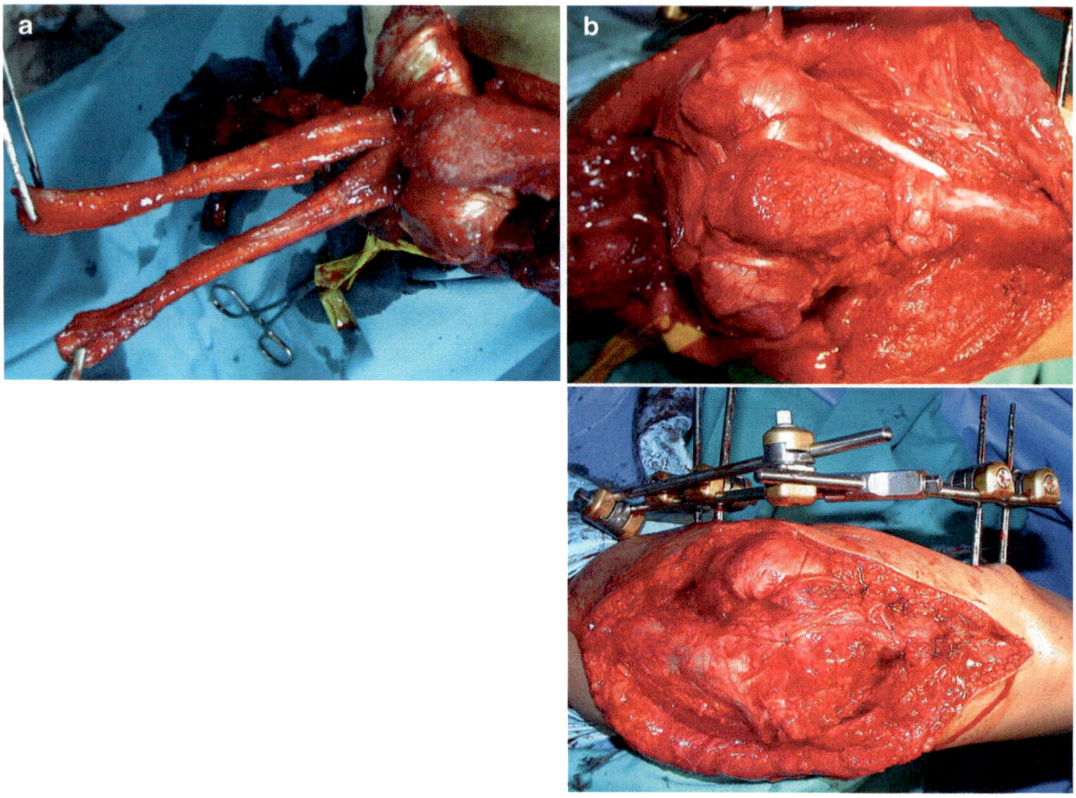

Fig. 18.4 Interposition arthroplasty has unpredictable results with risks of late deterioration (**a**) Interposition arthroplasty with Achilles tendon allograft (**b**) ligaments reconstruction and external fixator distraction

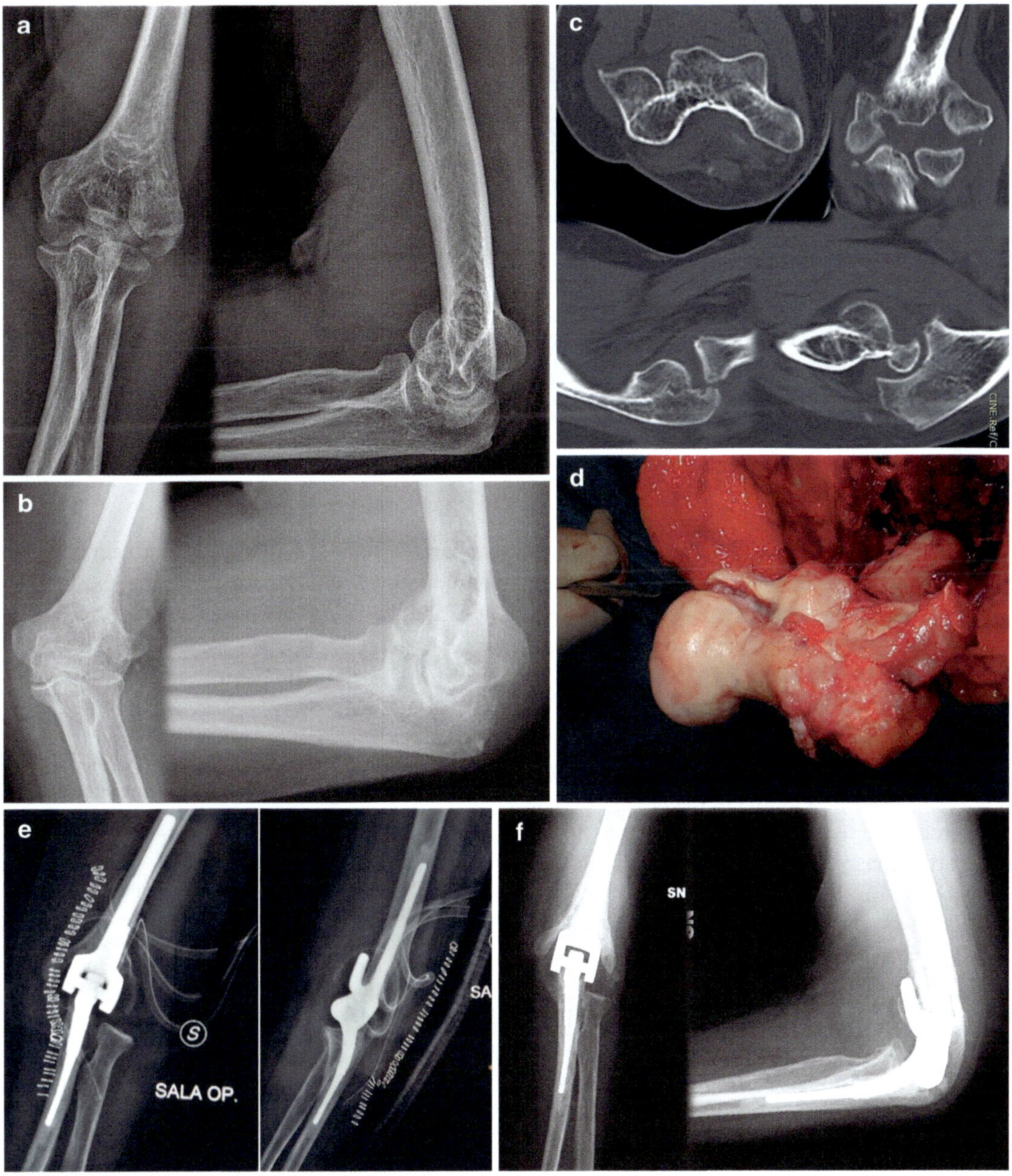

Fig. 18.5 (**a–g**) A 68-year-old female, retired, right hand dominant, left elbow, no other pathology, closed distal humeral articular fracture treated with a cast (**a**). X-ray at 2 months (**b**). CT scan at 3 months (**c**). Intraoperative image with severe deformity of the articular deformity (**d**). Coonrad-Morrey total elbow replacement (linked semiconstrained design) postoperative X-ray (**e**). X-rays at 6 years of follow-up (**f**). Range of motion at 6 years of follow-up (**g**)

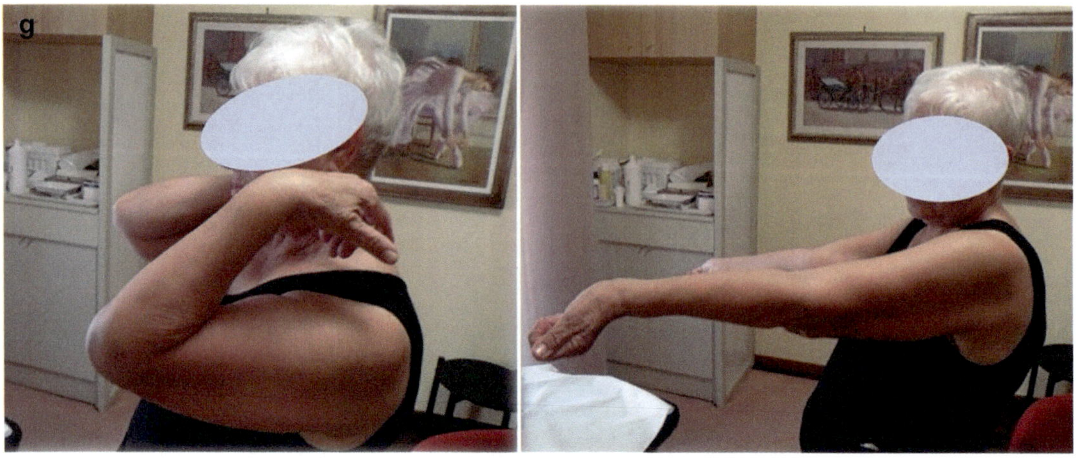

Fig. 18.5 (continued)

include triceps-sparing exposures, implantation of components with better-than-expected wear performance, ulnar nerve management, prevention of infection, and the development of successful cementless components [23–26]. TEA has the potential to improve pain, function, and quality of life for many patients with joint destruction secondary to degenerative arthropathy or trauma. Continued advances in this field are key to make this procedure as reliable and lasting as hip or knee arthroplasty.

18.7 Conclusion

TEA is performed in extreme cases as a salvage procedure, namely if painless motion and stability cannot be restored with other surgical procedures. Implant failure is the most common complication after TEA in younger patients. Linked semiconstrained designs have a dominant role in this field, as they afford recovery of joint stability through implant design. We feel that persistent instability (subluxation or dislocation) after fracture–dislocation or intra-articular bone deformity for malunion or nonunion is the main indication for elbow replacement in patients with post-traumatic elbow stiffness. Alternatively, distal humeral hemiarthroplasty may be performed in younger patients who need management of malunion, intra-articular avascular necrosis, and unreduced shear fracture involving the capitellum and the lateral trochlea [27].

References

1. Schrumpf MA, Lyman S, Do H, Schreiber JJ, Gay DM, Marx R, et al. Incidence of postoperative elbow contracture release in New York State. J Hand Surg Am. 2013;38:1746–52.
2. Evans PJ, Nandi S, Maschke S, Hoyen HA, Lawton JN. Prevention and treatment of elbow stiffness. J Hand Surg Am. 2009;34:769–78.
3. Bauer AS, Lawson BK, Bliss RL, Dyer GS. Risk factors for posttraumatic heterotopic ossification of the elbow: case-control study. J Hand Surg Am. 2012;37:1422-9.e1–6.
4. King GJ, Faber KJ. Posttraumatic elbow stiffness. Orthop Clin North Am. 2000;31:129–43.
5. Mansat P, Morrey BF. Semiconstrained total elbow arthroplasty for ankylosed and stiff elbows. J Bone Joint Surg Am. 2000;82-A:1260–8.
6. Moro JK, King GJ. Total elbow arthroplasty in the treatment of posttraumatic conditions of the elbow. Clin Orthop Relat Res. 2000;370:102–14.
7. Peden JP, Morrey BF. Total elbow replacement for the management of the ankylosed or fused elbow. J Bone Joint Surg (Br). 2008;90-B:1198–204.
8. Celli A, Morrey BF. Total elbow arthroplasty in patients forty years of age or less. J Bone Joint Surg Am. 2009;91(6):1414–8.
9. Celli A, Bonucci P. The anconeus-triceps lateral flap approach for total elbow arthroplasty in rheumatoid arthritis. Musculoskelet Surg. 2016;100(Suppl 1):73–83. Epub 2016 Nov 30

10. Bryan RS, Morrey BF. Extensive posterior exposure of the elbow. A triceps-sparing approach. Clin Orthop. 1982(166):188–92.
11. Prokopis PM, Weiland AJ. The triceps-preserving approach for semiconstrained total elbow arthroplasty. J Shoulder Elb Surg. 2008;17(3):454–8.
12. Alonso-Llames M. Bilaterotricipital approach to the elbow. Its application in the osteosynthesis of supracondylar fractures of the humerus in children. Acta Orthop Scand. 1972;43(6):479–90.
13. Little CP, Carr AJ, Graham AJ. Total elbow arthroplasty: a systematic review of the literature in the English language until the end of 2003. J Bone Joint Surg Br. 2005;87(4):437–44.
14. Celli A, Paroni C, Bonucci P, Celli L. Total elbow arthroplasty for acute distal humeral fractures with humeral condyle resection or retention: a long-term follow-up study. JSES Int. 2021;5(4):797–803.
15. Quenneville CE, Austman RL, King GJ, Johnson JA, Dunning CE. Role of an anterior flange on cortical strains through the distal humerus after total elbow arthroplasty with a latitude implant. J Hand Surg Am. 2008;33(6):927–31.
16. Levy JC, Loeb M, Chuinard C, Adams RA, Morrey BF. Effectiveness of revision following linked versus unlinked total elbow arthroplasty. J Shoulder Elb Surg. 2009;18(3):457–62.
17. Blaine TA, Adams R, Morrey BF. Total elbow arthroplasty after interposition arthroplasty for elbow arthritis. J Bone Joint Surg Am. 2005;87(2):286–92.
18. Schneeberger AG, Adams R, Morrey BF. Semiconstrained total elbow replacement for the treatment of post-traumatic osteoarthrosis. J Bone Joint Surg Am. 1997;79(8):1211–22.
19. Sanchez-Sotelo J. Total elbow arthroplasty. Open Orthop J. 2011;5:115–23.
20. Kim JM, Mudgal CS, Konopka JF, Jupiter JB. Complications of total elbow arthroplasty. J Am Acad Orthop Surg. 2011;19(6):328–39.
21. Peden JP, Morrey BF. Total elbow replacement for the management of the ankylosed or fused elbow. J Bone Joint Surg Br. 2008;90(9):1198–204.
22. Mansat P, Morrey BF. Semiconstrained total elbow arthroplasty for ankylosed and stiff elbows. J Bone Joint Surg Am. 2000;82(9):1260–8.
23. Bauer AS, Lawson BK, Bliss RL, Dyer GS. Risk factors for posttraumatic heterotopic ossification of the elbow: case-control study. J Hand Surg. 2012;37(7):1422-9 e1–6.
24. Welsink CL, Lambers KTA, van Deurzen DFP, Eygendaal D, van den Bekerom MPJ. Total elbow arthroplasty: a systematic review. JBJS Rev. 2017;5(7):e4.
25. Throckmorton T, Zarkadas P, Sanchez-Sotelo J, Morrey BF. Failure patterns after linked semiconstrained total elbow arthroplasty for posttraumatic arthritis. J Bone Joint Surg Am. 2010;92(6):1432–41.
26. Booker SJ, Smith CD. Triceps on approach for total elbow arthroplasty: worth preserving? A review of approaches for total elbow arthroplasty. 1. Shoulder Elbow. 2017;9(2):105–11.
27. Celli A, Ricciarelli M, Guerra E, Bonucci P, Ritali A, Cavallo M, Rotini M, Rotini R. Elbow hemiarthroplasty for acute distal humeral fractures and their sequelae: medium- and long-term follow-up of 41 cases. J Shoulder Elb Surg. 2022;31(5):1015–25.

19 Nerve Entrapment in Elbow Stiffness

Raffaele Garofalo, Angelo De Crescenzo, and Andrea Celli

19.1 Introduction

The elbow is a joint extremely susceptible to stiffness, even after a trivial trauma [1]. Up to 5% of patients with elbow injury can develop an ankylosis [1], whereas 10–15% of patients may need an additional surgery to manage joint contracture [2]. As for other joints, several factors can generate stiffness such as immobilization, joint incongruity, heterotopic ossification, adhesions, or pain. Prolonged joint immobilization, pursued to assure bony and ligamentous healing, represents the most acknowledged risk factor for joint stiffness. Consequently, increasing efforts have been channeling to achieve as much as possible elbow stability, thereby avoiding unfavorable prolonged immobilization. Nonetheless, immobilization time as well as energy of incipit trauma cannot predict the degree of joint stiffness suggesting as other elements may play significant role in contracture development.

The elbow is a common site of nerve entrapment syndromes. The reasons are multifactorial but peculiar elbow anatomy and biomechanics play a role. Passing from the arm into the forearm, the ulnar, median, and radial nerves run at the elbow in close rapport with the joint and fibrous arches and through narrow fibro-osseous tunnel. Here, pulleys and sheaths promote a smooth gliding throughout range of motion. The elbow joint, in fact, has a large range of flexion which expose nerves lying posterior to the axis of rotation to traction and those anterior to compression. The ulnar nerve, which is subjected to traction during elbow flexion, has an excursion of 5.1 mm from 10–90° of elbow motion [3]. In the same range of motion, 8.8 mm of nerve excursion is needed for the radial nerve [4]. Even though not sufficient to compromise nerve function, these anatomical features when coupled with factors restricting excursion can result in repetitive traction and friction of the nerve. In this way, capsule and ligaments thickening as well as adhesions and heterotopic ossifications following a trauma can play a role in the pathophysiology of a mechanical neuropathy.

Nerve irritation can trigger and exacerbate connective tissue fibrosis and heterotopic ossification development as an attempt to reduce joint motion otherwise further detrimental on nerve conduction [1]. However, preoperative electromyography (EMG) studies can show the absence of abnormality even though nerve can be narrowed, inflamed and grayish [5]. On the other hand, soft tissue and bone surgical release for

R. Garofalo · A. De Crescenzo
Ospedale "F. Miulli", Department of Orthopaedic and Traumatology Surgery, Shoulder and Elbow Unit, Acquaviva delle Fonti, Bari, Italy

A. Celli (✉)
Department of Orthopaedic and Traumatology Surgery Shoulder and Elbow Unit, Hesperia Hospital, Modena, Italy

L. Pederzini et al. (eds.), *Stiffness of the Elbow, Wrist and Related Pathologies*,
https://doi.org/10.1007/978-3-031-81381-8_19

elbow stiffness can have significant consequences on nerve conduction especially in severe contracture. In spite of a normal preoperative neurological condition, preventive nerve release and tunnel decompression must be considered when addressing surgically an elbow contracture. The significant motion recover can indeed decrease nerves "paths volume turning symptomatic a neuropathy that was subclinical [6]".

In the setting of a congruent joint without heterotopic ossification or joint arthrosis, joint contracture is regarded as the main reason of loss motion. From a histological point of view, studies have revealed an increased myofibroblast numbers as for other fibroproliferative conditions [7]. These are a specialized lineage of fibroblast with an increased expression of alpha smooth muscle actin (α-SMA), which provides contractile properties. These cells play a crucial role in stiffness development as suggested by the inverse proportion observed between flexion–extension arc of motion and number of myofibroblasts [8]. At the same time, a disorganized extracellular matrix (ECM), with an increased deposition of collagen types I and III, is typically found in these conditions [1, 9].

However, other cells can act a significant and synergic role in the fibroproliferative conditions. In the last decades, a growing interest has been observed in mast cells, which are significantly increased in different fibrotic diseases such as scleroderma, hypertrophic wound healing, or myocardial fibrosis [1]. Producing important mediators like basic fibroblast growth factor (bFGF), platelet-derived growth factor (PDGF), and transforming growth factor beta (TGF-b); mast cells can deeply influence fibroblast to become myofibroblasts increasing production of collagen and α-SMA [10].

Mast cells seem to represent the link by which neurogenic pathways can trigger soft tissue fibrosis. The neuroinflammatory process as root of post-traumatic or surgical joint contracture has been evidently acknowledged, even though without a distinct mechanism. Neuropeptides like substance P and calcitonin-gene-related peptide (CGRP) are neurotransmitters and paracrine factors playing an important role in connective tissue healing. Synthesized in the dorsal root ganglia, these are released because of noxious stimuli (e.g., traumatic injury) and growth factors (e.g., NGF). In this scenario, these molecules promote beneficial and effective local responses such as vasodilation, cellular proliferation, and matrix production. In a physiological setting, this cellular activation decreases as bone and soft tissue healing is going to be achieved. In patients with an ongoing joint stiffness, the constant mechanical and/or chemical stimuli provide a chronic mast cells and fibroblasts activation. As a result, an overactivation of myofibroblasts leads to a connective tissue fibrosis characterized by ECM shortening and disorganized collagen deposition.

Thus, neuropathy can be the upstream event which leads to secondary tissue remodeling and following joint stiffness. Consequently, surgical management for elbow stiffness should evaluate the potential neurological role as root of joint contracture. Scar tissues and heterotopic ossification surgical release could be otherwise unsuccessful.

19.2 Ulnar Nerve

19.2.1 Anatomy

The ulnar nerve (UN) arises as an extension of the medial cord of brachial plexus lying medial to the brachial artery. The ulnar nerve travels in the medial aspect of the arm between the coracobrachialis laterally and the medial head of the triceps posteriorly. Then, the nerve pierces the intermuscular septum at the level of distal insertion of coracobrachialis, at approximately 10 cm above the medial epicondyle, to enter the posterior compartment of the arm. Here, the nerve can travel inside the Arcade of Struthers, which is an occasional fascia enveloping the ulnar nerve at approximately 8 cm proximal to the medial epicondyle [11]. This arcade is a thickening of the deep fascia found 8–10 cm proximal to the medial epicondyle and it is an infrequent structure since it is present in about 70% of anatomical specimens [12]. The ulnar nerve then crosses the elbow posteriorly entering the cubital tunnel,

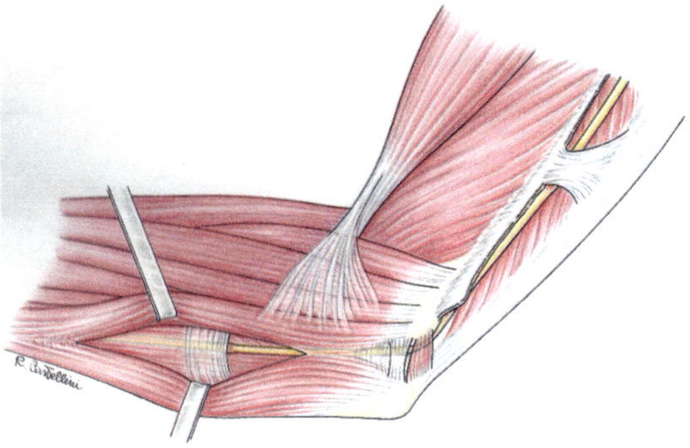

Fig. 19.1 The ulnar nerve and possible compression points around the elbow

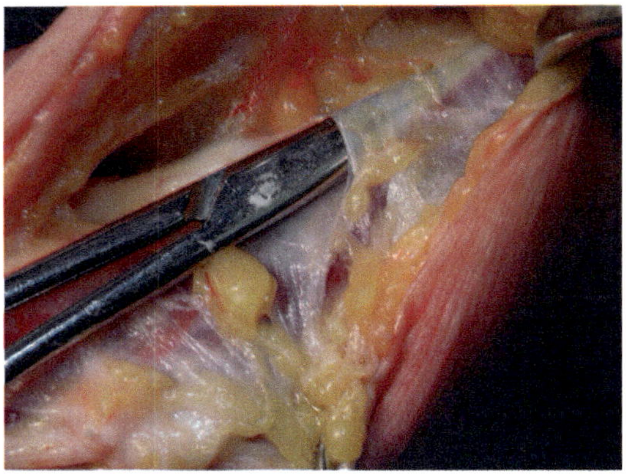

Fig. 19.2 The arcade of Struthers

which is defined anteriorly by the posterior surface of medial epicondyle and posteriorly by the retinaculum. At this point, as the nerve travels more distally, it is in close relationship with the medial collateral ligament (MCL), and in particular its posterior band (pMCL). Here, a sensitive branch arises for the capsule and the first motor branch for the flexor carpi ulnaris (FCU) (Fig. 19.1). As a matter of fact, multiple branches can arise, with some degree of anatomical variation, from 4 cm proximal to 10 cm distal to the medial epicondyle [11]. Muscular branches for flexor digitorum profundus (FDP) usually arise at 4–5 cm distal to the medial epicondyle [11].

19.2.2 Sites of Compression

19.2.2.1 The Arcade of Struthers

The arcade of Struthers is the most proximal side of potential primary UN entrapment in the elbow as well as secondary when it is not released during an anterior transposition. This should not be confused with the arcade of Struthers which is a facial band of variable thickness and width observed in less than 1% of specimens (Fig. 19.2) [12–14]. This ligament extends from the humeral supracondylar process to the medial epicondyle and the proximal insertion of pronator teres muscle and may compress median nerve [13, 14]. The arcade of Struthers is a thickening of the deep fascia of the arm observed in about 70% of anatomical specimens, 8–10 cm proximal to the medial epicondyle [12]. However, the studies on the anatomical features are limited and their finding contrasting. If in some studies this has been described as a fibrous canal with an average length of 5.7 cm through which the ulnar nerve passes 8–10 proximal to the medial epicondyle [15], in others it has been described as a fascial condensation spanning from the medial head of triceps to the medial intermuscular septum [16].

19.2.2.2 Medial Intermuscular Septum

This is an area of special interest for the surgeon approaching to the ulnar nerve. Dividing the anterior from the posterior compartment, this septum is remarkably thicker in the inferior supracondylar region, whereas its superior portion is thinner and with the less distinct attachment to the ulnar nerve. The ulnar nerve is firmly bound to the underlying triceps and then to the posterior aspect of the tick medial septum and the dorsal surface of the medial epicondyle. A complete resection of the distal 3.5 cm of septum is mandatory when an anterior never transposition is performed since it may otherwise represent a tenacious and predictable site of nerve kinking and compression (Fig. 19.3).

19.2.2.3 Anconeus Epitrochlearis Muscle

The anconeus epitrochlear is a rudimental muscle present in about 4–34% of population [17]. Although it is a rare finding, this muscle is a well-established cause of ulnar neuritis secondary to static compression. The muscle arises from the

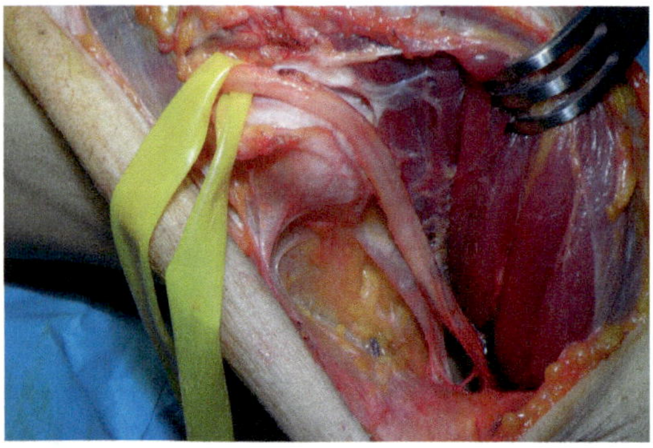

Fig. 19.3 The medial intermuscular septum

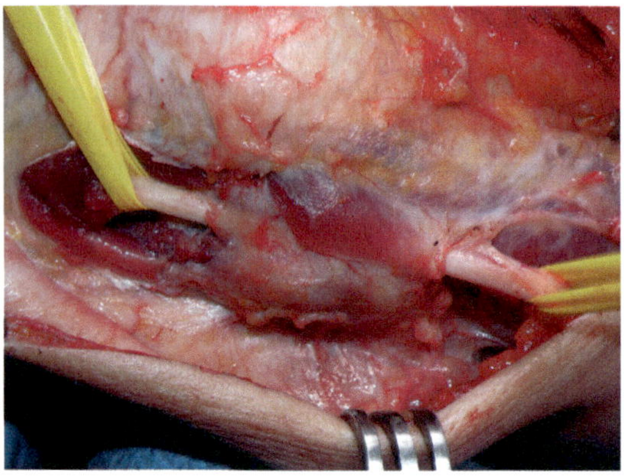

Fig. 19.4 The anconeus epitrochlearis muscle

medial border of the olecranon to insert into the medial epicondyle, and it can vary in shape from a very small band to a tick muscle to be even appreciated on physical examination (Fig. 19.4). However, an anconeus epitrochlearis ligament is more often observed instead of the muscle in about 70% of elbows. In case of an anconeus epitrochlearis muscle, the management suggested is an excision and a nerve anterior subcutaneous transposition.

19.2.2.4 Cubital Tunnel

The cubital tunnel is a fibro-osseous structure posterior to the medial epicondyle. The posterior portion of medial collateral ligament (MCL) and the overall medial aspect of humeroulnar capsule form the floor of this tunnel, whereas a thick fibrous layer between the epicondyle and the olecranon forms its roof (Fig. 19.5). In 1991

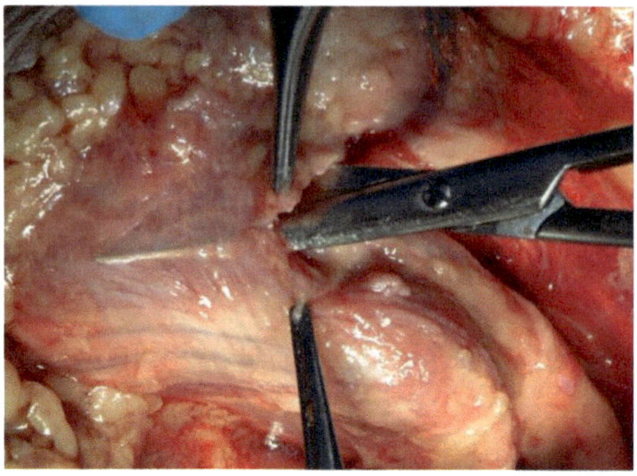

Fig. 19.5 The cubital tunnel

O'Driscoll and colleagues, studying 27 specimens, defined the roof of the cubital tunnel formed by the cubital tunnel retinaculum (CTR) and the flexor carpi ulnaris (FCU) aponeurosis. The CTR, likely a remnant of the anconeus epitrochlearis muscle, is a 4 mm wide fibrous band that forms the entrance to the cubital tunnel. This band tightens during elbow flexion preventing ulnar nerve dislocation. The FCU deep aponeurosis also known as Osborne's band is a fibrous arcade formed from the fusion of the deep FCU fascia and the antibrachial fascia. As the UN enters the anterior forearm compartment through the interval between the humeral and ulnar origin of the FCU muscle, it can be compressed by this fascial arcade of varying thickness.

The first portion or entrance of the cubital tunnel is composed by the medial epicondyle, the medial border of the olecranon, and the CTR. The latter, as described by O'Driscoll, presents four times of anatomical variance according to their potential of UN compression [18]: when the CTR is absent, it is defined as type 0; type 1A is considered the normal type, it is thin and becomes taut with elbow flexion; when the band is taut inducing nerve compression and chronic neuropathy, it is defined 1B type; type 2 is defined as presence of the anconeus epitrochlearis muscle [18]. The second portion of the capital tunnel is characterized by the presence of the Osborne's band which connects the ulnar and humeral head of the FCU muscle.

19.2.2.5 Deep Flexor–Pronator Aponeurosis

The compression of the ulnar nerve at the common flexor–pronator aponeurosis (CFA) is uncommon, but it can be a secondary point of compression when it is transposed anteriorly. The CFA lies between the flexor–pronator region and the flexor digitorum superficialis muscle (FCS) (Fig. 19.6). When the ulnar nerve enters the forearm between the two ads of FCU, it runs into an elliptical tunnel on the anterior medial edge of the CFA. In a cadaveric study, CFA was observed in all elbows and the average length was 2.9 cm [19]. In the surgical nerve release, the ulnar nerve should be thoroughly exposed removing all the anatomical structure potentially cause of compression till the deep flexor–pronator fascia aponeurosis.

The cubital syndrome represents the second most frequent peripheral neuropathy of upper limb. Ulnar nerve can be compressed in several points around the elbow. However, cubital tunnel is the most frequent site for the ulnar nerve compression. The nerve crosses a narrow cubital tunnel with a diameter of 6 ± 1.9 mm, whereas the ulnar nerve diameter is 4.9 ± 1.3 mm [20]. In addition, the cubital tunnel is subjected to a dynamic variation during elbow motion. As the flexion increases, the distance between the humeral and ulnar insertions of the cubital tunnel retinaculum (CTR) increases with flexion, leading to tightening of the band [18, 21] and a decrease in the volume of the cubital tunnel [22].

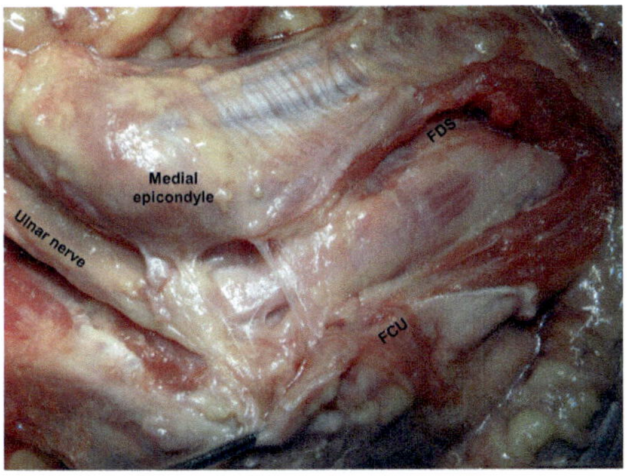

Fig. 19.6 The deep flexor–pronator aponeurosis

In particular, with elbow flexion the cross-sectional contour of cubital tunnel narrows by about 55%, changing from smooth and circular shape to flattened triangle [22]. Coupled with nerve traction, the reduction in the volume increases the intraneural pressure as the elbow flexes, exacerbating ulnar nerve neuropathy [18, 23]. Cadaver studies have demonstrated an inter-neural ulnar nerve pressure at the tunnel of 7 mm Hg with full extension, whilst with 90° of flexion intramural pressure increases to 11–24 mm Hg [24]. Moreover, shoulder abduction, elbow flexion, and wrist extension increase the intraneural pressure at least sixfold. This suggests the traction on the ulnar nerve as additional cause of increased intraneural pressure and neuropathy [23].

Considering the peculiar anatomy promoting nerve compression, even subtle anatomical modification can further promote ulnar neuropathies. Thus, the nerve can be exposed to be compressed when the fibrous bands, such as CTR or the Osborn's band, are thickened by pathological conditions or when space-occupying lesions lead to a reduction in the tunnel volume [22]. Similarly, pathologic conditions affecting the medial collateral ligament, the floor of the cubital tunnel, have also been reported to decrease the size of the tunnel [18]. Moreover, ulnar nerve can be compressed in the area between the two heads of FCU in patients with a significant hypertrophy of the two muscles when engaged in powerful exercises. At the same time, pathologic conditions, like absence of fibrous bands (type 0 CTR) or patient with generalized fibrous tissue laxity, can be predisposed to excessive friction due to subluxation or dislocation leading to subsequent ulnar neuritis.

19.2.3 Clinical Findings

The compression on the nerve can lead to different clinical scenario on the prevalence of which kind of fibers are compressed if sensitive or motor. However, the topography and intraneural anatomy of the fibers composing the ulnar nerve in the cubital tunnel can in some way predict which are the most frequent clinical manifestations. Sunderland and colleagues have studied the intraneural topography and the branches that take off from the nerve into cubital tunnel [25]. Sensory fibers and intrinsic motor axons of the hand lay superficial under the cubital tunnel retinaculum, while in the deeper a central area the motor fibers to the FCU and the flexor digitorum profundus (FDP) can be found. This organization explains the early onset of sensory symptoms in the hand and why weakness of the long flexor tendons occurs usually later with more significant compression. In the cubital tunnel, the ulnar nerve usually gives off branches to the two heads of FCU within or at approximately 3 cm from the medial epicondyle. The deep branches for the FDP take off the nerve at 5 cm distance to the medial epicondyle.

The clinical presentation of UN compression can be variable. The initial phase is usually characterized by a reported "cotton wool" feeling involving the two last fingers and pain along the medial side of proximal forearm. With the same cutaneous distribution, intermittent paresthesia and progressive sensory loss are thereafter observed. Symptoms are usually worse at the night likely due to the loss of muscle pump and following pooling of interstitial fluids. The motor symptoms usually reveal later and after the sensory deficit even though sometimes they can be observed in the initial phases. Motor deficits show up initially with the feeling of clumsiness in the hand with daily living activities such as hair drying, brushing hair, and telephone use aggravated by elbow flexion. Atrophy of the intrinsic muscle with the clawing of the last two fingers due to weakness of the third palmar interosseous muscle and all the lumbricals innervated by the UN are the typical presentation of patient with severe and persistent motor and sensory deficits.

19.2.4 Surgical Technique

Several techniques have been described to manage ulnar nerve neuropathy due to an entrapment at the elbow. These techniques aim to release and free the nerve from any kind of compression or restraint along all its course and throughout the elbow range of motion. The methods so far known are the following: 1. In situ nerve decompression; 2. Medial epicondylectomy; 3. Anterior subcutaneous transposition; 4. Anterior intramuscular transposition; and 5. Submuscular transposition.

These five methods can be divided into two groups on basis of the rationale used to manage the nerve compression. The in-situ decompression and the medial epicondylectomy decompress the nerve suffering while preserving the deep attachment without affecting its blood supply and general local environment. Conversely, the transposition techniques involve a more aggressive approach necessarily needed to release all the potential secondary nerve compression sites and create and new pathway for the ulnar nerve. These techniques are suggested when a plain or subtle instability in the epicondylar groove is detected at the end of nerve release throughout range of motion. Even though instability with subsequent neuropathy can be in this way prevented, a more aggressive approach on the nerve can determine itself a tissue damage known as "double crush phenomenon" [26–30].

19.3 Median Nerve

19.3.1 Anatomy

The median nerve (MN) travels in the arm anteromedially to the humerus and laterally to the brachial artery without any muscular branches. Approaching the elbow, the rapport with the brachial artery change becomes medial to it. At the cubital fossa, it is covered by the lacertus fibrosus (LF) and then proceed between the two heads of pronator teres. The anterior interosseous nerve (AIN) arises from posterolateral aspect of MN immediately after the superior border of flexor digitorum superficialis (FDS) about 4 cm distal to the medial epicondyle. The AIN is a pure motor nerve to flexor digitorum profundus (FDP) of the index and middle finger, flexor pollicis longus (FPL), and pronator quadratus (PQ).

The median nerve (MN) may be compressed in predictable anatomical sites at elbow and proximal forearm leading to two pathologic conditions (Fig. 19.7): the pronator tunnel syndrome and the anterior interosseous nerve (AIN) compression. The potential anatomical sites are from proximal to distal as follows: the supracondylar process and the ligament of Struthers; a fibrous thickening of the bicipital aponeurosis; hypertrophic pronator teres (PT) muscle with or without an abnormal fibrous band between the two heads; the fibrous arch of the flexor digitorum superficialis (FDS); and the Gantzer's muscle which is an accessory head of the flexor pollicis longus (FPL).

19.3.2 Sites of Compression

19.3.2.1 Supracondylar Process and Ligament of Struthers

Described in 1848 by Struthers, the supracondylar process is an abnormal congenital bone structure arising from the medial aspect of the humerus at approximately 3.5 cm above the medial epicondyle (Fig. 19.8) [13, 14]. This process gives attachment to a band of connective tissue, the ligament of Struthers, that inserts distally to the medial epicondyle. When present, the process and the ligament create with the medial aspect of the humerus a tunnel where the brachial artery and the median nerve travel. Sometimes these structures received insertion of the brachialis muscle or an anomalous superficial head of the

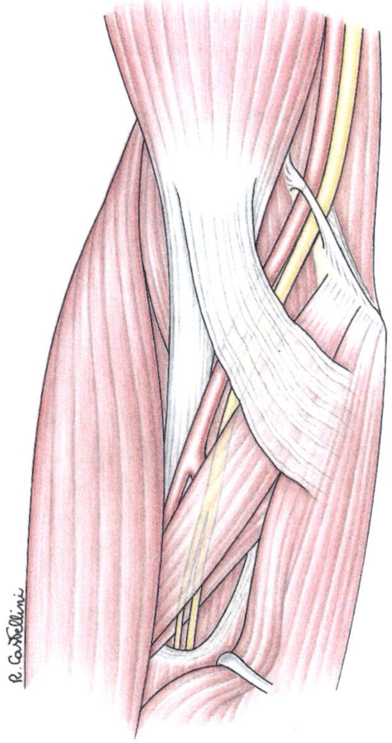

Fig. 19.7 The median nerve may be compressed in predictable anatomical sites at elbow and proximal forearm leading to two pathologic conditions: the pronator tunnel syndrome and the anterior interosseous nerve compression

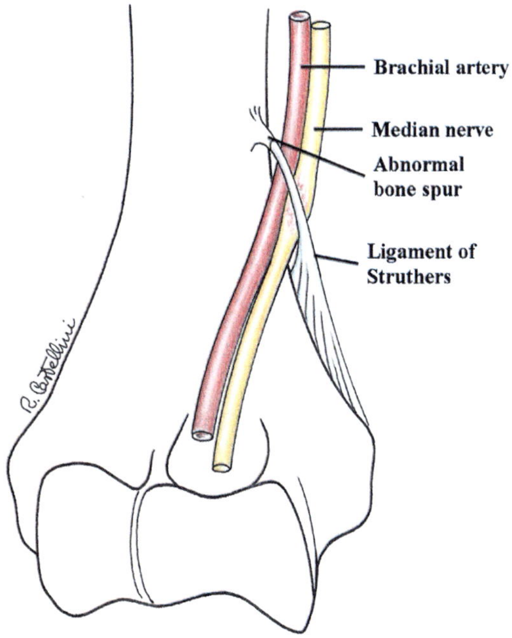

Fig. 19.8 The supracondylar process and ligament of Struthers

PT. These are usually easy to diagnose both with the palpation that reveals the process and thereafter with an X-ray confirming its presence. Clinical findings are similar to pronator syndrome except for elbow flexion and forearm pronation that are often painful and associated with paresthesia.

19.3.2.2 Fibrous Thickening of Lacertus Fibrous

The lacertus fibrosus (LF) is normally a thin fibrous band but sometimes it is prominent, becoming a substantial structure that may cause an entrapment of MN, known by some authors as "lacertus fibrosus syndrome" (Fig. 19.9) [31]. The symptoms are usually triggered by elbow flexion and supination [32]. The MN compression can be found in the presence of anatomical variation such as anomalous accessory bicipital aponeurosis [33], abnormal flexor muscle origin, or an anomalous PT that uncovers the nerve and exposes it directly to LF compression [34]. This space, dubbed by Hager "lacertus tunnel," is bounded medially by the PT and laterally by the brachialis muscle, while the roof is formed by the LF and the floor by the medial humeral trochlea [31]. In this point, it is evident the close relationship that the MN has with the anterior capsule and significant consequences that abnormal bony or fibrous connective tissue can have on it. Another condition that can increase the pressure of the MN in this narrow space is the distal biceps pathology. In particular, an acute compression has been described as a complication of partial complete rupture of the distal biceps tendon insertion with or without formation of any hematoma or compressive bursa [35]. In patients with the distal biceps' tendon rupture and an intact LF, the muscle retraction displaces the LF proximally and laterally. This situation creates a secondary compression site when the elbow is actively flexed or passively extended with the forearm supinated. When the brachial artery is compressed as well, the nerve entrapment syndrome is associated with the intermittent radial and ulnar nerve pulse loss during passive elbow hyperextension and forced forearm supination [36]. This aspect represents a crucial condition to be considerate in the management of the elbow stiffness. In patients with the long-standing elbow stiffness with the extension contracture (>60°), the LF becomes fibrotic and retracted reducing the tunnel space and placing the MN and the brachial artery at risk of compression in patient undergoing surgical release to increase elbow extension. For this reason, to avoid an acute compression on the MN, the LF release and the PT insertion tenotomy are mandatory in this scenario and when a significant lengthening of the biceps tendon and the brachialis muscle is performed in cases with long-standing elbow flexion contracture without posterior joint impingement.

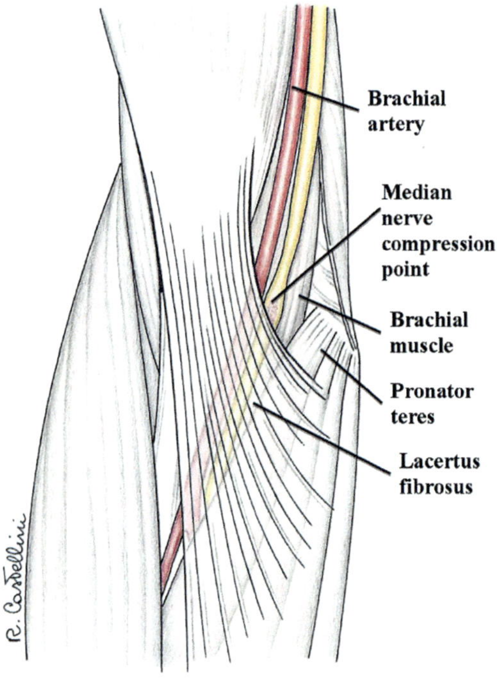

Fig. 19.9 The fibrous thickening of lacertus fibrous

19.3.2.3 Pronator Teres Muscle

The most common site of MN compression is the narrow muscle space between the two heads of the PT. Here, the humeral head may vary extremely in size and sometimes also in type of origin (Fig. 19.10). There are several conditions linked to the pronator teres (PT) muscle that can generate entrapment of the MN. Direct compression may occur when the nerve passes through the humeral and ulnar head of the PT, for exam-

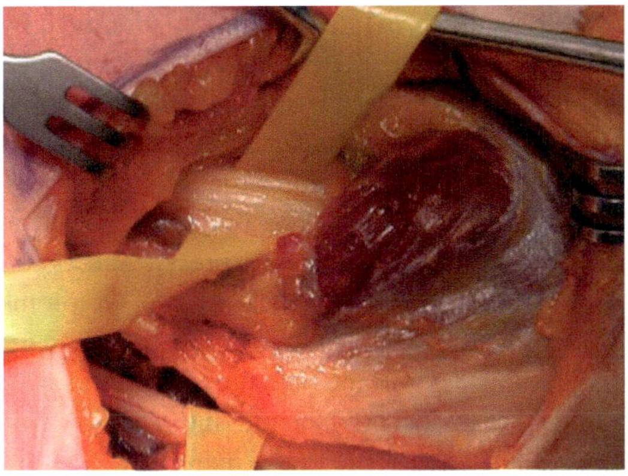

Fig. 19.10 The pronator teres muscle

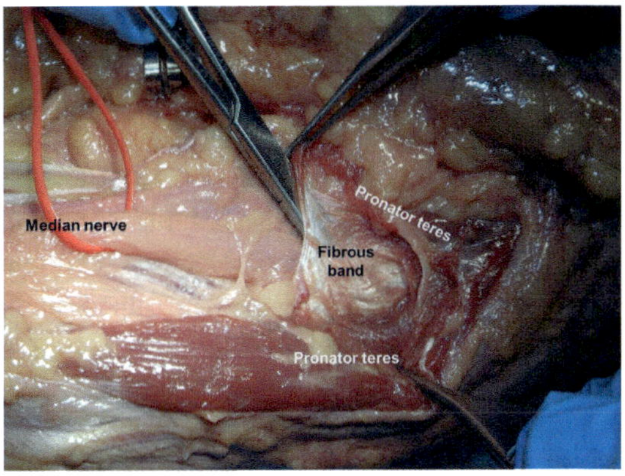

Fig. 19.11 The fibrous arcade of the flexor digitorum superficialis

ple, for an hypertrophic muscle [32]. Repetitive pronation and supination with elbow flexed can induce increased muscle volume and strengthening with the subsequent myostatic contracture. The nerve compression can also be secondary to the presence of abnormal structures that hamper nerve mobility during joint motion and medial epicondylar muscle contraction. For example, intramuscular fibrous structure or fascial bands between the superficial and deep head of pronator teres or vascular leashes can predispose to dynamic muscle compression [37]. The MN runs between the two heads of the PT in more than 80% of patients, whereas in 8–22% the ulnar head is absent [38]. Other causes of nerve compression are represented by anatomical variants of the PT ulnar head, which may arise from the FDS so that the MN may pierce the PT humeral head [37]. At the same time, also an abnormal insertion of the humeral head could represent a potential source of nerve compression, as a very proximal fibrous insertion can push the nerve anterior to the medial epicondyle favoring nerve entrapment [39]. Moreover, an accessory muscle, that is the accessory PT humeral head, can predispose to MN neuropathy. As described in a case report [40], this accessory muscle starting from this medial intermuscular septum and reaching the human head of the PT covers the brachial artery and the MN.

The relationship of the MN branches with the humeral and ulnar heads varies in relation to their location and number. The MN provides to the PT one to three or more muscular branching originating from the medial aspect of the nerve with the most proximal branch originating about 1–7 cm above the interepicondylar line and the distal 2–3 cm below the epicondyle in 90% of cases [41].

19.3.2.4 Fibrous Arcade of the Flexor Digitorum Superficialis

The MN and the ulnar artery enter the forearm passing under a fibrous arch formed by the radial and the humeroulnar head of the FDS. This is a common site of MN entrapment, which is also particularly predisposed by anatomical variants (Fig. 19.11) [39]. Anatomical variability can interest the origin of the heads of the FDS with the ulnar head that can be found in not more than 32% of specimens [42], but more importantly the variation can be observed in the arch of the FDS. This can be found as a tendinous arcade, called “sublime bridge” by Tubbs et al., or as muscular arcade [43]. The prevalence of the fibrous arcade is extremely variable in the studies thus far published with the 75% described by Tubbs et al. and a 36% by Dellon and Mackinnon [16].

19.3.2.5 Gantzer’s Muscle

Described in 1813 by Gantzer, this is an accessory head of the flexor pollicis longus (FPL) or the FDP and it is considered one of the causes of AIN entrapment and paralysis. Observed in

45–74% of dissected the forearms [42], its origin is variable with the most frequent site being the coronoid process of ulna and the medial epicondyle of the humerus [44]. Then assuming a spindle shape, the muscle inserts distally with a tendon into the ulnar border of the FPL and sometimes in the FDP muscle. Despite a certain variability, this accessory muscle runs usually anteriorly to the AIN and posteriorly to the MN. However, the mechanism determining the AIN or MN syndrome is not well known. Among the different authors describing cases of these rare syndromes, the most plausible mechanism is the direct compression of a hypertrophic muscle as the cause of neuropathy. Nonetheless, the majority of the Gantzer's muscles are asymptomatic [42, 44].

19.3.3 Clinical Findings

The MN neuropathy at the elbow can show up with the two clinical presentations that are the "pronator tunnel syndrome," with the similar but not identical findings to the carpal tunnel syndrome, and the "AIN syndrome" or Kiloh–Nevin syndrome with specific impairment in the ability to pinch with the thumb and the index finger due to palsy of the FPL muscle, FDP to the index finger and pronator quadratus muscle.

Described the first time in the 1951 by Seyffarth and Henry [45], "pronator tunnel syndrome" is a MN neuropathy due to the entrapment usually between the two heads of the PT or less commonly by the arch of the FDS. In patients with PT muscle overuse, which are those involved with the manufacturing jobs, weightlifting or sport like tennis, the nerve can be dynamically compressed when it passes between the two heads of the PT. The symptoms can be triggered by prolonged or repetitive forearm pronation associated with forced elbow and finger flexion. The other above-mentioned causes of nerve compressions, such as beneath the LF or the Gantzer's muscle, are markedly less common.

Patients with pronator tunnel syndrome typically report an aching pain with subtle onset localized in the volar region of proximal forearm and elbow and proximal irradiation, prompted by forceful pronation. The pain is usually associated with the weakness in grip and pinching small objects during manual tasks. Using the comparison with the asymptomatic hand, clinical examination shows specifically weakness of pronation, in the FPL, abductor pollicis brevis, and opponens pollicis muscles. Generally, the symptoms of pronator syndrome often overlap with those of carpal tunnel syndrome both are characterized by pain and paresthesia in the radial three and a half digits but exacerbated by increased forearm activity and relieved by rest. Unlike the carpal tunnel syndrome, the symptoms of pronator syndrome are indeed absent at the night. Moreover, patients can complain of forearm muscle cramping spasms associated with the repetitive pinching movements, such as writing that are reported as "writer's cramp."

Several provocative tests or maneuvers can be useful to confirm the diagnosis on the basis of the specific site of nerve compression. For instance, when the MN is compressed at the level of the bicipital aponeurosis, lacertus fibrosus test which consists in elbow flexion and forearm supination against the resistance would exacerbate the symptoms of the neuropathy. Similarly, pronator teres test and the flexor digitorum superficialis test trigger pain or paresthesia. The former is reproduced by pronation against resistance in full elbow extension or with the elbow flexion and progressive elbow extension. The latter is performed with the flexion only of the proximal interphalangeal joint against resistance of the middle to isolate the FDS activity. To diagnose the site of the MN compression at the elbow, other tests can be used such as the median nerve stretch test and the scratch collapse test. However, diagnosis is often delayed because of the vague and poorly defined findings.

The anterior interosseous nerve is a terminal branch of the MN exiting from it on the lateral or anterolateral aspect running on the interosseous membrane between and below the FDP and the FPL. The etiology of the AIN syndrome is unclear and includes both inflammatory and mechanical causes. As described by Spinner [46], the compression neuropathy can be determined by both

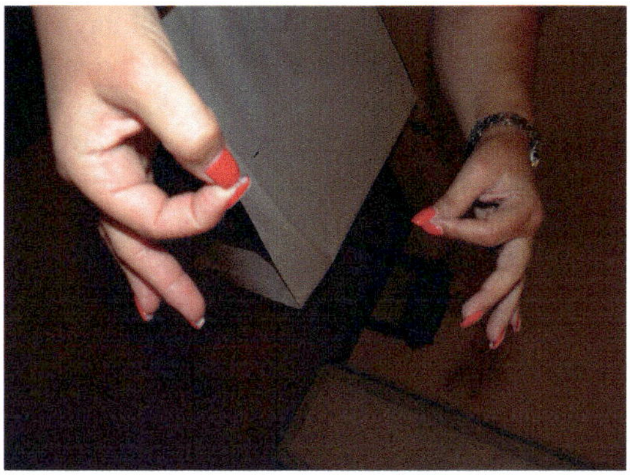

Fig. 19.12 The OK sign test

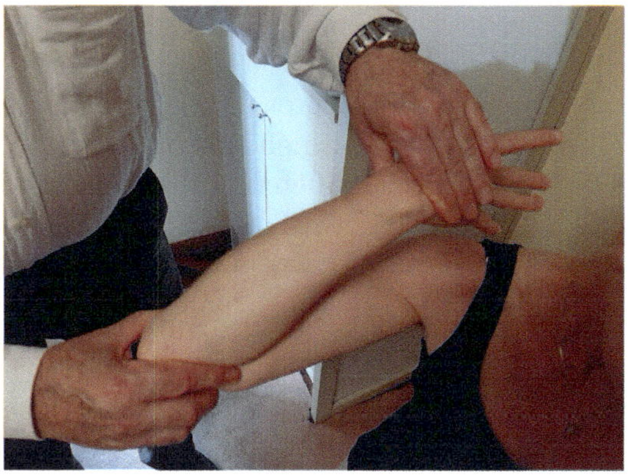

Fig. 19.13 The pronator quadratus test

spontaneous palsy and trauma. A fibrous band originating from the deep head of the PT and the fibrous band from the arch of the FDS are detected in the most cases of spontaneous palsy [46]. Among the trauma related causes of the AIN palsy, supracondylar fracture and the iatrogenic injury due to open reduction in internal fixation of radius fracture have to be reported [47]. The AIN is more susceptible to the MN to suffer palsy after supracondylar fracture being less mobile in the proximal forearm. This nerve supply motor innovation to the FDP of the index finger and the FPL and the pronator quadratus (PQ) whereas the medial portion of the FDP is supplied by the UN.

Accordingly, the AIN compression is a pure motor neuropathy resulting in weakness and paralysis of the FPL and FDP to the index combined with PQ involvement. The patients cannot typically make the pincer movement and they present a characteristic pinch deformity where the interphalangeal joint of the thumb and the distal interphalangeal joint of the index collapsed in extension [46]. Thus, the "OK sign test" results positive since the patients cannot make the OK sign but rather a narrow, oval pinch grip (Fig. 19.12). To evaluate the PQ function, Spinner proposed the pronator quadratus test which evaluates the pronation resistance with the elbow completely flexed and the arm stabilized by the examiner to avoid shoulder rotation. With the elbow flexion the effect of the humoral head of PT is removed, leaving only the pronating strength to the ulnar head that is approximately the 25% (Fig. 19.13) [46].

A thorough knowledge of the course of the MN is the of the utmost importance to perform correct diagnosis and definition of the site of compression to avoid muscle and nerve injuries during surgery. For instance, physical examination is crucial to understand if the MN compression is between the two PT heads. In this situation weakness can be found in all the muscle innervated by the MN except for the PT which receives its innervation proximal to the humeral head.

19.3.4 Surgical Technique

The surgical nerve decompression can be performed with both the limited and the extensive approach. If clinical diagnosis suggests a compression in the proximal part of the MN at the elbow, a limited approach can be performed to release the MN within the LF and the PT. Conversely, a traditional approach with an extensive S-shaped or zigzag incision is recommended when the all the potential compression sites are to be released [46, 47].

19.4 Radial Nerve

If the nerve compression syndromes are generally well-described conditions with usually a specific motor and sensory deficits, the radial nerve syndrome does not show itself with an easy pattern. To further complicate its diagnosis, radial nerve compression syndrome represents up to 2% of the upper limb peripheral syndromes [48, 49]. This significant difference, if compared to other conditions like carpal or cubital tunnel, can reflect the real incidence of this conditions but also the difficulty in making an accurate diagnosis. Despite a usually more straightforward differential diagnosis with median and ulnar nerve compression's syndromes, the radial nerve entrapment is less clear because a severe compression causing major nerve and motor disfunction is rare. The close relationship with the radiocapitellar joint capsule and other fibrous and muscles structures bounding the narrow radial tunnel make the radial nerve significantly vulnerable to be compressed or kinked after a trauma and surgical approaches.

The most frequent site of nerve compression is the arcade of Frohse [50–52]. In an anatomical study, Clavert et al. found a tendinous arcade in approximately 80% of cases [53]. At this site, superficial head of supinator muscle exerts a pressure of 40–50 mm Hg over the posterior interosseous nerve (PIN), which increases almost fourfold with active muscle contraction [54]. Since reduction in nerve venous blood flow can occur at 20–30 mm Hg and ischemia at 60–80 mm Hg, Werner et colleagues hypothesized that chronic and dynamic compression can lead to perineural abnormal changes [54]. With epineural vessels compressions, epineural edema followed by fibrosis can induce mechanical sensitivity of nerve fibers resulting in typical symptoms.

19.4.1 Anatomy

The radial nerve (RN) represents termination of the posterior cord of the brachial plexus and carries the fibers for the nerve at C6, C7, and C8. As it takes origin in the axilla, it descends behind the brachial artery and anterior to the subscapularis muscle and the insertion of the teres major and the latissimus dorsi tendon. At this point, it crosses the posterior aspect of the humerus close to the bone without the interposition of any muscle fibers into a spiral groove between the medial and long head of the triceps muscle, accompanied by the deep brachial artery and veins. The radial nerve gives origin to three cutaneous nerves and several muscular branches in the axilla and the arm. As the nerve reaches the lateral border of the medial head of the triceps, the RN pierces the intermuscular septum at around 10–12 cm proximal to the lateral epicondyle. Then, it runs distally in the flexor compartment between the brachioradialis and the brachial muscle. Anteromedially to the lateral epicondyle and under the brachioradialis and the extensor muscles within 3 cm of the elbow joint proximally or distally, the RN bifurcates into a superficial sensory and a deep motor (posterior interosseous nerve, PIN) branch. The superficial radial nerve then runs superficial to that supinator muscle and continues distally under the brachioradialis to pierce the fascia and became superficial in the subcutaneous tissue at approximately 7 cm above the wrist. The posterior interosseous nerve (PIN), instead, runs directly over the radiocapitellar joint before entering into the radial tunnel (Fig. 19.14). Even though always considered a completely motor radial nerve branch, some sensory nervous fibers for pain and proprioceptive innervation of posterior wrist capsule are included explaining some relatively uncommon vague dorsal wrist pain.

The radial tunnel extends for about 5–10 cm from radiocapitellar joint to the distal edge to supinator muscle. It is delimited medially by the

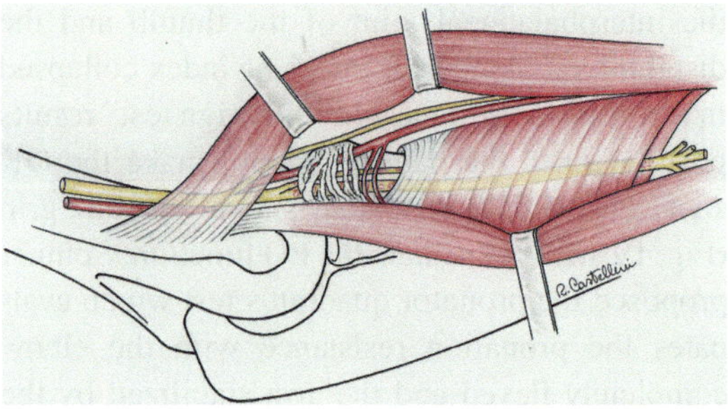

Fig. 19.14 The posterior interosseous nerve (PIN), instead, runs directly over the radiocapitellar joint before entering into the radial tunnel

brachialis and distal biceps tendon; anterolaterally by the mobile wad of the brachioradialis, extensor carpi radialis longus (ECRL), and extensor carpi radialis brevis (ECRB); posteriorly by the capitellum of the humerus, the capsule of the radiocapitellar joint and the deep head of supinator distally; and anteriorly by the radial recurrent vessels and superficial supinator head [55].

Even though it is not a real tunnel, the PIN can be compressed in four different points as follows: (1) at the entrance of the tunnel where the narrow is in close relationship with the radiocapitellar joint, which can become more significant and associated with risky adhesions after thickening or fibrous reaction; (2) anterior to the radial neck, a fan-shaped leash of vessels, both arteries and veins (the radial recurrent arteries and veins) described by Henry crosses anterior to the PIN; (3) at the level of tendinous edge of the ECRB medial proximal border, which may be abnormally thickened and compress the nerve during wrist flexion and forearm rotation [50]; and (4) at the fibrous proximal edge of the superficial head of supinator (arcade of Frohse) which forms a ligamentous band on the anterior aspect of the supinator, as the PIN runs between the two heads of the muscle [56] (Fig. 19.15).

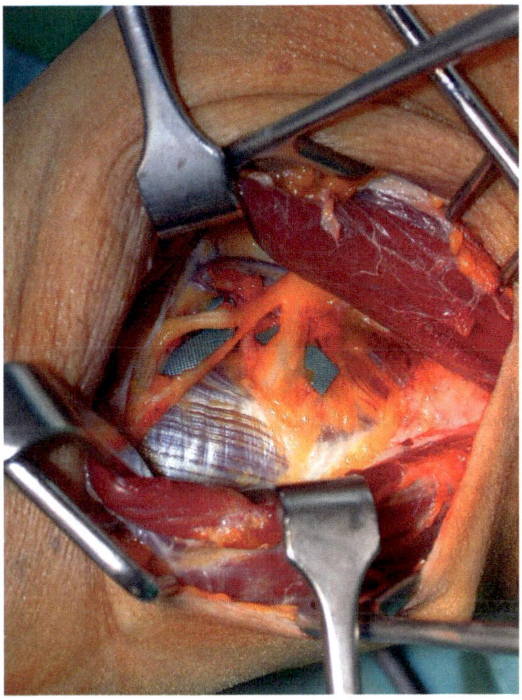

Fig. 19.15 The arcade of Frohse

The PIN compression in the radial tunnel may present with or without loss of motor function. Most of time, the compression syndrome shows up without motor deficits but mainly with persistent pain over the lateral aspect of the elbow typically distal to the lateral epicondyle [55, 57, 58]. A vague wrist pain may be infrequently associated. This condition defined "Radial tunnel syndrome" (RTS), can be considered the consequence of a neurapraxia leading to pain due to intermittent and mild compression. Conversely, a most severe compression as to induce a clear and evident motor disfunction is known posterior interosseous nerve (PIN) syndrome and is characterized by various degrees of weakness in wrist and digits extensors [59]. Compared to the other nerve compression syndromes such as carpal tunnel and cubital tunnel syndrome, the pathophysiology is less easy to comprehend. Many surgeons believe that the compression is not enough severe to cause distinct motor and sensory symptoms but with pain as nerve irritation and compression on unmyelinated (Group IV) and small myelinated (Group IIA) afferent fibers from the muscles along its distribution [60]. The large, myelinated fibers for motor activity of the PIN remain normal, explaining the normal electromyography (EMG).

19.4.2 Clinical Findings

On the clinical examination, patient with RTS reports a dull pain in the lateral forearm which usually worsens with forearm rotation and activities. In the details, the pain is elicited by firm compression at approximately 3–5 cm distally to the elbow with supination. This specific point where the pain may be elicited can be at the level of the arcade of Frohse in the proximal edge of the supinator that is at approximately 5 cm distal to the epicondyle or when the nerve emerges from the two heads supinator muscle at the junction of the proximal middle third of the forearm [55]. The pronation should release the pain since the nerve moves away from the pressure point. According to the rule-of-nine test in which the volar surface of proximal forearm is divided into nine squares, the pain is classically located in squares one and two that overlay the course of the radial nerve at the most radial and proximal portions of the forearm [61]. Moreover, these patients report pain and grip weakness without motor or sensory loss, since weakness is likely elicited by the pain rather than a real motor nerve dysfunction [62]. The pain typically increases with certain activities and diminishes with the rest, because the pain is caused by a dynamic nerve compression that is induce by both the passive pronation and wrist flexion or active supination and resisted wrist dorsiflexion [63]. In these situations, both ECRB and the supinator muscle are placed under tension eliciting pain that is increased when the elbow is extended.

The most frequent differential diagnosis for the RTS is the lateral epicondylitis (LE) and the radiocapitellar disease which usually is different for pain location and clinical findings. RTS and LE may coexist, but the pain site location is generally different. Lister has compared the pain elicited by digital pressure on three areas lying at same distance from one another in the proximal forearm: the lateral epicondyle with the ECRB insertion and the radio-capitellar joint and the PIN course [55]. However, it is always useful to compare the physical findings with the uninvolved side to establish whether the tenderness is significant. Hagert et al. defined three elements that suggest a PIN entrapment at the arcade of Frohse, rather than a lateral epicondylitis: night pain, tenderness at about 5 cm distal to the lateral epicondyle, and pain elicited by supination against resistance [52]. Lister, instead, described three pathognomonic signs: severe tenderness in the mobile wad just distal to the radial head, which is elicited by resisted middle finger extension (Maudsley's test) and similarly by supination against resistance with elbow extended [55]. For the latter sign, some controversies can be observed among different authors. Although some authors sustain elbow extension to neutralize supination force of biceps brachii [64], others suggest to perform the resisted supination with elbow flexion of 90° and full pronation to trigger the pain with the compression of PIN by proximal edge of supinator [65].

When the nerve compression becomes worse, motor deficiencies may show up with specific losses based on the location of the entrapment. Thus, a nerve compression in the radial tunnel, that is distal to the radial nerve bifurcation, can reveal with lateral arm pain, weakness of finger extension, no weakness of wrist extension, and potential dorsal wrist pain.

Electrodiagnostic studies are usually normal and without any specific finding in patients with RTS on both nerve-conduction velocity (NCV) and electromyography (EMG) studies. With a conductive slowing, the motor symptoms are likely observed then excluding the diagnosis of RTS. Even though most of the electrodiagnostic studies result negative even with forced supination, resisted supination can significantly increase the occurrence of latency prolongation in the PIN in patients with RTS when compared with control patients [51, 64]. However, electrodiagnostic studies can help to rule out other conditions such as cervical radiculopathies when clinical findings are not diriment. Selective and ultrasound-guided injection of local anesthetic can be helpful and sometimes extremely conclusive in the diagnosis process.

19.4.3 Surgical Technique

Surgical exploration and decompression are the same for both the PIN entrapment in RTS and nerve palsy in PIN syndrome. Carried out along the course of the nerve, the surgical release of the PIN consists in freeing the nerve at the level of the arcade of Frohse or along its entire course between the two heads of the muscle, from the tendinous edge of the ECRB insertion including the fibrous tissue anterior to the radiocapitellar joint and from ecstatic vessels which may develop and compress the nerve. Even though most of nerve compression are due to the arcade of Frohse, the tendinous edge of the ECRB must be considered in the surgical treatment of the neuropathic compression of the radial nerve. In spite of

Nayak et al. described the presence of tendinous edge in 29.1% of its specimens [66], Vergara-Amador and Ramírez found a fibrous arch in the anteromedial border of the muscle in 95.1% of cases [67]. This represents the medial thickened edge of the aponeurosis found in the undersurface of the ECRB of all the specimens analyzed [67]. The nerve can be exposed through several surgical approaches within the radial tunnel, including extensive anterolateral, limited anterior, and limited anterolateral approaches [57, 68–71].

19.5 Lateral Cutaneous Nerves of the Forearm

19.5.1 Anatomy

The compression neuropathy of the lateral cutaneous nerve is a relatively new syndrome and it could be an aggravating element for elbow stiffness. In 1976, Hale reported a case of lateral cutaneous nerve of the forearm (LCNF) compression at the elbow as handbag paresthesia [72].

The lateral antebrachial cutaneous nerve is the terminal branch of musculocutaneous nerve (MCN) and supplies cutaneous sensation to the anterolateral and anteromedial surfaces of forearm. It pierces the brachial fascia at approximately 3 cm proximal to the lateral epicondyle and then crosses the cubital fossa at 4.5 mm medial to the lateral epicondyle [73]. Being in close relationship with the biceps tendon, the forearm pronation increasing the tension of the lateral free edge of the bicipital aponeurosis applies tension on the LCNF. In addition, the sharp border of the biceps tendon becomes tighter when the elbow is extended and contracts against resisted flexion and pronation. Conversely, the nerve is stretched and may be compressed against the biceps tendon when the forearm is passively pronated with the elbow extended (Fig. 19.16a–c) [74]. In these conditions, the nerve is compressed between the biceps tendon and the brachialis fascia. With elbow contracture, this mechanism can easily be exacerbated and the nerve decompression should be taken into account in the surgical procedure.

19.5.2 Clinical Findings

The patients with the compression of the LCNF can show acute or chronic conditions characterized by pain in the lateral aspect of the elbow and radial forearm paresthesia [74]. These symptoms are usually induced by repetitive forceful movement with the elbow in extension and the forearm pronated. This mechanism is typical of overhead and backhand strokes in tennis, where the elbow extends shifting from supination to pronation with the actively resisted hyperextension. In the chronic setting, the pain is more an aching discomfort in the antecubital fossa usually with the paresthesia.

For the diagnostic process, Tinel's sign is elicited by tapping the side of the nerve injury that is where the nerve crosses the biceps tendon. This point is generally lateral to the tendon at the level of the elbow crease. The patient may experience some limitation in elbow extension especially with the forearm pronated, since the supination makes the biceps tendon more relaxed, and the joint can also extend completely. In chronic cases, LCNF compression may be confused with the resistant tennis elbow, cervical radiculopathy, bicipital tendinosis, or compression of the anterior interosseous nerve or median nerve.

The nonsurgical treatment could help to rule out other conditions. This involves anti-inflammatories, rest, and often splitting to prevent extension and pronation. The diagnosis could also be completed with injection of corticosteroids and local anesthetic under the lateral margin of the biceps tendon.

19.5.3 Surgical Technique

The patient is in a supine position with the arm on a specific support with the tourniquet for the ischemia. A short zig zag skin incision is made over the antecubital fossa and the LCNF is eas-

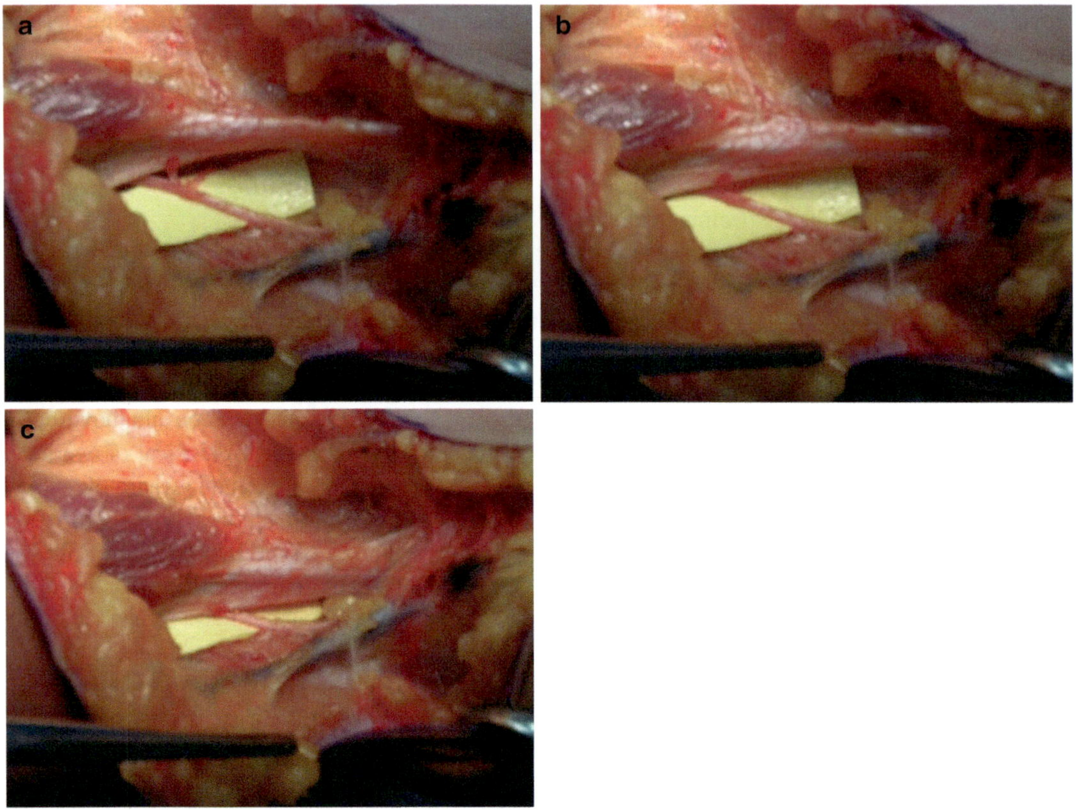

Fig. 19.16 (**a**–**c**) The nerve is stretched and may be compressed against the biceps tendon when the forearm is passively pronated with the elbow extended

ily identified at about 2 cm lateral to the biceps tendon at the level of the medial condyle. In the elbow crease, the nerve lies between the cephalic and the median cubital vein which are important landmarks to locate it. The compression may be demonstrated by passive forearm pronation with the elbow in extension [75]. A tight portion of antebrachial fascia could be demonstrated intraoperatively with elbow motion be the responsible of nerve tethering. At this point, a triangular wedge of the biceps aponeurosis and tendon of approximately 1 × 3 cm is removed (Fig. 19.17a, b). Then, the complete nerve decompression is established with the forearm pronation and supination with the elbow extended.

Another approach has been described by Gillingham and Mack which involves an oblique incision in the lateral margin of the biceps tendon with creation of a triangular flap that is reflected medially and sutured back to the remaining tendon [76]. After the decompression of the LCNF, the elbow is splinted postoperatively for 2 weeks and then full activity is gradually allowed.

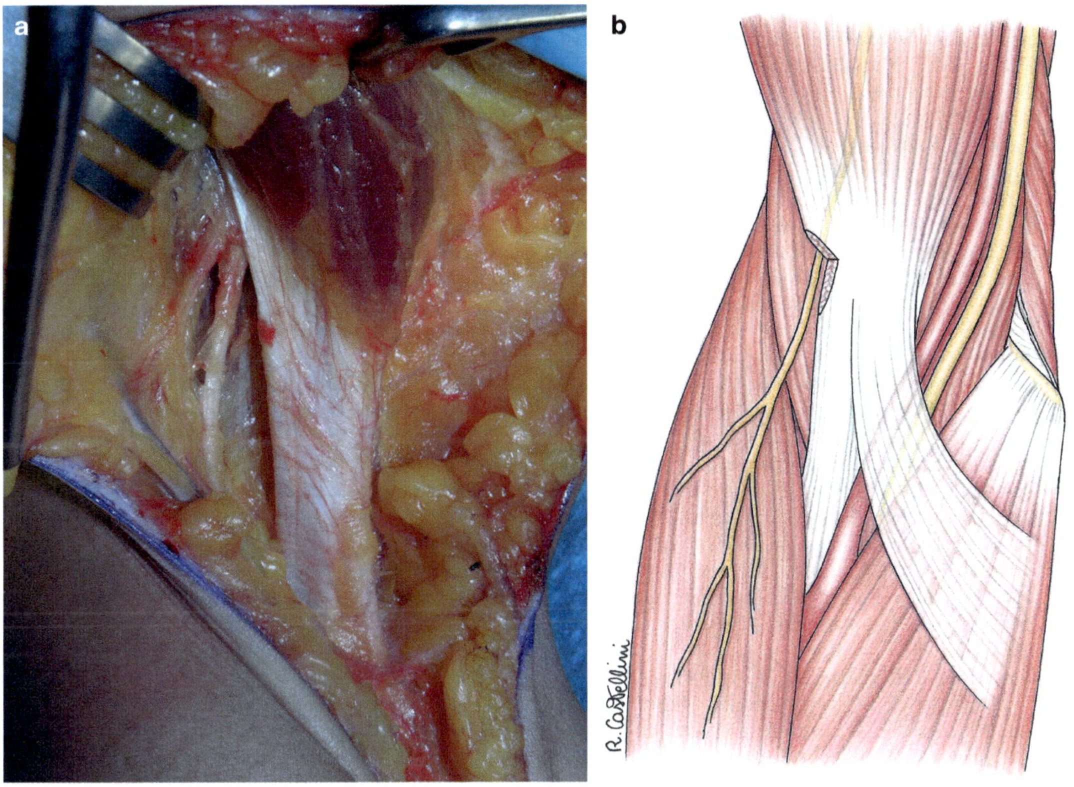

Fig. 19.17 (**a** and **b**) The triangular wedge of the biceps aponeurosis and tendon of approximately 1 × 3 cm is removed

References

1. Monument MJ, Hart DA, Salo PT, Befus AD, Hildebrand KA. Posttraumatic elbow contractures: targeting neuroinflammatory fibrogenic mechanisms. J Orthop Sci. 2013;18:869–77.
2. Myden C, Hildebrand K. Elbow joint contracture after traumatic injury. J Shoulder Elb Surg. 2011;20:39–44.
3. Wright TW, Glowczewskie F Jr, Cowin D, Wheeler DL. Ulnar nerve excursion and strain at the elbow and wrist associated with upper extremity motion. J Hand Surg Am. 2001;26:655–62.
4. Wright TW, Glowczewskie F Jr, Cowin D, Wheeler DL. Radial nerve excursion and strain at the elbow and wrist associated with upper-extremity motion. J Hand Surg Am. 2005;30:990–6.
5. Buchthal F, Rosenfalck A, Trojaborg W. Electrophysiological findings in entrapment of the median nerve at wrist and elbow. J Neurol Neurosurg Psychiatry. 1974;37:340–60.
6. Blonna D, Huffmann GR, O'Driscoll SW. Delayed-onset ulnar neuritis after release of elbow contractures: clinical presentation, pathological findings, and treatment. Am J Sports Med. 2014;42:2113–21.
7. Hildebrand KA, Zhang M, van Snellenberg W, King GJ, Hart DA. Myofibroblast numbers are elevated in human elbow capsules after trauma. Clin Orthop Relat Res. 2004;419:189–97.
8. Germscheid NM, Hildebrand KA. Regional variation is present in elbow capsules after injury. Clin Orthop Relat Res. 2006;450:219–24.
9. Cohen MS, Schimmel DR, Masuda K, Hastings H 2nd, Muehleman C. Structural and biochemical evaluation of the elbow capsule after trauma. J Shoulder Elb Surg. 2007;16:484–90.
10. Skold CM, Ohkuni Y, Liu XD, Numerof R, Rennard SI. Co-cultured human mast cells stimulate fibroblast-mediated contraction of collagen gels. Inflammation. 2001;25:47–51.
11. Khoo D, Carmichael SW, Spinner RJ. Ulnar nerve anatomy and compression. Orthop Clin North Am. 1996;27:317–38.
12. Spinner M. Management of nerve compression lesions. Instr Course Lect. 1984;33:498–512.
13. Struthers J. On a peculiarity of the humerus and humeral artery. J Hand Surg Eur. 2007;32:54–6.
14. Struthers J. On some points in the abnormal anatomy of the arm. Br Foreign Med Chir Rev. 1854;13:523–33.

15. al-Qattan MM, Murray KA. The arcade of Struthers: an anatomical study. J Hand Surg Br. 1991;16:311–4.
16. Dellon AL. Musculotendinous variations about the medial humeral epicondyle. J Hand Surg Br. 1986;11:175–81.
17. Dahners LE, Wood FM. Anconeus epitrochlearis, a rare cause of cubital tunnel syndrome: a case report. J Hand Surg Am. 1984;9:579–80.
18. O'Driscoll SW, Horii E, Carmichael SW, Morrey BF. The cubital tunnel and ulnar neuropathy. J Bone Joint Surg Br. 1991;73:613–7.
19. Green JR Jr, Rayan GM. The cubital tunnel: anatomic, histologic, and biomechanical study. J Shoulder Elb Surg. 1999;8:466–70.
20. Li MX, He Q, Hu ZL, Chen SH, Lv YC, Liu ZH, Wen Y, Peng TH. Applied anatomical study of the vascularized ulnar nerve and its blood supply for cubital tunnel syndrome at the elbow region. Neural Regen Res. 2015;10:141–5.
21. Vanderpool DW, Chalmers J, Lamb DW, Whiston TB. Peripheral compression lesions of the ulnar nerve. J Bone Joint Surg Br. 1968;50:792–803.
22. Apfelberg DB, Larson SJ. Dynamic anatomy of the ulnar nerve at the elbow. Plast Reconstr Surg. 1973;51:76–81.
23. Gelberman RH, Yamaguchi K, Hollstien SB, Winn SS, Heidenreich FP Jr, Bindra RR, Hsieh P, Silva MJ. Changes in interstitial pressure and cross-sectional area of the cubital tunnel and of the ulnar nerve with flexion of the elbow. An experimental study in human cadavera. J Bone Joint Surg Am. 1998;80:492–501.
24. Pechan J, Julis I. The pressure measurement in the ulnar nerve. A contribution to the pathophysiology of the cubital tunnel syndrome. J Biomech. 1975;8:75–9.
25. Sunderland S. The anatomy and physiology of nerve injury. Muscle Nerve. 199013(9):771-84. https://doi.org/10.1002/mus.880130903. PMID: 2233864
26. O'Driscoll SW, Jaloszynski R, Morrey BF, An KN. Origin of the medial ulnar collateral ligament. J Hand Surg Am. 1992;17:164–8.
27. Eaton RG, Crowe JF, Parkes JC 3rd. Anterior transposition of the ulnar nerve using a non-compressing fasciodermal sling. J Bone Joint Surg Am. 1980;62:820–5.
28. Kleinman WB, Bishop AT. Anterior intramuscular transposition of the ulnar nerve. J Hand Surg Am. 1989;14:972–9.
29. Learnmonth J. A technique for transplanting the ulnar nerve. Surg Gynecol Obstet. 1942;72:92–5.
30. Dellon AL, Coert JH. Results of the musculofascial lengthening technique for submuscular transposition of the ulnar nerve at the elbow. J Bone Joint Surg Am. 2004;86-A Suppl 1:169–79.
31. Hagert E. Clinical diagnosis and wide-awake surgical treatment of proximal median nerve entrapment at the elbow: a prospective study. Hand (NY). 2013;8:41–6.
32. Idler RS, Strickland JW, Creighton JJ Jr. Pronator syndrome. Indiana Med. 1991;84:124–7.
33. Spinner RJ, Carmichael SW, Spinner M. Partial median nerve entrapment in the distal arm because of an accessory bicipital aponeurosis. J Hand Surg Am. 1991;16:236–44.
34. Eversmann WW. Proximal median nerve compression. Hand Clin. 1992;8:307–15.
35. Seitz WH Jr, Matsuoka H, McAdoo J, Sherman G, Stickney DP. Acute compression of the median nerve at the elbow by the lacertus fibrosus. J Shoulder Elb Surg. 2007;16:91–4.
36. Bassett FH 3rd, Spinner RJ, Schroeter TA. Brachial artery compression by the lacertus fibrosus. Clin Orthop Relat Res. 1994;(307):110–6.
37. Gurses IA, Altinel L, Gayretli O, Akgul T, Uzun I, Dikici F. Morphology and morphometry of the ulnar head of the pronator teres muscle in relation to median nerve compression at the proximal forearm. Orthop Traumatol Surg Res. 2016;102:1005–8.
38. Nebot-Cegarra J, Perez-Berruezo J, Reina de la Torre F. Variations of the pronator teres muscle: predispositional role to median nerve entrapment. Arch Anat Histol Embryol. 1991;74:35–45.
39. Bilecenoglu B, Uz A, Karalezli N. Possible anatomic structures causing entrapment neuropathies of the median nerve: an anatomic study. Acta Orthop Belg. 2005;71:169–76.
40. Verma S, Sakthivel S. A case report on unilateral accessory humeral head of pronator Teres. J Clin Diagn Res. 2016;10:AD01–2.
41. Olehnik WK, Manske PR, Szerzinski J. Median nerve compression in the proximal forearm. J Hand Surg Am. 1994;19:121–6.
42. Caetano EB, Sabongi JJ, Vieira LA, Caetano MF, Moraes DV. Gantzer muscle. An anatomical study. Acta Ortop Bras. 2015;23:72–5.
43. Tubbs RS, Marshall T, Loukas M, Shoja MM, Cohen-Gadol AA. The sublime bridge: anatomy and implications in median nerve entrapment. J Neurosurg. 2010;113:110–2.
44. al-Qattan MM. Gantzer's muscle. An anatomical study of the accessory head of the flexor pollicis longus muscle. J Hand Surg Br. 1996;21:269–70.
45. Seyffarth H. Primary myoses in the M. Pronator teres as cause of lesion of the N. Medianus (the pronator syndrome). Acta Psychiatr Neurol Scand Suppl. 1951;74:251–4.
46. Spinner M. The anterior interosseous-nerve syndrome, with special attention to its variations. J Bone Joint Surg Am. 1970;52:84–94.
47. Warren JD. Anterior interosseous nerve palsy as a complication of forearm fractures. J Bone Joint Surg Br. 1963;45:511–2.
48. Weitbrecht WU, Navickine E. [Combined idiopathic forearm entrapment syndromes]. Z Orthop Ihre Grenzgeb. 2004;142:691–6.
49. Stanley J. Radial tunnel syndrome: a surgeon's perspective. J Hand Ther. 2006;19:180–4.
50. Naam NH, Nemani S. Radial tunnel syndrome. Orthop Clin North Am. 2012;43:529–36.

51. Werner CO. Lateral elbow pain and posterior interosseous nerve entrapment. Acta Orthop Scand Suppl. 1979;174:1–62.
52. Hagert CG, Lundborg G, Hansen T. Entrapment of the posterior interosseous nerve. Scand J Plast Reconstr Surg. 1977;11:205–12.
53. Clavert P, Lutz JC, Adam P, Wolfram-Gabel R, Liverneaux P, Kahn JL. Frohse's arcade is not the exclusive compression site of the radial nerve in its tunnel. Orthop Traumatol Surg Res. 2009;95:114–8.
54. Werner CO, Haeffner F, Rosen I. Direct recording of local pressure in the radial tunnel during passive stretch and active contraction of the supinator muscle. Arch Orthop Trauma Surg. 1978;1980(96):299–301.
55. Lister GD, Belsole RB, Kleinert HE. The radial tunnel syndrome. J Hand Surg Am. 1979;4:52–9.
56. Spinner M. The arcade of Frohse and its relationship to posterior interosseous nerve paralysis. J Bone Joint Surg Br. 1968;50:809–12.
57. Roles NC, Maudsley RH. Radial tunnel syndrome: resistant tennis elbow as a nerve entrapment. J Bone Joint Surg Br. 1972;54:499–508.
58. Moradi A, Ebrahimzadeh MH, Jupiter JB. Radial tunnel syndrome, diagnostic and treatment dilemma. Arch Bone Joint Surg. 2015;3:156–62.
59. Sharrard WJ. Posterior interosseous neuritis. J Bone Joint Surg Br. 1966;48:777–80.
60. Lin YT, Berger RA, Berger EJ, Tomita K, Jew JY, Yang C, An KN. Nerve endings of the wrist joint: a preliminary report of the dorsal radiocarpal ligament. J Orthop Res. 2006;24:1225–30.
61. Loh YC, Lam WL, Stanley JK, Soames RW. A new clinical test for radial tunnel syndrome - the Rule-of-Nine test: a cadaveric study. J Orthop Surg (Hong Kong). 2004;12:83–6.
62. Strohl AB, Zelouf DS. Ulnar tunnel syndrome, radial tunnel syndrome, anterior interosseous nerve syndrome, and pronator syndrome. Instr Course Lect. 2017;66:153–62.
63. Erak S, Day R, Wang A. The role of supinator in the pathogenesis of chronic lateral elbow pain: a biomechanical study. J Hand Surg Br. 2004;29:461–4.
64. Barnum M, Mastey RD, Weiss AP, Akelman E. Radial tunnel syndrome. Hand Clin. 1996;12:679–89.
65. Lutz FR. Radial tunnel syndrome: an etiology of chronic lateral elbow pain. J Orthop Sports Phys Ther. 1991;14:14–7.
66. Nayak SR, Ramanathan L, Krishnamurthy A, Prabhu LV, Madhyastha S, Potu BK, Ranade AV. Extensor carpi radialis brevis origin, nerve supply and its role in lateral epicondylitis. Surg Radiol Anat. 2010;32:207–11.
67. Vergara-Amador E, Ramirez A. Anatomic study of the extensor carpi radialis brevis in its relation with the motor branch of the radial nerve. Orthop Traumatol Surg Res. 2015;101:909–12.
68. Henry AK. Extensile exposure. Edinburgh/New York: Churchill Livingstone; 1995.
69. Thompson JE. Anatomical methods of approach in operations on the long bones of the extremities. Ann Surg. 1918;68:309–29.
70. Sponseller PD, Engber WD. Double-entrapment radial tunnel syndrome. J Hand Surg Am. 1983;8:420–3.
71. Hall HC, MacKinnon SE, Gilbert RW. An approach to the posterior interosseous nerve. Plast Reconstr Surg. 1984;74:435–7.
72. Hale BR. Handbag paraesthesia. Lancet. 1976;2:470.
73. Adams JE, Steinmann SP. Nerve injuries about the elbow. J Hand Surg Am. 2006;31:303–13.
74. Bassett FH 3rd, Nunley JA. Compression of the musculocutaneous nerve at the elbow. J Bone Joint Surg Am. 1982;64:1050–2.
75. Davidson JJ, Bassett FH 3rd, Nunley JA 2nd. Musculocutaneous nerve entrapment revisited. J Shoulder Elb Surg. 1998;7:250–5.
76. Gillingham BL, Mack GR. Compression of the lateral antebrachial cutaneous nerve by the biceps tendon. J Shoulder Elb Surg. 1996;5:330–2.

Part V

Elbow Stiffness Rehabilitation

20 Principles of Elbow Stiffness Rehabilitation

Aleksandra Królikowska, Robert Prill,
Maciej Kentel, and Paweł Reichert

20.1 Elbow Stiffness from the Perspective of a Rehabilitation Specialist

A joint contracture is a stiff joint in a defined position lacking specific active and passive motion. There are various etiologies of elbow joint contractures, which have already been discussed in previous chapters. Elbow contracture is most often the result of an injury. It has been estimated that after trauma, up to 12% of all elbows are left with a decreased range of motion that requires surgical release, but the etiopathogenesis remains largely unknown [1]. Other contracture causes apart from injury include osteoarthritis, surgery, large surgical scars, burns, spasticity, and congenital conditions. Soft tissue contracture is often accompanied by, for example, periarticular ossification, which limits the range of motion and may lead to stiffening of the elbow joint [2].

Still, one of the most common causes of elbow joint contracture is improper treatment, including prolonged immobilization of the joint in a plaster cast or orthosis. Since elbow stiffness is a common complication, for example, after posterior luxation, early mobilization should be considered instead of plaster immobilization, since it allows recovery with better elbow function without inducing joint instability or recurrence [3].

Elbow contracture is commonly categorized according to the direction of movement restriction and depending on the location of the cause of the contracture, as introduced by Morrey. Corresponding to the direction of limitation, elbow contractures are divided into flexion contracture (elbow lacks extension), extension contracture (lacks flexion), pronation contracture (lacks supination), and supination contracture (lacks pronation). Elbow flexion contractures are more common than extension contractures and are generally less limiting in functionally and easier to manage with surgical treatment. Pronation contractures are more common than

A. Królikowska (✉)
Physiotherapy Research Laboratory, University Centre of Physiotherapy and Rehabilitation, Faculty of Physiotherapy, Wroclaw Medical University, Wroclaw, Poland
e-mail: aleksandra.krolikowska@umw.edu.pl

R. Prill
Center of Orthopedics and Traumatology, University Hospital Brandenburg/Havel, Brandenburg Medical School Theodor Fontane, Brandenburg an der Havel, Germany

Faculty of Health Sciences Brandenburg, Brandenburg Medical School Theodor Fontane, Brandenburg an der Havel, Germany

M. Kentel
eMKaMED Medical Center Traumotology and Ortopaedic Department, Wroclaw, Poland

P. Reichert
Department of Orthopedics, Traumatology and Hand Surgery, Faculty of Medicine, Wroclaw Medical University, Wroclaw, Poland

Clinical Department of Orthopedics, Traumatology and Hand Surgery, Jan Mikulicz-Radecki University Hospital, Wroclaw, Poland

L. Pederzini et al. (eds.), *Stiffness of the Elbow, Wrist and Related Pathologies*,
https://doi.org/10.1007/978-3-031-81381-8_20

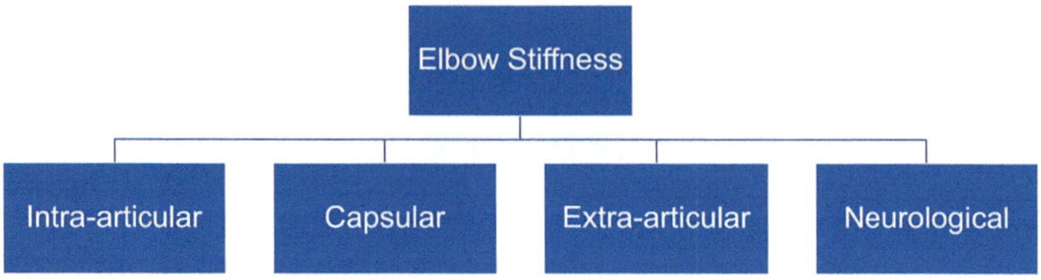

Fig. 20.1 Classification of elbow contractures according to Ref. [6]

supination contractures, but on the other hand, loss of pronation is more manageable to compensate than the loss of supination. According to the localization of pathology limiting elbow motion, elbow contractures are divided into extrinsic contracture (pathology exists outside the joint complex), intrinsic contracture (exists within the joint complex), and mixed contracture (both extrinsic and intrinsic pathologies) [4]. This classification, developed by Morrey, is especially helpful for making decisions on surgical or non-surgical treatment for elbow stiffness [4]. A significant proportion of extrinsic contractures respond well to rehabilitation. However, some contractures caused by extrinsic pathologies must be treated with surgical resection. Range of motion continues to improve up to 1 year after injury, but failure to progress 3 months after injury suggests impending elbow joint contracture [1]. Regarding intrinsic contractures, rehabilitation will be successful only after surgical correction of the articular anatomy. In almost all cases of intrinsic contracture, some extrinsic pathologies exist, since limited motion caused by within-joint factors leads to the adaptive shortening of soft tissues [5]. Treatment for this includes arthroscopically assisted or open-release surgery [2].

From the point of view of physiotherapy, the most useful classification is that introduced by Bain, who advanced the classification of elbow contractures to include the capsular group [6–8]. Bain considered that capsular contractures form a separate category, since they have a different etiology, treatment, and prognosis. This group of contractures covers pathologies related to ligaments, the capsule, and congruity. The causes of capsular contractures include ligament deficiency and ligament tears, capsulitis, and capsule contracture, as well also elbow incongruity, including subluxation and dislocation. This important group of contractures responds well to rehabilitation with nonoperative treatment. As presented in Fig. 20.1, apart from capsular contractures, the mentioned pathoanatomical classification comprised intra-articular, extra-articular, and neurological contractures. In intra-articular contractures, the cause is located within the articular surface, the subchondral layer, or the synovium. In extra-articular contractures, the pathology covers muscles, tendons, and bursa. Other extra-articular causes include fractures, heterotopic ossification, malignancy, and skin contracture. Neurological contractures may be the result of disorders affecting the central nervous system, the upper and lower motor neurons, or the sensory and autonomic nervous systems.

Decisions concerning surgical intervention for a stiff elbow are based on the functionality of the affected joint. The physiological range of motion varies from the so-called functional range of motion, and the physiological range of elbow extension and flexion exceeds 0–145°. The forearm supination and pronation amount to 85 and 75°, respectively, although to perform most activities in daily life, we do not need full extension in the elbow joint [9]. According to Morrey et al. (1981), a range of up to 30° of deficit of extension is enough. The functional capacity of flexion amounts to 130°. Also, a 100° arc from 50° of forearm supination to 50° of forearm pronation is sufficient. However, more recently, Sardelli et al. highlighted that for computer mouse, keyboard, or mobile phone usage, there needs to be pronation beyond 50° and flexion of more than 130° [10]. Therefore, it is extremely important that each patient be treated individually with their age, profession, hand dominance, and level of physical activity taken into consideration.

20.2 The Principles of Rehabilitating Elbow Stiffness

When considering a rehabilitation program, one must remember that the elbow joint needs sufficient range of motion, stability, comfort, and strength to fulfill its essential function, providing stability for power and precision tasks in open and closed kinetic chain activities. The elbow joint links the upper arm and the forearm and plays a crucial role in positioning the hand in the space [11].

Put simply; we can say that the aim of physiotherapy in patients with elbow stiffness is to regain an elbow that is stable, functional, and free of pain. The treatment needs to start with the reduction in edema and pain. Consecutively, it addresses increasing the range of motion and learning proper muscle tension. Specifically, contracted muscles need to be relaxed, and weakened muscles activated and strengthened. The treatment then aims to restore muscle endurance and joint proprioception. Finally, the patient should be prepared to return to work and sports activities.

Physiotherapy after surgical intervention is similar to non-surgical treatment. The elbow joint is not immobilized, and the treatment is focused on exercise therapy. The eventual use of splints or corrective orthoses is only for a short time after surgery, mainly when the patient is sleeping at night, and aims to maintain the correction of the operated contracture. A more detailed discussion of splints is provided in the following chapter.

20.2.1 Reducing Swelling and Pain

In the acute phase after injury or surgery, treatment for patients with a stiff elbow is focused primarily on reducing swelling, pain, and hematoma.

It should be mentioned that patients with elbow stiffness experience pain at rest and throughout the available range of motion mainly only in the acute posttraumatic or post-surgical phase. In contrast, a common complaint concerns pain that occurs at the end of ranges of motion, which negatively affects increasing limited elbow mobility [12]. The increase in pain intensity directly translates into more significant anxiety, while this increased anxiety leads to a further increase in pain intensity and results in pain-related fear of movement [13]. Due to pain-related fear of movement, patients with posttraumatic elbow stiffness may develop behavioral avoidance of movements and disuse [14].

To reduce swelling, cold therapy, which is a treatment based on lowering tissue temperature, is used. Depending on the method applied, tissues are cooled by having their thermal energy conducted or transferred to the cooling environment of a sufficiently low temperature used in a given method. Cold compresses, ice packs, ice massage, and cold water can be used several times daily. A few days after injury or surgery, the mentioned physical modalities can be replaced with local cryotherapy. Cold therapy will also reduce pain since it effectively lowers sensory nerve conduction velocity at a physiological level sufficient to induce a hypoalgesic effect [15].

A crucial physiotherapeutic modality to reduce swelling is lymphatic drainage massage, which gently manipulates specific areas of the affected limb to facilitate lymph movement to an area with working lymph vessels. Lymphatic drainage does not use techniques that increase the temperature of tissues; therefore, it can be used in an acute condition. A therapist can perform drainage, although the patient can also be taught to perform self-drainage. Additionally, the patient should be encouraged to elevate the positioning of the swollen limb to slightly above the level of the heart several times a day. Lymph drainage is also supported by frequently performed active exercises of the fingers and wrist.

Another physical modality that might be useful for the reduction in inflammation and pain with elbow stiffness is ultrasound therapy. This is a method of treatment using mechanical vibrations with a frequency exceeding the limit of human audibility (ultrasounds), causing mainly local changes related to the mechanical and thermal effects of ultrasounds and their impact on the reactions and chemical processes occurring in the tissue. Because of the thermal changes that occur during the application of ultrasound and as a result of the heat generated in the tissues, therapy is not allowed in acute inflammation. Nevertheless, the treatment can be used after the injury or following surgery in the subacute phase. Ultrasound therapy might be applied alone or with topical nonsteroidal anti-inflammatory drugs in a gel base [16].

It is worth considering graded motor imagery (GMI) training when planning physiotherapeutic procedures. This method has already been proven effective as an adjunct to exercise programs for patients with posttraumatic elbow stiffness [17]. GMI is a motor-cognitive intervention consisting of three consecutive stages: left–right discrimination (implicit motor imagery), motor imagery (explicit motor imagery), and mirror therapy (tricking the brain with a mirror) [18]. The basis of the method lies in the evidence that the sensorimotor and cortical representations of the immobilized and non-used limb disorganize and decrease [19–22]. Training for GMI aims to increase the activation of the cortex and therefore beneficially affects cortical plasticity. The method is also intended to reverse the effect of learned disuse of the involved limb and improve the disturbed body schema. In the first stage of GMI training, to train the left/right discrimination ability, the patient needs to judge a pictured limb quickly and accurately as belonging to the left or right side of the body. According to the authors of GMI training, the method should aim for 80% accuracy or better, a response time of around 1.5 to 2.0 s, and approximately equal results for the left and right limbs. Once the goal is reached, the patient will continue the treatment program with motor imagery. At this stage, the patient must imagine moving the body into a predefined position and comfortably returning to the original position. Before progressing to the final stage of GMI training, the patient must have become comfortable with the imagined movements, which usually take about 2 weeks [23]. When performing mirror therapy, patients can use the movements they have remembered from the motor imagery training. A so-called mirror box, or a regular mirror set at an angle of 90°, is needed to perform mirror therapy. It is essential that the patient cannot see the affected limb during treatment; rather, they should always look at the mirror image and have the impression that the movements are being performed simultaneously and symmetrically in both limbs. Wristwatches and any jewelry should be removed before the therapy. Also, the table must be "cleaned" so that nothing disturbs the image in the mirror. In the first phase of mirror therapy, only the unaffected limb is exercised. If possible, bilateral exercises are introduced after about 2 weeks. In the final stage of mirror therapy, the bilateral exercises are performed with different devices, including those used in daily activities. The GMI program applied to patients with elbow stiffness reduces pain and fear of movement-related pain and improves function, active range of motion, and muscle strength [17].

20.2.2 Increasing Range of Motion

Restricted elbow joint motion can profoundly affect a person's life, and it influences the capacity of the entire upper limb. Since the other joints in the upper limb cannot compensate for the loss of function of the elbow, the restriction of motion in this joint significantly reduces the hand's ability to reach its objectives [24]. Even a slight improvement in the range of motion can be significant in view of regaining function, so every degree is worth the effort. In the case of postoperative rehabilitation, it is necessary to maintain the surgically restored range of motion, or at least have as little loss of it as possible.

When the acute phase is over in patients with elbow stiffness, heat therapy is recommended to relax and prepare contracted tissues before massage at the beginning of a physiotherapeutic session [16]. Heat therapy provides heat to the body for therapeutic purposes by conduction, convection, or radiation.

Next to heat, another physical modality that might be useful in patients with elbow stiffness is ultrasound therapy, which is intended for reducing muscle contracture and increasing the elasticity of connective tissue in scars, contractures, and fibrotic changes in muscles and joint capsules. The therapy is recommended because of the heat generated in the tissues and the mechanical changes that occur locally during the procedure. These changes are caused by the pressure difference in the course of the longitudinal ultrasonic waves and are also referred to as micro-massage. It is good to remember that if we use heat therapy in the affected area before ultrasound therapy, the energy of the waves will be absorbed mainly by the surface of the skin, which places intense congestion. In contrast, if we use a cold treatment before ultrasound therapy, the hyperemia will occur actively in deeper tissues, resulting in the absorption of ultrasounds at a greater depth [16].

Massage is a form of therapy that primarily uses mechanical stimuli; that is, pressure is exerted on tissues by the therapist's hands or some massage device. Massage is also defined as the conscious impact of mechanical energy in the form of elastic deformation on soft tissues and organs. Among the many available types of massage, the classic massage, characterized by its five primary techniques (stroking, rubbing, kneading, vibrating, and patting), is the most frequently used. The local mechanical impact of this massage to increase blood flow in a specific direction increases the supply of nutrients, and accelerates the removal of metabolic products, thereby optimizing the working conditions of the muscle. Massage should be performed before manual therapy and post-isometric relaxation (PIR) before treatments to increase the range of motion. Since massage increases the temperature of tissues, it cannot be used in the acute inflammation phase of elbow stiffness. To obtain the optimal effect, a classic massage should be performed according to the following six basic principles. The intensity of the massage should increase gradually as the nervous system becomes used to the increased stimulus. Superficial anatomical structures should be processed first, followed by structures lying in deeper layers. To treat a specific muscle, the skin in the area of the muscle and the fascia underlying it must be treated first, followed by the muscle belly itself. Muscles should be massaged in order of the activity they perform. In the case of patients with elbow stiffness, the muscles responsible for flexing and supinating the forearm should be massaged first, followed by the forearm extensors and pronator muscles. The massage should be performed in the direction from the distal to the proximal part of the limb. The final rule addresses the order of treating muscles and periarticular structures. To begin with, the resting tension of all muscles acting on the elbow joint should be normalized, and then the periarticular structures, including ligaments and the elbow joint capsule, should be massaged. Massage of the periarticular structures aims to improve the physiological processes, ensuring the normal function of tissues and preserving their biological, chemical, and physical properties, which helps improve joint function [25].

Even though there is currently little evidence in the literature proving its effectiveness, manual therapy is one of the primary treatments that physiotherapists use to increase the range of motion in patients with elbow stiffness [26]. Also, according to the authors of this chapter, based on their many years of experience, it is a crucial element of therapy in this group of patients. Manual therapy is mainly related to biomechanical and arthrokinematic ideas of joint movement for the mobilization of range of motion. Manual therapy is indicated in patients with elbow stiffness because of pain, changes in range of motion, and tissue changes. Absolute contraindications to manual therapy include pain related to the acute phase, pain during the treatment, and lack of initial muscle tension. In addition, manual therapy should not be performed in patients who do not feel comfortable with it. Relative contraindications include bone-weakening processes and circulatory disorders. Manual therapy techniques are mostly passive for the patient. They either aim to stretch the capsule anatomically or rehydrate this tissue for better movement and eventually to re-program the central nervous system (motor learning) to use a more extensive range of motion. Before an intervention, a specific manual therapy examination should be carried out.

In light of using manual therapy in patients with elbow stiffness, it must be remembered that the elbow joint complex consists of three anatomically separate joints covered by a common joint capsule, but not all of these are functionally related to each other. Because of this, in cases of limited extension and flexion movements of the forearm, techniques are used to mobilize the joints of the humerus with the forearm bones. Therefore, manual therapy techniques should be introduced to improve translational movements (gliding, traction) in the humeroulnar and humeroradial joints. Aiming to increase the rotational movements of the forearm, techniques of mobilization of the connection of the ulna with the radius are selected precisely for the proximal and distal ulnar–radial joints. According to the Kaltenborn method, force should be applied in stages II and III of joint capsule tension to perform adequate traction and sliding mobilization. The duration of mobilization should be at least 7 s and preferably about 1.5 min, and in the case of good tolerance toward the procedure by the patient, more than 1.5 min [27]. To improve the range of motion in patients with elbow stiffness, traction should be performed in the maximum position while the mobilization is in the submaximal position of the maximal range of a given movement. Apart from static joint mobilization, it is worth adding mobilization with movement, according to Mulligan [28]. It may be helpful after manual therapy sessions to use local cryotherapy to slow the return of the joint capsule to the initial length. In addition, it is crucial for patients to carry out homework for manual therapy mobilization since the capsule crimp will always be likely to return to its previous position within a few hours of a therapy session. Patients are asked to try to reach the new joint position on an hourly basis until the next therapy session.

A therapeutic modality that can be effectively used to improve the stiff elbow's range of motion through the release of hypertonic musculature is post-isometric muscle relaxation (PIR). PIR is a muscle energy technique used to treat muscle contractures and states of increased muscle tension by utilizing an isometric contractual phase followed by gentle stretching of the same muscle, as presented in Fig. 20.2 [29–31]. In PIR, the following sequence is performed: slow stretching of the muscle to the limit of the muscle's extensibility (Fig. 20.2a), stabilization in this position, attempting to move back against the resistance with a slow inhale (Fig. 20.2b), relaxation with a slow exhale, and attempting to stretch the muscle further to the next limit of its extensibility (Fig. 20.2c). The move back against resistance constitutes an isometric contraction lasting 4–6 s. After a series of repetitions, when it can be seen that the maximal limit of extensibility of the muscle has been reached (Fig. 20.2d, e), it is essential to end the treatment with an antagonist muscle contractual phase to activate antagonist muscles in the newly gained range of motion (Fig. 20.2f). The PIR technique provides an opportunity to avoid direct painful contraction of a muscle that requires lengthening. Although there have been few studies on the use and effectiveness of PIR, the authors can recommend it from their own experience of working with patients with a stiff elbow.

A stretching technique combined with a structured exercise program that seems to be more effective than static stretching in regaining range of motion in posttraumatic elbow stiffness is the hold–relax (HR) technique, which belongs to proprioceptive neuromuscular facilitation (PNF) stretching [32]. It must be highlighted that stretching techniques rooted in PNF are intended to stimulate sensory receptors that provide information about body position and movement to facilitate a desired motion. When using such techniques, one must remember that the main pillars of the concept constitute the basic principles and procedures of PNF involving patterning [33]. HR stretching aims to increase the passive range of motion and decrease pain. In this technique, restricting or contracted muscles called antagonists are lengthened passively by the therapist or actively by the patient to the end of the passive or pain-free range of motion. The patient then isometrically contracts the antagonistic muscles against the resistance provided by the therapist. Muscle contraction during the HR technique should be performed with an emphasis on rotation. Consecutively, both the patient and

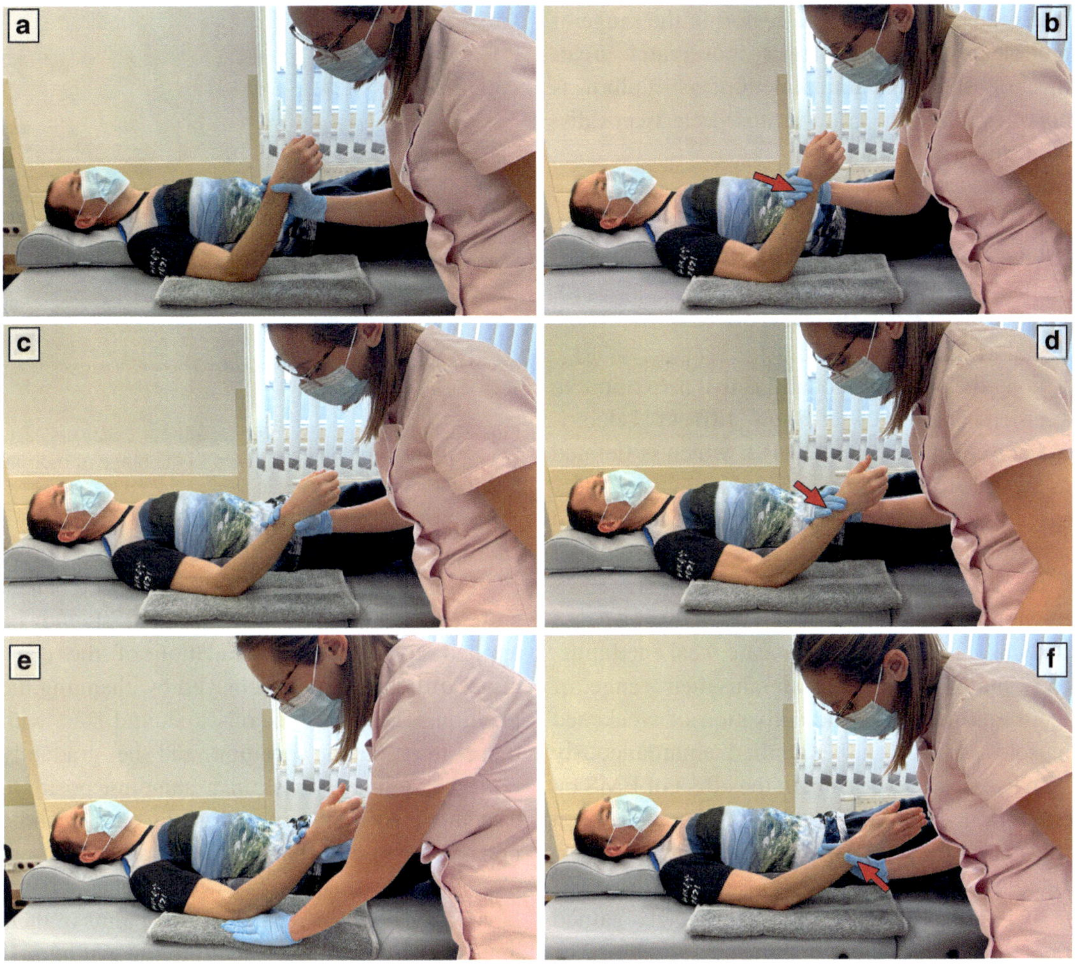

Fig. 20.2 Scheme of performing post-isometric relaxation. The red arrows indicate the place and direction of resistance provided by the therapist

the therapist relax and again the muscles are lengthened to the new limit of the range. The procedure then repeats at the new end of the motion [33]. The position and resistance cannot cause pain for the patient; if the patient experiences pain, one should exit this position and move back to one that does not cause pain. Furthermore, to avoid pain, the resistance should be increased slowly. If the patient still feels pain, the indirect HR technique based on resisting the synergistic muscles of the opposite pattern constitutes an alternative. Another PNF stretching method is the control–relax (CR) technique, which focuses on increasing the passive range of motion. The difference between the HR and CR techniques lies in the type of antagonist muscle contraction. In the CR technique, resisted isotonic contractions are used [33]. Other PNF techniques that aim to facilitate the increment of the range of motion are dynamic reversals (active range of motion), stabilizing reversals (active range of motion), rhythmic stabilization (passive and active range of motion), and repeated stretching from the beginning of the range, also called repeated initial stretching (initiation of motion and active range of motion) [33].

Exercises that increase the range of motion include passive and assisted active exercises, including self-assisted exercises. The effectiveness of using passive exercises, especially continuous passive motion, in restoring the range of motion in patients as part of conservative treatment or after surgical treatment of a stiff elbow is controversial [34, 35], and this issue is not discussed in this chapter.

20.2.3 Improving Strength, Endurance, and Proprioception

Among the physical modalities that help improve strength in patients with elbow stiffness is electrical muscle stimulation (EMS), which is defined as the induction of muscle contraction using electric impulses [16] and is strongly recommended for patients with elbow stiffness and concomitant nerve injuries. In this group of patients, EMS might prevent or retard muscle atrophy as a cause of disuse. It will help re-educate weakened muscles and increase or maintain their range of motion. To improve the activation of weakened muscles, EMS can be applied simultaneously with exercises. Even though the effect of EMS on accelerating nerve regeneration has not been proven, it still slows down the atrophy of denervated muscles [16].

It is essential to reinforce the newly gained range of motion using manual therapy alone or followed by post-isometric relaxation range of motion through proper exercises. Therefore, any so-called end of (new) motion exercise will be good. It is best to start with isometric contractions of the muscles' antagonists to contracted ones (Fig. 20.3), and then some active exercises should be introduced, including resistance exercises at the end of the motion. Figure 20.4 illustrates active exercise with resistance for elbow extensors. The ball provides an external focus. A band with gradual resistance allows the therapist to precisely adjust the resistance to the patient's capabilities. The patient should extend the elbow quickly and slowly return to the starting position. Therapists should remember to put something under the patient's elbow when exercises in the supine position are being performed to make the position comfortable.

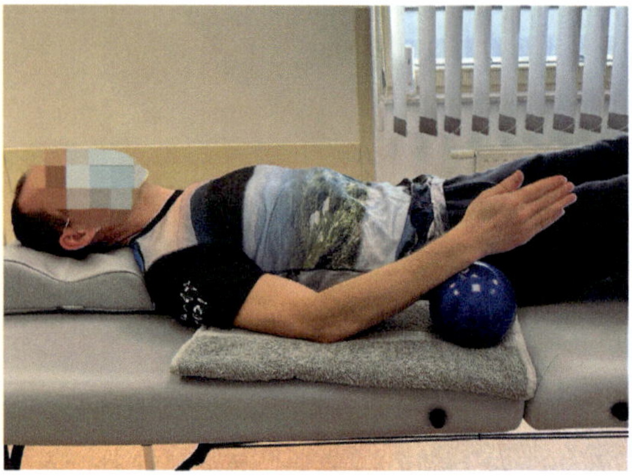

Fig. 20.3 Isometric exercise for elbow extensors. The size of the ball should be adjusted to the range of motion. The ball provides an external focus

To increase strength, active exercises, active exercises with progressive resistance with bands, and active exercises with weights should be applied consecutively. Gradation of the exercises' difficulty can be achieved by changing the position. The elbow exercises should start with those in a supine position and be gradually replaced with exercises in a standing position. The therapist must not lose sight of the whole person whose elbow they are treating. Consequently, it is necessary to evaluate patients beyond the affected area. One of the aims of therapy is to avoid a limitation of motion and muscle weakness in unaffected joints.

In patients with elbow stiffness, it is worth using not only PNF techniques aiming to increase the range of motion but also those focused on improving strength and proprioception, although there is no scientific evidence to support this [33]. PNF is a treatment concept with its philosophy based on the assumption that every human being has intact life potential. PNF is a method of neuromuscular re-education based on such physiological phenomena as a summation of afferent stimuli, irradiation, successive induction, and opposing innervation [36]. For this purpose, various techniques are used. Exercises are carried out according to movement patterns using special techniques of this method.

Based on their experience, this chapter's authors strongly advise carrying out exercise therapy in patients with elbow stiffness in line

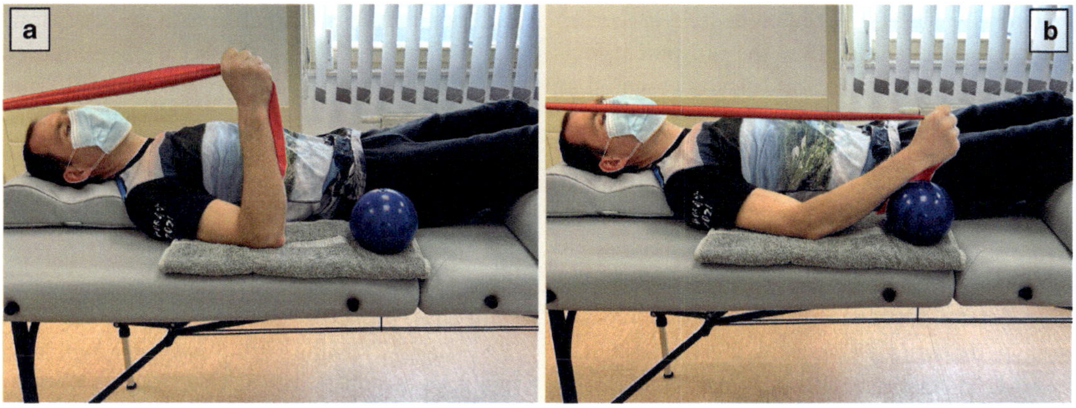

Fig. 20.4 Active exercise with resistance for elbow extensors. The ball provides an external focus

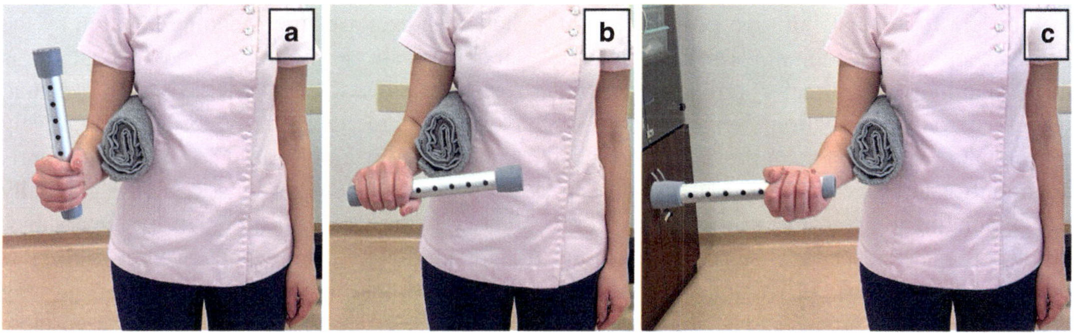

Fig. 20.5 Active exercise of pronation and supination. When pronation or supination is limited, the exercises of forearm rotation should be performed with the fixed arm. The stick in the hand provides an external focus. The activity should be performed in front of the mirror to provide visual feedback. Over time, a long bar can be used, and it can increase the rotation movement passively, depending on the place of grip

with the principles of the motor learning concept, which emerges from interactions between the individual, the task, and the environment [36, 37]. First, the need for a given action, function or movement should be created by defining the goal. It is better to use a randomized sequence of exercises. Also, using an external focus of attention for instruction is more effective than an internal focus. Internal focus refers to the patient thinking about something inside their body, such as a muscle or a bone, whereas external focus means that the patient thinks about something outside their body when performing a specific movement (Fig. 20.5). For example, when the patient actively exercises elbow flexion and supination, it is worth having them hold a ball in their hand; thus, our instruction would be, "*Try to touch your shoulder with the ball*," rather than "*Flex your elbow as much as you can*." In addition, the therapist should provide exercises crossing the midline of the patient's body. That is why it is worth adding an exercise with the command, "*Try to touch the other (contralateral) shoulder with the ball*." Bilateral exercises are also effective. Training activities should be repeated many times in changing conditions. The feedback should be delayed and not provided during exercise but after one or two exercises. Also, intrinsic feedback is more effective than extrinsic feedback. External sources provide extrinsic feedback during or after a performance. This is crucial, since someone watching the skill can observe and explain what needs to be done to correct it. In contrast, intrinsic feedback is the physical feel of the movement as it is being performed. In other words, it is what patients feel as they execute a skill or performance. Understanding how the movement feels from feedback from the muscles is essential so that patients can spot their errors. Intrinsic feedback should be developed so the patient is not reliant on others. Finally, the trained motor task needs to be incorporated into activities of daily living so that the specific function will be maintained. For example, forearm rotation exercises for a patient may include collecting a coin and turning the hand to see it. Other examples of exercises integrated with everyday activities to improve forearm rotation include carrying a tray or plate in one hand or turning a key in a lock.

Other critical exercises that need to be used in therapy are those that improve proprioception. Proprioception of the joint plays an essential role in its stability and normal coordination during movement and protection against injurious movements [38]. The term proprioception most commonly addresses the conscious proprioception belonging to somatosensory senses composed of kinesthesia, the sensation of joint position, and the sense of tension or force [39]. On the other hand, unconscious proprioception refers to neuromuscular control. The conscious sensation of the joint's position is defined as joint position sense, which constitutes a separate entity from kinesthesia, the conscious sensation of joint motion [40]. The two sensations differ in their central processing and interpretation in the brain [41].

Proprioception exercises should be provided from an early stage of rehabilitation; however, they need to be adjusted to a patient's current state. These exercises should begin with less difficult ones (Fig. 20.6) and progress to harder ones (Fig. 20.7). Changing from a bigger ball to a smaller one will make the exercises more difficult, but still safe, for the patient. Initially, exercises that put minimal pressure on the elbow joint are performed. Therefore, the therapist should start with exercises in a standing position by the table or wall (Fig. 20.8). Once the patient is ready, exercises are provided on the mat. Exercises are then introduced consecutively using partial weight-bearing. The therapist starts with two-handed exercises and gradually increases the weight-bearing. In the final stages of rehabilitation, one-handed weight-bearing is introduced, with the exercises always beginning on a stable surface, following which, an unstable surface is provided. A Swiss ball, dura disc, Pilates ring, or Pilates ball can be used for pro-

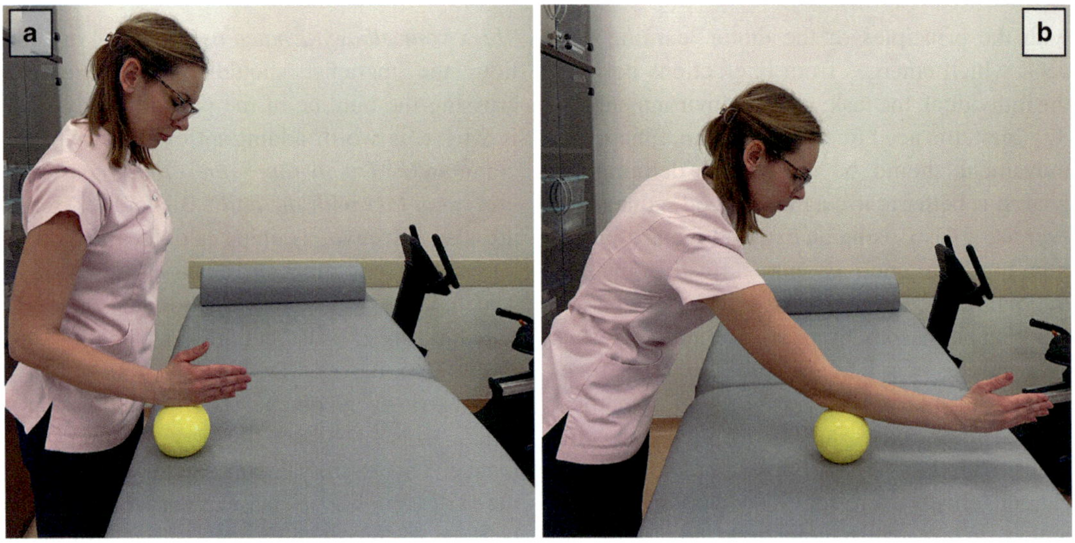

Fig. 20.6 An example of upper limb proprioception exercise that can be easily used by patients with a stiff elbow, even at the early stages of rehabilitation

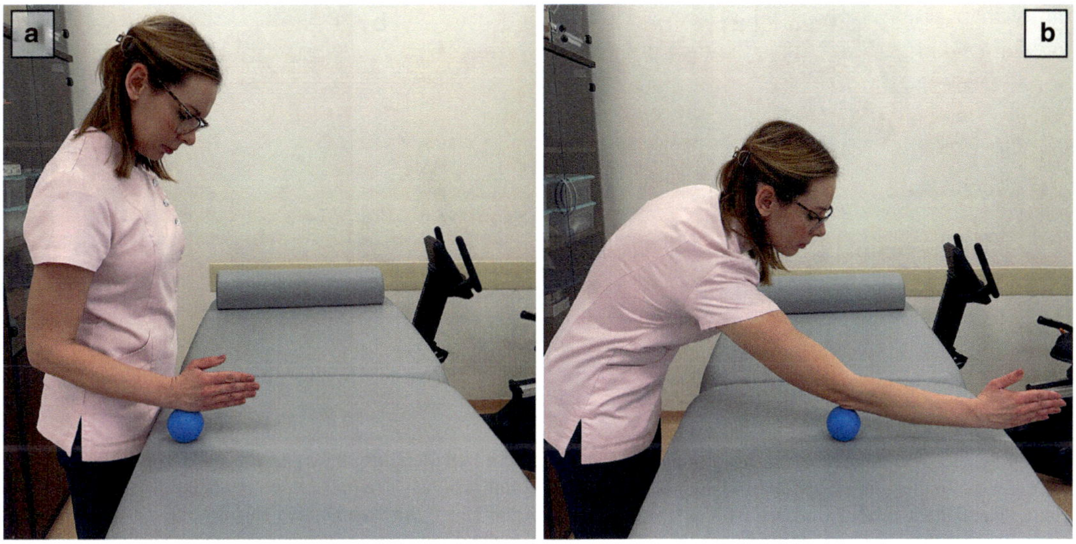

Fig. 20.7 An example of upper limb proprioception exercise that can be easily carried out by patients with a stiff elbow, even at the early stages of rehabilitation. Changing from a bigger ball to a smaller one raises the difficulty of the exercise

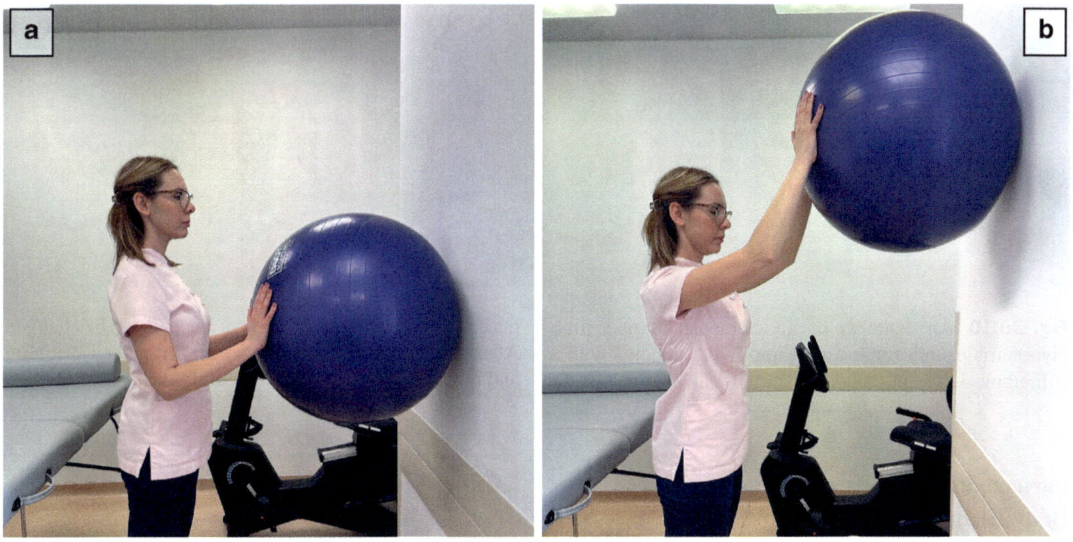

Fig. 20.8 An example of an upper-limb proprioception exercise useful in the rehabilitation of patients with a stiff elbow. Besides rolling the ball on the wall, pushing the ball at different angles of elbow flexion needs to be applied

prioception exercise purposes. Also, devices primarily used for wrist proprioception purposes, such as wooden disk stackers, tilt mazes, and a power ball, are helpful [39]. Applications installed on smartphones or tablets constitute a valuable option [42]. For joint position reproduction exercises, a standard goniometer is used. The so-called dynamic inertial resistance exercises incorporated into the strength and conditioning program should be applied, although this is not limited to patients returning to sports activities. The specific training is based on the oscillatory

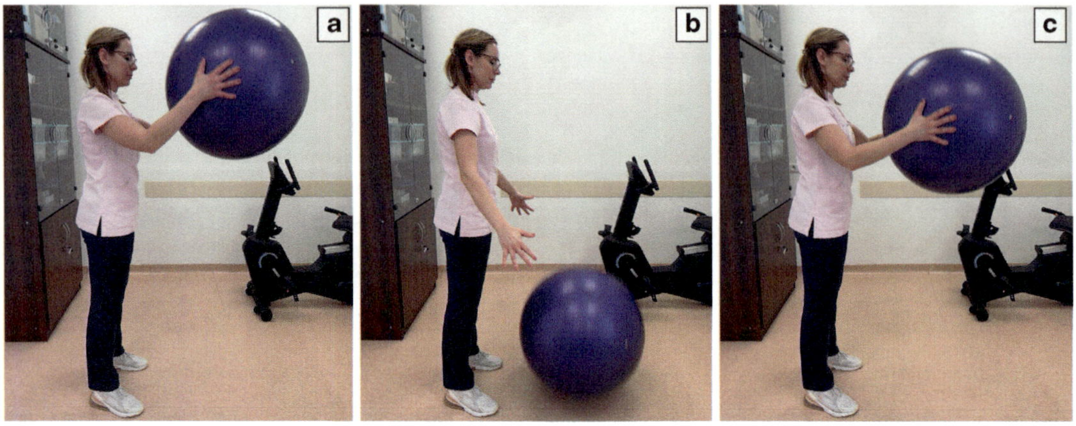

Fig. 20.9 An example of an elementary upper-limb plyometric exercise that can be applied in patients with a stiff elbow. The patient needs to throw a ball and catch it on its return. When the therapist wants to make the exercise more challenging, they can use balls with different sizes and weights. The ball can be bounced off a trampoline. It can start with two-handed throws and move on to one-handed throws

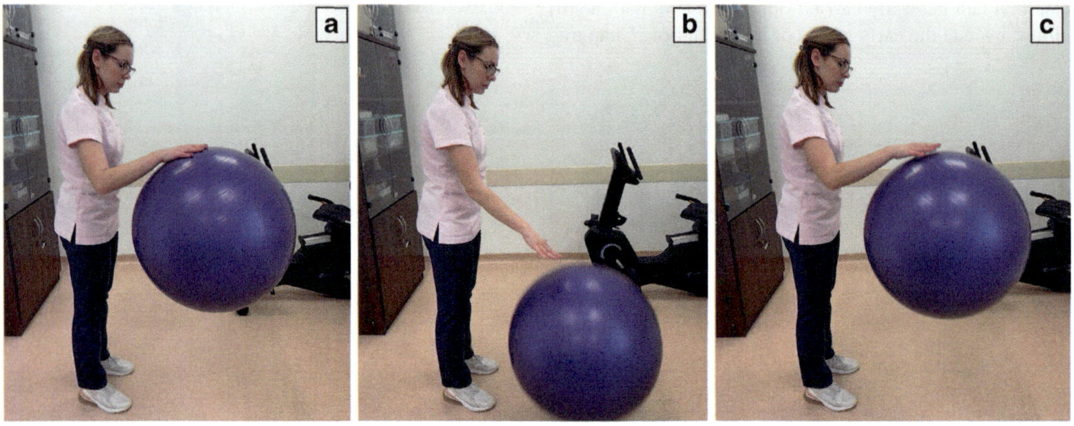

Fig. 20.10 An example of an elementary upper-limb plyometric exercise that can be applied in patients with a stiff elbow. Dribbling might be started with a large ball. To make it more complex, the size of the ball can be changed. Also, the training can begin with two-handed dribbling and move on to one-handed dribbling

movements of devices such as the Body Bar or Body Blade.

In the end, special attention should be given to plyometric exercises. Plyometric training is a quick, powerful movement involving a system of reactive exercises and explosive movements. Plyometrics can include exercises such as throwing (Fig. 20.9), dribbling (Fig. 20.10), and eventually pushups.

20.3 General Comments

The education of patients with elbow stiffness is a crucial element of their rehabilitation. First, we must inform the patient that rehabilitation can be a long-term process. It will not always be successful in terms of what the patient wants to achieve. Also, performing the exercises with a therapist in an outpatient clinic is not enough;

when recommending home exercises to the patient, try to order a maximum of two to three exercises that the patient knows well from the therapy session. We must encourage and educate the patient to use the affected elbow in daily activities.

Another essential rule during therapy for patients with stiffness in an elbow is avoiding pain. It must be clearly stated that pain with treatment means that injury is occurring. Injuring tissue using painful force or a passive range of motion can result in irreversible damage. Ignoring objective signs of tissue intolerance is irresponsible and highly unprofessional. We need to educate our patients that the so-called "no pain, no gain" attitude delays or eliminates opportunities to upgrade therapy not only by slowing the healing process but, in the case of patients with a stiff elbow, also by fostering more scarring and stiffness. Even how we address our patients matters; instead of saying, "*Exercise to the point of pain*," or the very common "*Go to pain*," we should use expressions such as "*Avoid pain when exercising*."

The entire therapeutic team shares the same goal, which is to improve the patient's physical aspect and psychological adaptation and for them to return as closely as possible to the pre-injury level of life. To achieve this goal, it is first necessary for all team members to know and accept it. It is essential to cooperate within a team to implement the principle of the so-called unity of influence. When it comes to the patients with a stiff elbow who we treat in outpatient clinics, the interdisciplinary therapeutic team will mainly consist of a medical doctor, a physiotherapist, the patient, and of course the patient's family and loved ones. It needs to be emphasized that patients with posttraumatic elbow stiffness exhibit significant depression and anxiety symptoms [13].

20.4 Specific Comments Regarding Patients with Concomitant Nerve Injury

If a patient with elbow stiffness also has a nerve injury, attention should be paid to several crucial elements of physiotherapy. The physiotherapeutic procedure additionally aims to accelerate the regeneration of the injured nerve (sensory and/or motor fibers). The patient needs to be educated on how to secure the limb from re-injury. Sometimes, the patient needs to be supported with an orthosis.

The first phase, the acute phase, lasts about 3 weeks after nerve injury, during which time the injured nerve must be protected from compression and stretching. Treatments focused on analgesic and anti-swelling effects need to be used as they would in patients with no nerve injury, albeit with one significant exception. It should be remembered not to use any kind of cold therapy in patients with elbow stiffness and concomitant nerve injury. As mentioned earlier, cold therapy modalities have been proven to reduce motor and sensory nerve conduction. In contrast, in patients with nerve injuries, therapy should be concentrated on promoting nerve conduction and inducing peripheral nerve regeneration [15]. Another specific and vital issue against cold treatment in this group of patients is cold intolerance remaining after nerve injury [43].

The second stage, the re-innervation phase, is the period of regeneration of the nerve fiber within the peripheral section of the nerve. The stage lasts until the appearance of the first arbitrary muscle contractions or the return of superficial sensation. When the acute phase is over, heat therapy is recommended, since heat promotes regeneration in the case of an injured nerve [12]. The therapy also needs to prevent contractures of the muscles and joints supplied by the damaged nerve. In addition, the therapy should avoid muscle atrophy and the formation of incorrect movement stereotypes.

If sensory disorders are present, sensory re-education should be involved. The therapy includes so-called sensory baths with products of various sizes, textures, and weights. Also, brushing is crucial. In rehabilitation, all types of small objects with different textures and the so-called acupressure circles are also helpful. In addition, special kits with different textures, such as texture dominoes, are often used; these serve to restore sensation and are used in tactile memory exercises.

The third and final phase begins after the appearance of the first arbitrary contractions or the return of superficial sensation. The therapy then focuses on gradually increasing muscle strength, neuromuscular coordination, muscle endurance, and power.

References

1. Myden C, Hildebrand K. Elbow joint contracture after traumatic injury. J Shoulder Elbow Surg. 2011;20:39–44. https://doi.org/10.1016/j.jse.2010.07.013.
2. Zhang D, Nazarian A, Rodriguez EK. Post-traumatic elbow stiffness: pathogenesis and current treatments. Shoulder Elbow. 2018;12:38–45. https://doi.org/10.1177/1758573218793903.
3. Rafai M, Largab A, Cohen D, Trafeh M. Luxation postérieure pure du coude chez l'adulte: Immobilisation ou mobilisation précoce: Étude prospective randomisée sur 50 cas. Ann Chir Main Memb Super. 1999;18:272–8. https://doi.org/10.1016/S0753-9053(99)80040-4.
4. Morrey BF. Post-traumatic contracture of the elbow. Operative treatment, including distraction arthroplasty. J Bone Joint Surg Am. 1990;72:601–18.
5. Altman E. Therapist's management of the stiff Elbow. In: Skirven TM, editor. Rehabilitation of the hand and upper extremity. Mosby: Elsevier; 2011.
6. Bain GI, Clitherow HDS. The pathogenesis and classification of shoulder stiffness. In: Itoi E, Arce G, Bain GI, Diercks RL, Guttmann D, Imhoff AB, Mazzocca AD, Sugaya H, Yoo Y-S, editors. Shoulder stiffness: current concepts and concerns. Berlin: Springer; 2015. p. 3–19.
7. McGuire DT, Luchetti R, Atzei A, Bain GI. Arthroscopic arthrolysis. In: Geissler WB, editor. Wrist and elbow arthroscopy: a practical surgical guide to techniques. New York: Springer; 2015. p. 165–75.
8. Watts AC, Bain GI. New techniques in elbow arthroscopy. In: AANA advanced arthroscopy: the elbow and wrist. Philadelphia, PA: Saunders-Elsevier; 2010. p. 124–31.
9. Morrey BF, Askew LJ, Chao EY. A biomechanical study of normal functional elbow motion. J Bone Joint Surg Am. 1981;63:872–7.
10. Sardelli M, Tashjian RZ, MacWilliams BA. Functional elbow range of motion for contemporary tasks. J Bone Joint Surg Am. 2011;93:471–7. https://doi.org/10.2106/jbjs.I.01633.
11. Nandi S, Maschke S, Evans PJ, Lawton JN. The stiff elbow. Hand. 2009;4:368–79. https://doi.org/10.1007/s11552-009-9181-z.
12. Dávila SA, Johnston-Jones K. Managing the stiff elbow: Operative, nonoperative, and postoperative techniques. J Hand Ther. 2006;19:268–81. https://doi.org/10.1197/j.jht.2006.02.017.
13. Liu W, Sun Z, Xiong H, Liu J, Lu J, Cai B, Wang W, Fan C. What are the prevalence of and factors independently associated with depression and anxiety among patients with posttraumatic elbow stiffness? A cross-sectional, multicenter study. J Shoulder Elbow Surg. 2022;31:469–80. https://doi.org/10.1016/j.jse.2021.11.014.
14. Osumi M, Sumitani M, Nishi Y, Nobusako S, Dilek B, Morioka S. Fear of movement-related pain disturbs cortical preparatory activity after becoming aware of motor intention. Behav Brain Res. 2021;411:113379. https://doi.org/10.1016/j.bbr.2021.113379.
15. Herrera E, Sandoval MC, Camargo DM, Salvini TF. Motor and sensory nerve conduction are affected differently by ice pack, ice massage, and cold water immersion. Phys Ther. 2010;90:581–91. https://doi.org/10.2522/ptj.20090131.
16. Bauer A, Wiecheć M. Przewodnik metodyczny po wybranych zabiegach fizykalnych (Methodological guide to selected physical procedures). 3rd ed. Wroclaw: Markmed Rehabilitacja s.c.; 2012. p. 445.
17. Birinci T, Kaya Mutlu E, Altun S. The efficacy of graded motor imagery in post-traumatic stiffness of elbow: a randomized controlled trial. J Shoulder Elbow Surg. 2022;31:2147–56. https://doi.org/10.1016/j.jse.2022.05.031.
18. Butler DS, Moseley GL. Explain pain. 2nd ed. Adelaide, SA: Noigroup Publications; 2013.
19. Lissek S, Wilimzig C, Stude P, Pleger B, Kalisch T, Maier C, Peters SA, Nicolas V, Tegenthoff M, Dinse HR. Immobilization impairs tactile perception and shrinks somatosensory cortical maps. Curr Biol. 2009;19:837–42. https://doi.org/10.1016/j.cub.2009.03.065.
20. Langer N, Hänggi J, Müller NA, Simmen HP, Jäncke L. Effects of limb immobilization on brain plasticity. Neurology. 2012;78:182–8. https://doi.org/10.1212/WNL.0b013e31823fcd9c.

21. Liepert J, Tegenthoff M, Malin JP. Changes of cortical motor area size during immobilization. Electroencephalogr Clin Neurophysiol. 1995;97:382–6. https://doi.org/10.1016/0924-980x(95)00194-p.
22. Avanzino L, Bassolino M, Pozzo T, Bove M. Use-dependent hemispheric balance. J Neurosci. 2011;31:3423–8. https://doi.org/10.1523/jneurosci.4893-10.2011.
23. Moseley GL, Butler DS, Beames TB. The graded motor imagery handbook. Adelaide, SA: Noigroup Publications; 2019.
24. Jones V. Conservative management of the post-traumatic stiff elbow: a physiotherapist's perspective. Shoulder Elbow. 2016;8:134–41. https://doi.org/10.1177/1758573216633065.
25. Kassolik K, Andrzejewski W. Masaż klasyczny (Classic Massage). In: Śliwiński Z, Sieroń A, editors. Wielka fizjoterapia (Great physiotherapy), vol. 1. Wroclaw: Elsevier Urban & Partner sp. z o. o.; 2014. p. 341–4.
26. Dvořák J, Gilliar W. Musculoskeletal manual medicine: diagnosis and treatment. Stuttgart: Thieme; 2008.
27. Kaltenborn FM, Evjenth O, Kaltenborn TB, Morgan D, Vollowitz E. Manual mobilization of the joints: the Kaltenborn method of joint examination and treatment. Oslo: Norli; 2002.
28. Hing W, Hall T, Rivett D, Vicenzino B, Mulligan B. The Mulligan concept of manual therapy - eBook: textbook of techniques. Amsterdam: Elsevier; 2014.
29. Lewit K, Simons DG. Myofascial pain: relief by post-isometric relaxation. Arch Phys Med Rehabil. 1984;65:452–6.
30. Wright P, Drysdale I. A comparison of post-isometric relaxation (PIR) and reciprocal inhibition (RI) muscle energy techniques applied to piriformis. Int J Osteopath Med. 2008;11:158–9. https://doi.org/10.1016/j.ijosm.2008.08.015.
31. Khan ZK, Ahmed SI, Baig AAM, Farooqui WA. Effect of post-isometric relaxation versus myofascial release therapy on pain, functional disability, rom and qol in the management of non-specific neck pain: a randomized controlled trial. BMC Musculoskelet Disord. 2022;23:567. https://doi.org/10.1186/s12891-022-05516-1.
32. Birinci T, Razak Ozdincler A, Altun S, Kural C. A structured exercise programme combined with proprioceptive neuromuscular facilitation stretching or static stretching in posttraumatic stiffness of the elbow: a randomized controlled trial. Clin Rehabil. 2019;33:241–52. https://doi.org/10.1177/0269215518802886.
33. Adler SS, Beckers D, Buck M. PNF in practice. An illustrated guide. 3rd ed. Berlin: Springer; 2008. p. 300.
34. Lindenhovius AL, Van de Luijtgaarden K, Ring D, Jupiter J. Open elbow contracture release: postoperative management with and without continuous passive motion. J Hand Surg Am. 2009;34:858–65. https://doi.org/10.1016/j.jhsa.2009.01.003.
35. O'Driscoll SW, Giori NJ. Continuous passive motion (CPM): theory and principles of clinical application. J Rehabil Res Dev. 2000;37:179–88.
36. Horst R. Therapiekonzepte in der Physiotherapie-PNF (Therapy concepts in physiotherapy PNF). Stuttgart: Thieme; 2008.
37. Newell KM. Motor skill acquisition. Annu Rev Psychol. 1991;42:213–37. https://doi.org/10.1146/annurev.ps.42.020191.001241.
38. Riemann B, Lephart S. The sensorimotor system, part I: the physiologic basis of functional joint stability. J Athl Train. 2002;37:71–9.
39. Hagert E. Proprioception of the wrist joint: a review of current concepts and possible implications on the rehabilitation of the wrist. J Hand Ther. 2010;23:2–17. https://doi.org/10.1016/j.jht.2009.09.008.
40. Proske U, Gandevia SC. Kinesthetic senses. Compr Physiol. 2018;8:31157–83.
41. Riemann BL, Lephart SM. The sensorimotor system, part II: The role of proprioception in motor control and functional joint stability. J Athl Train. 2002;37:80–4.
42. Algar L, Valdes K. Using smartphone applications as hand therapy interventions. J Hand Ther. 2014;27:254–6.; quiz 257. https://doi.org/10.1016/j.jht.2013.12.009.
43. Novak CB. Cold intolerance after nerve injury. J Hand Ther. 2018;31:195–200. https://doi.org/10.1016/j.jht.2018.01.003.

21 Elbow Brace and Rehabilitation

A. Marinelli, M. Riva, L. Ferra, and R. Rotini

21.1 Introduction

Braces can be effective devices in different phases of elbow rehabilitation and their use, especially if integrated with other modalities of physical therapies, can improve the recovery in many elbow disorders. In clinical practice, elbow braces are generally preferred over casts, because they are more comfortable for the patients and more practical for the caregivers, allowing control of the swelling and skin conditions and to start an early and protected rehabilitation. We can distinguish various categories of braces, articulated or non-articulated, custom-molded or prefabricated. The shapes and materials used to fabricate the elbow braces are very different and depend mostly on the specific function. On the basis of the function, we can identify two different types of braces: the protection braces and the mobilization braces. *The protection braces* are devices which prevent excessive stress on the articular surface, on the capsule, ligaments, or tendons; they are used after trauma, reconstructive surgeries, or in cases of inflammatory or degenerative situations. However, the *mobilization braces,* used to treat elbow stiffness, are mechanical devices exerting forces to stretch the retracted tissue stimulating the recovery of the elbow movement. It is important to underline that the elbow brace should not be thought as an alternative to the physical therapist. On the contrary, the use of the elbow brace should be included in a global rehabilitation program shared between the orthopedic and the physical therapist. The compliance of the patient with the brace program instruction is fundamental and the patient must be carefully instructed on how to wear and use the brace.

A. Marinelli (✉) · M. Riva · L. Ferra · R. Rotini
Shoulder and Elbow Unit, Istituto Ortopedico Rizzoli, Bologna, Italy
e-mail: alessandro.marinelli@ior.it

21.2 Elbow Brace Classification

We can identify two different types of brace with different functions: the protection braces and the mobilization braces (Table 21.1). Each type includes a great variety of braces, produced with different shapes and materials.

21.2.1 Protection Brace

The role of the protection elbow brace is to protect the damaged structures of the joint or, in some cases, immobilizing or restricting the range of motion (ROM), permitting healing and allowing an early but protected mobilization. The most common clinical situations are as follows:

L. Pederzini et al. (eds.), *Stiffness of the Elbow, Wrist and Related Pathologies*,
https://doi.org/10.1007/978-3-031-81381-8_21

Table 21.1 Elbow brace classification

Elbow braces	Protection brace	Mobilization brace
Types of braces	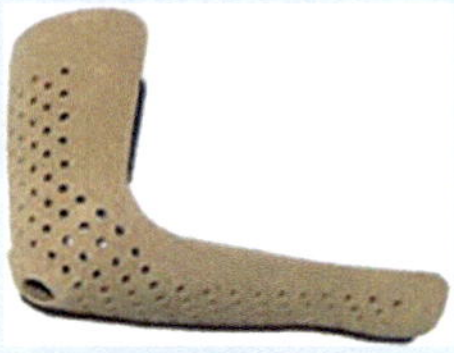 • Non-articulated 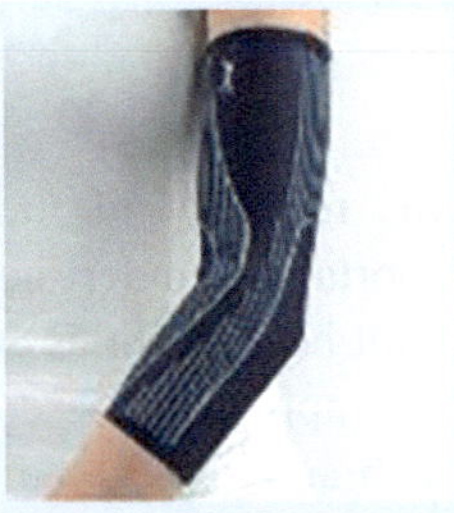 • Sleeve 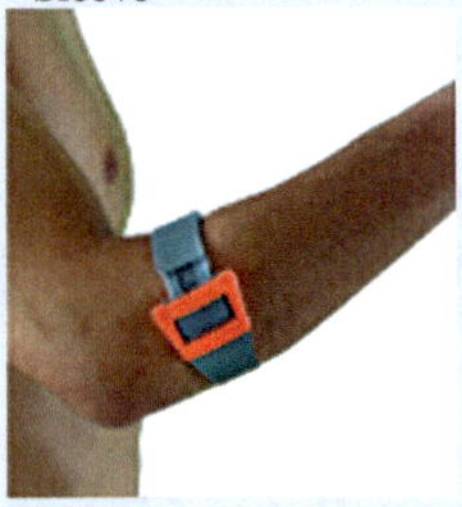 OR • Forearm strap 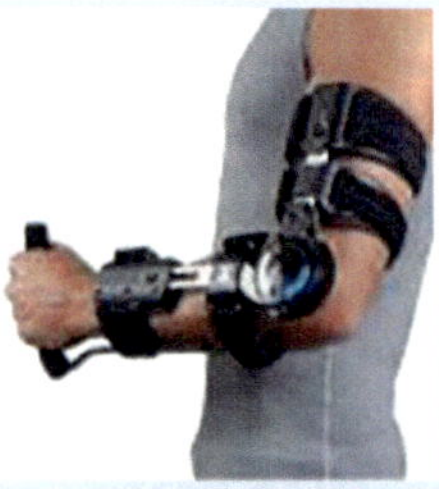 • Articulated	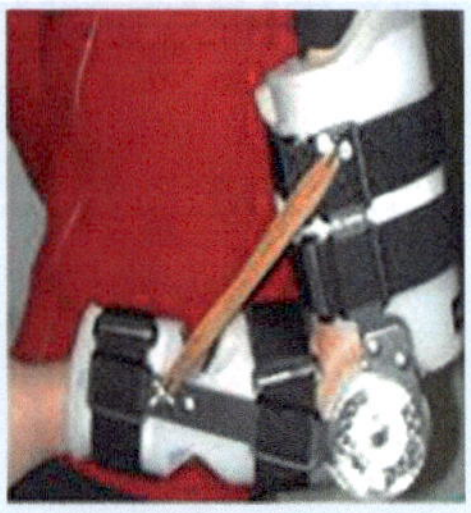 • Dynamic • Elastic or spring mechanism • Static progressive: • Turnbuckle type 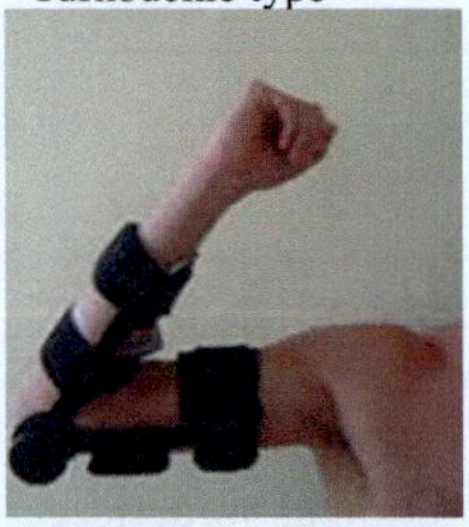 • Gear hinge mechanism 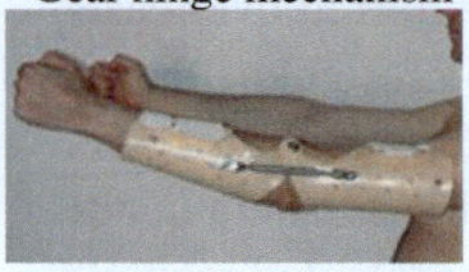
Indications	• Acute trauma • After a surgery • Inflammatory/degenerative situations	• Conservative treatment of a post-traumatic elbow stiffness • Post-operative course after a surgical arthrolysis

a) The conservative treatment of an acute trauma, such as a simple elbow dislocation, collateral ligament lesion, or an un-displaced elbow fracture;

b) The conservative treatment of degenerative or inflammatory situations, like lateral epicondylitis or degenerative/rheumatic elbow disorders;

c) The postoperative care after bone fixation (distal humeral fractures, radial head fractures, olecranon fractures, coronoid process fractures) or after tendon repair (biceps or triceps), collateral ligament reconstruction or surgeries that might jeopardize the joint stability (e.g., radial head removal).

Among the protection braces, we can recognize some different types.

1. ***Non-articulated braces***: The purpose of these braces is purely to protect the elbow by completely restricting its movement. The non-articulated braces are made of rigid and usually light materials, moldable, and adjustable on the patient. The non-articulated braces are indicated in the initial phase after trauma or surgery, when an early movement cannot be allowed.
2. ***Sleeve brace or Forearm strap brace***: They present different shapes, usually are made with stretch elastic materials.

   The sleeve braces are designed to manage the pain in many elbow disorders, like mild instability, minor trauma, arthritis (degenerative or inflammatory), olecranon bursitis and lateral or medial epicondylitis. Some models present pads to place higher pressure on the lateral and/or medial epicondyle or to protect the olecranon from repetitive trauma.

   *The forearm strap braces***,** also called counterforce braces**,** can be included in elbow braces, because they are prescribed for a specific elbow disorder: the lateral epicondylitis. These orthoses are designed to protect the tendon-to-bone insertion over the lateral epicondyle.
3. ***Articulated***: The design of these braces has greatly improved in recent years. Many companies are now producing articulated braces that are lighter, easier to apply, and more comfortable with respect to the past. The movement is guaranteed by a hinge, with the possibility to set the ROM, usually allowed from 0 to 120° of flexion–extension, with increments of 10 or 15°.

   The articulated braces present a great versatility of use, according to the needs: they can protect the joint when the locking mechanism is fully locked; they can be adjusted to enable controlled movement when the system is partially locked; or they can help in maintaining the ROM obtained with the surgery or physical therapy if the locking mechanism is locked in full flexion or full extension.

21.2.2 Mobilization Brace

21.2.2.1 Mobilization Brace

The mobilization elbow braces are designed to exert distractive forces on the retracted soft tissues to increase the range of movement of the elbow after a traumatic elbow stiffness or a surgical release.

The use of the mobilization brace is indicated in two clinical situations:

a) The conservative treatment of post-traumatic elbow stiffness to exert a progressive distraction force with the aim of stretching the retracted capsular tissue and subsequently increasing the range of movement.
b) The post-operative course after a surgical arthrolysis, with the aim of avoiding the soft tissue contracture relapse and maintaining the range of motion achieved in the operating room.

There are two types of mobilization elbow braces [1]:

- Dynamic braces that work with an adjustable elastic or spring mechanism;
- Static progressive brace that acts with distractive forces with a turnbuckle or a continuous gear hinge.

Both types of braces (dynamic or static progressive) can be "custom made" or ready to use.

The mobilization braces exploit the viscoelastic properties of the soft tissues and their use, together with physical therapy, can induce a physiological lengthening of the collagen fibers.

The main difference between dynamic and static progressive braces is the different force applied [1].

The dynamic splinting uses low-load progressive stretching exerted by elastics or springs; the static progressive splinting uses a load alternated to stress-relaxation by progressive hinges, turnbuckle, or gears to statically position the joint as close to end range as possible. With static progressive splint, the soft tissues, between two successive phases of progressive stretching, although remaining in tension, have the time to relax. Over time, a biological adaption of the tissue can be obtained.

The viscoelastic characteristics of the soft tissues and the possibility therefore to be modeled substantially have been known since ancient times and are still exploited in some populations. Such populations show us how, with stretching, a notable lengthening can be achieved through slow, gradual, and progressive phases of relaxation alternated with phases in which the tissues, despite remaining under stress, have time to adapt.

The rational principle of the method is to obtain a small amount of gradual stretching to be maintained for long periods of time.

The static progressive mobilization braces present a micrometric regulation system managed by a knob or a turnbuckle to precisely adapt the tension applied and set minimal progressive adjustments (Fig. 21.1).

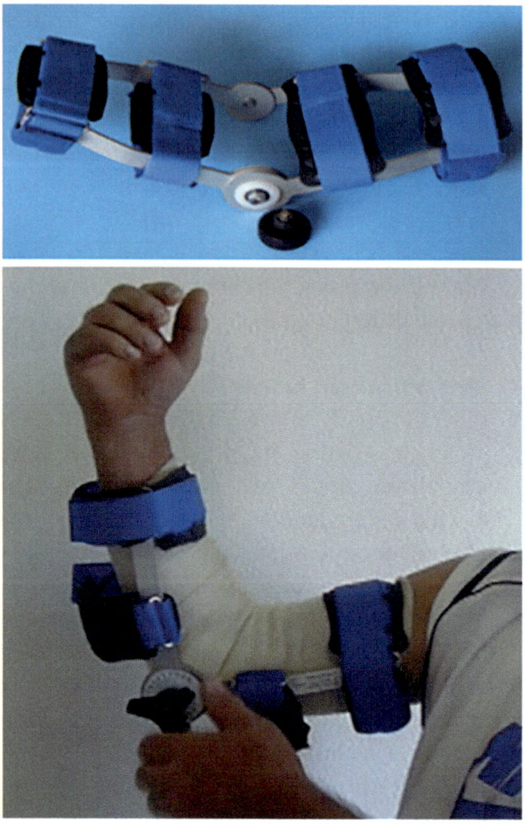

Fig. 21.1 Static progressive mobilization brace-knob type

Even if the protective articulated brace can also be locked in a forced flexion or extension position to apply tension on the soft tissues, the fixed gap of 10–15° between one point of adjustment and the other makes these types of braces less functional in gaining motion than the progressive mobilization brace which, on the contrary, presents a continuous spectrum of regulations.

Independently from the mobilization brace used (dynamic or static progressive, turnbuckle or with a gear hinge, custom made or prefabricated) problems like malposition, skin hyper pressure, difficulties in reaching the last degrees of movement are common.

In the literature, there is no definitive data to support the use of dynamic or static progressive mobilization braces [2, 3].There is a systematic review [4] reporting good results in the treatment of elbow stiffness with both braces, without significant differences. However, most of the authors prefer the use of a static progressive brace that can be adjusted incrementally by the patient, setting the appropriate tension and minimizing the risk of overstretching and damaging the tissues.

Mobilization braces for pronation–supination stiffness have received less attention until now, but the recovery of the forearm rotation is as important as the movement in flexion–extension and equally difficult to recover.

There are mobilization braces that can exert distraction in flexion–extension, and if needed, a rotational device can be applied distally to the brace to stretch the tissues also in pronosupination (Fig. 21.2).

If the stretching in pronosupination is the only one required, it is possible to use a custom-made

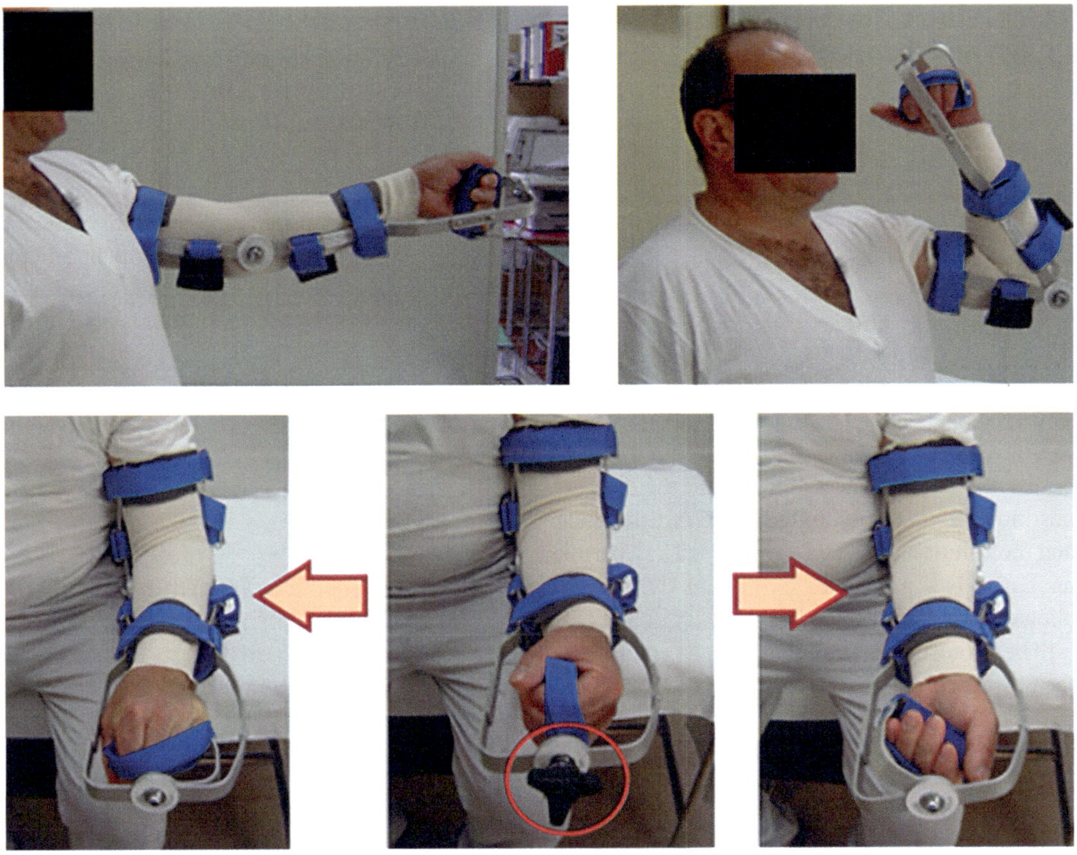

Fig. 21.2 Static progressive mobilization brace to exert flexion–extension and pronosupination stretching forces

Fig. 21.3 Thermoplastic brace for forearm rotation stretching

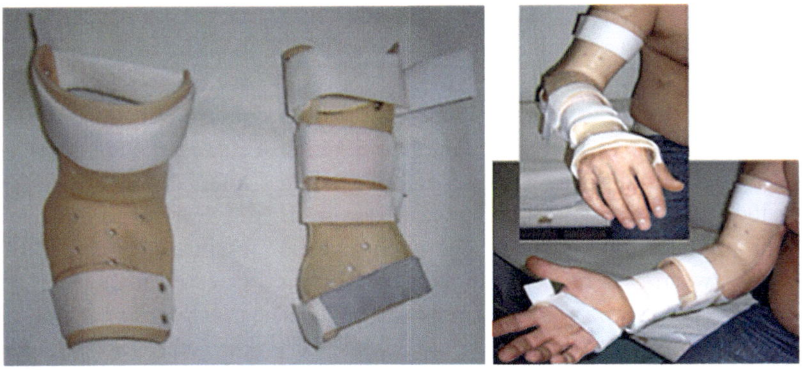

thermoplastic brace that can exert specifically pronosupination forces (Fig. 21.3).

Pronation–supination forces are applied by rotating the distal part on the first one and the position reached is fixed using Velcro straps. The main drawbacks of pronosupination braces are that they are bulky, difficult to put on, impractical for carrying out even an easy routine task and uncomfortable for use at night.

21.3 Elbow Braces: Indications and Protocols

We can identify four main situations where the brace can have a specific indication in elbow rehabilitation. In the first two cases, the protective braces are used, whereas the mobilization braces are used in the final 2.

21.3.1 Acute Trauma

The elbow brace, after fracture or dislocation, can have both protective and rehabilitation purposes, allowing the stress forces and the dangerous movements to be limited to permit the bone and the soft tissues to heal correctly. They permit an early but protected movement within an allowed range of motion.

The protective articulated brace is, therefore, the most used in these situations.

After a simple elbow dislocation, for example, a protective articulated brace is kept locked at 90° of flexion–extension for the first 5–15 days depending on the severity of the damaged structures. The aim of the brace is to prevent dangerous degrees of movement, to avoid the dangerous varus stress on the lateral collateral ligament produced by the shoulder abduction and to permit early passive and active movement in the allowed range of motion.

The protection articulated brace can also be indicated for the conservative treatment of radial head or coronoid fractures. Based on the healing of the damaged elbow stabilizers, the range of motion can be progressively improved and the patient, wearing the brace, can start performing many everyday tasks. The use of the brace is usually discontinued at rest after 3–6 weeks, and during weight lifting after 4–8 weeks, to be evaluated case by case.

21.3.2 Postoperative Course After Fracture Fixation or Ligament/Tendon Repair or Reconstruction

In the first period after distal humerus, olecranon or radial head fracture fixation, after an elbow or radial head replacement or ligament/tendon reconstruction or repair, elbow immobilization is useful; in a second phase an articulated protection brace is generally used.

The brace protocol and the physical therapy have to be personalized according to the fixation strength, ligament stability, pain, and risk of stiffness.

21.3.3 Conservative Treatment of Elbow Stiffness by Brace

The idea of treating elbow stiffness with devices that allow progressive distraction of soft tissues goes back centuries, as testified by a woodcut dated 1517 showing a static progressive splint very similar to the modern turnbuckle braces currently used.

Before considering the brace as treatment for elbow stiffness, we have to assess the type of stiffness (intrinsic or extrinsic), the type of end point of motion (rigid or springy), the degree of stiffness (mild, moderate, severe and very severe), the duration of stiffness, and some of the patient's characteristics such as age, expectations, and motivations.

The indications and contraindications for the treatment of elbow stiffness with a brace are summarized in Table 21.2.

At present, there is a lack of consensus among the authors about how many hours a day the brace should be used and the bracing protocol varies from three sessions a day for 30 min for a period

Table 21.2 Indications and contraindications for bracing in elbow stiffness

Indications	Contraindications
• Extrinsic stiffness	• Intrinsic stiffness
• Moderate grade (ROM between 60–90°)	• Severe stiffness (rom between 30 and 60°) or very severe (ROM < 30°)
• Springy end-point of motion	• Presence of significant heterotopic ossifications
• Onset not longer than 6–8 months before treatment	• Onset longer than 6 months for an adult, 1 year for a child.
• Patient highly motivated	• Poor patient compliance or impossibility to follow the patient
• Good skin condition	• Poor skin condition
• No ulnar nerve neuropathy	• Ulnar nerve neuropathy

to 1–4 months to 15 h a day for an average of 5 months [2]. In the clinical practice, it is also important to consider the initial degree of contracture, the splint tolerance, the personal circumstances, the compliance, the rate of progression, and the possibility of integrating the brace with other modalities of rehabilitation treatment.

21.3.3.1 Tips

- If the stretching action is performed too quickly the tissues will be damaged, resulting in antalgic contracture, bleeding, an increase in scarring, heterotopic ossifications, and worsening of the stiffness. It is, therefore, fundamental to inform the patient that when the brace is worn a tolerable level of tension and mild-to-moderate stretching sensation should be felt.
- In case of skin problems or ulnar nerve symptoms onset, the patient should be instructed to contact the doctor promptly.
- The brace should be applied in both directions (flexion–extension) to ensure that motion gained in one direction is not lost in the other.
- During the night the splinting extension is suggested, because the flexion position does not allow the majority of the patients to sleep.
- The bracing program is suspended gradually, checking that the range of movement achieved is not going to decrease, and encouraging the patient to keep performing range-of-motion exercises to maintain the improvements.

Our preference of bracing protocol is to prescribe the brace at least for 4–6 h during the day, with at least 4 sessions a day 1 h each and combining the time of the brace with those for the physical therapy (massages, gentle manipulation, hydrokinesitherapy). During the night, we suggest wearing the splint in extension, because in our experience the flexion position does not allow the majority of the patients to sleep.

Most improvement is noted in the first weeks of treatment. The use of the brace is usually discontinued after 3–6 months, when there is no further improvement in the range of motion for a period of 1 month.

With correct indications, our experience shows that the mobilization elbow brace is a useful device, perhaps sometimes unjustly underappreciated and underutilized [3].

The few studies present in the literature confirm the good results obtainable with the mobilization brace, reporting a total improvement in the flexion–extension ranging from 20 to 40° [3] with a low rate of complications: 10% heterotopic ossification, ulnar nerve neuropathy 7% (only 50% of them required a surgical nerve decompression), no improvement 7% [4].

21.3.4 Mobilization Brace After Soft Tissue Release

One of the greatest difficulties after surgical release in the treatment of stiff elbow is to maintain the range of movement obtained in the operating room in the following post-operative phase. In fact, after soft tissue release, the elbow stiffness has the tendency to recur in four phases: bleeding, edema, granulation tissue, and fibrosis. Such phases develop within hours, days, weeks, and months, respectively (Fig. 21.4).

To decrease the bleeding and edema phases, it is possible to set the limb extended and unloaded, to use a compressive bandage, and prescribe non-steroidal anti-inflammatory drugs (NSAIDs) and continuous passive mobilization. Compression

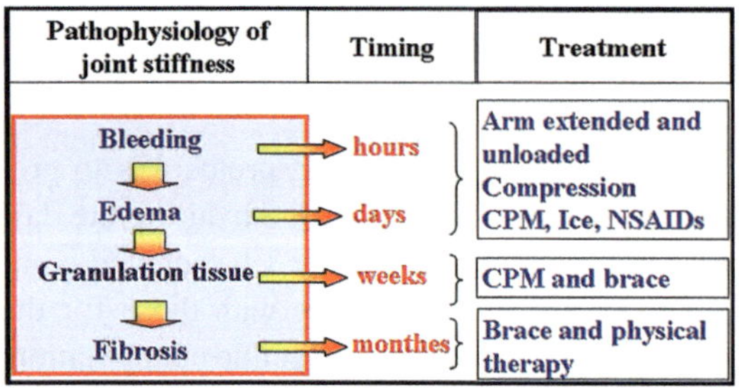

Fig. 21.4 Pathophysiology of soft tissue contraction and its treatment

ice systems, with gentle squeezing to augment venous and lymphatic return, can be useful in this phase.

Continuous passive motion (CPM), together with the brace, is also used during the following granulation phase, with the aim of reducing swelling and preventing the formation of scar tissue. Depending on the machine, CPM can be applied for flexion–extension and/or forearm rotation ROM recovery.

CPM is useful in the prevention and reduction of swelling and maintains the movement already present (e.g., obtained with a surgical release), but by itself does not induce any increase; squeezing the soft tissues at the end of the flexion and extension movements reduces the soft tissue elbow swelling and helps to maintain the full range of motion [5].

To increase the movement through the stretching of the retracted soft tissue, the only effective tools are mobilization braces or joint manipulation. Braces and physical therapy are in fact specifically indicated in the last phase, where the fibrosis formation occurs with the following natural tendency of the soft tissue to shorten and retract.

In our experience, the mobilization braces are useful devices especially in more severe stiffness cases after having obtained with surgical arthrolysis more than 50–60° of improvement in ROM. The protocol we use consists in alternating the extension and flexion position every 60 min 3–4 times a day and using CPM machine 2–3 times a day for 20–30 min in the time free from the brace.

In the fibrosis phase, it is useful to combine brace treatment with exercise consisting of passive and active movement assisted by a physical therapist. The physical therapist should be informed on the range of motion gained in the operating room and on the risk of instability. In case of skin problems or ulnar nerve symptoms onset, the patient should be instructed to contact the doctor promptly.

21.4 Manual Physical Therapy and Instrumental Techniques

Very often in elbow stiffness bracing rehabilitation program is complemented by self-assisted exercises and manual physical therapy performed by therapists that are one of the key points of rehabilitation for elbow stiffness. It's important to underline that the exercises must be continuously modeled and calibrated on the specific situation of the patient: swelling, pain, improvements, neurological symptoms, skin conditions, and X-rays. In particular, the strength of the manual technique, stretching, and mobilization is adjusted based on the therapist's sensation of "end point" and on the pain referred by the patient, taking into consideration that significant pain should be avoided. Overhead exercises are useful especially if a partial joint instability is suspected. At a later stage, perceptive and proprioceptive rehabilitation exercises are also useful to recover the normal elbow function. Among instrumental techniques, one of the most used is Tecar therapy which can be useful in preparing tissues to the following stretching. With the same aim, ultrasounds can be employed. High-power laser therapy, such as Nd-YAG laser, has an anti-inflammatory, anti-edema, and bio-stimulating action as well as an analgesic effect. Also, the possibility to act on the nervous pathways of pain by TENS can be considered. Cryotherapy, compression, and functional taping are other modalities to improve the rehabilitation program.

Through an infraclavicular or axillary block with continuous infusion of local anesthetic and also the possibility to plan boluses, it is possible to achieve appropriate analgesia of the elbow region in the postoperative period to allow effective rehabilitation therapy.

21.5 Mobilization Braces: Limits and Alternative Treatments

It is important to know that braces, particularly the mobilization ones, present several limits: the braces are expensive, they need to be carefully adapted to the patient's arm, and they do not always fit correctly. The brace is time consuming for the related caregivers and, at least for the first phases, frequent follow-up exams are usually necessary. In fact, as the brace is a removable device, managed for a long time at home, complete information, a total understanding and full collaboration of the patient is mandatory. Ulnar nerve irritation is possible, and the presence of skin damage is possible especially after surgery. Moreover, the brace may need to be modified during this time, according to modifications of swelling, pain, and progress made.

Despite the improvement in the design and in the material obtained in the last years, elbow braces can make some daily activities difficult to perform, and are often are felt cumbersome and heavy to wear by the patients.

Alternative treatments for elbow stiffness are as follows:

- Occupational and/or physical therapy without bracing under the supervision of the physical therapist to avoid that an uncontrolled therapy may exacerbate pain and inflammation, inhibiting rather than facilitating mobilization.
- CPM: Its use is indicated only in the first phases. If the stiffness is already structured, its use is not indicated.
- Serial casting: The treatment is time consuming and this technique was used mostly in the past, poorly tolerated by the patients because it immobilizes the arm, interferes with the performance of daily activities, and may cause stiffness in the opposite direction.
- Examination or forced manipulation under anesthesia: We have concerns about the possible associated complications such as fractures, ulnar nerve injuries, instability, and development of heterotopic ossification. Based on our experience, a gentle examination under narcosis can be occasionally indicated to solve a moderate stiffness in a stable and centered elbow after few weeks from a surgical treatment (e.g., external fixator removal).
- Surgical release, performed open or arthroscopically.

21.6 Conclusion

Rehabilitation of elbow stiffness can be challenging. Self-assisted exercises and manual physical therapy performed by expert therapists play the key role in recovering the elbow ROM. However, other rehabilitation modalities can be combined to optimize the final outcome. In particular, elbow brace are effective devices in the rehabilitation of many elbow disorders. They are usually better tolerated by the patient with respect to the heavy casts used in the past. With respect to casts, braces can allow the permitted movements of the elbow, protecting it from dangerous ones, in this way reducing the risk of stiffness, venous stasis, and reflex sympathetic dystrophy.

In elbow rehabilitation, the brace constitutes a possible device to contrast the risk of instability or stiffness. In elbow stiffness, the brace is a therapeutic device that makes it possible, in selected cases, to treat elbow contractures conservatively. Also, after soft tissue release, the brace can be useful to maintain the range of motion gained in the operating room. In order to ensure that the rehabilitative treatment with the brace is successful, it is almost always necessary to combine many competencies at the same time: the orthopedic or physiatrist for the correct prescription, the pain control and the follow-up, the orthopedic technician to build or adapt the cast, the physical therapist to combine the brace with the physical therapy. For this reason, it is important that the brace is not thought of as an alternative to the physical therapist. On the contrary, the use of the elbow brace should be included in a global rehabilitation program shared between the patients and the caregivers involved. The authors think that the new classification they propose can simplify the communication between the different professional figures involved (Table 21.1).

Despite the improved design and materials, for many patients the discomfort caused by a brace that does not always fit perfectly, the long periods it has to be worn, the difficulty in sleeping and carrying out daily activities wearing the brace, do not infrequently decrease their compliance and therefore the effectiveness of the brace. Other limitations of the braces in elbow physical therapy are that they are expensive and are time consuming, requiring frequent follow-up exams.

Despite these limitations in our experience, the use of the brace in elbow physical therapy has improved results in our patients.

In the future, 3D-printing technology will permit to create personalized casts and braces that will be lighter, less bulky, water-friendly making more comfortable their long-term wear.

References

1. Morrey BF. Splints and bracing the elbow. In: Morrey BF, Sanchez-Sotelo J, editors. The elbow and its disorders. 4th ed. Philadelphia: Saunders Elsevier; 2009. p. 164–72.
2. Gelinas JJ, Faber KJ, Patterson SD, King J. The effectiveness of turnbuckle splinting for elbow contractures. J Bone Joint Surg Br. 2000;82(1):74–8.
3. Marinelli A, Bettelli G, Guerra E, Nigrisoli M, Rotini R. Mobilization brace in post-traumatic elbow stiffness. Musculoskelet Surg. 2010;94 Suppl 1:S37–45.
4. Veltman ES, Doornberg JN, Eygendaal D, van den Bekerom MP. Static progressive versus dynamic splinting for posttraumatic elbow stiffness: a systematic review of 232 patients. Arch Orthop Trauma Surg. 2015;135(5):613–7.
5. O'Driscoll SW, Giori NJ. Continuous passive motion (CPM): theory and principles of clinical application. J Rehabil Res Dev. 2000;37(2):179–88. Review. Erratum in: J Rehabil Res Dev 2001 Mar-Apr;38(2):291.

Part VI

Wrist: General and Diagnostic Considerations

22 Stiff Wrist Assessment: General Consideration, Etiology of the Wrist Stiffness

Panai Laohaprasitiporn and Gregory I. Bain

22.1 Definition of Wrist Stiffness

The authors propose that the phrase "restriction of both active and passive wrist motion," thereby impeding daily activities, is the most suitable explanation for wrist stiffness. While joint stiffness has been extensively documented in various joints such as shoulder, knee, elbow, and ankle, the characterization of wrist joint stiffness remains relatively sparse. Wrist mobility encompasses three principal planes of motion: flexion–extension, radial–ulnar deviation, and pronation–supination. The range of motion of the wrist varies among individuals; therefore, a standard range has been suggested, including flexion 80°, extension 70°, radial deviation 20°, ulnar deviation 30°, and both pronation and supination 80° [1].

The wrist joint plays a pivotal role in positioning the hand for optimal efficiency while minimizing energy expenditure. Thus, suboptimal wrist motions below functional thresholds can significantly impair daily activities. Various task may elicit distinct patterns of wrist motion. Carpentry and housekeeping activities primarily involve extension of the wrist, whereas secretary tasks predominantly involve wrist flexion. Certain activities involve a combination of wrist motion planes, often referred to as "dart thrower's motion"; examples include combing hair, wringing a washcloth, and pouring water. The functional range of motion for the wrist is suggested to be flexion 5°, extension 30°, radial deviation 10°, ulnar deviation 15°, and both pronation and supination 50° [2]. It is noteworthy that most routine activities do not necessitate the entire range of motion for functional fulfillment. The majority of hand placement and wrist range of motion required for performing daily activities could be achieved using 70% of the maximum range of motion of the individual's wrist [3].

22.2 Etiology

Wrist stiffness often occurs after trauma or surgical procedures involving the wrist joint. Additionally, inflammatory conditions affecting the wrist joint, such as degenerative and rheumatoid arthritis, septic arthritis, or infection around the joint, can lead to stiffness. Abnormal bony alignment, malunion of the previous fractures, and carpal ligament instability contribute to abnormal motion of the joint which ultimately culminates in wrist stiffness.

P. Laohaprasitiporn (✉)
Department of Orthopaedic Surgery, Faculty of Medicine Siriraj Hospital, Mahidol University, Bangkok, Thailand
e-mail: panai.lao@mahidol.edu

G. I. Bain
Department of Orthopedic Surgery, Flinders University of South Australia and Flinders Medical Centre, Adelaide, Australia
e-mail: greg@gregbain.com.au

L. Pederzini et al. (eds.), *Stiffness of the Elbow, Wrist and Related Pathologies*,
https://doi.org/10.1007/978-3-031-81381-8_22

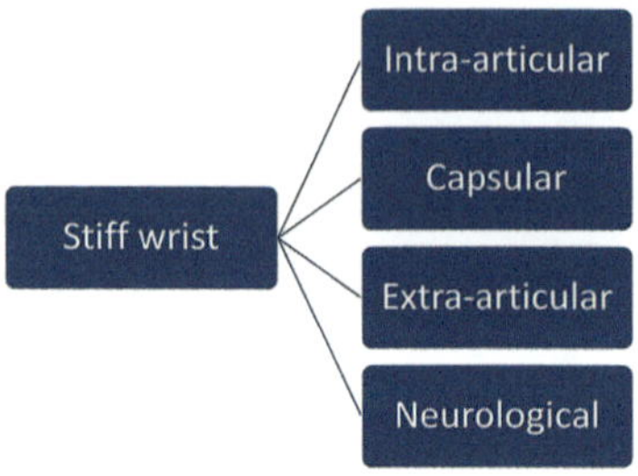

Fig. 22.1 Etiology of wrist stiffness according to anatomical location of pathology

Table 22.1 Etiology of wrist stiffness according to anatomical location of pathology

Intra-articular	Capsular	Extra-articular	Neurological
Intra-articular adhesion or arthrofibrosis	Capsular contracture from prolong immobilization	Extra-articular malunion of distal radius	Nerve injury (median nerve, superficial branch of radial nerve, etc.)
Synovitis from inflammation or infection	Ligament contracture, calcification	Carpal instability adaptive	Complex regional pain syndrome (type I)
Intra-articular malunion of distal radius, humpback deformity of scaphoid	Carpal ligament injury (scapholunate, lunotriquetral dissociation)	Heterotopic ossification	Spastic paralysis
Osteoarthritis of wrist joint		Muscle/Tendon contractures	Dystonia
Avascular necrosis of carpal bone (Kienbock's disease)		Skin/Scar contracture	Charcot arthropathy

Modified from Alessandro M. et al. [4]

The causes of wrist stiffness can be classified based on the location of the pathology into intra-articular, capsular, extra-articular, or neurological categories (Fig. 22.1 and Table 22.1).

22.3 Pathogenesis of Wrist Stiffness

There is limited research available regarding the pathogenesis and cellular mechanisms underlying wrist stiffness. Nevertheless, extensive investigations into organ fibrosis are imperative for comprehending of arthrofibrosis, which is one of the causes of wrist stiffness. Arthrofibrosis, as a variant of fibrosis, shares common pathogenic mechanisms observed in organ and tissue fibrosis. Indeed, fibrosis represents a fundamental aspect of the human tissue healing process. However, excessive fibrosis can lead to functional disturbances within the affected tissue.

Fibrosis arises from complex dysregulation of both innate and adaptive immune responses, which are implicated in the pathogenesis of numerous chronic inflammatory conditions. Injury, whether acute or repetitive, triggers oxidative stress and inflammatory cascade, inducing the production of pro-inflammatory cytokines and transforming growth factor beta (TGF-β) [5]. This sequence of events prompts an influx of mast cells, macrophages, and lymphocytes to the injured sites, facilitating fibroblast proliferation while concurrently reducing vascularization. Diminished autophagy within fibrotic tissues contributes to the accumulation of defective mitochondria and oxidative stress. This positive feedback loop exacerbates immune cell dysregulation. However, the severity of fibrosis does not necessarily correlate with the extent of inflammation. Even minimal inflammation can persist over prolonged periods and precipitate fibrotic processes. Ordinarily, inflammatory cytokine levels are downregulated over time. However, sustained presence of these inflammatory cytokines and mediators can induce a pro-inflammatory state in tissues, potentially leading to the onset of fibrosis.

The dysregulation in the equilibrium between the synthesis and breakdown of the extracellular matrix (ECM) arises from the influence of profibrotic cytokines, resulting in disproportionate of matrix protein synthesis. Among these, collagen type I predominates as a main component of ECM proteins. Collagen type I has a high tensile strength which prevents normal stretching of the tissue. Fibrotic tissue manifests an elevated collagen type I to elastin ratio compared to normal tissues, which contributes to its diminished flexibility. Additionally, fibrotic ECM exhibits intricate cross-linking, rendering its degradation process.

Insufficient comprehension of the inflammatory mechanisms involved in arthrofibrosis may prompt excessively vigorous physical therapy interventions. However, such aggressive exercises can trigger an inflammatory reaction, characterized by elevated levels of inflammatory cytokines, increased collagen synthesis, and dysregulated TGF-β signaling, all of which are implicated in fibrotic processes.

22.4 Classification of Wrist Arthrofibrosis

At present, there is no standard consensus upon classification system for wrist arthrofibrosis. However, any proposed classification should include the following details to enhance comprehension of the patient's pathology and potentially guide treatment strategies.

22.4.1 Phases of Arthrofibrosis

Most patients with arthrofibrosis typically experience painful stiffness, although some may exhibit painless stiffness. Kayley et al. proposed a classification scheme distinguishing between two types of arthrofibrosis [6]:

1. Active arthrofibrosis: This type involves ongoing processes of ECM formation and inflammation within the joint.
2. Residual arthrofibrosis: The joint's restricted range of motion results from pre-existing ECM deposition, while active inflammation and further ECM deposition have subsided.

22.4.2 Planes of Limited Motion

The unique requirements of wrist motion vary among individuals in accordance with their daily activities or occupational demands. Consequently, limitations in motion experienced by one individual in a particular position may not necessarily impede the functionality of others in the same position, and vice versa. The wrist operates within three principal planes of motion:

- Flexion–extension
- Radial–ulnar deviation
- Pronation–supination

22.4.3 Locations of Pathology

It is crucial to accurately identify the specific location responsible for wrist stiffness to guide appropriate treatment. However, it is noteworthy that the pathology underlying wrist stiffness may involve more than one location. Wrist stiffness pathology can be categorized into the following locations:

- Intra-articular
- Capsular
- Extra-articular
- Neurologic

22.4.4 Severity of Wrist Contracture

Severity assessment should encompass various dimensions of disability, including the degree of pain, range of motion compared to the unaffected contralateral wrist, limitations in daily activity, and restrictions or issues with movement in adjacent joints. For example, a patient experiencing wrist stiffness may be unable to use the tenodesis effect to assist in finger motion. Consequently, if the fingers are also stiff, the disability will be more pronounced.

22.5 Risk Factors

Arthrofibrosis represents a multifactorial etiology, wherein numerous associated factors collectively contribute to the manifestation of wrist arthrofibrosis.

- Early onset osteoarthritis: This pathological state can serve as a predisposing factor or predictive marker for the onset of arthrofibrosis after trauma or surgical procedures. Individuals afflicted with osteoarthritis often exhibit fibrotic alterations within the synovial tissue [7] Notably, an elevated presence of fibroblasts within the synovium is observed, which can exacerbate the inflammation and undergo further activation after the surgery [8].
- Pre-existing injury: Injuries to the joint induce inflammatory responses, which can precipitate the development of arthrofibrosis. Subsequent surgical interventions following the initial injury exacerbate inflammatory cascades, thereby heightening the likelihood of arthrofibrosis.
- Having undergone more than two previous surgeries also constitutes a risk factor for postoperative arthrofibrosis, suggesting a cumulative effect or "memory" of each surgical insult.
- Reconstructive surgeries involving artificial implants or ligaments: Implantation of prosthetic devices initiates fibrotic tissue formation, as the body's response aims to encapsulate the foreign substances [9–11].
- Depression: Patients with depression exhibit an elevated susceptibility to arthrofibrosis. However, it's crucial to acknowledge that the inflammatory mechanisms inherent in active fibrosis can reciprocally precipitate depressive symptoms [12].
- Inadequate adherence to rehabilitation protocols: Prolonged immobilization and suboptimal compliance with postoperative rehabilitation can lead to capsular contracture and thickening. Scar tissues, resulting from prolonged immobilization, tend to contract and become progressively challenging to mobilize over time [13].
- Pre-existing inflammatory or autoimmune diseases, as well as type II diabetes mellitus, are associated with propensity for pro-inflammatory physiological states [14, 15].

22.6 Pathological Responses to Injury of the Wrist Joint

22.6.1 Primary Insult

The insult to the wrist joint can result in an injury that initiates an inflammatory response within the wrist. This injury spectrum spans from minor soft tissue contusions to more significant occurrences such as distal radius fractures, carpal bone fractures, or ligament tears. These injuries can elicit varying degrees of inflammatory response within the joint.

22.6.2 Response to the Insult

The typical physiological response of the body to an insult involves efforts to repair and remodel the affected structures, aiming to restore them to their pre-injury state.

A pathological reaction to the injury arises when tissue ischemia and necrosis occur, leading to excessive inflammation within the wrist joint. The typical response is for edema and inflammation, followed by fibrous scar tissue, which naturally shortened, and this predisposes to joint contracture. The response to injury varies among individuals and is influenced by their pre-existing factors, as well as the type and severity of the pathological insult.

22.6.3 Secondary Insult

Following the healing phase, a secondary insult may occur, which may involve avascular necrosis, infection, nonunion, degenerative arthritis, or even interventions such as surgery, all of which can further impact the progression of wrist arthrofibrosis.

22.7 General Considerations

Clinical assessment should target understanding the primary cause of wrist stiffness, which may result from pathological effects on various anatomical structures, and this condition may evolve over time. A thorough evaluation, including a detailed history, physical examination, and appropriate investigations, is essential for effective management of wrist stiffness.

22.7.1 History

The assessment should encompass details regarding the initial onset and progression of stiffness and pain. Additionally, it should include significant past medical conditions, prior injuries or surgeries, any accompanying symptoms beyond pain and stiffness, the extent of functional impairment, previous treatments and response to the treatments, and the patient's adherence to the treatment. This comprehensive approach offers valuable insights into the primary pathology underlying the entire clinical presentation.

Factors to consider when evaluating wrist stiffness include:

1. Patient:
   (a) Age
   (b) Comorbidities
   (c) Patient's needs and expectations
   (d) Previous treatment and response to the treatment
   (e) Compliance
2. Wrist
   (a) Range of the motion
   (b) Duration of stiffness
   (c) Effect of physiotherapy
   (d) Stability/Congruency
   (e) Pain
   (f) Neurologic symptoms
   (g) Prior surgery/hardware presence
   (h) Skin condition
3. Adjacent joints
   (a) Hand, elbow, shoulder, neck

22.7.2 Physical Examination

The assessment should commence with observation of the affected wrist compared to the contralateral wrist, noting any differences in swelling, scars from prior injuries or surgeries, and the resting posture of the wrist. Palpation should be performed at points of tenderness to pinpoint the specific location of the issue. Both active and passive motions of the wrists, including flexion–extension, radial–ulnar deviation, and pronation–supination should be measured. Additionally, evaluating finger motions and elbow motion is crucial for gaining insight into the patient's functional disturbances. The physical examination should also include an assessment of motor and sensory functions of the nerves to identify any concomitant nerve injuries. This evaluation is essential for a comprehensive understanding of the patient's condition and to guide appropriate management strategies.

22.7.3 Investigation

The necessity for imaging studies is determined by the findings from the patient's history and physical examination.

22.7.3.1 Plain Radiographs

Plain radiographs are the mainstay of initial imaging modality, offering a comprehensive view of wrist pathology regarding osseous structures and articular alignment Figs. 22.2, 22.3, 22.4, 22.5.

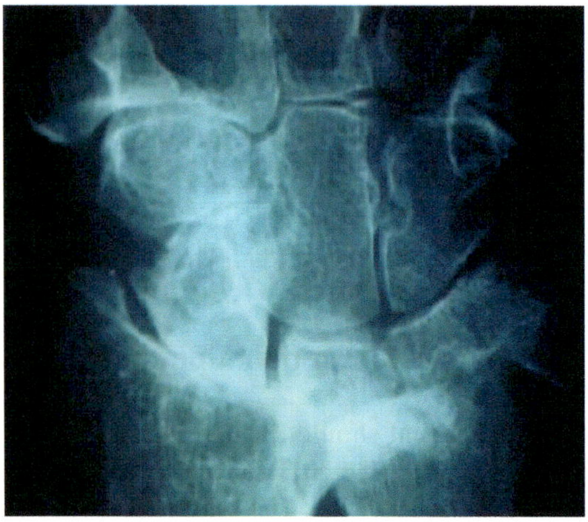

Fig. 22.2 Plain radiograph of rheumatoid arthritis of the wrist joint, with radiocarpal arthritis and ulnar translocation of the carpus. However, the midcarpal joint is preserved (Copyright Dr. Gregory Bain)

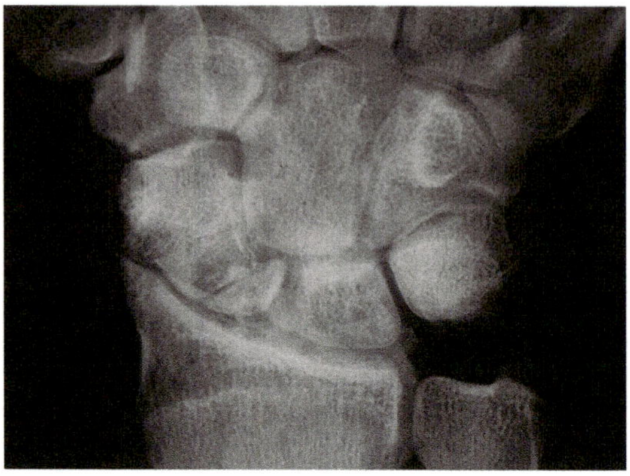

Fig. 22.3 Plain radiograph of wrist showing scaphoid proximal pole nonunion with degenerative arthritis over the radial styloid. This is scaphoid nonunion advanced collapse (SNAC). The osteophytes will likely restriction the motion (Copyright Dr. Gregory Bain)

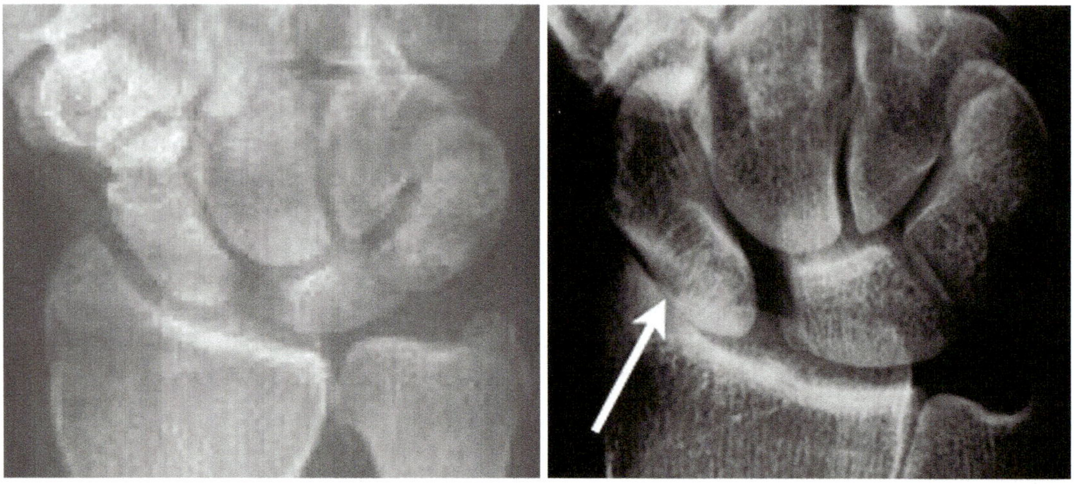

Fig. 22.4 Scapholunate instability. (**a**) Plain radiograph of scapholunate diastasis, (**b**) Plain radiograph of scapholunate diastasis and scapholunate advanced collapse (SLAC 2), with narrowing of the radioscaphoid joint space narrowing (Copyright Dr. Gregory Bain)

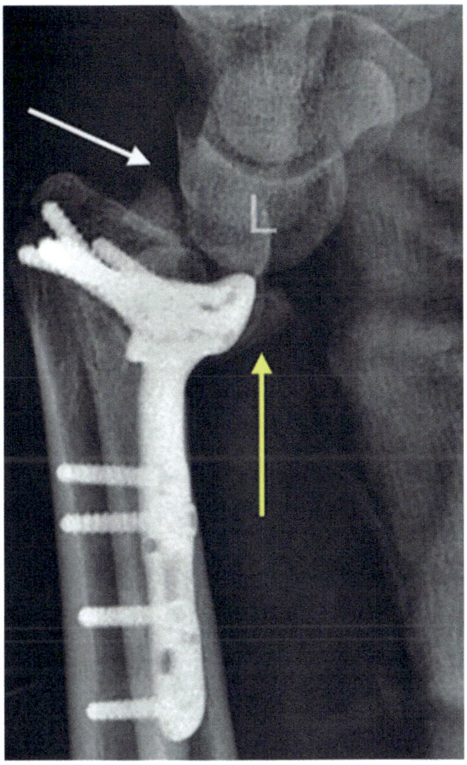

Fig. 22.5 Fragment escape after surgical fixation of the volar rim. This is often due to the fragment not being adequately contained and/or captured by the fixation. A lateral X-ray of a distal radius fracture internally fixed with a volar distal radius plate. There is fragment escape of the volar ulnar corner fragment (yellow arrow) and associated volar translation of the lunate (L) and carpus (white arrow) (Copyright Dr. Gregory Bain)

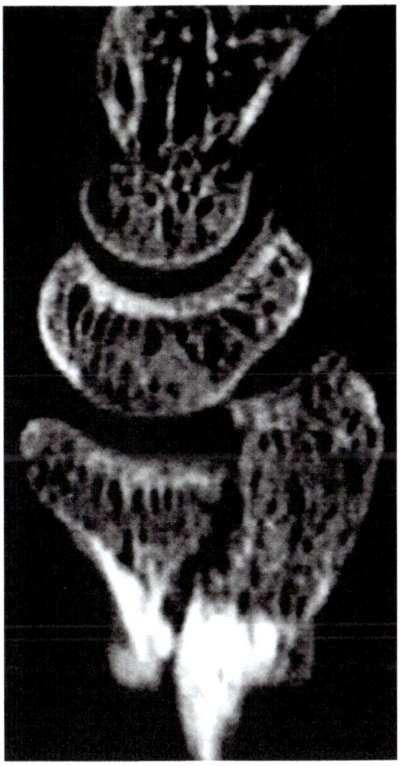

Fig. 22.6 CT scan showing intra-articular lunate facet fracture subluxation of distal radius (Copyright Dr. Gregory Bain)

22.7.3.2 Computed Tomography (CT Scan)

CT scan is utilized for enhanced visualization of bony structures, especially in cases of articular pathology such as intra-articular distal radius malunion (Fig. 22.6), humpback deformity of scaphoid bone, bony impingement due to excessive callus formation, and extra-articular malunion (Fig.22.7). This imaging modality offers detailed three-dimensional reconstructions and precise delineation of structural abnormalities, aiding in accurate diagnosis and treatment planning. Moreover, four-dimensional reconstruction CT scan of the wrist is a dynamic imaging technique, by capturing the wrist's motion over time, which offers enhanced visualization of bony impingement areas and provides deeper understanding of wrist kinetics and kinematics [16–18].

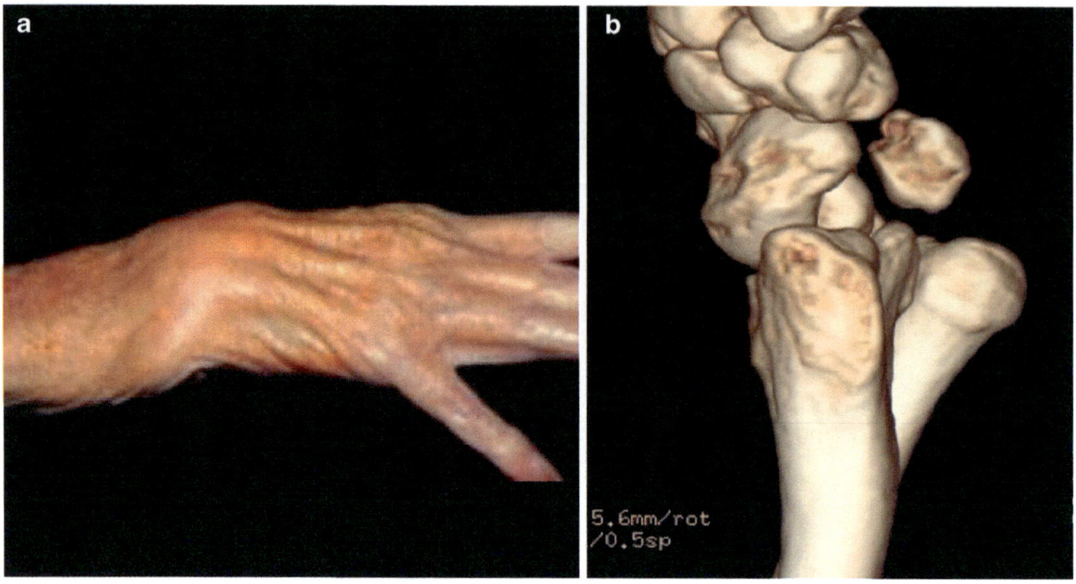

Fig. 22.7 Clinical picture and CT scan showing extra-articular malunion with DRUJ instability. (**a**) Clinical picture of the wrist deformity after extra-articular malunion of the distal radius, (**b**) CT scan showing a dorsally tilted malunion of the distal radius and a volarly dislocated DRUJ. (Copyright Dr. Gregory Bain)

22.7.3.3 Magnetic Resonance Imaging (MRI)

This imaging modality provides detailed visualization of soft tissues, including ligaments, tendons, cartilage, and synovium, enabling accurate assessment of soft tissue abnormalities such as tears, inflammation, and degeneration.

22.7.3.4 Wrist Arthroscopy

Intra-articular pathology can be both visualized and treated simultaneously through arthroscopy of the wrist (Fig. 22.8). Conditions such as torn ligaments (Fig. 22.9), cartilage lesions (Fig. 22.10), intra-articular fibrosis (Fig. 22.11), and capsular pathology (Fig. 22.12) can be effectively addressed using wrist arthroscopy, which allows for precise surgical intervention while minimizing trauma to surrounding tissues [13, 19, 20].

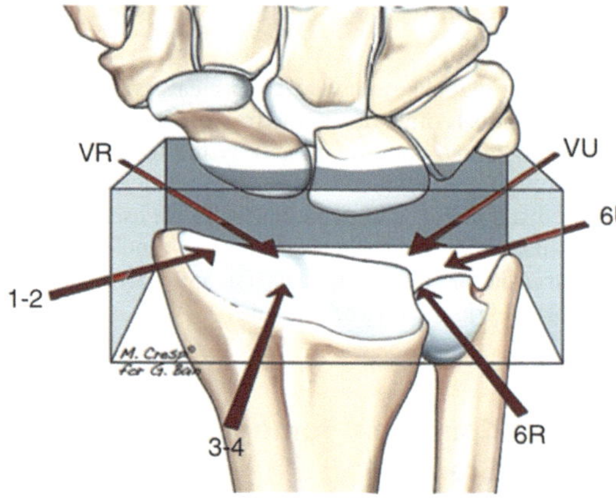

Fig. 22.8 Wrist arthroscopy portals. Through 2 dorsal (3–4, 6R), 2 volar (VR, VU), 1 radial (1–2), and 1 ulnar (6 U) portals, complete visualization of the wrist is possible. The multiple portals enable optimal viewing and instrumentation of the joint (Copyright Dr. Gregory I. Bain and Max Crespi)

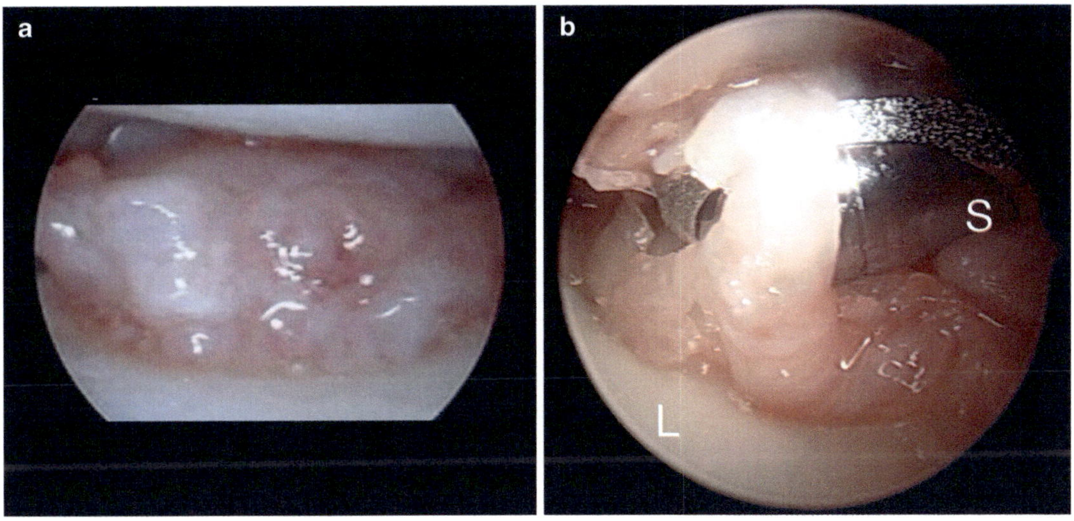

Fig. 22.9 (**a**) Wrist arthroscopy showing intra-articular view of avulsed volar carpal ligaments, with adjacent granulation tissue. (**b**) Debridement of osteochondral debris from the capitate caught between the scaphoid and lunate (Copyright Dr. Gregory Bain)

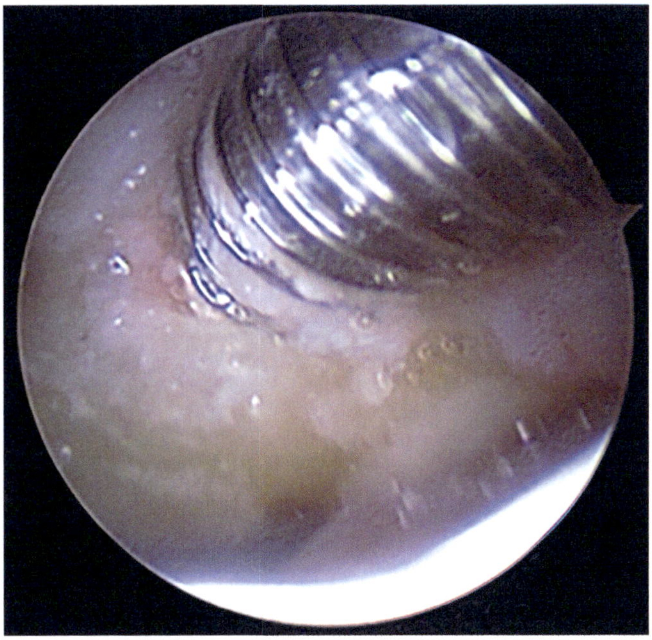

Fig. 22.10 Wrist arthroscopy showing intra-articular screw penetration following internal fixation of a distal radius fracture (Copyright Dr. Gregory Bain)

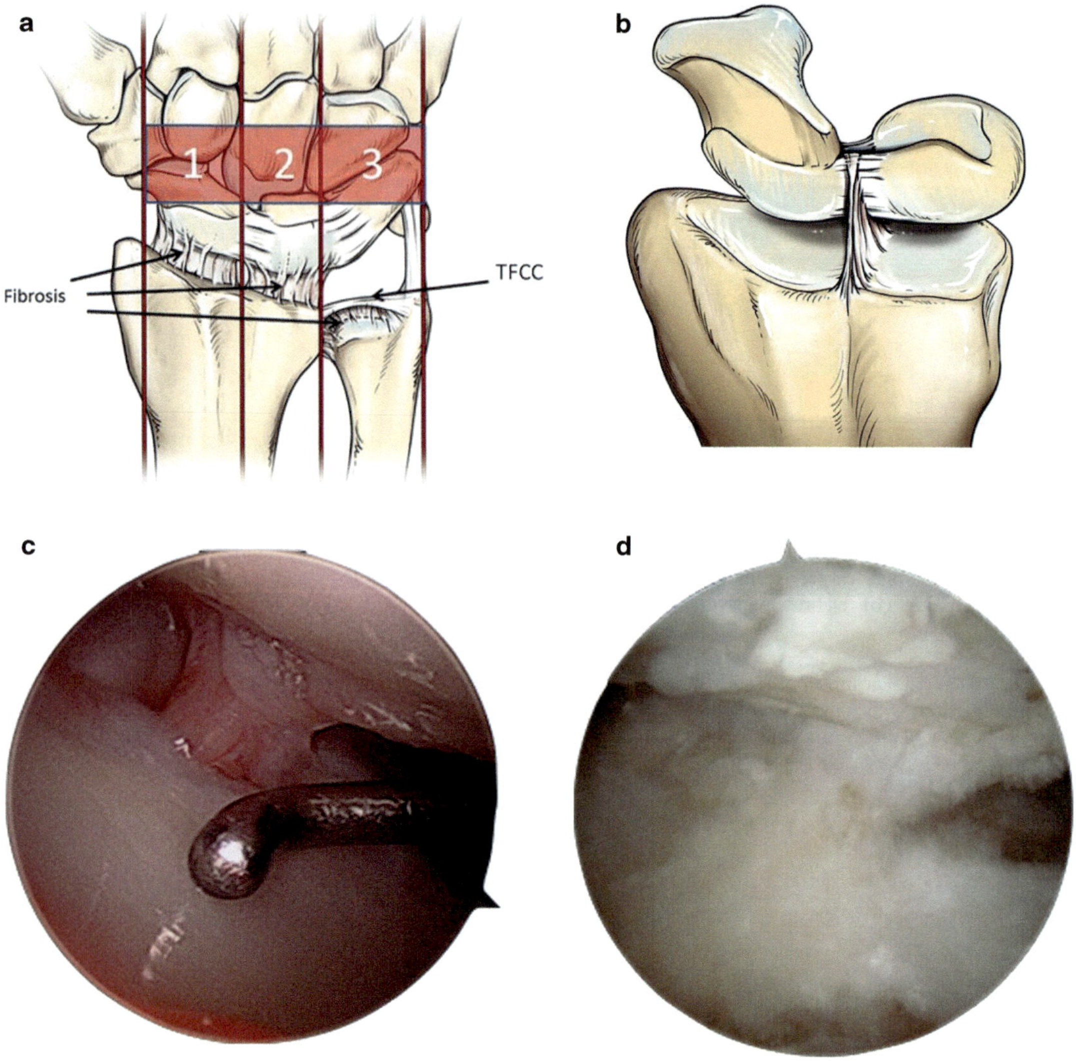

Fig. 22.11 (**a**) Illustration showing intra-articular fibrosis within three parts of the radiocarpal joint, the radioscaphoid, radiolunate, and ulnocarpal joints. The ulnocarpal joint is rarely involved. In this drawing, the fibrosis is located in the radiocarpal joint, the distal radioulnar joint (DRUJ), and under the triangular fibrocartilage complex (TFCC) [21]. (**b**) Illustration showing "synechia", a fibrotic adhesion between scapholunate ligament and sagittal ridge of previous fracture of distal radius [21]. (**c**) Wrist arthroscopy showing normal radiocarpal joint (Copyright Dr. Gregory Bain). (**d**) Wrist arthroscopy showing scarred articular cartilage with thickened arthrofibrosis (Copyright Dr. Gregory Bain)

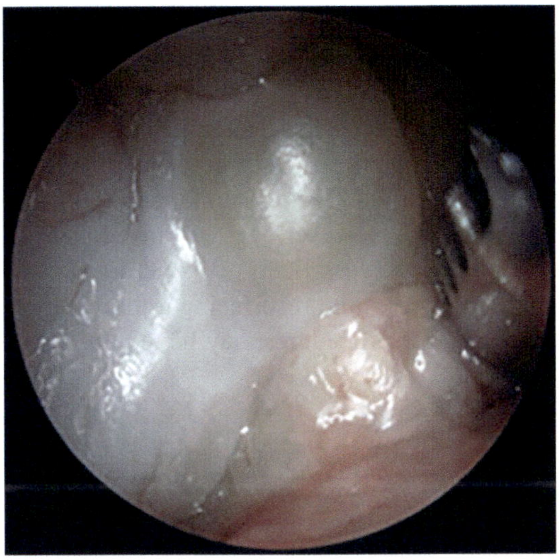

Fig. 22.12 Wrist arthroscopy image showing a ganglion cyst (Copyright Dr. Gregory Bain)

22.8 Approach to Wrist Stiffness

The treatment algorithms of wrist arthrofibrosis can be evaluated through an inside-out approach. This involves initially assessing the intra-articular pathology, followed by examination of bony and ligamentous pathology, and finally addressing any soft tissue contractures and nerve injuries. This systematic approach allows for comprehensive management of wrist arthrofibrosis, targeting each component of the condition in a strategic manner (Table 22.2). However, it is important to note that some patients with wrist stiffness might present with multiple pathologies contributing to their condition.

Table 22.2 Approach to wrist arthrofibrosis and its treatment options

Location	Pathology	Treatment options
Intra-articular	Arthritis	Mild to moderate: Arthroscopic debridement. Severe: Proximal row carpectomy, limited fusion, total wrist fusion, wrist arthroplasty
	Ligament instability	Ligament repair/reconstruction, limited fusion
	Intra-articular fibrosis	Arthroscopic/open arthrolysis
Capsular	Capsular contracture	Arthroscopic/open capsular release, physiotherapy
Extra-articular	Malunion/nonunion	Corrective osteotomy, open reduction, and internal fixation, vascularized/non-vascularized bone grafting
	Tendon contracture	Physiotherapy, splinting, tendon lengthening procedures
	Skin contracture	Scar revision, local/free flap coverage
Neurological	Nerve injury	Nerve repair, neurolysis, neuroma excision
	Complex regional pain syndrome	Medications, physiotherapy

The clinical manifestations of the disorders are dependent upon the impact of the pathological alterations within each anatomical structure. These may undergo changes over time. The prognosis is determined by the pathological progression and the extent to which it has compromised the anatomical structures.

22.8.1 Intra-articular Pathology

Intra-articular structures can be addressed through articular surgical interventions. These encompass procedures such as arthroscopic or open arthrolysis, arthroscopic synovectomy, and the removal of chondral flaps and loose bodies [19, 22]. Injuries to the interosseous ligaments should be corrected or reconstructed to restore normal kinetics and kinematics of the wrist joint. However, in advanced stages, debridement is less likely to yield success. In such instances, joint resurfacing arthroplasty or other salvage procedures may be required (Fig. 22.13).

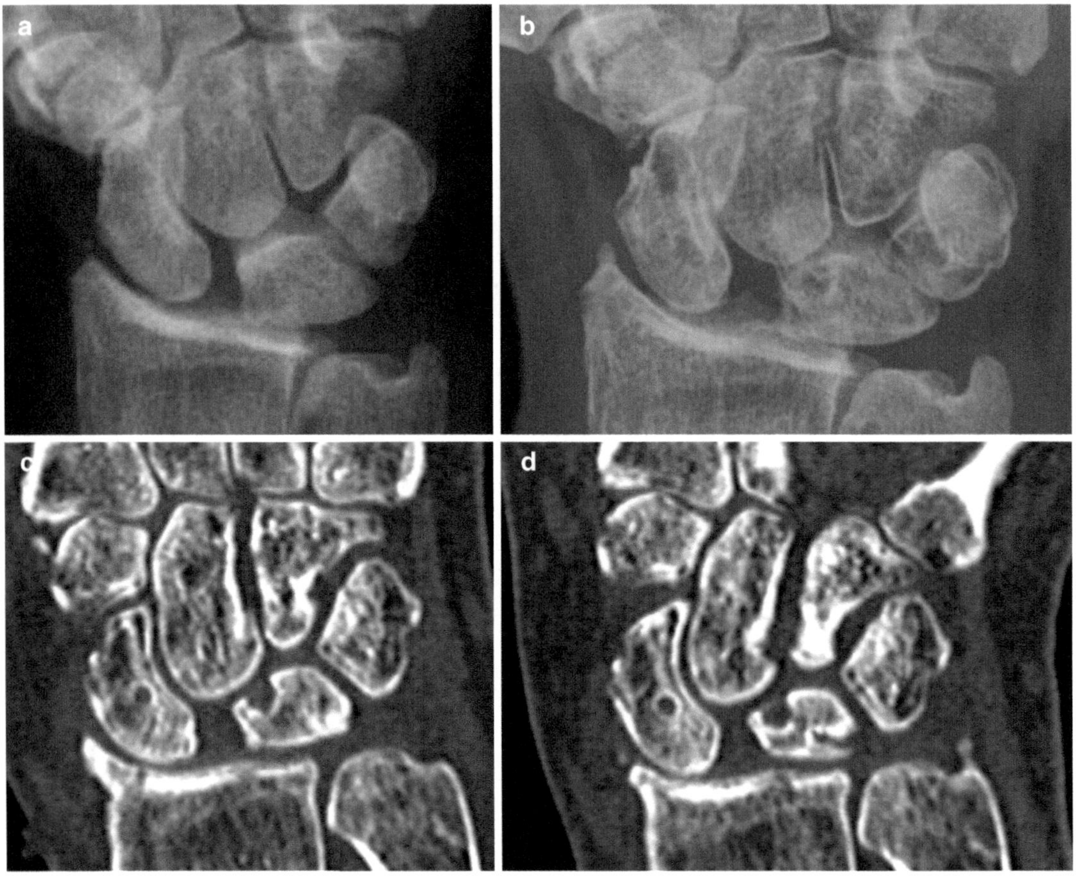

Fig. 22.13 Scapholunate reconstruction. (**a**) Wrist radiograph showing scapholunate diastasis. (**b**) Wrist radiograph following scapholunate ligament reconstruction with trans-osseous tunnels, using flexor carpi radialis (FCR) tendon and suture. However, the scapholunate diastasis persists. (**c**) Wrist stiffness following SL ligament reconstruction. Coronal CT image during radial deviation position. Note the cortical disruption of the midcarpal lunate, and the degenerative arthritis over the radial styloid. (**d**) Coronal CT image during ulnar deviation. (**e**) Fragmented lunate at time of proximal row carpectomy. The tendon has not healed to the cancellous bone of the lunate. (**f**) Histology of lunate with birefringent suture material, inflammatory cells, and giant cells. (Copyright Dr Gregory Bain)

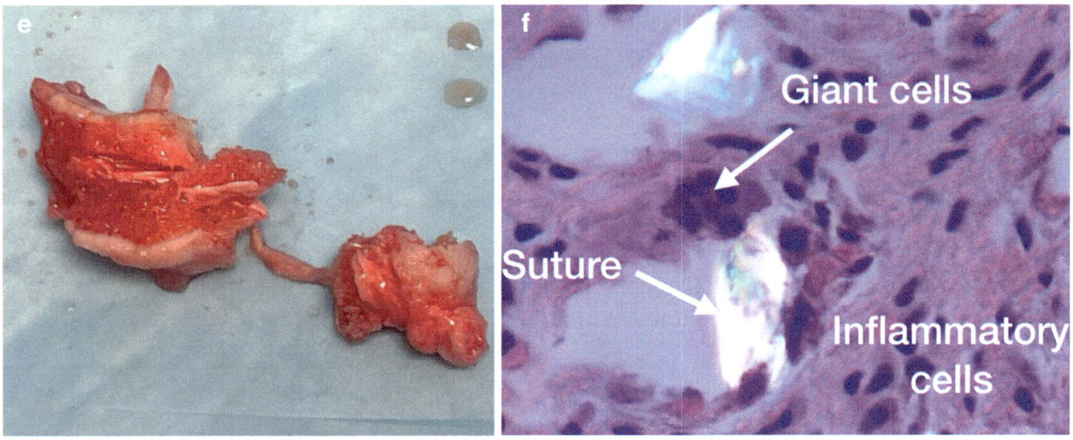

Fig. 22.13 Continued

22.8.2 Capsular Pathology

Capsular contracture can be solved through release or resection, which may be conducted via open or arthroscopic techniques [13, 20, 23]. When the condition is an isolated pathology, the prognosis is generally favorable. However, caution must be exercised to avoid excessive capsular release, as this could potentially jeopardize joint stability. Viegas's findings suggest that the sectioning of the radioscaphocapitate and radiolunate ligaments does not result in substantial ulnar translocation of the carpus. Instead, either the volar ulnar ligament or the dorsal ulnar ligament complex alone is sufficient to prevent such translation. During arthroscopic capsulectomy, the preservation of the volar ulnar ligament and dorsal ulnar ligament complex maintains this stability [24]. It is crucial to preserve the integrity of the primary ligamentous stabilizers, and if compromised, they may necessitate repair or reconstruction.

22.8.3 Extra-articular Pathology

Extra-articular structures can be addressed through open or endoscopic procedures involving resection or release of the offending structures. This may involve removing heterotopic bone or excessive bone which impinge the joint such as dorsal rim of the distal radius. Prognosis depends upon the pathological process. Release or resection of the extra-articular tissues typically results in recovery of much of the passive range of motion. However, surgical intervention targeting muscles and tendons may potentially impact the strength of active motion. Scarring of the skin and soft tissues over the wrist can contribute to wrist stiffness. Flexible skin and soft tissue covering the wrist facilitate the smooth gliding of the tendons and enable a full motion of the wrist joint.

22.8.4 Neurological

Treatment for neurological causes should target the underlying primary neurological disorder. Additionally, secondary effects may also require treatment.

It is interesting that nerve pathology can contribute to wrist stiffness. Therefore, we would like to provide further details on this issue. The assessment and management of patients experiencing nerve-related pain and stiffness can pose challenges. It is unfortunate that complex regional pain syndrome (CRPS) is often a common diagnosis in such cases. The diagnostic criteria for CRPS include the absence of any other diagnosis that better explains the signs and symptoms. However, based on our experience, a significant number of cases presenting with severe pain and labelled as CRPS ultimately reveal underlying medical conditions that provide a more accurate explanation. We acknowledge Dr. Paco Pinal for his critical work to break this travesty of medical care in the wrist [25–28]. His work has shed light on surgically correctable conditions previously misdiagnosed as CRPS. Additionally, we acknowledge Dr. Shawn O'Driscoll, who is pioneering a similar approach in understanding elbow pain and stiffness attributed to ulnar nerve entrapment [29].

Dr. Pinal has reported that most diagnoses of CRPS are made by clinicians and non-clinicians who provide this label, which, emotionally cripples the patient and makes them a target of inappropriate care. The most common causes of patients labelled as CRPS include poor initial care (40%), carpal tunnel syndrome (40%), malingering/psychogenic (10%), and causalgia/CRPS type II (10%) [26]. The poor initial care includes cases of distal radius fractures which have not been reduced or had screw left in the joint. The group of patients exhibiting symptoms related to carpal tunnel pathology presents with a distinct presentation that differs from typical carpal tunnel syndrome. Dr. Pinal has introduced the term "irritative carpal tunnel syndrome" to describe this condition. Patients with this condition often experience pain localized to the radial side of the hand, which can disrupt sleep patterns. They may exhibit swelling of the hand and wrist and difficulty in making a full fist.

In many cases, the severity of pain experienced by patients can overshadow their awareness of nerve-related symptoms. However, from our experience, persistent, burning pain that subsides in the nerve is highly indicative of nerve involvement. Patients in this group often struggle to articulate their symptoms clearly due to the overwhelming nature of their pain. Engaging in rational discussions with both the patient and their family can be challenging. Once the cause is pinpointed, surgical intervention may be an effective option, especially if the issue is surgically correctable.

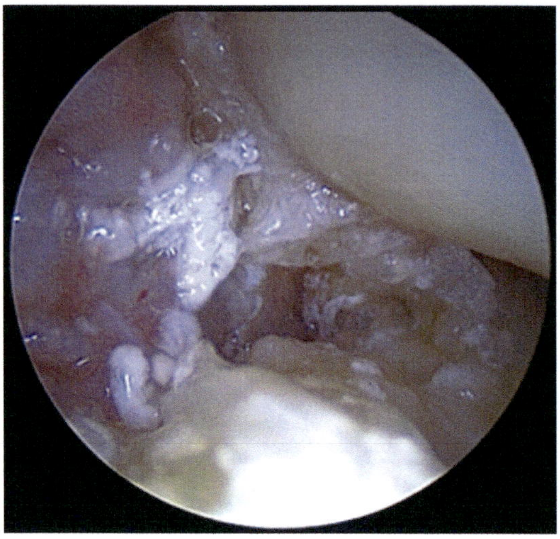

Fig. 22.14 Crystal arthropathy. Pseudogout is an important cause of the stiff wrist in the older patient. Note the crystal deposition throughout the capsule, ligaments and on the articular cartilage (Copyright Dr. Gregory Bain)

22.8.5 Systemic Disorders

Systemic causes can impact individual anatomical structures differently. For instance, rheumatoid arthritis and crystal arthropathy affect intra-articular synovium and overlying cartilage of the joint (Fig. 22.14), Dupuytren's contracture and diabetes mellitus affect the capsule, and muscular dystrophy affects the muscles. While treating these conditions, systemic factors should be considered and addressed accordingly.

Wrist stiffness can arise from common local pathological factors like trauma and infection, as well as systemic conditions such as rheumatoid arthritis, diabetes mellitus, spastic cerebral disorder, and muscular dystrophy. These diverse pathological aspects collectively contribute to the surgical sieve, impacting various anatomical components of the wrists. Factors such as the timing of the insult, the response of the patient from previous treatment, adjacent joint problems, and secondary insults further influence the presentation of patients with stiff wrist.

22.9 Summary

Wrist arthrofibrosis, commonly referred to as wrist stiffness, presents as pain accompanied by limitations in both active and passive wrist movement, hindering daily activities. While the characterization of wrist joint stiffness remains relatively sparse compared to other joints, its impact on functionality is significant. Various factors contribute to wrist stiffness, including trauma, surgical procedures, inflammatory conditions, abnormal bony alignment, and ligament instability. Pathological responses to injury involve inflammation, fibrosis and subsequent tissue remodeling, often leading to chronic stiffness if left untreated. Understanding the etiology, pathogenesis, and classification of wrist arthrofibrosis is crucial for accurate diagnosis, proper investigation, and effective management. Treatment options may include conservative measures such as physiotherapy or more invasive interventions such as arthroscopy and open surgery, depending on the severity and underlying causes of stiffness. A comprehensive clinical assessment is essential for personalized treatment plans tailored to individual patients. Considering the multifactorial nature of wrist stiffness, a systematic inside-out approach is recommended to address all contributing pathologies and optimize patient outcomes.

References

1. Yu H, Chase R, Strauch B. Terminology for functions and movements of the hand. Atlas of hand anatomy and clinical implications. St. Louis, MO: Mosby; 2004. p. 30–42.
2. Palmer AK, Werner FW, Murphy D, Glisson R. Functional wrist motion: a biomechanical study. J Hand Surg Am. 1985;10(1):39–46.
3. Ryu JY, Cooney WP 3rd, Askew LJ, An KN, Chao EY. Functional ranges of motion of the wrist joint. J Hand Surg Am. 1991;16(3):409–19.
4. Marinelli A, Guerra E, Bain G. Classification of elbow stiffness. J Isakos. 2023;9:234.
5. Liu RM, Gaston Pravia KA. Oxidative stress and glutathione in TGF-beta-mediated fibrogenesis. Free Radic Biol Med. 2010;48(1):1–15.
6. Usher KM, Zhu S, Mavropalias G, Carrino JA, Zhao J, Xu J. Pathological mechanisms and therapeutic outlooks for arthrofibrosis. Bone Res. 2019;7:9.
7. Remst DF, Blaney Davidson EN, van der Kraan PM. Unravelling osteoarthritis-related synovial fibrosis: a step closer to solving joint stiffness. Rheumatology (Oxford). 2015;54(11):1954–63.
8. Snelling SJ, Bas S, Puskas GJ, Dakin SG, Suva D, Finckh A, et al. Presence of IL-17 in synovial fluid identifies a potential inflammatory osteoarthritic phenotype. PLoS One. 2017;12(4):e0175109.
9. Jerosch J, Aldawoudy AM. Arthroscopic treatment of patients with moderate arthrofibrosis after total knee replacement. Knee Surg Sports Traumatol Arthrosc. 2007;15(1):71–7.
10. Ries MD, Badalamente M. Arthrofibrosis after total knee arthroplasty. Clin Orthop Relat Res. 2000;380:177–83.
11. Schiavone Panni A, Denti M, Franzese S, Monteleone M. The bone-ligament junction: a comparison between biological and artificial ACL reconstruction. Knee Surg Sports Traumatol Arthrosc. 1993;1(1):9–12.
12. Bufalino C, Hepgul N, Aguglia E, Pariante CM. The role of immune genes in the association between depression and inflammation: a review of recent clinical studies. Brain Behav Immun. 2013;31:31–47.
13. Bain GI, Munt J, Turner PC, Bergman J. Arthroscopic dorsal capsular release in the wrist: a new technique. Tech Hand Up Extrem Surg. 2008;12(3):191–4.
14. Huang YP, Fann CY, Chiu YH, Yen MF, Chen LS, Chen HH, et al. Association of diabetes mellitus with the risk of developing adhesive capsulitis of the shoulder: a longitudinal population-based follow-up study. Arthritis Care Res (Hoboken). 2013;65(7):1197–202.
15. Schiavone Panni A, Cerciello S, Vasso M, Tartarone M. Stiffness in total knee arthroplasty. J Orthop Traumatol. 2009;10(3):111–8.
16. Bain GI, Krishna SV, MacLean S, Carr R, Slavotinek J. "Locked" Scapholunate instability diagnosed with 4D computed tomography scan. J Wrist Surg. 2019;8(4):321–6.
17. Carr R, MacLean S, Slavotinek J, Bain GI. Four-dimensional computed tomography scanning for dynamic wrist disorders: prospective analysis and recommendations for clinical utility. J Wrist Surg. 2019;8(2):161–7.
18. MacLean SBM, Bain GI. Kinematics of the wrist in Kienböck's disease: a four-dimensional computed tomography study. J Hand Surg Eur. 2021;46(5):504–9.
19. Luchetti R, Atzei A, Fairplay T. Arthroscopic wrist arthrolysis after wrist fracture. Arthroscopy. 2007;23(3):255–60.
20. Schmidle G, Benedikt S, Kastenberger T, Kaiser P, Arora R, Gabl M. Arthroscopic debridement of the dorsal capsule in intraarticular distal radius fractures: does it provide superior outcomes? Arch Orthop Trauma Surg. 2022;142(4):691–9.

21. Luchetti R. The role of arthroscopy in postfracture stiffness. In: Piñal F, Luchetti R, Mathoulin C, editors. Arthroscopic management of distal radius fractures. Berlin/Heidelberg: Springer; 2010. https://doi.org/10.1007/978-3-642-05354-2_12.
22. Guidi M, Luchetti R, Besmens I, Rothenfluh E, Calcagni M. Wrist Arthrolysis: a systematic review of open and arthroscopic techniques. J Wrist Surg. 2021;10(6):543–50.
23. Kamal RN, Ruch DS. Volar capsular release after distal radius fractures. J Hand Surg Am. 2017;42(12):1034.e1–6.
24. Viegas SF, Patterson RM, Ward K. Extrinsic wrist ligaments in the pathomechanics of ulnar translation instability. J Hand Surg Am. 1995;20(2):312–8.
25. Del Piñal F. Editorial. I have a dream … reflex sympathetic dystrophy (RSD or Complex Regional Pain Syndrome - CRPS I) does not exist. J Hand Surg Eur Vol. 2013;38(6):595–7.
26. Del Piñal F. Reflex sympathetic dystrophy (RSD)/CRPS/Sudeck does not exist. Ezine (IFSSH). 2019;9:22–31.
27. Del Piñal F. Diagnosis and outcomes of 225 consecutive cases of complex regional pain syndrome of the hand. Plast Reconstr Surg. 2023;152(4):807–16.
28. Piñal FD. Hand allodynia, lack of finger flexion, and the need for carpal tunnel release. J Hand Surg Am. 2023;48(4):370–6.
29. Jupiter JB, O'Driscoll SW, Cohen MS. The assessment and management of the stiff elbow. Instr Course Lect. 2003;52:93–111.

23 The Stiff Wrist: Physical Exam

Christian M. Lozano

23.1 Introduction

Understanding the complex anatomy of the normal wrist, added to its biomechanics and pathologies that can affect it, represents a challenge for the upper extremity surgeon.

The evaluation of a stiff wrist is a complex process in which the identification of the possible intrinsic and extrinsic factors that could have caused this condition is extremely important in order to reach an adequate etiological diagnosis for optimal treatment and maximum possible results [1].

Wrist stiffness can be caused by a variety of problems including overuse injuries, wound sequelae, joint pain, injuries, and nerve compression. In order to identify the source of the pain and stiffness of the wrist, we will have to perform a thorough physical examination, which is essential in this type of entity [2].

We will review in the following lines the procedures for a careful physical examination of the stiff wrist.

C. M. Lozano (✉)
Clínica Anglo Americana, Lima, Peru

23.2 Background

When doing a physical examination of a stiff wrist, it is crucial to collect as much history as possible regarding this condition. To begin with and above all, the evaluating doctor must create a comfortable and pleasant environment for the patient throughout the examination [2].

The patient's clinical history, reporting any previous surgery or injury, as well as any problem related to the intake of medications or some type of drug that may affect the examination, must also be taken into account by the evaluating physician in order to be able to carry out the clinical examination in the best way and reduce the possible biases that could occur during it [2].

23.3 Range of Motion

The first step in a physical examination for wrist stiffness is to assess the range of motion of this joint. The evaluating physician will ask the patient to move the wrist in several directions, such as flexion, extension, radial and ulnar deviation, as well as supination and pronation. Special attention should be paid to observing the range of motion and noting any limitations, pain, or crepitus. It is important to note that some people may have natural limitations in the range of motion of the wrist, so the clinician should compare the

L. Pederzini et al. (eds.), *Stiffness of the Elbow, Wrist and Related Pathologies*,
https://doi.org/10.1007/978-3-031-81381-8_23

patient's range of motion with what is considered normal for the patient's age and gender [3, 4].

The goniometer is the recommended instrument for measuring the hand and wrist range of motion.

An optimal result is full range of motion in all directions without pain or crepitus, while an unfavorable result would be limited range of motion or severe pain with movement [3].

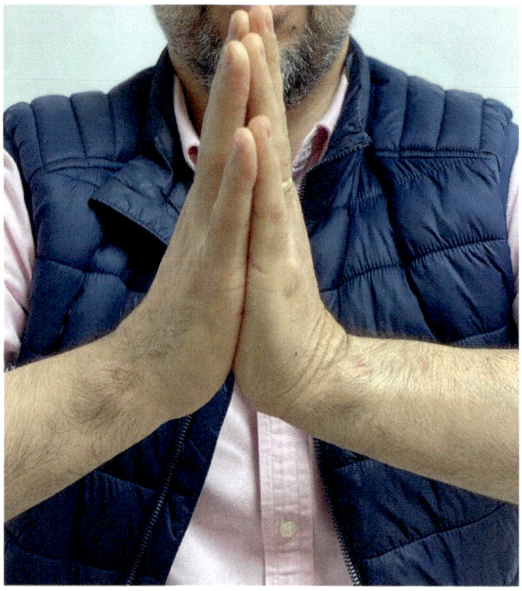

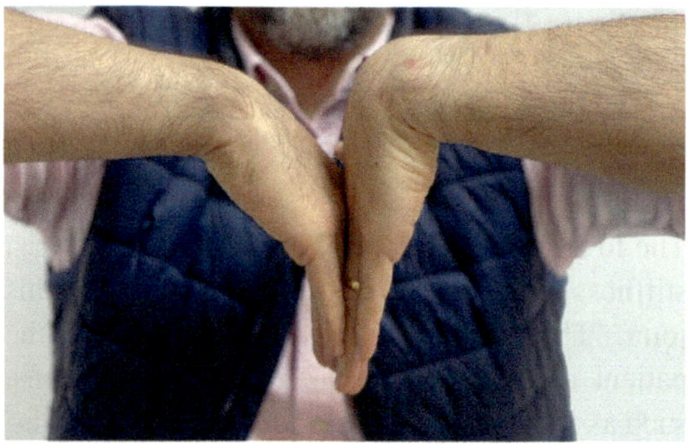

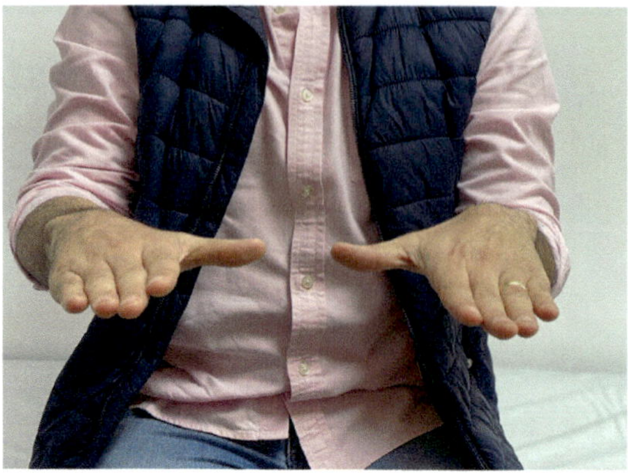

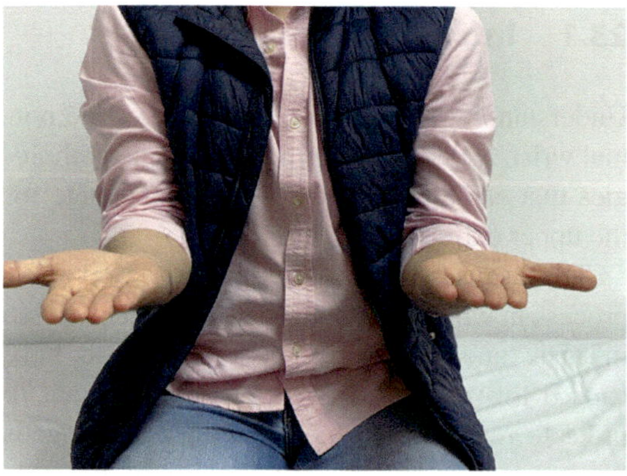

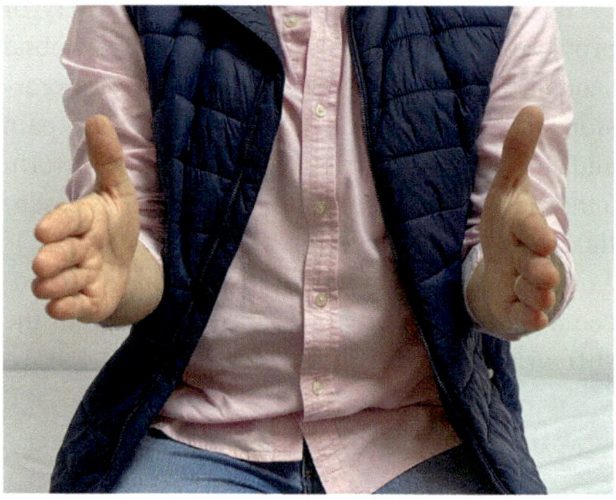

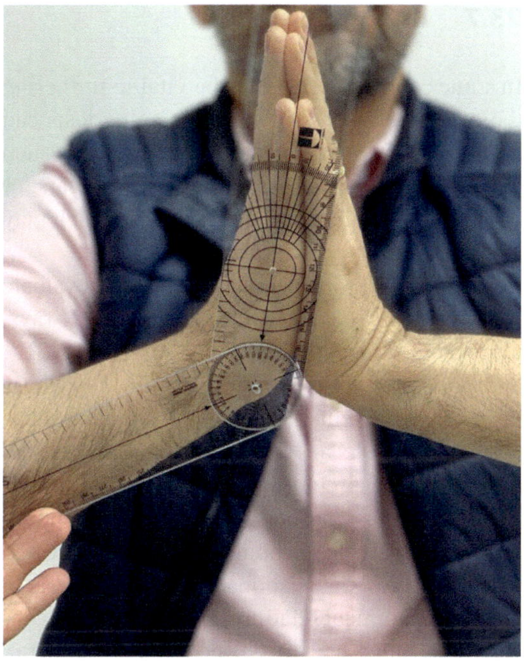

23.4 Strength

It is extremely important to assess joint quality by testing the strength to perform different tasks, such as holding, squeezing, and pushing different objects. The physician should observe the patient's ability to perform these tasks and note any deficiencies or difficulties in performing them [5].

It is important that the evaluating physician compares the strength of the stiff wrist with that of the unaffected wrist. An ideal outcome would be the ability to perform all tasks without difficulty, while an adverse outcome would be a serious deficiency in strength or severe limitation in executing agreed upon orders.

Additionally, to assess strength, examiners may perform grip strength tests, such as asking the patient to squeeze a dynamometer or asking the patient to perform functional tasks that require neck strength, arms and hands, such as opening a bowl or lifting weights. Weakness or asymmetry in grip strength may indicate a muscle or nerve problem that requires further evaluation [6, 7].

23.5 Stability

The strength and stability of the wrist joint will also be evaluated by the evaluating physician. Various tests should be performed, such as the drawer test, to assess ligament weakness. In addition, the doctor can test stability against resistance by applying weight to the wrist joint. An optimal outcome might be a stable wrist joint with no deficits or laxity, while an adverse outcome would be weakness or extreme difficulty with weight [8, 9].

23.6 Special Tests

Depending on the initial findings, the doctor may perform special tests to help evaluate the stiff wrist. These tests may require instruments, such as a goniometer or an ultrasound machine [4]. The most used are as follows:

23.6.1 Watson Test

Assesses for scapholunate instability.

Scaphoid shift test.

Procedure

Place thumb over scaphoid tubercle and index finger over dorsal aspect of scapholunate joint.

Apply dorsally directed force with thumb against distal pole of scaphoid while passively moving wrist from ulnar to radial deviation.

Positive Test

Sudden, dyskinesia of scaphoid with dorsal wrist pain.

"Catch-up Clunk".

Pathoanatomy

Instability at the scapholunate joint interferes with normal flexion–extension motion of the scaphoid during wrist radial–ulnar avoidance.

23.6.2 Lunotriquetral Shuck/Shear

Assesses for lunotriquetral instability.

Procedure

Grasp lunate between the thumb and index finger of one hand.

Grasp triquetrum/pisiform between the thumb and index finger of second hand.

Shift the two grasping hands in opposite directions.

Positive Test

Reproduction of pain.

Lunotriquetral excursion greater than 2 mm.

Pathoanatomy

Instability/ligamentous insufficiency at lunotriquetral articulation.

23.6.3 Distal Radioulnar Joint Instability

Assesses for dorsal–volar instability.

Procedure

Grasp distal radius and ulna between thumb and index of opposite hands 3–4 cm proximal to wrist.

Translate radius relative to ulna in neutral, supination and pronation.

Positive Test

Crepitus.

Translation >5 mm.

The next step after assessing the range of motion of the stiff wrist is to assess the quality of the muscles in the wrist and hand. This point is crucial, as it provides data on the intrinsic and extrinsic motion of the entire wrist and hand. This evaluation can detect any entities that contribute to wrist stiffness [4, 8].

Care must be taken when performing these tests to avoid further injury or discomfort to the patient. The examiner should start with light pressure and gradually increase the pressure to avoid causing additional pain or joint damage. It is also important to ensure that the patient is relaxed and comfortable during the examination.

23.7 Imaging Studies

In some cases, imaging may be vital in furthering the evaluation of a stiff wrist. Imaging tests can help to recognize particular basic problems, such as ruptures of various structures, tendon tears, or damage to specific areas of the joints, which may be contributing to stiffness [8].

The images considered to be used to evaluate the soundness of the wrist incorporate X-rays, ultrasound, magnetic resonance imaging (MRI), and computed tomography (CT). Each of these tests has its benefits, indications, and contraindications. The relevance of requesting images will depend on the circumstances of each patient.

Radiographs can be a commonly used imaging test to evaluate the bony anatomy of the wrist, since fractures, dislocations, and/or alterations of normal anatomical relationships as well as degenerative changes can be discovered. In general, they are quick and non-invasive, making them perfect to start with in conjunction with external inspection for wrist stability [8].

MRI is commonly used to evaluate soft tissue structures such as tendons and ligaments. These types of images can provide detailed data on the degree of tissue damage and may be sufficient together with the clinical examination to plan a surgical intervention. MRI is a non-invasive method, but the test can be lengthy and requires patient peace of mind for a longer or shorter period of time [2, 4].

A CT scan uses X-rays to create images of your hand from various perspectives. The evaluating physician can obtain a variety of information about the bone structures, joints, and soft tissues of the wrist from these images. Broken bones or other bone problems can occasionally be visible on CT scans. However, some people may be concerned because the radiation from the CT scan is much stronger than regular X-ray radiation.

Remember that a CT scan is not always necessary and that the choice to have one will depend on the specific circumstances. In most cases, a clinical examination and the patient's history are sufficient to provide physicians with the knowledge they need to make a diagnosis.

An accurate and clear image of the wrist showing any problems that may be causing stiffness would be the ideal result for imaging studies. An image that is not clear or inconclusive and requires additional imaging studies or other diagnostic tests would be a terrible result [2, 4].

Because radiation exposure can be harmful to a developing fetus, it is important to take precautions when performing imaging studies, including making sure the patient is not pregnant. Detailed instructions about the test should also be given to the patient, including how to prepare for the test and what to expect during the procedure. Before any contrast material is administered, it is crucial to obtain a complete medical history because some patients may react negatively to the contrast material used in some imaging studies.

23.8 Conclusion

A person's daily life can be significantly affected by the disabling nature of a m stiff wrist. A crucial step in the diagnostic process for a stiff wrist is a physical examination, which can help determine the underlying cause of the stiffness. Each step of the physical examination should be systematic and complete, based on the knowledge gathered in the previous step.

Although imaging tests may be necessary in some circumstances, a complete clinical examination is often sufficient to make a diagnosis. Treatment for a stiff wrist is aimed at reducing discomfort, improving function, and regaining range of motion. Depending on the underlying cause of the stiffness, the best treatment may be a combination of surgical and non-surgical interventions.

It is important to remember that the best results for patients with a stiff wrist require early intervention.

References

1. Castro WH, Jerosch J, Grossman TW. Examination and diagnosis of musculoskeletal disorders. New York: Thieme; 2001.
2. Finney A, Thwaites C. Rheumatoid arthritis.1: background, symptoms and ensuring prompt diagnosis and treatment. Nurs Times. 2010;106(9):22–4.
3. Van de Pol RJ, van Trijffel E, Lucas C. Inter-rater reliability for measurements of passive physiological range of motion of upper extremity joints is better if instruments are used: a systematic review. J Physiother. 2010;56(1):7–17.
4. Adams I, Greene L, Topoozian E. Clinical assessment recommendations. Am Soc Hand Ther. 1999;2:56–70.
5. Gates DH, Walters LS, Cowley J, Wilken JM, Resnik L. Range of motion requirements for upper-limb activities of daily living. Am J Occup Ther. 2016;70(1):7001350010p1–7001350010p10.
6. Carter TI, Pansy B, Wolff AL, Hillstrom HJ, Backus SI, Lenhoff M, Wolfe SW. Accuracy and reliability of three different techniques for manual goniometry for wrist motion: a cadaveric study. J Hand Surg Am. 2009;34(8):1422–8.
7. Barakat MJ, Field J, Taylor J. The range of movement of the thumb. Hand (N Y). 2013;8(2):179–82.
8. McRae R. Capitulo 6 Muñeca. In: En: McRae R. Ortopedia y Fracturas. Madrid: Marban; 2006. p. 57–67.
9. Kapandji IA, Capitulo IV, Muñeca L. Kapandji IA Cuadernos de fisiologia articular I. 4th ed. Barcelona: Masson; 1989. p. 138–71.

Diagnostic Imaging of the Stiff Wrist

24

Toshiyasu Nakamura

24.1 Introduction

Loss of the range of motion (ROM) of the wrist due to the wrist contracture or stiff wrist indicates severe restriction in activity of daily life [1]. Diagnosis of wrist contracture or stiff wrist normally depends on the physical examination. Image diagnosis of stiff wrist helps for its diagnosis and decision making of treatment strategy.

24.2 Image Diagnosis of Wrist Contracture

24.2.1 Radiographs

Diagnosis of wrist contracture itself is normally easy, where the patient indicates loss of wrist motion due to the wrist problems. The radiographs of the wrist indicate narrowing of the joint space either the radiocarpal joint (RCJ) (Fig. 24.1) or midcarpal joint (MCJ) (Fig. 24.2) or both, suggesting problems of the surrounding soft tissue of the wrist. Narrowing of the joint space suggests the osteoarthritic situation partially or totally in the RCJ or MCJ. Causes of the narrowing of the joint or partial osteoarthritis are due to rheumatoid arthritis, idiopathic osteoarthritis [1], stage 2 and 3 of the scapholunate advanced collapse (SLAC) wrist [2] (Fig. 24.3), or scaphoid nonunion advanced collapse (SNAC) wrist (Fig. 24.4). Avulsion of the scapholunate interosseous ligament (SLIL) later indicates advanced degeneration of the RCJ or MCJ, which is known as the SLAC wrist and nonunion of the scaphoid shows similar osteoarthritic changes on the RCJ and MCJ in SNAC wrist. All of these pathologies indicate loss of flexion–extension and radial–ulnar deviation range of the wrist.

T. Nakamura (✉)
Department of Orthopaedic Surgery, School of Medicine, International University of Health and Welfare, Tokyo, Japan
e-mail: toshiyasu@ae.em-net.ne.jp

L. Pederzini et al. (eds.), *Stiffness of the Elbow, Wrist and Related Pathologies*,
https://doi.org/10.1007/978-3-031-81381-8_24

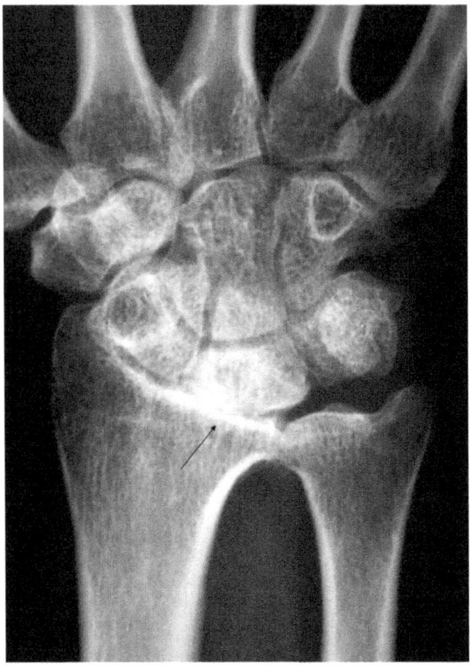

Fig. 24.1 Radiograph of stiff wrist. Arrow indicates narrowing of the radiolunate space at the radiocarpal joint are noted on posteroanterior radiograph

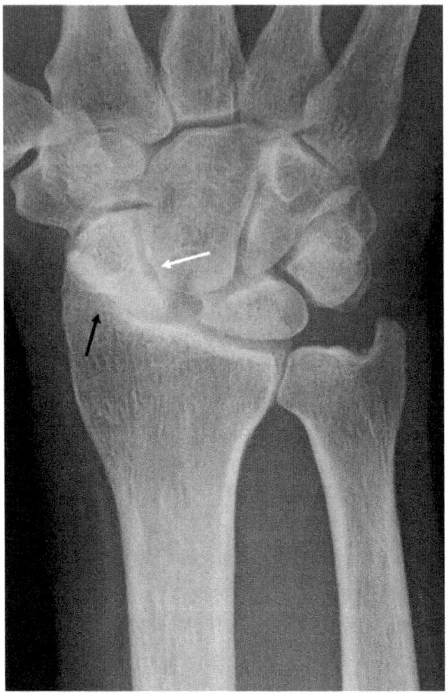

Fig. 24.3 Posteroanterior radiograph of SLAC wrist stage 3 indicating the severe joint space narrowing at the scaphoradial joint (white arrow) and slightly narrowing of the scaphocapitate joint interval (black arrow)

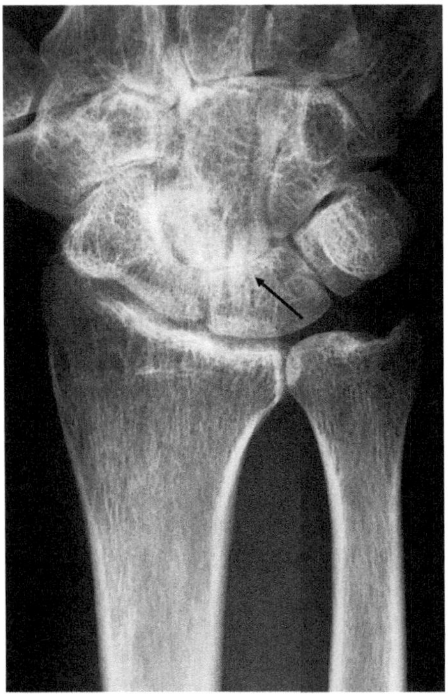

Fig. 24.2 Radiograph of stiff wrist. Narrowing of the midcarpal joint space is shown with black arrow

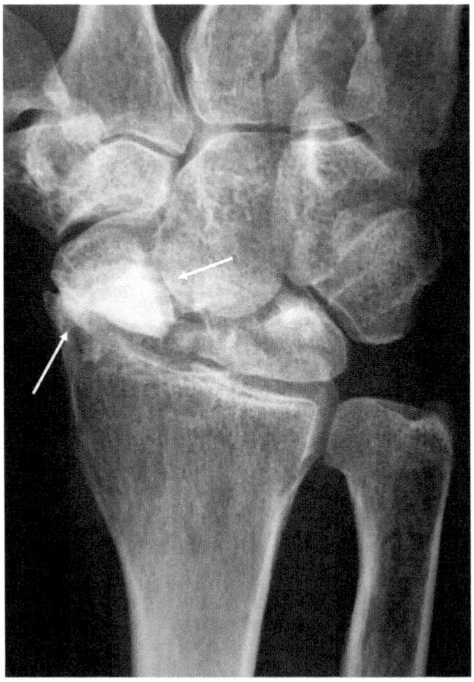

Fig. 24.4 Radiograph of SNAC wrist stage 3 demonstrates the severe joint space narrowing at the scaphoradial and scaphocapitate joint interval (white arrows)

24.2.2 Computed Tomography (CT)

CT demonstrates multiple planes of the wrist, such as coronal, sagittal, or axial views with three-dimensional (3D) reconstruction. It can demonstrate narrowing of the joint space in the specific part in the RCJ or MCJ in the stiff wrist, sometimes the coalition of the carpal bone(s). CT also demonstrates scaphoid nonunion in the SNAC wrist [3] and scapholunate gap in the SLAC wrist.

24.2.3 MRI

MRI is a noninvasive image modality. There are several pulse sequences for delineating the wrist well, such as gradient echo T2*-weighted image, proton-weighted image, or fat suppression T1- or T2-weighted image [4]. All images show low intensity in the bone marrow; thus, joint cartilage indicates high signal intensity and triangular fibrocartilage complex (TFCC) demonstrates low signal intensity. High contrast of low and high signals in these image modality [4, 5] and 3-T MRI [6] indicates details of small structure of the wrist. Normal T1- or T2-weighted images cannot demonstrate TFCC well. In the stiff wrist, MRI can indicate narrowing or defect of the joint hyaline cartilage (Fig. 24.5).

24.2.4 Arthrogram

Arthrogram is considered a classical image modality. Author still uses arthrogram for diagnosis of TFCC lesions. Radiologic dye is injected into the RCJ, MCJ, and/or DRUJ using 23G needle [7, 8]. In the stiff wrist, arthrogram directly indicates narrowing of the joint space with difficulty of dye intrusion to the space (Fig. 24.6).

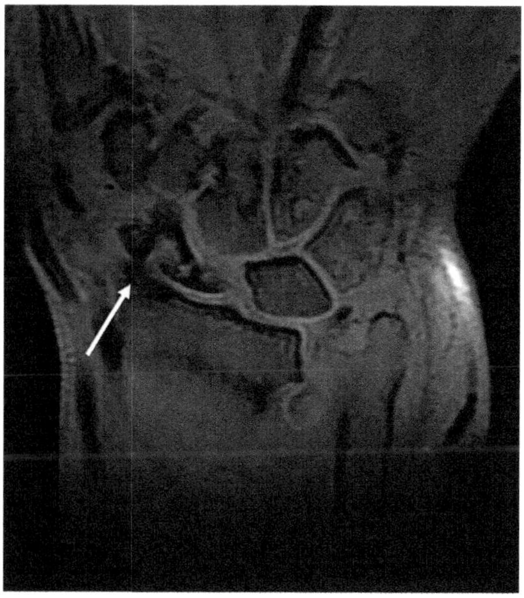

Fig. 24.5 Joint space narrowing and cartilage loss at the radiocarpal joint (white arrow) are noted on MRI of the SNAC wrist

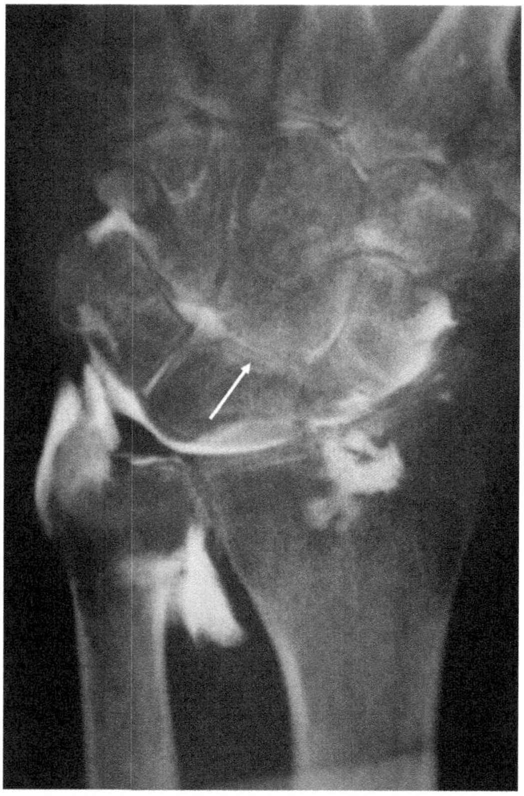

Fig. 24.6 Arthrogram of the wrist contracture indicates severe joint space narrowing and less radiographic dye intrusion in the midcarpal joint space (white arrow)

24.2.5 Arthro-CT Scan

Arthro-CT can be taken soon after the arthrogram. Radiologic dye is normally absorbed 2–3 h after the arthrogram, so it is necessary to take CT within this period. Detailed coronal, sagittal, or axial images are used for diagnosis [9, 10]. In the stiff wrist, narrowing of the joint space, less intrusion of the radiologic dye in the space, or defect of the joint cartilage is seen on arthro-CT (Fig. 24.7).

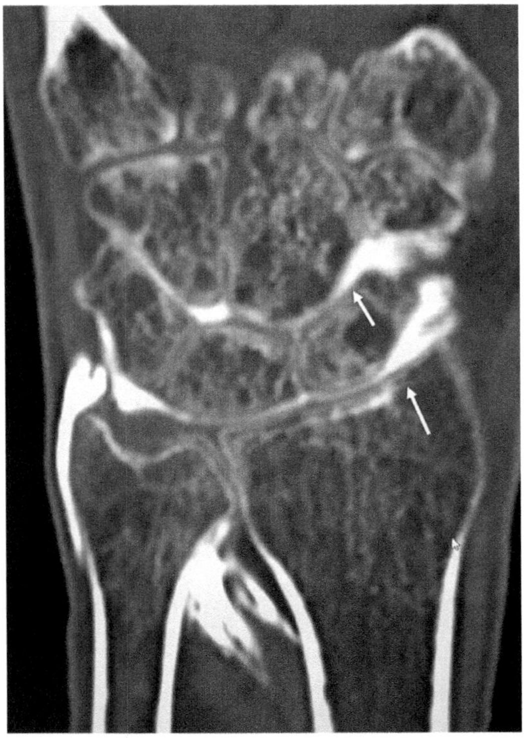

Fig. 24.7 Arthro-CT of the stiff wrist. Joint cartilage is lost at the radius scaphoid fossa, scaphoid, and capitate (white arrows)

References

1. Saffar P. Extrinsic and intrinsic causes of radiocarpal stiffness. In: Copeland SA, Gschwend N, Landi A, et al., editors. Joint stiffness of the upper limb. London: Martin Dunitz; 1997. p. 149–67.
2. Watson HK, Ballet FL. The SLAC wrist: scapholunate advanced pattern of degenerative arthritis. J Hand Surg. 1984;9A:358–65.
3. Miyamura S, Shiode R, Lans J, et al. Quantitative 3-D CT demonstrates distal row pronation and translation and radiolunate arthritis in the SNAC wrist. J Bone Joint Surg Am. 2023;105(17):1329–37. https://doi.org/10.2106/JBJS.22.01350.
4. Nakamura T, Yabe Y, Horiuchi Y. Fat suppression magnetic resonance imaging of the triangular fibrocartilage complex-comparison with spin echo, gradient echo pulse sequence and histology. J Hand Surg Br. 1999;24(1):22–6.
5. Tanaka T, Yoshioka H, Ueno T, et al. Comparison between high-resolution MRI with a microscopy coil and arthroscopy in triangular fibrocartilage complex injury. J Hand Surg Am. 2006;31(8):1308–14.
6. Magee T. Comparison of 3-T MRI and arthroscopy of intrinsic wrist ligament and TFCC tears. Am J Roentgenol. 2009;192(1):80–5.
7. Zinberg EM, Palmer AK, Coren AB, et al. The triple-injection wrist arthrogram. J Hand Surg Am. 1988;13(6):803–9.
8. Roth JH, Haddad RG. Radiocarpal arthroscopy and arthrography in the diagnosis of ulnar wrist pain. Arthroscopy. 1986;2(4):234–43.
9. Moritomo H, Arimitsu S, Kubo N, et al. Computed tomography arthrography using a radial plane view for the detection of triangular fibrocartilage complex foveal tears. J Hand Surg Am. 2015;40(2):245–51.
10. Belhaouane R, Lebeau N, Maes-Clavier C, et al. Reproducibility of X-rays and CT arthrography in SLAC, SNAC, SCAC wrists. Hand Surg Rehabil. 2016;35(6):393–400. https://doi.org/10.1016/j.hansur.2016.08.006.

Part VII

Surgical Treatment of Wrist Stiffness

25 Preoperative Planning (Soft Tissue and Bony Considerations)

Amanda I. Zeng, Stephanie T. Kha, and Jeffrey Yao

25.1 Introduction

Wrist stiffness represents a broad spectrum of pathologies that require a careful diagnostic and therapeutic approach to manage and treat appropriately. In wrist stiffness secondary to idiopathic osteoarthritis, post-traumatic arthritis (such as due to scapholunate advanced collapse [SLAC] and scaphoid nonunion advanced collapse [SNAC]), or rheumatoid arthritis (RA), the treatment algorithms include both nonoperative as well operative management. When patients have symptoms of significant limited range of motion in the wrist that causes substantial disability and have failed conservative management, physicians can discuss surgical treatment options. For surgical management of wrist stiffness, it is very important to be aware of soft tissue and bony considerations during the preoperative planning stage to optimize outcomes and achieve the desired result. In this chapter, we will review these soft tissue and bony considerations for the many different surgical treatment options for wrist stiffness secondary to degenerative arthropathies of the wrist.

A. I. Zeng
Stanford University, Stanford, CA, USA
e-mail: azeng@stanford.edu

S. T. Kha (✉) · J. Yao
Department of Orthopedic Surgery, Stanford University, Stanford, CA, USA
e-mail: skha@email.stanford.edu; skha@stanford.edu; jyao@stanford.edu

25.2 SLAC and SNAC Wrist

In SLAC wrist, the most common degenerative condition of the wrist, there are progressive deformity, instability, and arthritis that affect the radiocarpal and midcarpal joints of the wrist [1]. Decreased wrist range of motion and weaker grip strength lead to abnormal joint kinematics that can lead to symptoms of pain aggravated by heavy use of the wrist. Progression of SLAC wrist is staged by the Watson classification describing the location of arthritis [2]. In stage 1 SLAC wrist, there is arthritis between the scaphoid and the radial styloid. Surgical treatment includes radial styloidectomy and scaphoid stabilization, or posterior interosseous nerve (PIN) and anterior interosseous nerve (AIN) denervation. In stage 2 SLAC, progression of arthritis is now seen between the scaphoid and the entire scaphoid facet of the radius. Surgical treatment includes proximal row carpectomy (PRC). A radiographic example of PRC is demonstrated in Fig. 25.1. In stage 3 SLAC involving arthritis between the capitate and lunate, surgical treatment options include scaphoid excision and four-corner fusion or total wrist fusion. A radiographic example of scaphoid excision and four-corner fusion is demonstrated in Fig. 25.2.

L. Pederzini et al. (eds.), *Stiffness of the Elbow, Wrist and Related Pathologies*,
https://doi.org/10.1007/978-3-031-81381-8_25

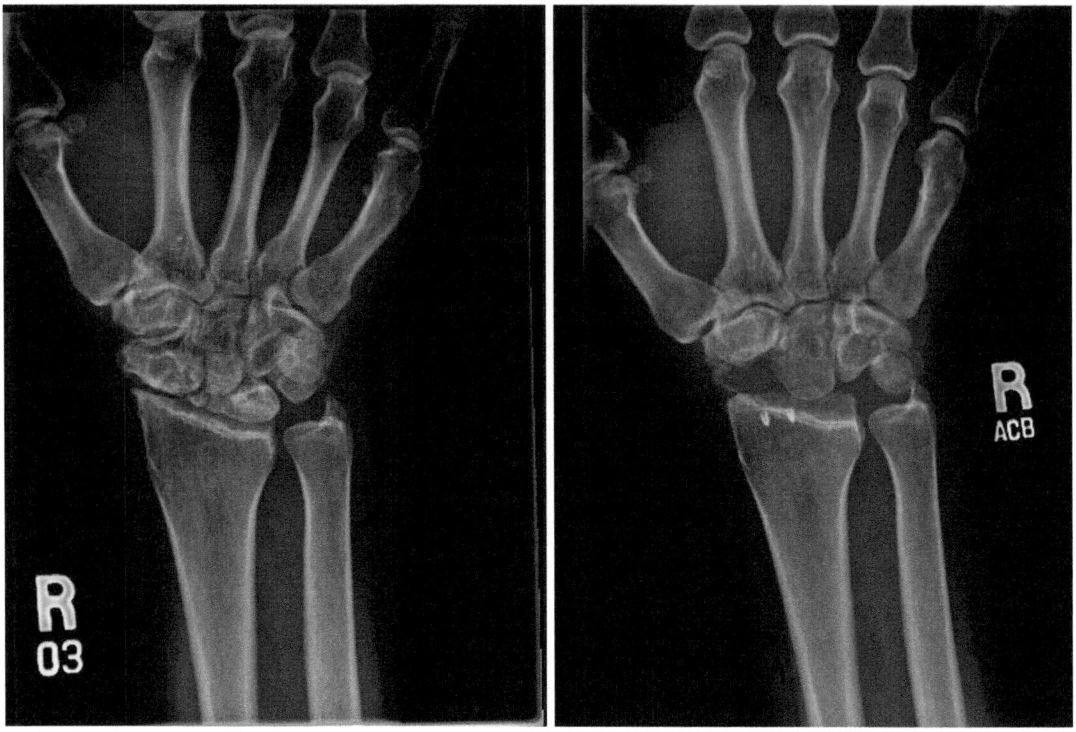

Fig. 25.1 Preoperative and postoperative radiographs of a patient who underwent proximal row carpectomy

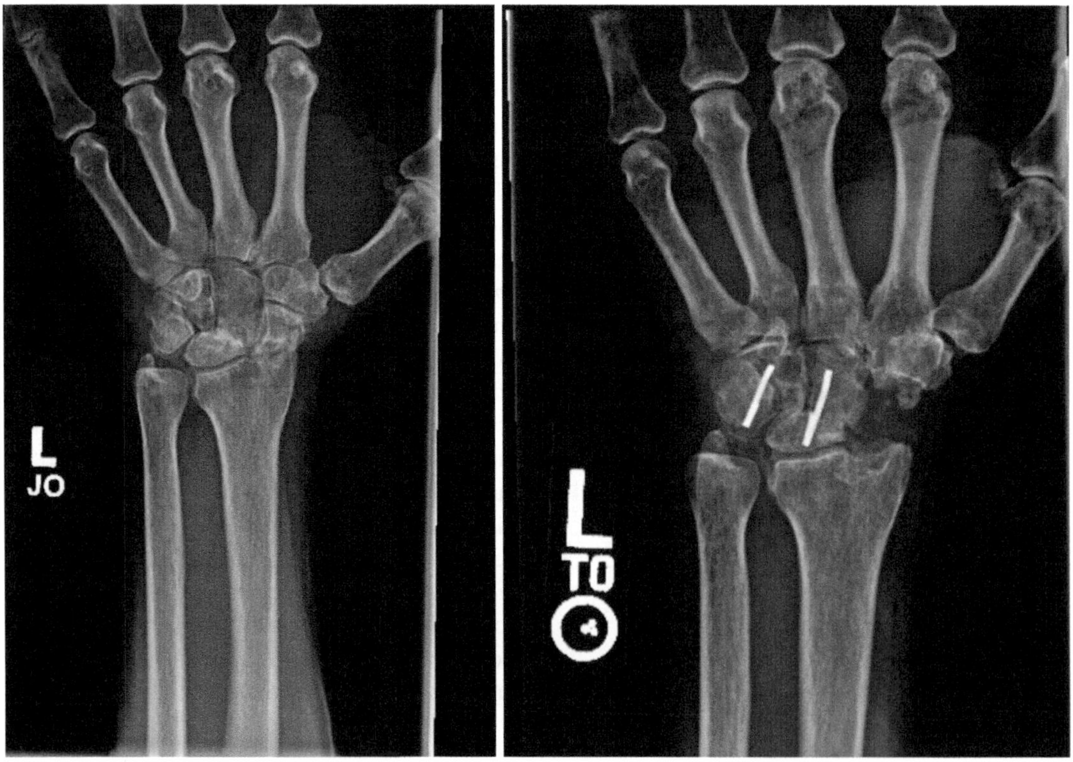

Fig. 25.2 Preoperative and postoperative radiographs of a patient who underwent scaphoid excision with four-corner fusion

Scaphoid nonunion advanced collapse (SNAC) is another common degenerative wrist condition in which scaphoid fracture and subsequent nonunion lead to disrupted joint kinematics in the wrist. Consequent joint deformities and biomechanical imbalances of the wrist will lead to the development of degenerative arthritis changes. SNAC mirrors SLAC in that it follows a similar progressive onset pattern of arthritis and can be treated similarly. Progression of SNAC wrist is classified by Vender et al. based on localized degenerative changes. In stage I SNAC wrist, there are preliminary arthritic changes to the radial styloid and distal scaphoid fragments. Surgical treatment includes radial styloidectomy plus scapholunate reduction and stabilization. Arthritic changes in stage II SNAC wrist progress and reach the proximal scaphoid capitate joint. Surgical treatment consists of proximal row carpectomy, four-corner fusion, or capitolunate arthrodesis. In stage III SNAC wrist in which arthritis changes involve the radioscaphoid, scaphocapitate and capitolunate joints, surgical treatment is partial or total wrist fusion.

For radial styloidectomy and scaphoid stabilization in stage I SLAC and stage I SNAC wrist, important preoperative considerations include type of approach (i.e., open vs. arthroscopic-assisted approach) and amount of resection in relation to carpal stability. Traditionally, radial styloidectomy was performed through an open incision directly over the radial styloid; however, arthroscopic techniques have been well-described in the literature and provide the benefit of direct visualization of the resection while visualizing and preserving volar ligaments necessary for wrist stability [3–6]. In a biomechanical study evaluating the implication of different millimeters of resection for the radial styloidectomy, Nakamura et al. found that the risk of carpal instability increased at 6 and 10 mm of radial styloidectomy, therefore recommending that the styloid resection be limited to 3–4 mm [7].

In the past, Wilhelm first recommended total wrist denervation for patients with chronic wrist pain. However, selective partial denervation procedures are being performed more commonly [8–10]. In fact, posterior interosseous nerve (PIN) and anterior interosseous nerve (AIN) denervation for stage II SLAC wrist can help alleviate pain while sparing motor and sensory function. The procedure is typically performed in conjunction with other midcarpal procedures including proximal row carpectomy and four-corner fusion; however, the denervation can also be performed as an isolated procedure. Preoperative considerations include use of a diagnostic nerve block, incisional technique (i.e., single dorsal incision vs. the more traditional multiple-incision technique), and location of incision. A preoperative diagnostic nerve block, which can be conducted by injecting 1% lidocaine localized 1 cm proximal to the dorsal head of the ulna, may be useful to determine which patients theoretically will benefit from denervation procedure [11, 12]. In terms of incisional technique, in a cadaveric study analyzing the anatomical considerations of AIN denervation, Berger et al. discovered that the close anatomical proximity of the PIN and AIN allows transection of PIN and AIN via a single dorsal incision [13]. However, Lin et al. suggest that Berger's AIN denervation via a 2-cm dorsal neurectomy technique poses risk to the motor branches to the pronator quadratus [8]. Although Berger's technique reduces the number of incisions and provides excellent visual exposure of the PIN, Lin et al. argue that the procedure lacks sufficient exposure of the motor branches to the pronator quadratus muscle during the AIN resection. To avoid denervating the pronator quadratus completely, Lin et al. suggest that the AIN resection be performed at the distal border of the pronator quadratus [8].

Significant preoperative considerations for proximal row carpectomy for stage II SLAC and stage II SNAC wrist include location of arthritis and efficacy of modified PRC techniques. In particular, patients with degenerative changes at the radioscaphoid articulation or avascular necrosis of the lunate are candidates for proximal row carpectomy (PRC) [14]. However, PRC is not suitable for patients with capitolunate arthritis [15, 16]. Articular surfaces, specifically the surface of the scaphoid, also need to be intact to facilitate sufficient bone support for proper articulation [14]. Proximal row carpectomy is advantageous given its technical simplicity and predictable results. However, Imbriglia et al. found that standard PRC alters the biomechanics of the wrist joint by creating a difference in radii of curvature between the capitate and lunate facet. This not only causes stress at the new articulation site, but also can lead to dorsal and volar instability with wrist flexion and extension [17]. To address this, some authors have recommended the placement of an interposition arthroplasty that aims to recreate anatomical radiocarpal pressures. Nanavati et al. found the insertion of a lateral meniscal interposition allograft in conjunction with PRC statistically restored pressures and areas that resemble the normal wrist [18]. Lee et al. found that PRC with interposition arthroplasty via a decellularized dermal allograft in wrists with degenerative changes at the capitate compares favorably with standard PRC on less arthritic wrists [19]. Lee et al. argue that interposition arthroplasty is effective in expanding the indications for PRC and can help avoid more invasive salvage procedures when more extensive arthritis is encountered [19].

Four-corner fusion with scaphoid excision is also a common surgical procedure to treat stage III SLAC and stage II SNAC wrist that involves the resection of the scaphoid bone and fusion of the lunate, capitate, humate, and triquetrum bones. Important preoperative considerations for four-corner fusion include type of approach (i.e., open vs. arthroscopic) and method of incision to maximize exposure of the carpus. Traditionally for the open approach, a dorsal midline incision localized over the third metacarpal-capitate-lunate-radius axis is used to expose the carpus [20]. This longitudinal incision may present inadequate exposure and could require excessive retraction of the soft tissue flaps. Alternatively, a T-shaped incision allows for increased exposure without extensive dissection [20, 21]. The transverse limb of the "T" lies over the midcarpal joint and the longitudinal limb extends 3–4 cm starting from the center of the transverse limb [21]. Meanwhile, arthroscopic-assisted four-corner fusion utilizes standard wrist arthroscopy setup and portals. The arthroscopic fusion procedure is technically demanding with a steep learning curve; however, it has potential to minimize surgical trauma, achieve shorter mobilization periods, and promote better range of motion and grip strength results [22]. Arthroscopic four-corner fusion should be performed by specialists who have overcome this learning curve to avoid the risk of revision surgeries.

Other essential preoperative considerations for four-corner fusion involve the method of fixation. The traditional technique for four-corner fusion uses Kirschner wires (K-wires), memory staples, or compression screws for midcarpal fixation. However, in 1999, circular plates were introduced which offered a simpler method of internal fixation and earlier mobilization of the wrist [23, 24]. While circular plate fixation has been shown to achieve better postoperative results regarding grip strength and range of motion, Vance et al. concluded that circular plate fixation resulted in higher complication, impingement, and nonunion rates than traditional fixation techniques [25]. In fact, Vance et al. reported that circular plate fixation in 27 patients resulted in a nonunion rate of 26% and a hardware impingement of 22% [25]. However, Ashmead found that out of 100 cases of four-corner fusion for SLAC wrist using Kirschner wires, only 3% of patients developed nonunion and 12% of patients showed signs of dorsal impingement [26]. To avoid impingement altogether, surgeons can consider using headless compression screws for midcarpal fusion. The containment of the headless screws within the outer dimensions of the carpal bones significantly reduces the risk of impingement while achieving proper alignment of the capitolunate relationship [27]. Shintani found that a triangle fixation technique using three headless screws resulted in a shorter splint immobilization period and more satisfactory results compared to the conventional K-wire technique [28].

Preoperative considerations for total wrist fusion for stage III SLAC and stage III SNAC wrist include the traditional open wrist versus arthroscopic approach and method of fixation. Arthroscopic-assisted total wrist arthrodesis presents superior cosmetic advantages and prevents high carpal tunnel syndrome rates and demand for bone grafts that are associated with the open surgical technique [29].

25.3 Rheumatoid Arthritis of the Wrist

Rheumatoid arthritis (RA) of the wrist is an autoimmune disease that attacks the lining of one's joints, cartilage, and bone. This chronic inflammatory disease is not only painful but can progress into bone erosion and joint deformity. Subsequently, these degenerative changes can disrupt the kinematics of the distal radioulnar joint (DRUJ). Alongside SLAC and SNAC, common symptoms of wrist RA include stiffness, loss of grip strength, and pain stimulated by forearm rotation. Simmen and Huber introduced a new classification of the type of destruction of rheumatoid arthritis based on its natural course [30]. In type I RA, there is a spontaneous tendency for stiffness and immobility of the joints and bones. Surgical treatment includes a Darrach procedure or dorsal wrist synovectomy [31, 32]. Type II RA is an arthritic type that resembles osteoarthritic changes. Surgical treatment involves a Darrach procedure, radiolunate fusion, or the Sauvé-Kapandji procedure [32]. Type III RA is a disintegrating process involving ligamentous destabilization, loss of carpal alignment, and total collapse of the carpal architecture. Surgical treatment consists of total wrist arthroplasty or wrist fusion [32].

The Darrach distal ulna resection procedure for type I and II RA wrist is an excision of the distal ulna to manage chronic DRUJ instability and provide pain relief. The procedure is generally performed using a dorsal approach through the fifth dorsal compartment. Once the joint is exposed, the distal ulna can be removed using oblique and straight cuts. Important preoperative considerations include the amount of ulna resected relative to carpal stability and the efficacy of supplementary procedures following the Darrach procedure. When resecting the ulna, it is important to minimize the amount of ulna removed. Tulipan achieved good success, carrying a success rate of 91% among his patients [33]. Yet, Tulipan stressed that the Darrach procedure be carried out with minimal bony resection and precise soft tissue reconstruction in order to avoid stump instability [33, 34]. While Tulipan achieved desired results with the isolated Darrach procedure, others recommend that the Darrach procedure be conducted in conjunction with ulnar stump stabilization procedures to avoid ulnar carpal drift [34–36]. In particular, Ishikawa recommended that the Darrach procedure be followed by a wrist extensor tendon transfer or partial radiocarpal fusion [37].

The primary preoperative consideration for the Sauvé-Kapandji procedure for type II RA is the amount of ulna resected relative to ulnar instability and methods of proximal ulnar stump stabilization. To minimize risk of ulnar translation, the Sauvé-Kapandji procedure aims to create a radioulnar fusion between the ulnar head and distal radius [34]. The procedure involves resecting a segment of the ulna, proximal to the arthrodesis site. While a minimum of 1 cm of ulna is typically removed to minimize risk of bony regrowth, Daecke et al. found that a shortening of the proximal stump of less than 35 mm is correlated with greater stability of the stump [34, 38]. The Sauvé-Kapandji is a suitable treatment option for DRUJ disorders, but can occasionally result in postoperative proximal ulnar stump and radioulnar convergence. To prevent these complications, Minami and Lamey found that tenodesis with the extensor carpi ulnaris tendon and flexor carpi ulnaris tendon can achieve good stump stabilization results [39, 40].

For synovectomy for type I or II RA wrists, an important preoperative consideration involves the efficacy of an open versus arthroscopic-assisted approach. Traditionally, an open synovectomy in RA of the wrist allows for more extensive inspection of all wrist compartments [41]. However, an arthroscopic-assisted synovectomy has been introduced that allows for easier access to radiocarpal and midcarpal areas and minimization of damage to the joint capsule and ligaments [41]. Arthroscopic synovectomy also serves as an opportunity to delay the demand for more complex procedures including wrist fusion or total wrist arthroplasty, thus making the procedure more suitable for RA wrists with less advanced arthritic changes. In particular, Park analyzed the results of arthroscopic synovectomy in 18 patients and found that the procedure was effective in achieving pain relief and wrist functionality for those in early stage RA wrist [42]. However, while arthroscopic synovectomy is less invasive, it is impossible to treat the extensor tendons or reconstruct the soft tissue. Hence, in a situation in which the extensor tendons are involved, open synovectomy is necessary prevent and address any potential tendon rupture and instability [43].

Preoperative considerations for radiolunate fusion for type II RA wrist include method of fixation via K-wires, plates, screws, compression screws, or staples. The procedure is typically performed through a standard dorsal approach. Prior to fusion, it is essential to fix the lunate to a neutral position relative to the radius. Extension of the lunate will limit wrist flexion. In a comparison study analyzing the implementation of Shapiro staples, plate, and obliques in radiolunate fusion, Gaulke et al. found that the miniplate and oblique screw achieved superior results over the staple fixation technique [44]. Plate and oblique screw fixation showed much greater flexibility than the staple fixation. Likewise, in a study looking just at Shapiro staples, Gaulke found that staple fixation of the radiolunate joint was associated with a high complication rate and evidence of early fusion loosening [45].

Significant preoperative considerations for wrist fusion for type III RA wrist include pin versus plate osteosynthesis and position of arthrodesis. There are two primary techniques of fixation: the Mannerfelt and AO-plate fixation method. As the most commonly used technique in treating RA wrist, Mannerfelt arthrodesis uses a Rush pin for fixation of the carpal bones. AO-plate fixation of wrist fusion also generates promising results and achieves good carpal stability. However, in a comparison study, Toma found that plate fixation had a 26% higher complication rate than the Mannerfelt technique, likely due to direct soft tissue irritation by the plate [46]. The position of the fused wrist is also an important consideration. The optimal position for fixation is slight extension of 10–20° and ulnar deviation of 5–10° [34, 47, 48]. In a study evaluating the long-term efficacy of wrist fusion, Barbier found that the average position of fusion was 8° extension and 9° ulnar deviation, and all patients experienced satisfactory pain relief [49]. Likewise, Lautenbach found that an arthrodesis using the Mannerfelt technique in a slightly extended position achieved the best patient ratings and postoperative results [47]. However, some authors recommend fusion in the neutral position, arguing that it allows for better pronosupination and stronger balancing of the extensor and flexor tendons [34, 46, 47].

For wrist arthroplasty in type III RA wrist, preoperative considerations primarily involve choice of implant design. These prostheses aim to replicate the natural center of motion to improve wrist balance and range of motion [50]. The early designs were silicone implants. However, due to a high incidence rate of implant breakage and prominent silicone synovitis, new metal designs were introduced. In particular, the BIAX total wrist prosthesis and universal total wrist implant attempted to minimize the amount of bone resection, but were correlated with complications regarding carpal stem breakout from the metacarpal and dislocation respectively [51]. Modern-day metal-polyethylene implants are designed to maximize bone stock and minimize carpal instability by being attached to the radius via bony ingrowth rather than cement interface [51].

There are three implant systems currently used in the United States that optimize clinical outcomes: the ReMotion Total Wrist System (Stryker, Kalamazoo, MI), the Universal 2 Implant System (Integra LifeSciences, Plainsboro, NJ), and the Maestro Total Wrist System (Biomet, Warsaw, IN). While all three prostheses offer improved postoperative results relating to grip strength, range of motion, pain, and performance measures, each technique has its own unique advantages. Herzberg found that the ReMotion prostheses achieved more favorable results and lower complication incidences than the older generation TWAs [52]. Likewise, in comparing the ReMotion prosthesis with the older BIAX implant and the Maestro implant, Sagerfors et al. noticed significant improvements in implant survival and postoperative measures in the modern-day designs [53, 54]. After 8 years, the cumulative implant survival rate was 81% for the Biax implant, 94% for ReMotion, and 95%

for Maestro implants [53]. Two percent of the Maestro implants experienced radiographic loosening compared to the 18% of those with ReMotion [53].

25.4 Capsular Contracture Release for Wrist Stiffness

Surgical arthrolysis is another surgical option for treating wrist stiffness. The procedure can be conducted openly or arthroscopically. Preoperative considerations when deciding between the two techniques include the joint associated with the limited range of motion and the origin of wrist stiffness. Localization of wrist stiffness depends on the damaged site, which typically involves the radiocarpal or DRUJ joint. Wrist arthrolysis is commonly performed on the radiocarpal joint to enhance flexion–extension and/or the DRUJ to improve pronosupination articular range of motion [55].

While arthroscopic arthrolysis is generally more minimally invasive than traditional open arthrolysis, arthroscopic arthrolysis of the DRUJ is technically demanding and holds a steep learning curve. Some authors advocate for open arthrolysis in severe conditions, where capsular contraction coupled with intra-articular tissue synovitis, fibrosis, and adhesions can obstruct visibility of the joint, leading to a lengthy and potentially more risky procedure if attempted arthroscopically [55–58]. Meanwhile, Verhellen et al. found that arthroscopic capsular contracture release of the radiocarpal joint is a safe and minimal invasive technique that provides noticeable improvements to wrist range of motion [59]. While relative indications may vary among providers, the arthroscopic approach for capsular contracture release may be more appropriate for wrists with capsular contracture as the origin of stiffness, normal articular cartilage and congruity, and no evidence of arthropathy of the joints [59]. Assessment of articular cartilage and arthritic changes can be evaluated with imaging modalities that include radiographs, computed tomography (CT), and/or magnetic resonance imaging (MRI) during the preoperative period.

25.5 Preoperative Imaging Considerations

Radiographs remain as a fundamental aspect of the evaluation of patients presenting with wrist stiffness [60, 61]. Radiographs can measure two-dimensional (2D) changes in angle or length of wrist bones through different motions (flexion, extension, radial or ulnar deviation) [62]. Fluoroscopy can also be valuable to examine dynamic pathology or instability of the wrist [60]. When evaluating patients with wrist arthritis and selecting the most appropriate surgical treatment, surgeons utilize radiographs to determine the degree of advanced arthritis in both the radiocarpal and midcarpal regions [61]. However, intraoperative assessment does not always correlate with radiographic findings; therefore, surgeons must be prepared to change operative course as needed based on intraoperative findings [63].

CT and MRI imaging are advanced imaging techniques that are certainly useful in understanding wrist pathology and evaluating bony and soft tissue anatomy. However, a recent scoping review by Baylosis et al. reported that most studies do not report specifically on how certain CT or MRI findings change the surgical decision-making process [61]. CT scans can help demonstrate carpal bone morphology when planning for any bony work or arthrodesis procedures. CT imaging also has better spatial resolution to capture subtleties in the articular surfaces between carpal bones, and 3D reconstruction techniques can allow surgeons to carefully evaluate bony alignment prior to surgery [62]. Meanwhile, MRI can allow for the evaluation of the integrity of extrinsic and intrinsic ligaments of the wrist which can act as secondary joint stabilizers that help to maintain carpal alignment. For example, the dorsal intercarpal and dorsal radiocarpal ligaments are stabilizers of the proximal carpal row during wrist motion, the radioscaphocapitate ligament helps to stabilize radiocarpal pronation and ulnar translocation, and the short and long radiolunate ligaments stabilize the wrist through restricting lunate motion [62]. Evaluating these ligaments ahead of time on MRI and understanding where they attach can be important in the preoperative planning period because changes in bony alignment during surgery or any injury to these ligaments intra-operatively can lead to destabilization of the wrist with particular motions.

Despite the recognized general usefulness of CT and MRI imaging modalities in understanding each patient's unique wrist anatomy, the utility of cross-section imaging during the preoperative period remains an area for future research opportunities to clearly define the role of these imaging techniques when planning surgical treatment for patients with wrist stiffness [61].

25.6 Conclusion

In summary, wrist stiffness secondary to degenerative arthropathies or rheumatoid arthritis has a broad range of surgical treatment options. Prior studies in the literature have helped surgeons better understand indications, contraindications, benefit and risk profiles, and technical pearls and pitfalls in order to optimize clinical outcomes for patients. Preoperative planning is critical. Radiographs remain a fundamental aspect of the imaging workup prior to any surgical treatment, and CT/MRI modalities allow for further evaluation of the carpal bones, articulations, and ligamentous stabilizers. Surgeons should be aware of these soft tissue and bony considerations during the preoperative planning stage in order to optimize outcomes and achieve the goals of surgery.

Funding/Grant Support This research did not receive any specific grant from funding agencies in the public, commercial, or not-for-profit sectors.

References

1. Lane R, Tafti D, Varacallo M. Scapholunate advanced collapse. In: StatPearls [Internet]. Treasure Island, FL: StatPearls Publishing; 2022. [cited 2022 Dec 30]. Available from: http://www.ncbi.nlm.nih.gov/books/NBK537124/.
2. McLean A, Taylor F. Classifications in brief: Watson and Ballet classification of Scapholunate advanced collapse wrist arthritis. Clin Orthop Relat Res. 2019;477:663–6.
3. Kalainov DM, Cohen MS, Sweet S. Radial styloidectomy. In: Geissler WB, editor. Wrist arthroscopy. New York, NY: Springer; 2005.
4. Plancher KD, Mangonon ML, Petterson SC. Wrist arthritis: arthroscopic techniques of synovectomy, abrasion chondroplasty, radial Styloidectomy, and Proximal row carpectomy of the wrist. In: Geissler WB, editor. Wrist and elbow arthroscopy with selected open procedures. Cham: Springer; 2022.
5. Herzberg G. Isolated arthroscopic radial styloidectomy: the three-portal approach. J Hand Surg. 2020;9:353–6.
6. Yao J, Osterman AL. Arthroscopic techniques for wrist arthritis (radial styloidectomy and proximal pole hamate excisions). Hand Clinics. 2005;21:519–26. Elsevier.
7. Nakamura T, Cooney WP III, Lui W-H, Haugstvedt J-R, Zhao KD, Berglund L, et al. Radial styloidectomy: a biomechanical study on stability of the wrist joint. J Hand Surg. 2001;26:85–93. Elsevier.
8. Lin DL, Lenhart MK, Farber GL. Anatomy of the anterior interosseous innervation of the pronator quadratus: evaluation of structures at risk in the single dorsal incision wrist denervation technique. J Hand Surg. 2006;31:904–7. Elsevier.
9. Chin KW, Engelsman AF, van Gulik TM, Strackee SD. Selective denervation of the wrist for chronic pain: a systematic literature review. J Hand Surg Eur Vol. 2020;45:265–72. SAGE Publications Sage UK: London, England.
10. Vanden Berge DJ, Kusnezov NA, Rubin S, Dagg T, Orr J, Mitchell J, et al. Outcomes following isolated posterior interosseous nerve neurectomy: a systematic review. Hand. 2017;12:535–40. SAGE Publications Sage CA: Los Angeles, CA.
11. Wilhelm A. Denervation of the wrist. Techniques in hand & upper extremity surgery. LWW. 2001;5:14–30.
12. Milone MT, Klifto CS, Catalano LW III. Partial wrist denervation: the evidence behind a small fix for big problems. J Hand Surg. 2018;43:272–7. Elsevier.
13. Berger RA. Partial denervation of the wrist: a new approach. Techniques in hand & upper extremity surgery. LWW. 1998;2:25–35.
14. Klausmeyer M, Fernandez D. Scaphocapitolunate arthrodesis and radial styloidectomy: a treatment option for posttraumatic degenerative wrist disease. J Wrist Surg. 2012;1:115–22. Thieme Medical Publishers.
15. Balk ML, Imbriglia JE. Proximal row carpectomy: indications, surgical technique, and long-term results. Oper Techn Orthop. 2003;13:42–7. Elsevier.
16. Matthew T. Scapholunate advanced collapse wrist: Proximal row carpectomy or limited wrist arthrodesis with scaphoid excision? J Hand Surg. 1994;19:134–42.
17. Imbriglia JE, Broudy AS, Hagberg WC, McKernan D. Proximal row carpectomy: clinical evaluation. J Hand Surg. 1990;15:426–30. Elsevier.
18. Nanavati VN, Werner FW, Sutton LG, Klena J. Proximal row carpectomy: role of a radiocarpal

interposition lateral meniscal allograft. J Hand Surg. 2009;34:251–7. Elsevier.
19. Lee S. Proximal row carpectomy using decellularized dermal allograft: preliminary results. J Wrist Surg. 2021;10:116–22.
20. Shin AMD. Four-corner arthrodesis. J Am Soc Surg Hand. 2001;1:93–111.
21. Dao KD, Shin AY, Berger RA. T incision for exposure of the distal radius and wrist. J Hand Surg Br. 2000;25:544–7. Elsevier.
22. Vihanto A, Kotkansalo T, Pääkkönen M. The learning curve and pitfalls of arthroscopic four-corner arthrodesis. J Wrist Surg. 2019;8(3):202–8.
23. Ahmadi AR, Duraku LS, van der Oest MJW. The never-ending battle between proximal row carpectomy and four corner arthrodesis: a systematic review and meta-analysis for the final verdict. J Plastic Reconstr Aesthet Surg. 2022;75:711–21.
24. Bedford B, Yang SS. High fusion rates with circular plate fixation for four-corner arthrodesis of the wrist. Clin Orthop Relat Res. 2010;468:163–8. Springer
25. Vance M. Complications and outcome of four-corner arthrodesis: circular plate fixation versus traditional techniques. J Hand Surg. 2005;30:1122–7.
26. Ashmead D IV, Watson HK, Damon C, Herber S, Paly W. Scapholunate advanced collapse wrist salvage. J Hand Surg. 1994;19:741–50. Elsevier.
27. Henry M. Internal headless compression screw method for 4-corner fusion. J Hand Microsurg. 2009;1:45–9. Thieme Medical and Scientific Publishers Private Ltd.
28. Shintani K, Kazuki K, Takamatsu K, Yoneda M, Uemura T. Limited wrist arthrodesis for scapholunate advanced collapse wrist: triangle fixation for four-corner fusion. J Hand Surg Asian Pac Vol. 2016;21:207–11. World Scientific.
29. Nazerani S, Nazerani T, Molayem A, Keramati MR. A modified surgical technique for minimally invasive arthroscopic total wrist fusion. J Wrist Surg. 2019;8:084–8. Thieme Medical Publishers.
30. Simmen BR, Huber H. Das Handgelenk bei derchronischen Polyarthritis-Eine neue Klassifizierung aufgrund des Destruktionstyps des naturlichen Verlaufes und deren Konsequenzen fur die chirurgische Therapie. Handchir Mikrochir Plast Chir. 1994;26:182–9. Stuttgart [Germany]: Hippokrates Verlag; 1982.
31. Flury MPMD, Herren DBMD, Simmen BRMD. Rheumatoid arthritis of the wrist: classification related to the natural course. Clin Orthop Relat Res. 1999;366:72–7.
32. Hodgson SP. The Wrightington classification of rheumatoid wrist X-rays: a guide to surgical management. J Hand Surg. 1989;14:451.
33. Tulipan DJ, Eaton RG, Eberhart RE. The Darrach procedure defended: technique redefined and long-term follow-up. J Hand Surg. 1991;16:438–44. Elsevier.
34. Rizzo M, Cooney WP. Current concepts and treatment for the rheumatoid wrist. Hand Clin. 2011;27:57–72. Elsevier.
35. Syed AA, Lam WL, Agarwal M. Stabilization of the ulna stump after Darrach's procedure at the wrist. Int Orthop (SICOT). 2003;27:235–9.
36. Tsai T-M, Shimizu H, Adkins P. A modified extensor carpi ulnaris tenodesis with the Darrach procedure. J Hand Surg. 1993;18:697–702. Elsevier.
37. Ishikawa H, Hanyu T, Tajima T. Rheumatoid wrists treated with synovectomy of the extensor tendons and the wrist joint combined with a Darrach procedure. J Hand Surg. 1992;17:1109–17. Elsevier.
38. Daecke W, Martini A-K, Schneider S, Streich A, N. Amount of ulnar resection is a predictive factor for ulnar instability problems after the Sauvé-Kapandji procedure: a retrospective study of 44 patients followed for 1–13 years, vol. 77. Acta Orthop; 2006. p. 290–7. Taylor & Francis.
39. Minami A, Iwasaki N, Ishikawa J, Suenaga N, Kato H. Stabilization of the proximal ulnar stump in the Sauvé-Kapandji procedure by using the extensor carpi ulnaris tendon: long-term follow-up studies. J Hand Surg. 2006;31:440–4. Elsevier.
40. Lamey DM, Fernandez DL. Results of the modified Sauvé-Kapandji procedure in the treatment of chronic posttraumatic derangement of the distal radioulnar joint. J Bone Joint Surg Am. 1998;80:1758–69.
41. Kim S-J, Jung K-A. Arthroscopic synovectomy in rheumatoid arthritis of wrist. Clin Med Res. 2007;5:244–50. Marshfield Clinic.
42. Park MJ, Ahn JH, Kang JS. Arthroscopic synovectomy of the wrist in rheumatoid arthritis. J Bone Joint Surg Br Vol. 2003;85:1011–5. The British Editorial Society of Bone and Joint Surgery.
43. Trieb K. Treatment of the wrist in rheumatoid arthritis. J Hand Surg. 2008;33:113–23. Elsevier.
44. Gaulke R, O'Loughlin PF, Probst C, Mommsen P, Oszwald M, Hildebrand F, et al. Comparative biomechanical analysis of two techniques of radiolunate fusion: Shapiro staples vs. plate and oblique screw. Technol Health Care. 2010;18:111–21. IOS Press.
45. Gaulke R, Suppelna G, Hildebrand F, Citak M, Hüfner T, Krettek C. Radiolunate fusion in the rheumatoid wrist with Shapiro staples: clinical and radiological results of 22 cases. J Hand Sur Eur Vol. 2010;35:289–95. Sage Publications Sage UK: London, England.
46. Toma CD, Machacek P, Bitzan P, Assadian O, Trieb K, Wanivenhaus A. Fusion of the wrist in rheumatoid arthritis: a clinical and functional evaluation of two surgical techniques. J Bone Joint Surg Br Vol. 2007;89:1620–6. The British Editorial Society of Bone and Joint Surgery.
47. Lautenbach M, Millrose M, Langner I, Eisenschenk A. Results of Mannerfelt wrist arthrodesis for rheumatoid arthritis in relation to the position of the fused wrist. Int Orthop. 2013;37:2409–13. Springer
48. Trieb K. Arthrodesis of the wrist in rheumatoid arthritis. World J Orthop. 2014;5:512. Baishideng Publishing Group Inc.

49. Barbier O, Saels P, Rombouts J-J, Thonnard J-L. Long-term functional results of wrist arthrodesis in rheumatoid arthritis. J Hand Surg. 1999;24:27–31. SAGE Publications Sage UK: London, England.
50. Adams BD. Wrist arthroplasty: partial and total. Hand Clin. 2013;29(1):79–89.
51. Halim A, Weiss AP. Total wrist arthroplasty. J Hand Surg Am. 2017;42(3):198–209.
52. Herzberg G. Prospective study of a new total wrist arthroplasty: short term results. Chir Main. 2011;30:20–5.
53. Sagerfors M, Gupta A, Brus O, Pettersson K. Total wrist arthroplasty: a single-center study of 219 cases with 5-year follow-up. J Hand Surg. 2015;40:2380–7. Elsevier.
54. Sagerfors M, Gupta A, Brus O, Rizzo M, Pettersson K. Patient related functional outcome after total wrist arthroplasty: a single center study of 206 cases. Hand Surg. 2015;20:81–7. World Scientific.
55. Guidi M, Luchetti R, Besmens I, Rothenfluh E, Calcagni M. Wrist Arthrolysis: a systematic review of open and arthroscopic techniques. J Wrist Surg. 2021;10:543–50.
56. Kleinman W. DRUJ Contracture Release. Tech Hand Up Extrem Surg. 1999;3:13–22.
57. Luchetti R, Atzei A, Fairplay T. Wrist arthrolysis. In: Geissler WB, editor. Wrist arthroscopy [internet]. New York: Springer; 2005. p. 145–54. [cited 2022 Dec 30]. Available from: http://link.springer.com/10.1007/0-387-27087-6_19.
58. Luchetti R, Bain G, Morse L, McGuire D. Arthroscopic arthrolysis. In: Arthroscopy. Cham: Springer; 2016. p. 935–51.
59. Verhellen R, Bain GI. Arthroscopic capsular release for contracture of the wrist: a new technique. Arthroscopy. 2000;16:106–10.
60. Wilson AJ, Mann FA, Gilula LA. Imaging the hand and wrist. J Hand Surg. 1990;15(2):153–67.
61. Baylosis BL, McQuiston AS, Bayne CO. Preoperative imaging for surgical decision-making and the frequency of wrist arthrodesis and carpectomy procedures: a scoping review. Skeletal Radiol. 2023;52:143–50.
62. Kamal RN, Starr A, Akelman E. Carpal kinematics and kinetics. J Hand Surg. 2016;41:1011–8. Elsevier.
63. Zinberg EM, Chi Y. Proximal row carpectomy versus scaphoid excision and intercarpal arthrodesis: intraoperative assessment and procedure selection. J Hand Surg. 2014;39:1055–62. Elsevier.

Open Management of the Stiff Wrist

26

Toshiyasu Nakamura

26.1 Introduction

Contracture of the wrist joint or stiff wrist indicates limited range of motion (ROM) actively and passively, and it typically is caused by fibrosis of the soft tissue including the capsule or supporting ligament around the joint [1]. The other causes are skin contracture, such as burn, and heterotopic ossification inside the wrist joint [2]. The wrist is the important joint between the elbow and the hand to achieve handling the object to the mouth, throwing, hammering, or writing. Loss of the range of motion (ROM) of the wrist caused by the wrist contracture induces severe restriction in activity of daily life.

Conservative treatment is normally selected in early phase of the stiff wrist or wrist contracture for 3 months, then forwarded to surgical treatments. Most popular surgery for stiff wrist nowadays is arthroscopic joint release [3–5], while some of the cases still require open release [6].

T. Nakamura (✉)
Department of Orthopaedic Surgery, School of Medicine, International University of Health and Welfare, Tokyo, Japan
e-mail: toshiyasu@ae.em-net.ne.jp

26.2 Anatomy of the Wrist

The wrist is the complex joint that consists of the radiocarpal joint (RCJ), midcarpal joint (MCJ) and distal radioulnar joint (DRUJ), achieving flexion–extension, radial–ulnar deviation, and pronation–supination [7]. In the radiocarpal joint, the proximal carpal row including the scaphoid, lunate, and triquetrum faces to the radius. The surface of the radius to the scaphoid is called the scaphoid fossa and the surface to the lunate is called the lunate fossa. The triquetrum attaches to the distal surface of the triangular fibrocartilage complex (TFCC), then the TFCC attaches to the ulnar head [8]. The midcarpal joint is the S-shaped joint consisting of the proximal row of the carpus (scaphoid, lunate, and triquetrum) and distal carpal row (trapezium, trapezoid, capitate, and hamate). The joint between the scaphoid and trapezium-trapezoid is named STT joint. In the distal radioulnar joint, the sigmoid notch of the radius faces to the ulna head [8]. Flexion and extension motion or radial–ulnar deviation motion is mainly occurred at the radiocarpal and midcarpal joint [7, 9]. Forearm pronation-supination motion (rotation) is achieved by the DRUJ and proximal radioulnar joint (PRUJ). If the fibrosis occurs at the radiocarpal or midcarpal (or both), flexion–extension motion and radial–ulnar deviation motion are restricted easily. If there is a contracture occurs at the DRUJ, patients indicate severe loss of forearm pronosupination.

L. Pederzini et al. (eds.), *Stiffness of the Elbow, Wrist and Related Pathologies*,
https://doi.org/10.1007/978-3-031-81381-8_26

The TFCC is the unique structure in the ulnar side of the wrist [8]. It locates between the radius, ulna, lunate, and triquetrum. Function of the TFCC is (1) inducing smooth wrist motion including flexion–extension, radial–ulnar deviation and pronosupination; (2) load distribution between the ulna and ulnar carpus; and (3) providing stability of the DRUJ and ulnocarpal joint. The TFCC consists of the triangular fibrocartilage (TFC, disc, disc proper), radioulnar ligament (RUL), ulnolunate ligament, ulnotriquetral ligament, and sheath floor of the extensor carpi ulnaris (ECU) tendon [8]. The key structure of DRUJ stability is the RUL, proximal component of the TFCC, arises from the fovea of the ulna to the dorsal and ulnar distal surface of the sigmoid notch of the radius [8]. The other key structure is the triangular fibrocartilage (TFC) providing load distributing function and supporting function of the TFCC itself [8].

There are many ligaments in the radiocarpal and midcarpal joints, which are classified to the extrinsic ligaments and intrinsic ligaments [10]. The intrinsic ligaments of the wrist are the scapholunate (SL) (interosseous) ligament and the lunotriquetral (LT) (interosseous) ligament. The SL ligament consists of dorsal, palmar, and membranous (proximal) portion, surrounding the scapholunate interval from dorsal, proximal to palmar and connecting the scaphoid and the lunate [10]. There is no connection on the distal surface of the scapholunate interval, showing C-shaped structure. The dorsal portion is the strongest part in the SL ligament [10]. The LT ligament demonstrates similar structure as the SL ligament, while the palmar portion is the strongest.

In the dorsal surface of the radiocarpal and midcarpal joint, there are the dorsal radiocarpal (DRC) ligament connecting the radius to the triquetrum and the dorsal intercarpal (DIC) ligament connecting the triquetrum to the scaphoid and lunate as the extrinsic ligaments [10]. Those ligaments demonstrate horizontal V-shape to allow smooth flexion–extension and radial–ulnar deviation. The extrinsic volar ligaments described by Berger [10] are radiocapitolunate, long radiolunate, short radiolunate on the radiocarpal joint and scapho-trapezium-trapezoid (STT) ligament, scaphocapitate, triquetrocapitate, and triquetrohamate ligaments. These ligaments show vertical double V-shape for radial–ulnar deviation.

26.3 Causes of Wrist Contracture

There are several causes of wrist contracture, such as due to burn on skin [2], tendon adhesion, surrounding soft tissue problem, fibrosis of the RCJ or MCJ itself or both, carpal coalition after trauma, bone tumor, and heterotopic ossification. Major causes of wrist contracture are surrounding soft tissue problem.

26.4 Symptom of Wrist Contracture

Wrist contracture demonstrates loss of flexion–extension and radial–ulnar deviation. Those symptoms are due to contracture of either the radiocarpal or midcarpal joint or both. Normal range of flexion is 70°, extension is 70°, radial deviation is 25°, and ulnar deviation is 45°. Treatment should be needed the range of less than 30° of extension, 30° of flexion, 10° of radial deviation, and 15° of ulnar deviation [7, 9].

Wrist contracture also includes loss of pronosupination mainly due to contracture of the DRUJ. If the DRUJ is intact, the pronosupination contracture maybe due to the contracture of the proximal radioulnar joint (PRUJ) or interosseous membrane problem. The details of pronosupination contracture are described in the different chapter.

26.5 Diagnosis of Wrist Contracture

Diagnosis of wrist contracture is easy, where the patient indicates loss of wrist motion or forearm pronosupination mainly due to the wrist. The burn is main cause of skin contracture, indicating serious scar formation on the dorsal or palmar side of the wrist. Iatrogenic scar formation on the wrist also demonstrates loss of wrist range of motion (ROM). If the appearance of the wrist is normal, radiographs of the wrist indicate narrowing of the joint space either the RCJ or MCJ (Fig. 26.1) or both suggesting problem of the surrounding soft tissue of the wrist. CT is also useful to demonstrates narrowing of the joint space or sometimes, local coalition of the carpal bone(s). Details of image diagnosis of wrist contracture have been described in the other chapter.

26.6 Treatments of Wrist Flexion–Extension or Radial–Ulnar Deviation Contracture

26.6.1 Conservative Treatments

Conservative treatments, such as gentle manipulation, work in the early stage of wrist contracture. Aggressive passive ROM exercise should be avoided not to produce iatrogenic ossification.

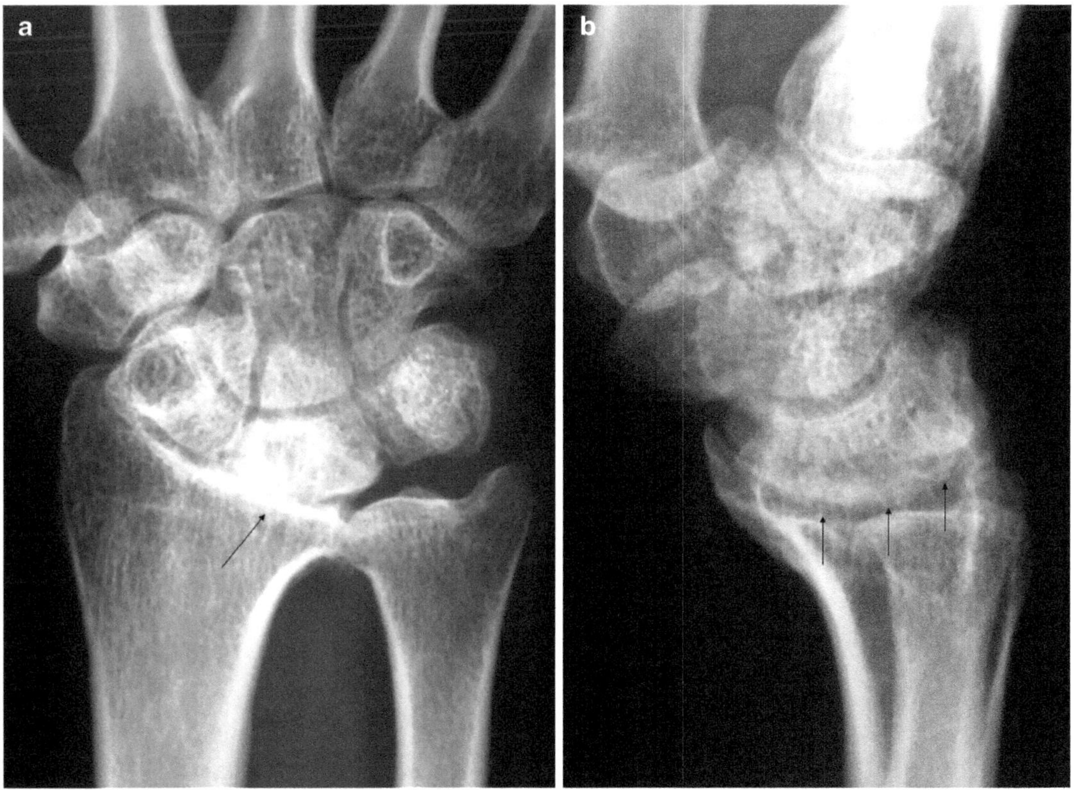

Fig. 26.1 Radiographs of stiff wrist. Narrowing of radiolunate space at the radiocarpal joint are noted on posteroanterior (**a**) and lateral (**b**) radiographs with arrows

26.6.2 Surgical Treatments

26.6.2.1 Skin Problems

Massive scar formation after burn, trauma, or surgery can introduce wrist contracture. Resection in the scar with skin graft is indicated for such skin problems.

26.6.2.2 Tendon Problems

Shortening of the flexors or extensor or both can reduce the wrist ROM. Surgical treatment, such as elongation of the tendon can increase wrist ROM. However, too many elongation decreases wrist ROM. Adhesion of the flexors or extensors or both to those floor(s) can decrease wrist ROM. Release of the tendons from the floor can increase the wrist ROM.

26.6.2.3 Soft Tissue Problems Around the Joint

Contracture of the extrinsic ligaments can cause wrist contracture. Especially, shortening of the short RL ligament is often seen after intraarticular fracture of the distal radius. In dorsal side, shortening of the DRC and DIC ligaments seldom occurs, while scar formation between the DRC and DIC shows restriction of wrist flexion. Arthroscopic or open release of the ligaments is indicated, while in chronic situation, fibrosis of the RCJ and/or MCJ is combined with surrounding ligament contracture.

26.6.2.4 Fibrosis of the Joint

Joint space narrowing of the RCJ and/or MCJ is obvious in this situation. Joint release either dorsal side or volar side or both is necessary. The author prefers to use an open release [6, 11] from the dorsal side using a Berger-Bishop incision [12], where the sectioning is along with the ligament in the direction ofon the DRC and DIC to open the window on the dorsal surface of the wrist (Fig. 26.2). Fibrotic tissues are removed or released with surgical knife or sharp elevator, then expansion of the joint space by elevator with manual force. Z-shape elongation of the DRC ligament is sometimes needed for increase of flexion range. Volar side release of the short RL ligament can be also done by sharp elevator [13]. Same procedure can be done in arthroscopic fashion [3–5, 14].

26.6.2.5 Other Problems

For bone tumor and heterotopic ossification, similar open procedure with joint fibrosis is done to remove bone tumor or resect heterotopic ossification.

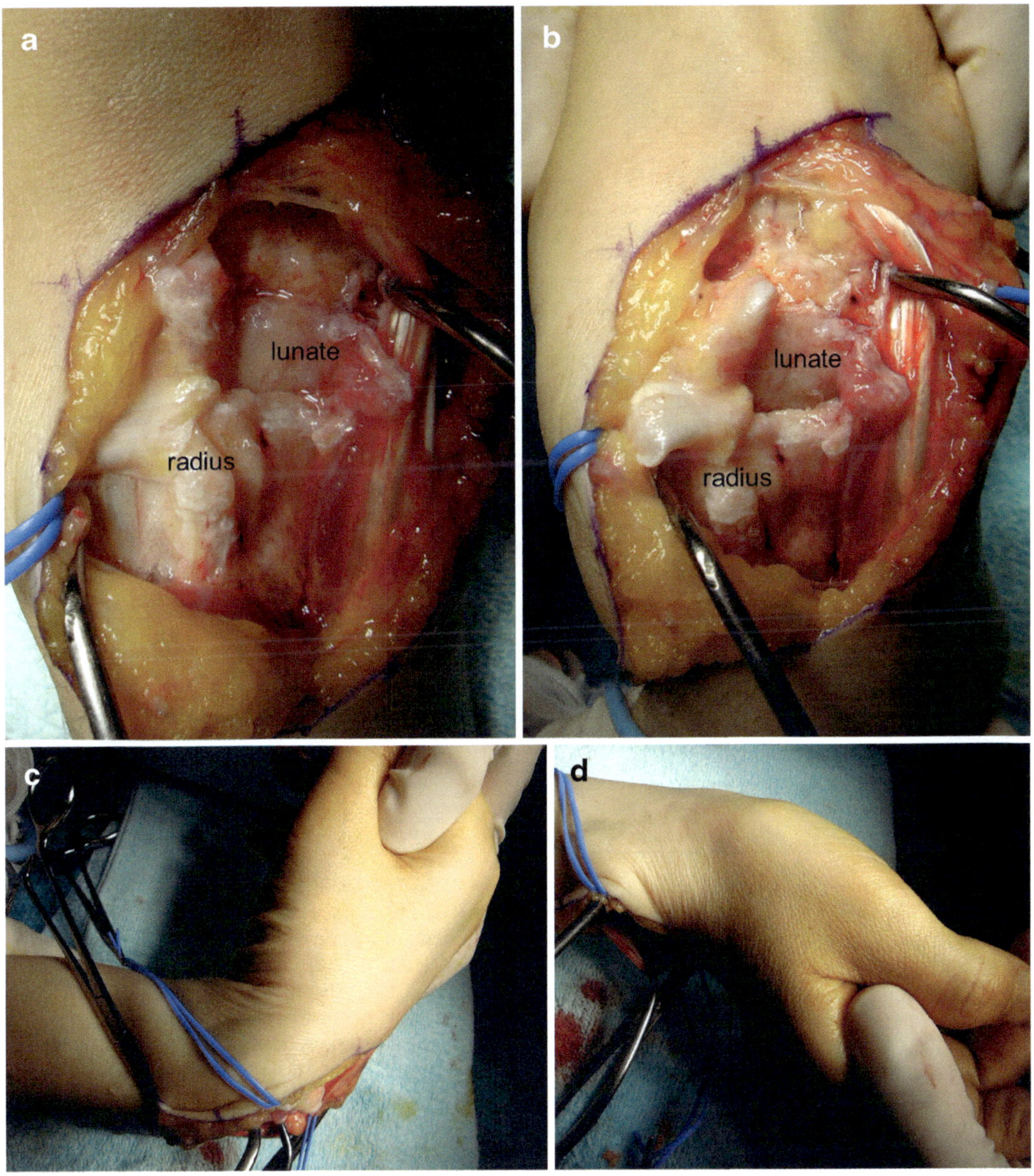

Fig. 26.2 Berger's open exploration of the radiocarpal joints indicates the narrow space of the radius–lunate interval on the same patient of Fig. 26.1 (**a**). After open release of the radiolunate joint (**b**), range of flexion (**c**) and extension (**d**) is expanded. Ten years after the release, posteroanterior radiograph shows space of the radiolunate interval. Suture anchor on the radiograph was used to reattach the radiocarpal ligament (**e**). Range of flexion (**f**) and extension (**g**) still are maintained 10 years after the surgery

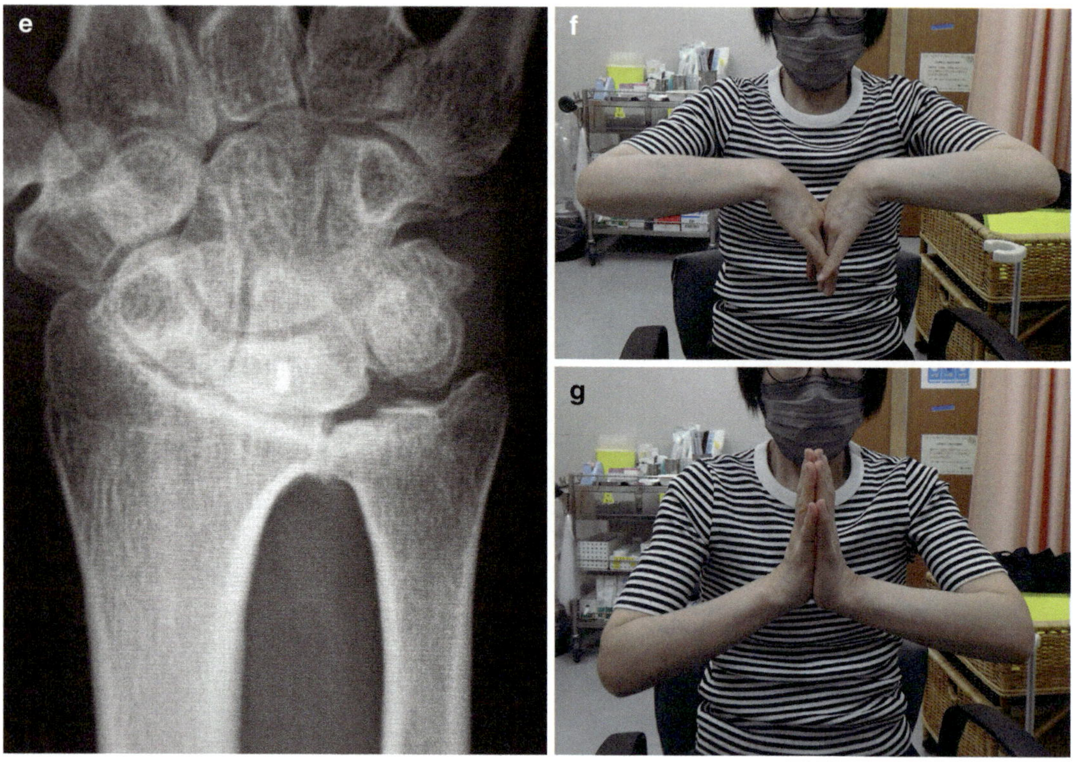

Fig. 26.2 (continued)

References

1. Saffar P. Extrinsic and intrinsic causes of radiocarpal stiffness. In: Copeland SA, Gschwend N, Landi A, et al., editors. Joint stiffness of the upper limb. London: Martin Dunitz; 1997. p. 149–67.
2. Brown M, Chung KC. Postburn contractures of the hand. Hand Clin. 2017;33(2):317–31.
3. Verhellen R, Bain GI. Arthroscopic capsular release for contracture of the wrist: a new technique. Arthroscopy. 2000;16(1):106–10.
4. Luchetti R, Atzei A, Fairplay T. Arthroscopic wrist arthrolysis after wrist fractures. Arthroscopy. 2007;23(3):255–60.
5. Luchetti R, Atzei A, Papini ZI. Arthroscopic wrist arthrolysis. Chir Main. 2006;25(S1):S244–53.
6. Della Rossa N, Colzani G, Petrella G, et al. Open release of stiff wrist: a medium to long term case series and literature review. Acta Biomed. 2022;93:e2022114. https://doi.org/10.23750/abn.v93iS1.10055.
7. Palmer AK, Werner FW, Murphy D, et al. Functional wrist motion: a biomechanical study. J Hand Surg Am. 1985;10(1):39–46.
8. Nakamura T, Yabe Y, Horiuchi Y. Functional anatomy of the triangular fibrocartilage complex. J Hand Surg Br. 1996;21(4):571–86. https://doi.org/10.1016/s0266-7681(96)80135-5.
9. Ryu JY, Cooney WP, Askew LJ, et al. Functional ranges of motion of the wrist joint. J Hand Surg Am. 1991;16(3):409–19.
10. Berger RA. The ligaments of the wrist. A current overview of anatomy with considerations of their potential functions. Hand Clin. 1997;13:63–82.
11. Voche P, Merle M. Arthrolysis of the wrist, indications and technique. Rev Chir Orthop Reparatrice Appar Mot. 1993;79(2):135–9.
12. Berger RA. A method of defining palpable landmarks for the ligament-splitting dorsal wrist capsulotomy. J Hand Surg Am. 2007;32(8):1291–5. https://doi.org/10.1016/j.jhsa.2007.07.023.
13. Babazadeh S, Puig de la Bellacasa I, Jamieson R, et al. Anteromedial release for posttraumatic flexion-pronation contracture of the wrist: surgical technique. Tech Hand Up Extrem Surg. 2019;23(4):170–5.
14. Del Pinal F, Klausmeyer M, Thams C, et al. Arthroscopic resection arthroplasty for malunited intra-articular distal radius fractures. J Hand Surg Am. 2012;37(12):2447–55.

Arthroscopic Arthrolysis of the Wrist

27

Luchetti Riccardo, Lucian Lior Marcovici, Marco Guidi, and Gregory I. Bain

27.1 Introduction

Wrist stiffness is a multifactorial and invalidating complication after wrist trauma or surgery. This condition can be as either intra-articular or extra-articular [1]. Capsular structures are frequently involved [2, 3]. Either large or minimal injury of the capsule may lead to wrist contracture [4]. Arthrofibrosis may be stimulated by intra-articular and capsular injuries as well as prolonged immobilization and this can be seen after conservative and surgical treatment (Table 27.1) [5, 6].

The first choice of management should be a conservative treatment with a good rehabilitation protocol. Wrist manipulation under anesthesia is a possible option when the rehabilitation regime has failed. However, this procedure can be harmful by causing chondral or osteochondral damage, traumatic ligamentous injuries, or even fractures. Surgical arthrolysis is a controlled option that can be performed via open or arthroscopic techniques [1, 7, 8]. The arthroscopic techniques are already a successful treatment solution in other joints [9–13]. Arthroscopic arthrolysis (AA) of the wrist treats the radiocarpal (RC), midcarpal (MC), and intercarpal joints, and distal radioulnar joint (DRUJ) while minimizing the capsular injuries and the risk of secondary damage to other articulations with an immediate postoperative mobilization [2, 3, 14–22].

Failure to reduce distal radius (DR) fractures is frequently a cause of a stiff and painful wrist. Intra-articular and extra-articular malunions should be accurately corrected with osteotomies to restore normal alignment of the distal radius [23].

Two main conditions can lead to painful limitation of range of motion (ROM) in wrist contractures after distal radius fractures:

1. Capsular contracture with intra-articular adhesions (capsule with fibrotic connection to the carpal bones and radiocarpal fibrotic bands).
2. Radiocarpal impingement due to either malunion of inter- and intra-facet fractures or malunion involving the dorsal and volar rim of the distal radius (Figs. 27.1a, b and 27.2a, b).

L. Riccardo (✉)
Rimini Hand and Upper Limb Surgery & Rehabilitation Center, Rimini, Italy

L. L. Marcovici
Hand & Microsurgery Unit, Jewish Hospital of Rome, Rome, Italy

M. Guidi
Department of Plastic Surgery and Hand Surgery, Cantonal Hospital, Aarau, Switzerland

G. I. Bain
Department of Orthopedic Surgery, Flinders University of South Australia and Flinders Medical Centre, Adelaide, Australia
e-mail: greg@gregbain.com.au

L. Pederzini et al. (eds.), *Stiffness of the Elbow, Wrist and Related Pathologies*,
https://doi.org/10.1007/978-3-031-81381-8_27

Table 27.1 Causes of wrist stiffness

Intra-articular	
	Post-traumatic • Intra-articular adhesions • Intra-articular fractures • SLI
	Degenerative disorders • Osteophytes, synovitis (OsteoArthritis (OA), Reuhmatoid Arthritis (RA), crystals)
	Post-surgery
Capsular[a]	
	Capsular tears Immobilization
Extra-articular	
	Heterotopic ossification Skin contracture Neuromuscular disorders (Carpal tunnel syndrome)

[a]Post-traumatic and degenerative conditions can also affect the capsular. We keep it as a separate category, as it can have different causes, treatment, and prognosis. Extra-articular conditions typically are managed with open procedures but could be managed with endoscopy

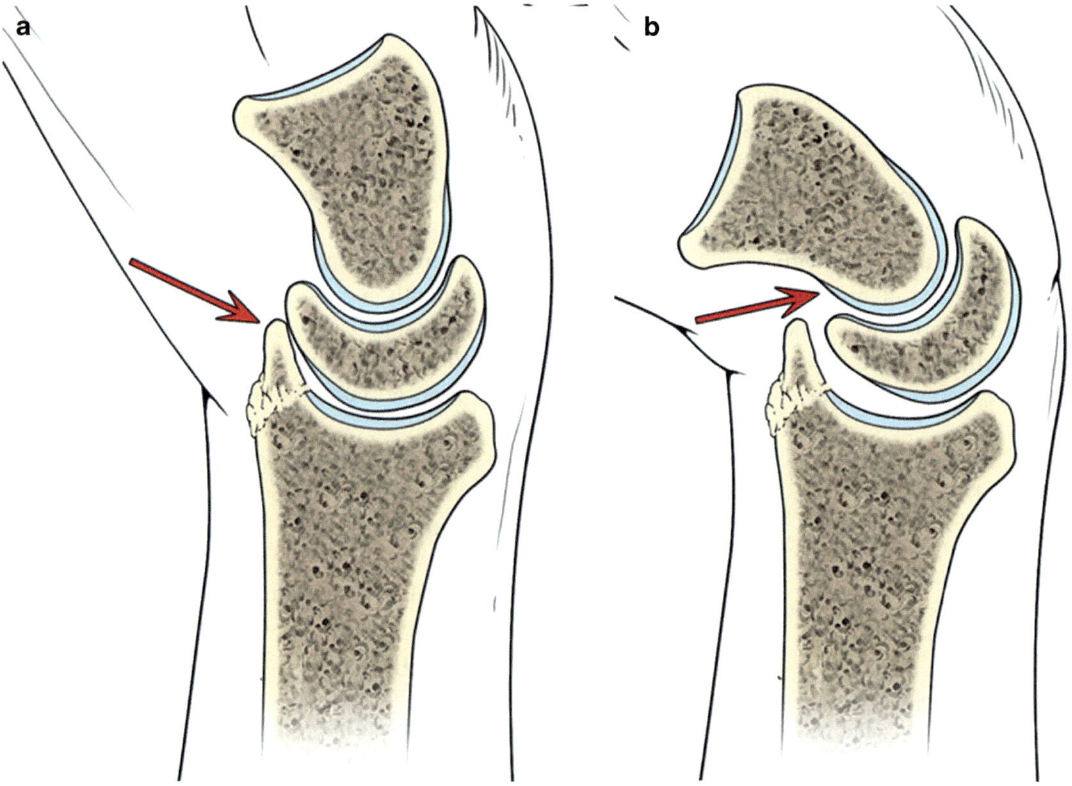

Fig. 27.1 Malunion of the dorsal rim of the distal radius (**a**). Note the impingement between the dorsal rim and the carpus (**b**). (Reproduced and modified with permission from [4])

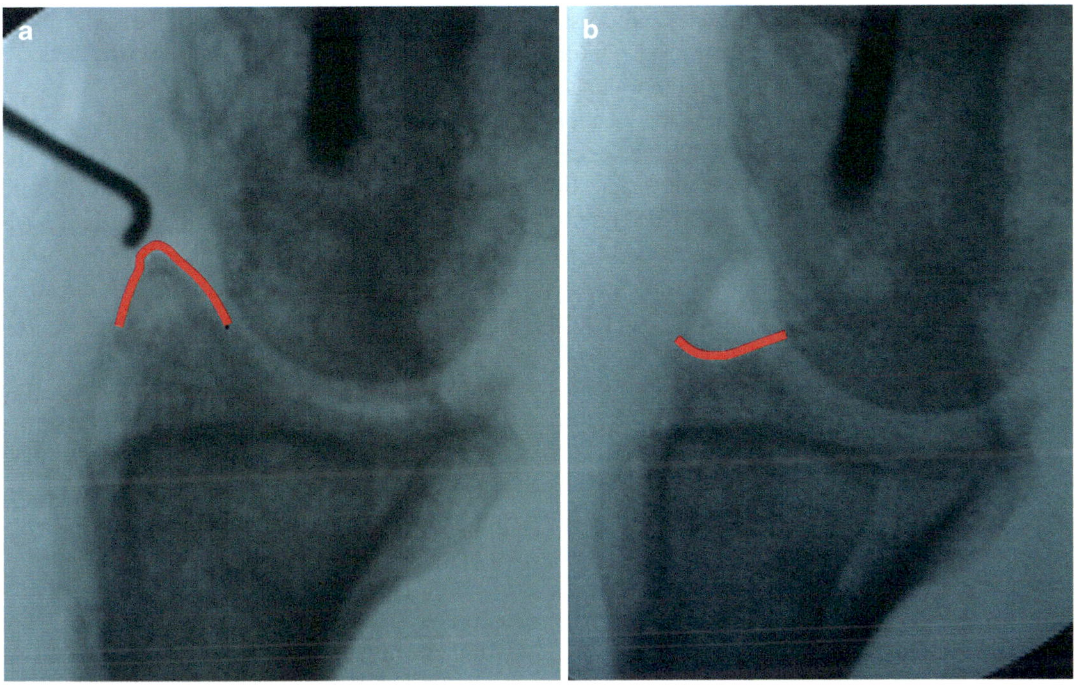

Fig. 27.2 Lateral radiograph of a wrist showing dorsal impingement of the distal radius malunion: (**a**) before and (**b**) after arthroscopic debridement. (Reproduced and modified with permission from [4])

These two conditions can sometimes affect the wrist at the same time and must be treated in the same procedure [24]. However, these injuries are usually first managed with a corrective osteotomy of the distal radius (DR) malunion followed by secondary open or arthroscopic arthrolysis [8]. Any procedure that would involve postoperative immobilization such as ligament reconstructions must be avoided. Immediate wrist mobilization after AA is mandatory.

In this chapter, we propose a step-by-step procedure of arthroscopic arthrolysis of the wrist (RC, MC, and DRUJ) that we defined "inside-out progressive technique." "Inside-out" concept begins with a procedure from the internal part or the joint, progressing toward the external to the joint through the capsule resection (volar and/or dorsal). "Progressive" means that after each arthroscopic step, the wrist mobility is assessed, and if adequate motion is not obtained, then the next step is performed, until adequate motion is obtained. This technique is adapted according to the arthroscopic findings.

27.2 Indications

The main indications for arthroscopic wrist arthrolysis are persistent wrist stiffness after a conservative rehabilitation program following a trauma, surgical treatment, and immobilization. The best indication for AA is the stiff joint that has minimal pain, with an intact articular surface. However, pain is frequently associated with wrist stiffness, and this could direct the surgeon to choose a different surgical treatment. DRUJ stiffness with normal ulnar head (UH) length and that is well centered in the sigmoid notch (SN) is a good indication for AA.

27.3 Contraindications

The main contraindications to the AA are complex articular cartilage defects, especially those involving the main loading across the joint. Examples include intra-articular step-off related to intra-articular distal radius malunion, osteochondral defects of the radius and carpal bone, and dorsal dislocation or unreducible ulnar-head. Intra-articular step-off of the scaphoid and/or lunate facet has to be managed in relation to the location of the defect. Intra-facet step-off will have benefit by corrective osteotomy and inter-facet by arthroscopic resection or corrective osteotomy [24]. Osteochondral defect centered on load-bearing joint will have a minimal advantage by AA. Wrist stiffness due to mal-positioned palmar plate needs an open surgery and plate removal. However, in some case, arthroscopy can be useful to explore the wrist, detect intra-articular screws, and perform a direct corrective osteotomy.

AA has a little chance to improve ROM in DRUJ stiffness if the UH is not centered to the sigmoid notch (SN). UH dorsal dislocation needs to be treated by different techniques through open surgery [21, 25, 26]. In DRUJ stiffness with normal position of the UH, AA can be useful. However, in cases with minimal dorsal subluxation, to improve the prono-supination the surgeon should evaluate the need to convert to open surgery.

Radiological findings with X-ray, computed tomography (CT) scan, and magnetic resonance imaging (MRI) have to be carefully evaluated concerning the articular surface condition of both the UH and the SN. Osteochondral defect and/or step-off of both articular surfaces are contraindications of the AA of the DRUJ.

27.4 Surgical Technique

27.4.1 Preoperative Planning

Preoperative planning passes through clinical evaluation, X-ray, arthrography [27], CT scan, and MRI [28, 29]. Clinical evaluation may help to understand injury dynamics and estimate the articular damage. X-ray and CT scan might show intra- and extra-articular abnormalities. MRI can put in evidence cartilage defects and ligament irregularities. Dynamic four-dimensional (4D) CT scans provide an assessment of the articulation, and how the joint moves in relation to the defect [30].

27.4.2 Patient Positioning, Portals, and Arthroscopic Instruments

The patient is positioned supine on the operation table with tourniquet applied on the affected arm. The arm is abducted at 90° and the elbow flexed at 90° allowing a vertical position of the forearm, wrist, and hand. Traditional vertical traction system is applied to the wrist through a second and third finger trap and counter-traction at the elbow [31, 32]. Surgeon should use a traction device, which allows free prono-supination of the wrist during arthroscopy [31, 32]. Surgeon should be able to pass from the vertical position to a traditional horizontal position to be able to check flexion–extension of the wrist obtained during the different phases of AA. We require vertical traction systems with counterweight (4 kg) that permit prono-supination check during arthroscopy. Traditional RC, MC, and DRUJ portals are used for AA of the wrist [2, 6, 18, 19].

Arthrolysis may be performed using a variety of instruments (Table 27.2). Dry arthroscopy is utilized more frequently for this condition as it has the benefit of avoiding fluid extravasation into the soft tissues and may permit a hybrid technique with open approach combined with and arthroscopic approach to the wrist [31, 33].

Small diameter wrist scopes are used (1.9 mm or 2.7 mm). If the wrist is very tight, a 1.9 mm scope is required (Fig. 27.3a, b).

Table 27.2 Instruments for arthroscopic arthrolysis

Motor powered
• Full radius blade
• Cutter blade/incisor
• Razor cut blade
• Barrel abrader
• Burr
Dissector
Mini-scalpel
Hook scalpel
Radiofrequency
Laser

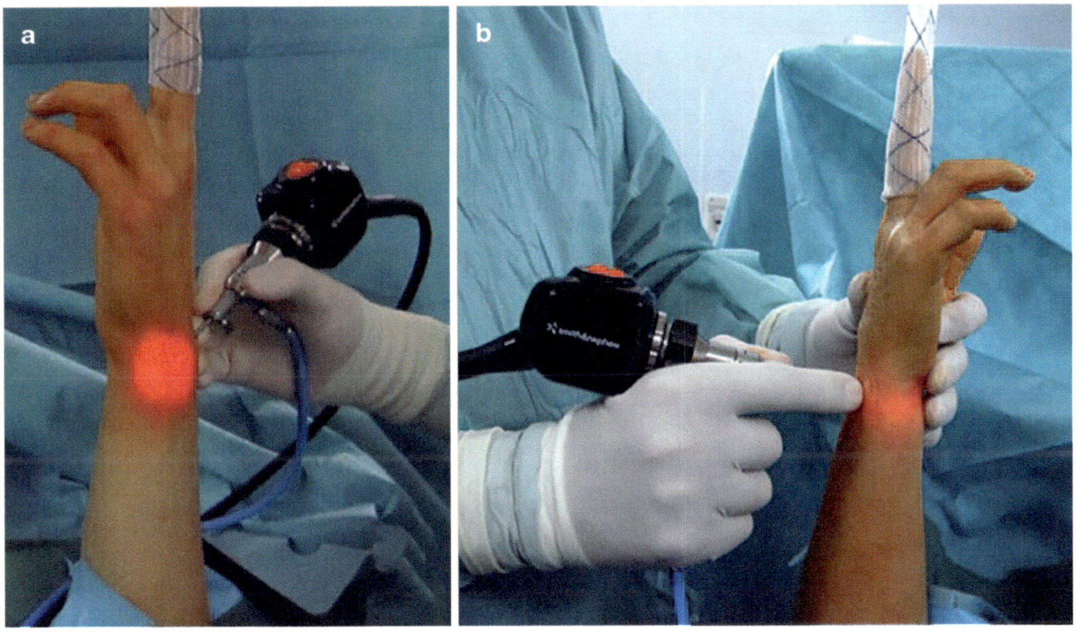

Fig. 27.3 (**a** and **b**) Technique of handling the 1.9 mm videoarthroscope. The tip of the second finger touches the dorsal wrist and the millimetric motion into the joint is determined by pushing with the tip of the finger on the skin without losing the objective (microsurgery = arthroscopic surgery)

27.4.3 Principles of the Technique

According to the "box concept" [14, 15], all dorsal RC portals (1–2, 3–4, 4–5, 6R, and 6U) and volar portals may be used (Fig. 27.4). Scope and working instruments can be interchanged between portals. Dry arthroscopy is the preferred one and regularly used by the authors. With this technique trocar inflow and outflow valves must be open permitting the entrance of air. Occasional use of saline solution may be used by 10/20 cc syringe introduced to the trocar portal in order to wash-out the joint. In this case shaver connected to aspiration will remove fluid, blood, and debris from the joint (Fig. 27.5). Radiofrequency is not used in our practice.

Joint contractures are usually due to a localized area of scarring and fibrosis. So, to use a systematic approach, we start from simple and central to the joint, and extend to more complex ligament and articular surface. So arthrolysis is divided in four steps.

1. Intra-articular fibrosis and fibrotic bands: These are often synovitis and congealed hematomas that are simple to divide or remove with arthroscopic instruments.
2. Capsular adhesion to the carpal bones: The scarred contractures that bridge ligament insertion into the carpal bone. By elevating and reflecting the ligament insertion with a Freer elevator, it allows the carpus to move more freely.
3. Capsule contracture: This is a scarred contracted ligament/capsule that prevents motion, despite the two previous debridements. It is less common and typically localized to one or two ligaments. The capsule is divided or resected in those cases of complex capsular contractures.
4. Articular and osseous step-offs/defects: Debridement of the chondral flaps and intra-articular fractures. For more severe cases, an intra-articular osteotomy is required.

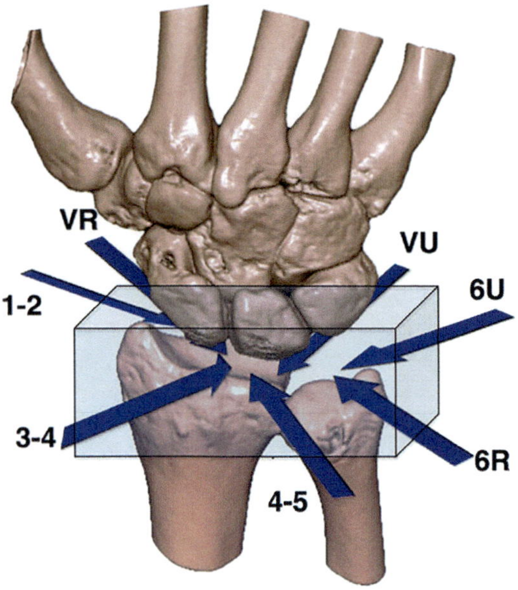

Fig. 27.4 Box concept. The wrist can be thought of as a box, which can be visualized from every perspective. Through a combination of arthroscopic portals, it is possible to have viewing and working portals that encircle the wrist. This enables the arthroscopic surgeon to modify the position of his scope to obtain an optimal view and then to ensure the working instruments are best positioned to perform their duties. The portals can be changed and adjusted for each aspect of the procedure [10]

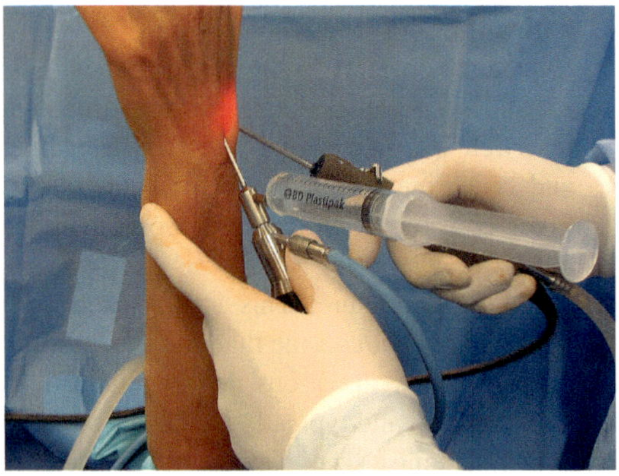

Fig. 27.5 Technique of dry arthroscopy changed in a temporary wet arthroscopy using a syringe attached to the sleeve of the arthroscope

27.4.4 Radiocarpal Joint

27.4.4.1 Step 1: Fibrosis and Fibrotic Band Resection

The procedure starts from the radial side of the RC joint (Fig. 27.6). Scope is introduced in the 3–4 portal and instruments are used through the 1–2 portal. However, during the procedure scope and instruments are frequently switched between the portals.

A 2.9 mm full radius or aggressive shaver is used initially to remove the fibrotic tissue. In the beginning of the procedure the adhesions and the scar tissue increase the difficulty of triangulation and intra-articular vision. One can use a small Freer dissector to create space (Fig. 27.7) and then point the shaver on the scope to be better oriented in the joint before turning it into action. At this point the shaver can be used in the 1–2 portal or be switched with the scope and used in the 3–4

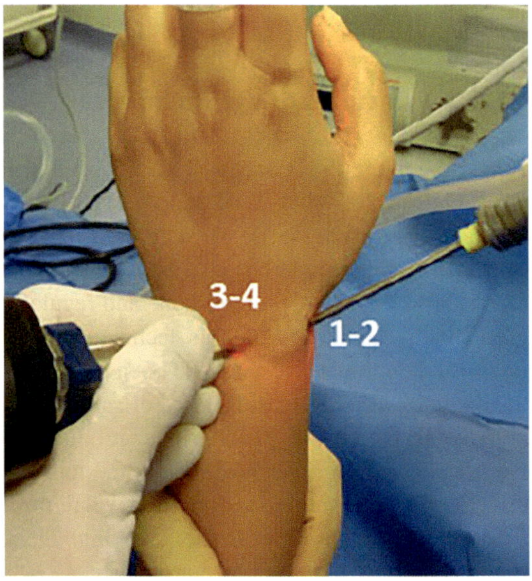

Fig. 27.6 Preferred portals to commence the arthroscopic wrist arthrolysis: 1–2 portal for the scope and 3–4 portal for the shaver or vice versa

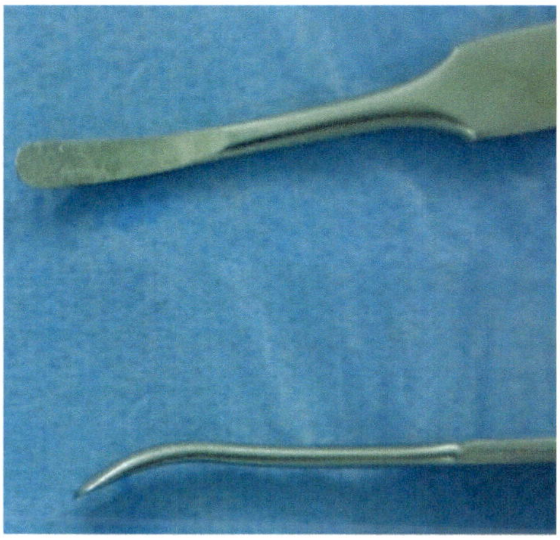

Fig. 27.7 Curved dissector (or periosteal osteotome) used to remove part of fibrosis in the wrist joint

portal till the radial part of the joint is cleared from the fibrotic tissue. Once fibrosis is completely removed from the radial side of the RC joint, the arthroscopic procedure is shifted to the ulnar side. The scope is introduced through the 3–4 portal and the shaver through the 6R. Visualization of the shaver is frequently limited by the presence of the fibrotic band (Fig. 27.8a, b). Traditionally the fibrotic band [6, 18, 19, 34] is localized between the scapholunate (SL) ligament and the ridge between the scaphoid and lunate facets of the distal radius (Fig. 27.9). It may be partial or complete fibrous band (Fig. 27.8a, b). When it is complete, it divides the radiocarpal joint into two separate spaces. The fibrotic band may be incised using an 18G needle

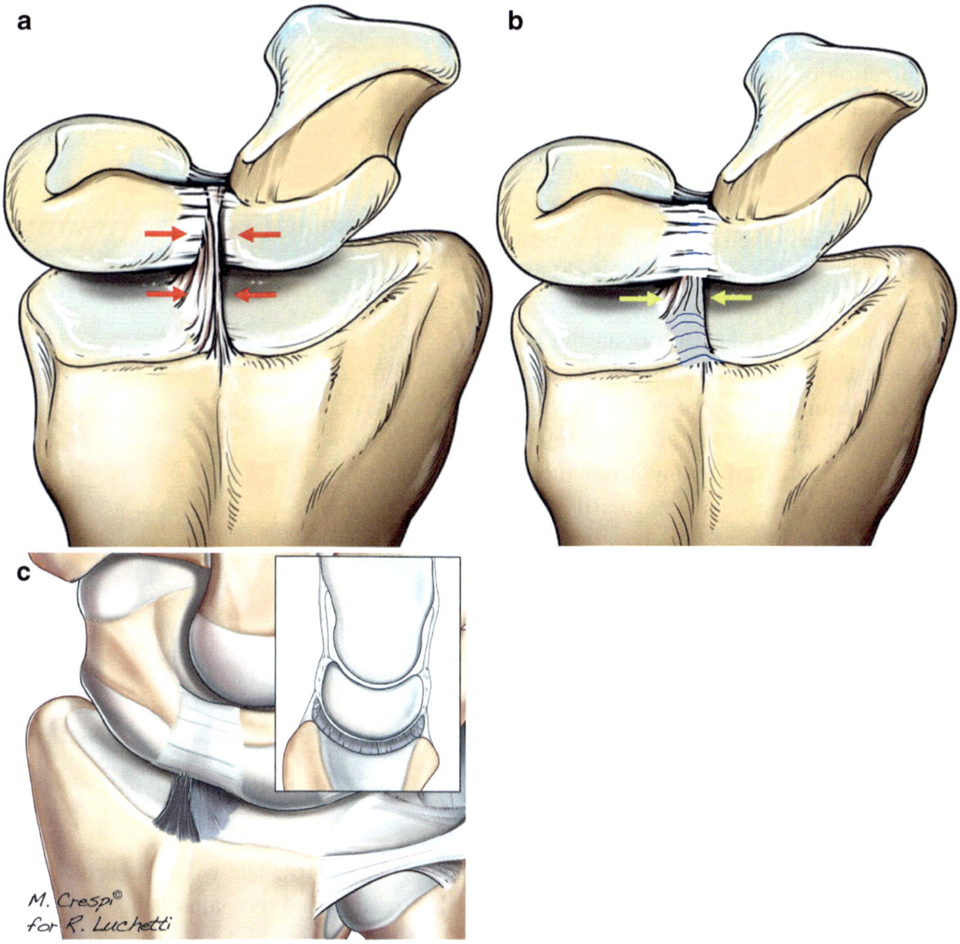

Fig. 27.8 Drawings of fibrotic bands located into the joint between the radius and scapholunate ligament. In the complete sheet divides the radiocarpal joint in two separate compartments: the radio-scaphoid and the radio-lunate joint. (**a**) Complete fibrotic band (red arrows). (**b**) Partial fibrotic band located mostly in the volar aspect; it is always in the same position (yellow arrows). (**c**) Sagittal plane view of the fibrotic band

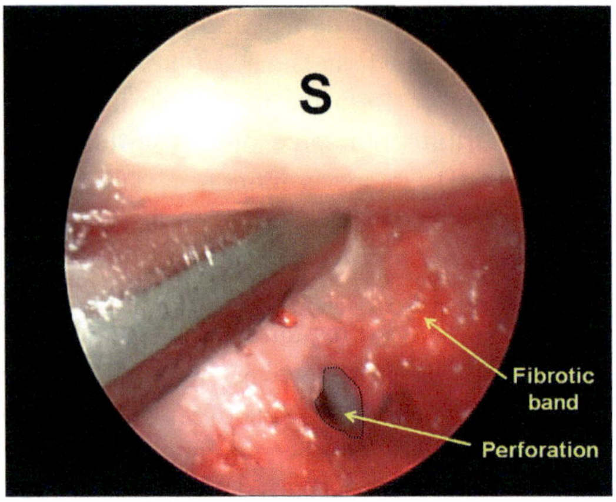

Fig. 27.9 Arthroscopic picture showing the fibrotic band with a small perforation through which it is possible to see the ulnar part of the radiocarpal joint: the radio-lunate joint. (Reproduced with permission from [4])

or small dissector introduced via the 6R portal in the direction of the scope or vice versa from the 3–4 portal when the scope is in 6R. The fibrotic band is carefully detached from the articular surface of the radius using the dissector, scalpel, or hook scalpel (Fig. 27.10a, b). The free parts of the fibrotic band may then be removed using a basket forceps (Fig. 27.11) or a shaver. To obtain a complete resection of the band, the scope and instruments must be switched to obtain the best view and instrument access. Multiple fibrotic bands may be encountered in a joint with osteochondral damage to the articular surface of the distal radius, with all of them originating from the articular defect. Rarely these bands may ossify and form a fibro-osseous band, and with progression may result in an ankylosis of the RC joint (Fig. 27.12).

When fibrosis in the ulnar side of the RC joint has been completely excised (Figs. 27.13 and 27.14), the procedure continues into the ulnocarpal (UC) joint (Fig. 27.15). This part of the wrist joint is rarely affected by fibrosis, and arthroscopy is often diagnostic only. Occasionally, peripheral Triangular FibroCartilage Complex (TFCC); tears may be found; however, the treatment should be limited to a debridement in order to avoid the DRUJ instability and due to the need for postoperative immobilization.

Before moving to the second step of the procedure, it is suggested to evaluate the wrist ROM

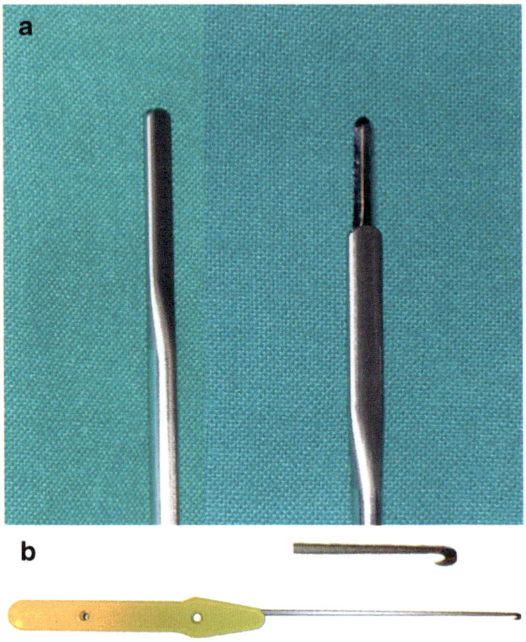

Fig. 27.10 (**a**) Special blades used for microsurgery or ophthalmic surgery. (**b**) Hook blade used for the trigger finger

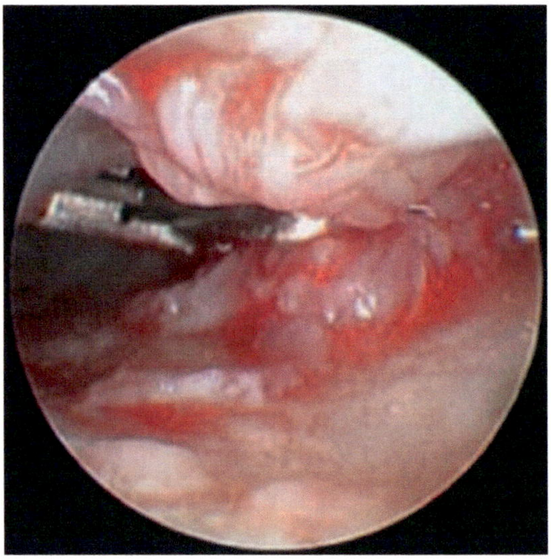

Fig. 27.11 Fibrotic band resected with scissor

(Fig. 27.16). The wrist showed be taken off from traction and the gain of motion is evaluated. The surgeon should decide if the wrist motion gained is sufficient and the procedure is finished or insufficient and the procedure continues to Step 2.

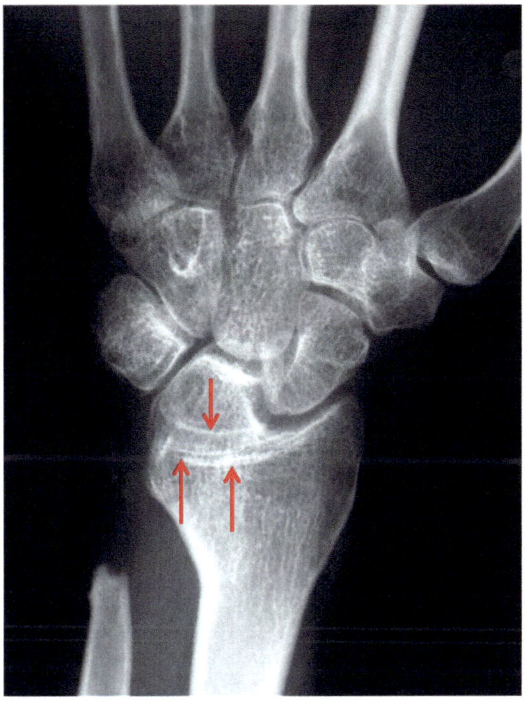

Fig. 27.12 X-ray of a wrist showing an ankylosis of the radio-lunate joint (red arrows) due to progression of an osteofibrotic band. (Reproduced with permission from [4])

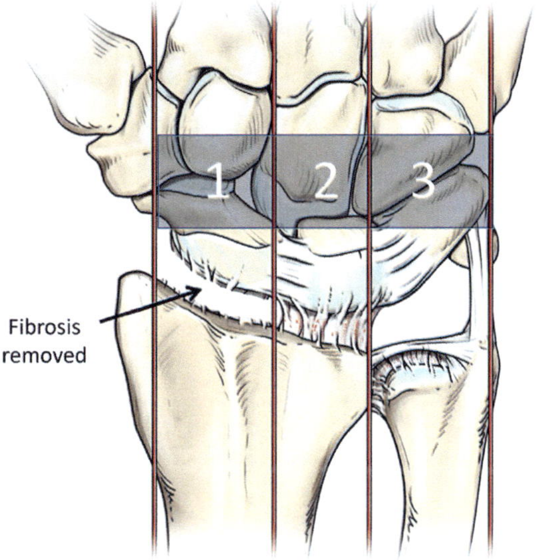

Fig. 27.14 Step 1: Drawing showing division of the radiocarpal joint into three parts, where fibrosis in the radial side has been removed. (Reproduced and modified with permission from [4])

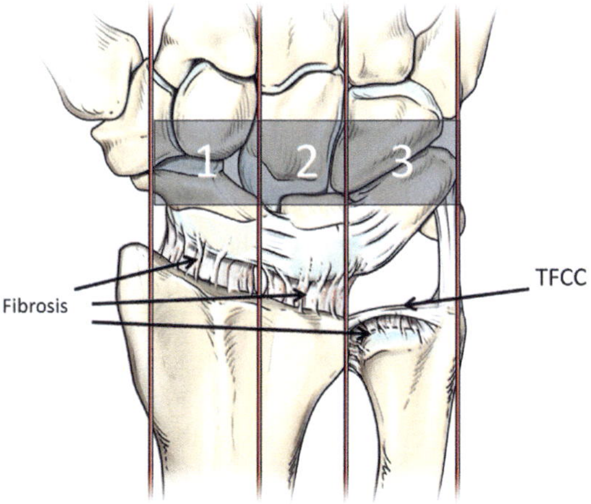

Fig. 27.13 Drawing showing the division of the radiocarpal joint into three parts. The proper radiocarpal joint is divided into two parts by a longitudinal line passing through the scapholunate joint. The ulnocarpal joint is separated from the radiocarpal joint by a longitudinal line through the medial border of the radius at the sigmoid notch. The ulnocarpal joint is rarely involved. In this drawing, fibrosis is located in the radiocarpal joint and in the DRUJ, under the TFCC ligament. (Reproduced and modified with permission from [4])

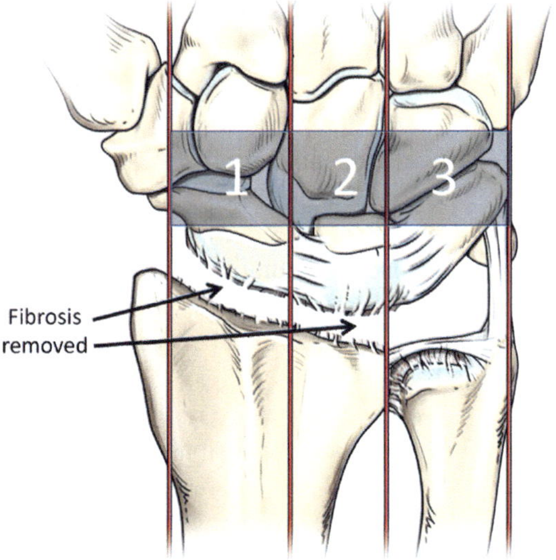

Fig. 27.15 Step 1 completed: Drawing showing complete resection of fibrosis in the radiocarpal joint. (Reproduced and modified with permission from [4])

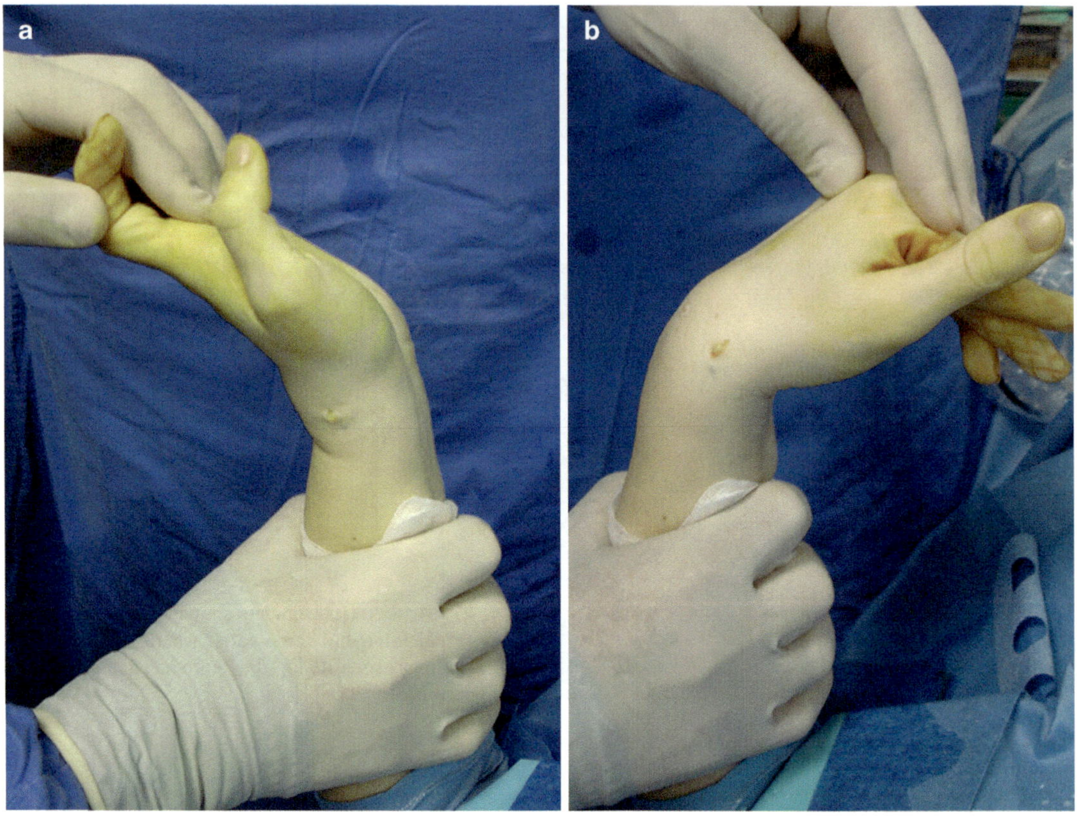

Fig. 27.16 Wrist ROM (**a** and **b**) evaluation after Step 1 of the arthroscopic arthrolysis. (Reproduced with permission from [4])

27.4.4.2 Step 2: Detachment of Volar and Dorsal Capsular Adhesion to the Carpal Bones

The wrist returns in traction; this part of procedure can be done in continuity with the previous one. A small Freer elevator is used to elevate and detach the scar tissue formed between the carpal bones and the capsule (Figs. 27.17a–c and 27.18a–c). A shaver is used to resect the fibrotic tissue [35]. For dorsal adhesions, the scope is introduced in the 1–2 portal to better visualize the dorsal capsule and the instruments are introduced in the 3–4 portal (Fig. 27.19a–c) [8]. The direction of movement of the Freer elevator is from the lunate to the scaphoid in a delicate manner to avoid damaging the cartilage.

The volar adhesions, frequently less important than the dorsal one, are detached positioning the scope in 6R and the Freer in 1–2 portal (Fig. 27.20a–c). As for the dorsal dissection, the tip of the Freer is introduced close to the volar radio-scaphoid border of the radius and, with gentle curved maneuver, starting from the radius proceeds dorsal to the scaphoid detaching the adhesions. After this passage the same maneuver is done volar to the lunate. The adhesions to the triquetrum are detached using the scope in the 3–4 portal and the dissector in 6U portal. In some occasions radiocarpal ligaments (volar and dorsal) may be detached. In our series this was never associated to postoperative instability.

As for the end of the previous step, the wrist is removed from the traction and range of motion is reassessed. If the improvement is satisfying the procedure is complete, if not it continues to Step 3.

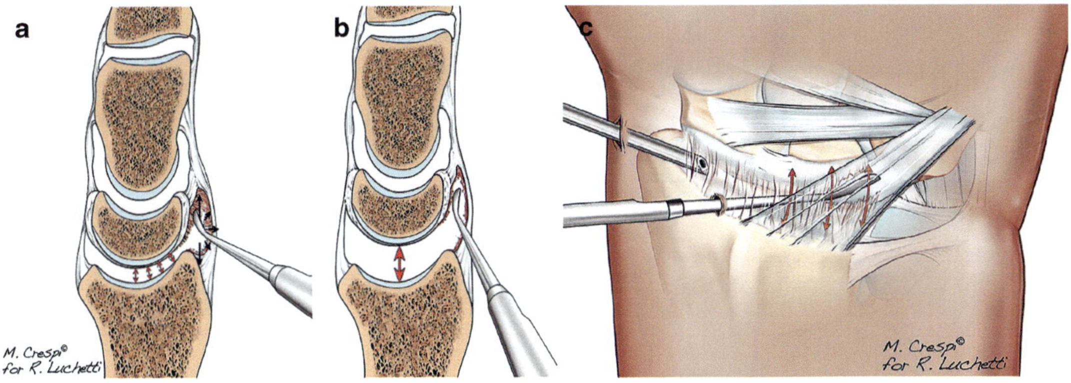

Fig. 27.17 Step 2: Drawings showing the detachment with a dissector of the fibrous adhesions between the capsule and the carpal bones (**a** and **b**). This permits a clear increase of the joint space (**b**: red arrow) and improvement of the wrist flexion. (**c**) Frontal view of the technique of dorsal fibrosis resection: the scope is in 1–2 portal and the dissector in 3–4 portal. The curved red arrows show the motion that the dissector required to release the fibrous adhesions

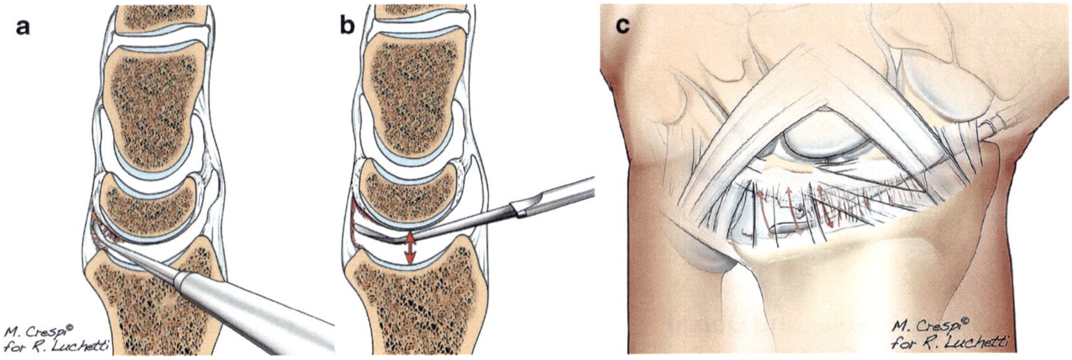

Fig. 27.18 Drawings showing the detachment of the fibrotic tissue between the capsule and the carpal bones using the same dissector (**a**). A clear increase of the joint space is obtained after the resection (**b**: red arrows). (**c**) Frontal view of the technique of volar fibrosis resection: the scope is in 3–4 portal and the dissector in 1–2 portal (the curved red arrows demonstrate the movement required by the dissector to detach the adhesions). It corresponds to the second step

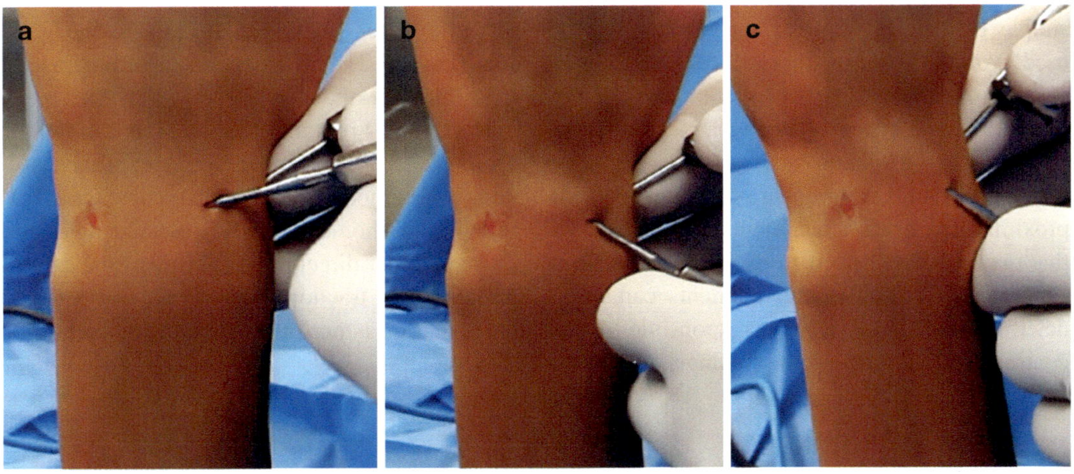

Fig. 27.19 Intraoperative pictures (**a**–**c**) showing the technique of dorsal fibrosis dissection (Step 2)

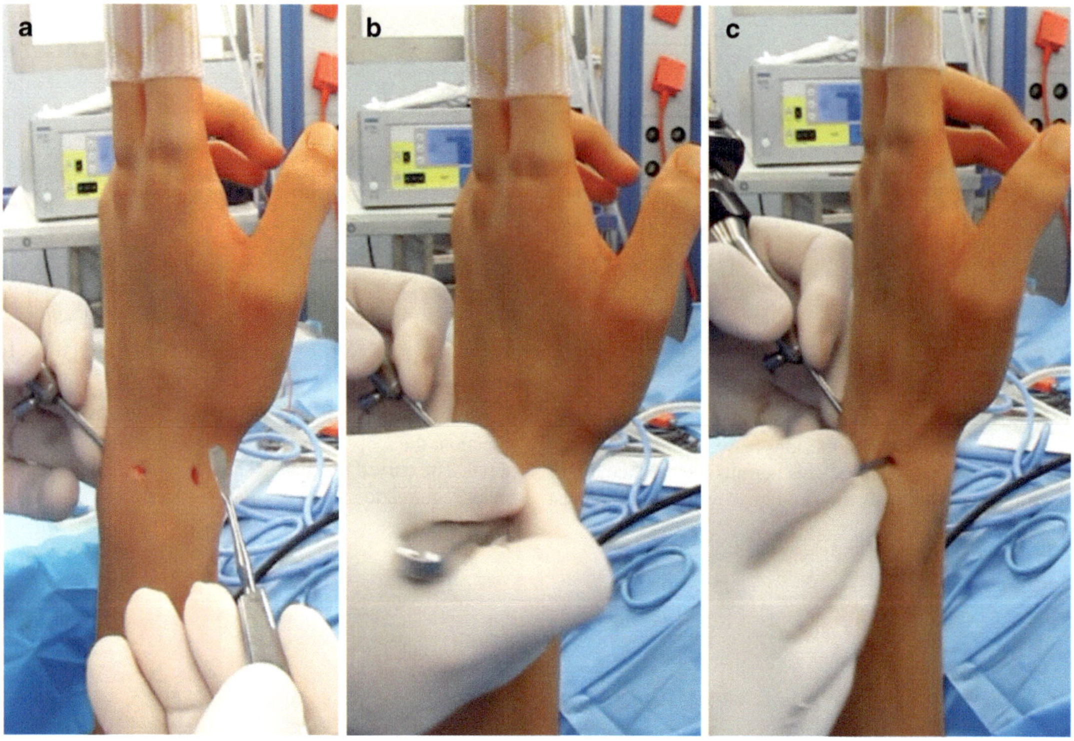

Fig. 27.20 Intraoperative pictures (**a**–**c**) showing the technique of volar fibrosis dissection (Step 2)

27.4.4.3 Step 3: Volar and Dorsal Capsule Contracture Resection

Wrist is put back into traction and the capsular contracture is assessed [3, 22]. Typically, it will be a one or two localized ligament contracture.

Instruments for resection of the capsule might be a mini-scalpel used in peripheral nerve surgery, micro-scalpel used for ocular surgery, or a simple 16G needle. Bipolar cautery can also be used. Volar capsule is approached first as it is easier to reach. Shaver is used to debride the intra-articular portion of the volar ligaments in order to have a clear visualization of the ligament. Care is taken to ensure that the ligament proximal and distal attachments are cleared, as this may avoid the need to divide the ligament. Close visualization of the ligaments can often determine the ligament that is responsible for the contracture. The responsible ligament is divided first (Fig. 27.21). Often one can encounter articular incongruency, which makes access difficult to some parts of the capsule. A burr can be used to smooth the articular surface, to allow access to the volar capsule [24]. The Radio-scapho-capitate and radio-lunate ligaments are resected at their base with the instruments in 1–2 portal and scope in 3–4 portal. If required the procedure then continues through to the ulnar side (Fig. 27.21) of the radius. Instruments are used through the 6R portal while the scope remains in 3–4 portal. The volar ulnar limit of the distal radius is the limit of volar capsule resection. Volar ulnocarpal (UC) ligament (Figs. 27.22 and 27.23) should never be resected as it will cause an ulnar direction instability of the carpus. At this point traction is removed, and a gentle manipulation is performed to control the gain in movement.

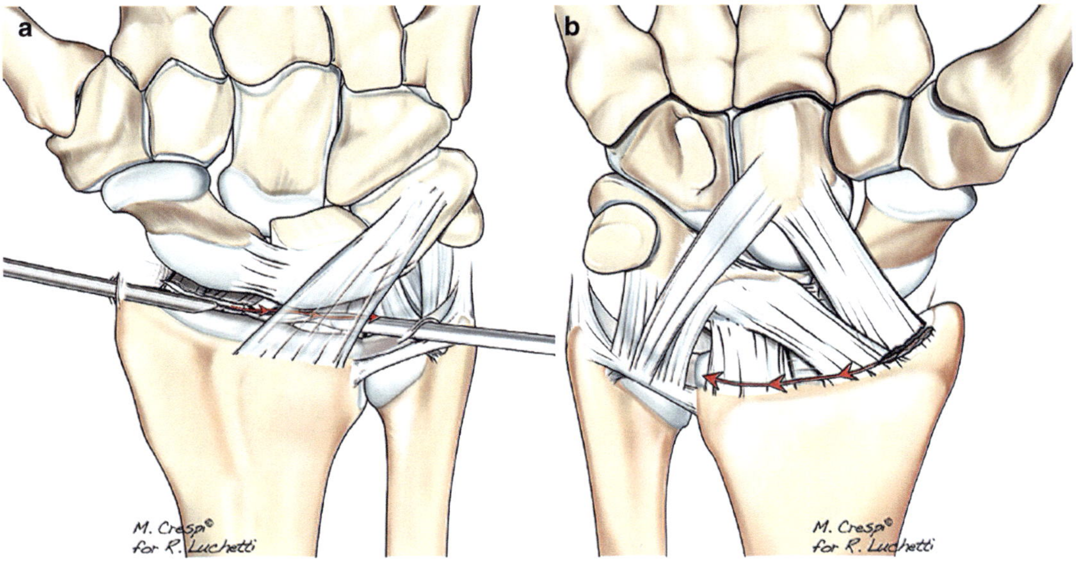

Fig. 27.21 Drawing illustrating the site of resection of the volar capsule and ligaments of the wrist (red arrows). Scope is in 1–2 portal and hook blade in the 6R portal. Only perform the release on the abnormal ligaments (Step 3) (**a** and **b**)

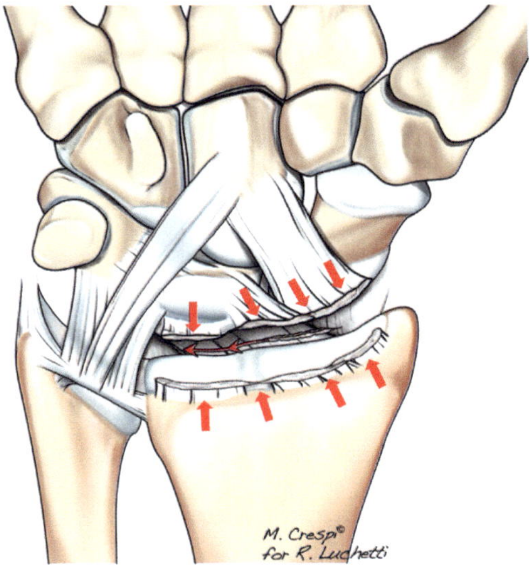

Fig. 27.22 Complete resection of the volar capsule and radiocarpal ligaments (Step 3)

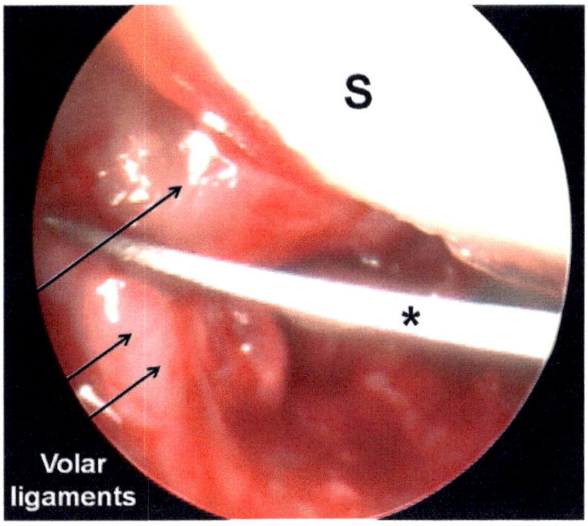

Fig. 27.23 Arthroscopic view of resection of the volar capsule and ligaments with blade (*) (Step 3). S: scaphoid. (Reproduced with permission from [4])

If there is restricted motion then the traction is re-applied, and the procedure continues with resection of the dorsal wrist capsule (Fig. 27.24a). Scope is positioned in the 1–2 portal and the instruments are introduced through the 6R portal. The central part of the dorsal capsule is first sectioned. The portals are switched with the instruments in 1–2 portal and scope in 6R portal. The intra-articular position of the 3–4 portal is located, and from this point the resection of the capsule starts by using a mini-scalpel, shaver, or radiofrequency with a hook tip (Fig. 27.25) or directly a hook scalpel (Fig. 27.10). The radial part of the dorsal capsule is easily resected through the 1–2 portal with the scope in the 6R portal. The ulnar part of the dorsal capsule contains the strong dorsal radiocarpal ligament

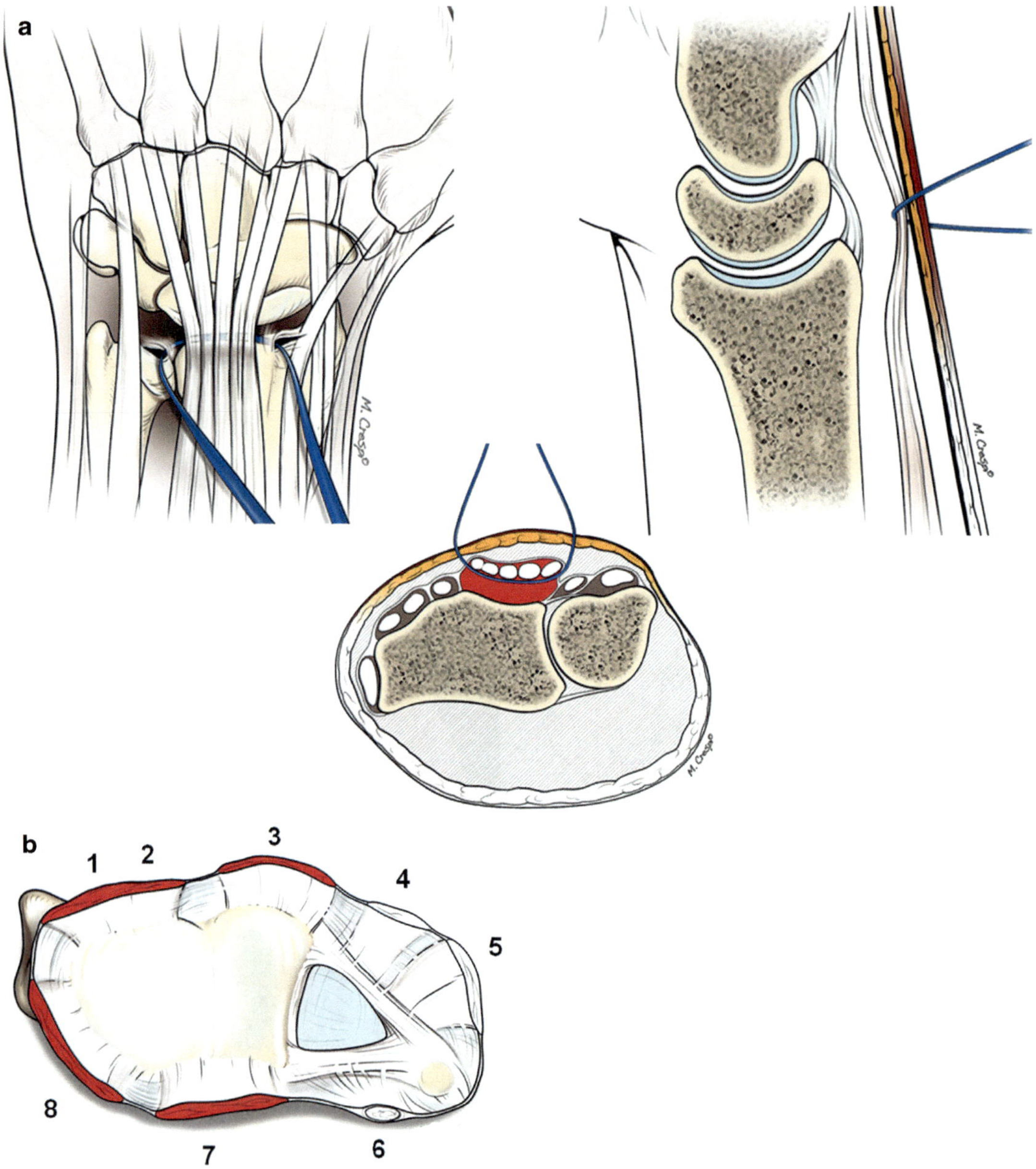

Fig. 27.24 (**a**) Drawings illustrating the use of nylon tape to retract the extensor tendons away from the dorsal wrist capsule. (**b**) Schematic drawing showing the extrinsic ligaments of the radiocarpal joint. (1) radio-scapho-capitate, (2) long radio-lunate, (3) short radio-lunate, (4) ulno-lunate, (5) ulno-triquetral, (6) ECU tendon, (7) dorsal radiocarpal, and (8) dorsal capsule. The ligaments (1–2–3–7) that can be sectioned during the arthroscopic volar and dorsal capsulotomy are shown in red (according to Bain et al. [14, 15] [9]). The ulnocarpal ligaments (4 and 5) must be preserved (Step 3). (Reproduced with permission from [4])

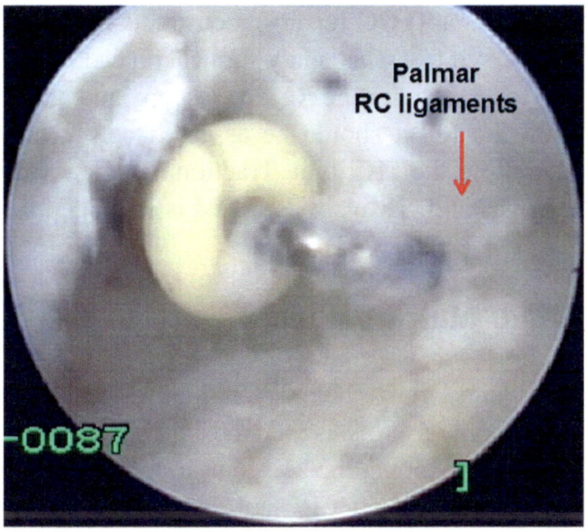

Fig. 27.25 Arthroscopic view of radiofrequency resection with a hook tip of the palmar radiocarpal (RC) ligaments using the wet arthroscopy (Step 3). (Reproduced with permission from [4])

(radio-triquetrum ligament). Here, the procedure becomes more difficult due to the firm consistency of this ligament. In this case, a volar radial portal may be used [36–38]. The volar radial portal is established with an inside-out technique, using a Wissinger rod [3], similar to that described with a Wissinger rod for the shoulder [32, 39] and elbow arthroscopy. Bain et al. [14, 15] have described a technique where a nylon tape is placed between the capsule and the extensor tendons, and is used to retractor the extensor tendons out of harm's way (Fig. 27.24a).

It is very important to remember that the volar UC ligaments and dorsal capsule of the UC joint must not be resected (Fig. 27.24b). The dorsal capsule of the UC joint is without a proper ligament but is reinforced by the floor of the Extensor Carpi Ulnaris (ECU) tendon sheath. The three volar UC ligaments are the ulno-lunate, the ulno-capitate, and the ulno-triquetral ligament. Moritomo et al. [40] showed that the volar UC ligaments insert into the volar aspect of the TFCC ligament and both run proximally attaching to the ulnar head. They demonstrated that a TFCC detachment produces both DRUJ and UC instability. Viegas et al. [41] reported that sectioning the radio-scapho-capitate and radio-lunate ligaments does not lead to significant ulnar translation of the carpus, and that either the volar ulnar ligament or the dorsal ulnar ligament complex alone can prevent ulnar translation. Therefore, the arthroscopic capsulotomy leaves the volar ulnar ligament and dorsal ulnar ligament complex intact.

If after this step gain of motion is still not satisfying the procedure continues to Step 4, otherwise, it finishes at this step.

27.4.4.4 Step 4: Step-Off and Bone Resection

Dorsal RC impingement secondary to malunion of a distal radius fracture may cause a limitation in wrist extension. In this case it is necessary to resect the dorsal rim of distal radius (Fig. 27.1) [24]. As the dorsal capsule in this phase is resected, the dorsal rim of the distal radius is easily exposed and resected by using a 2.9–3.5 mm burr introduced through the 6R or 1–2 portal. The most ulnar part of the distal radius dorsal rim is difficult to reach; it is resected mostly through the 6R or 6U portals.

Same procedure is used for volar margin and intra-articular step-off, when needed. For the volar margin the burr is introduced through the 1–2 portal, and scope in 6R portal. The most ulnar side of the volar margin of the radius is removed with burr in 6R or 6U portals. Fluoroscopy can be used in order to verify the articular step-off and dorsal/volar rim resection and position of the instrumentations.

Small articular steps (<1 mm) of the distal radius may be discovered at arthroscopy (Figs. 27.26 and 27.27). A 3.2 mm burr is used through the 6R portal while the scope in the 3–4 or 1–2 portal [24]. Larger steps can also be treated but this often results in fibrotic band recurrences and ongoing wrist pain with unsatisfying clinical results. The wrist motion is reassessed.

It is important to point out that in most cases the radiocarpal arthrolysis is limited to Steps 1 and 2. Step 3 is for advanced capsular contracture and Step 4 for articular incongruity. The procedure is determined by the articular findings in each case.

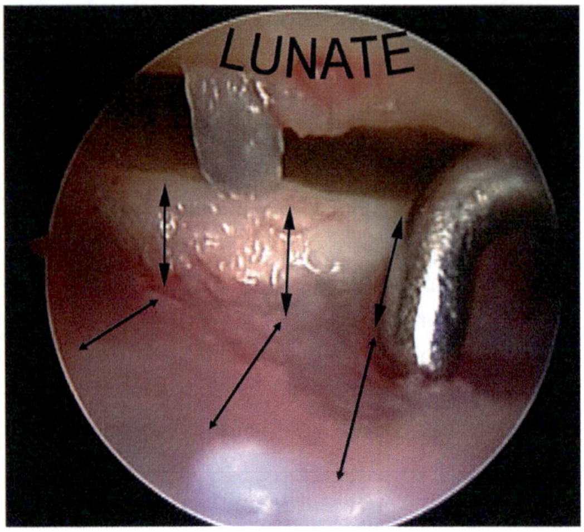

Fig. 27.26 Arthroscopic view showing an articular step of the distal radius that became evident during arthrolysis (Step 4). (Reproduced with permission from [4])

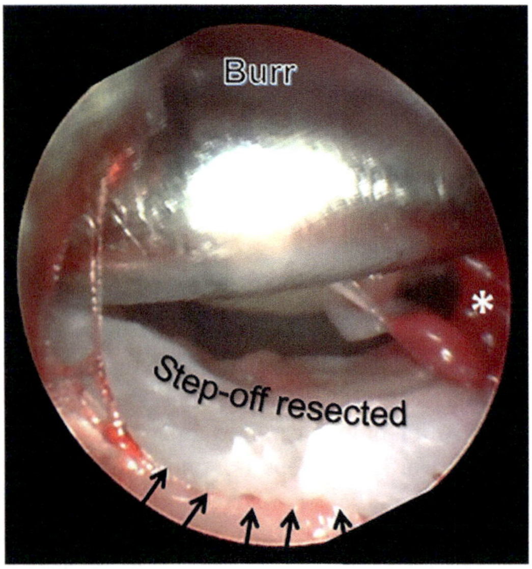

Fig. 27.27 Bone resection with reduction of the step-off (black arrows) (Step 4)

27.4.5 Ancillary Procedures

During arthroscopy one may identify other occult articular, DRUJ, or carpal bone pathologies. Some of these may be treated during the same procedure, such as debridement of central TFCC tears, arthroscopic wafer resection for positive ulnar variance, or removal of intra-articular loose bodies. Reconstructive procedures that require immobilization (e.g., TFCC repairs/reconstruction) should be reserved for a secondary surgical procedure.

This concludes the RC arthroscopy and at this point the ROM should be assessed before proceeding to the MC joint. Traction is temporarily removed and passive wrist ROM is evaluated.

27.4.6 Midcarpal Joint

MC joint must be explored always during arthroscopic arthrolysis even if the gained motion is satisfying. Scoping the MC joint becomes mandatory when ROM after RC arthrolysis is not fulfilling. There are two main portals for the MC joint: radial midcarpal (RMC) and ulnar midcarpal (UMC). Other portals may be used if necessary: trapezio-trapezoid (STT) and triquetro-hamate (TH). Scoping this joint is easier. Synovitis at STT joint or TH joint is usually the main finding. Cartilage damage of the capitate and hamate are commonly seen. These findings are more associated to pain than stiffness. Debridement of the MC joint is performed and may improve pain and ROM.

The same four steps are used for the MC joint contractures.

27.4.6.1 Step 1: Fibrosis and Fibrotic Band Resection

Fibrotic bands are less frequent in MC joint than RC; they are usually seen rising from the capitate hamate joint to the luno-triquetral joint (Fig. 27.28a, b). These bands do not permit the scope to pass from the ulnar part to the radial part of the joint. A dissector, shaver, or a 16G needle is introduced in MCR with scope in MCR and the band are cut and removed.

27.4.6.2 Step 2: Detachment of Dorsal Capsular Adhesion to the Carpal Bones

In some cases, MC joint arthroscopy requires adhesions resection between the dorsal capsule and the capitate (Fig. 27.29a, b). With the scope in MidCarpal Ulnar portal; (MCU) and a Freer in MidCarpal Radial portal (MCR), the dorsal capsule is detached from the capitate. Portals can be switched during the procedure.

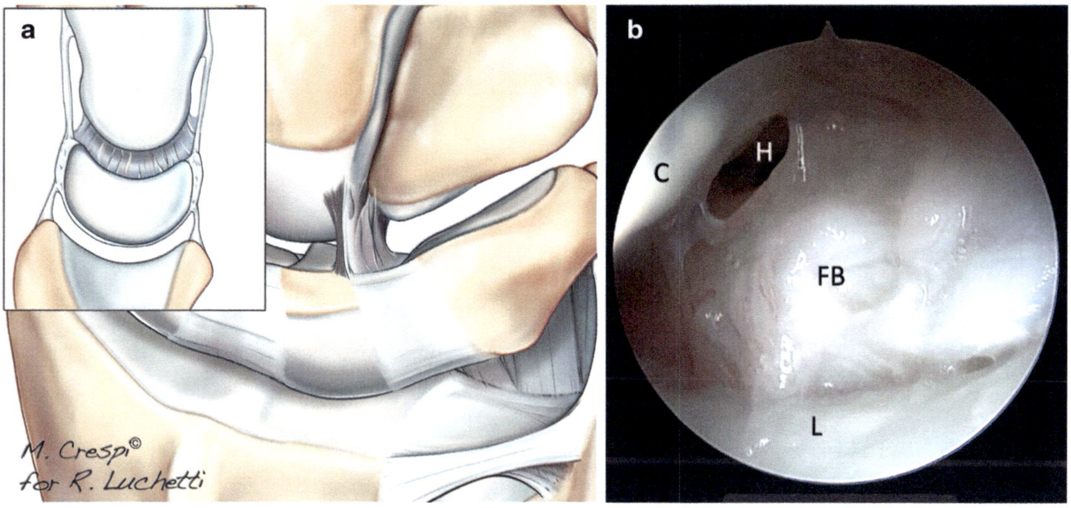

Fig. 27.28 Arthroscopic view (**a**) and drawing (**b**) showing fibrotic band (FB) rising from the capitate (C)–hamate (H) joint and inserting on the luno (L)–triquetral (T) joint

Fig. 27.29 Resection with a dissector of the fibrosis between the capsule and the capitate in the midcarpal joint (**a** and **b**) permitting a further increase of the wrist flexion

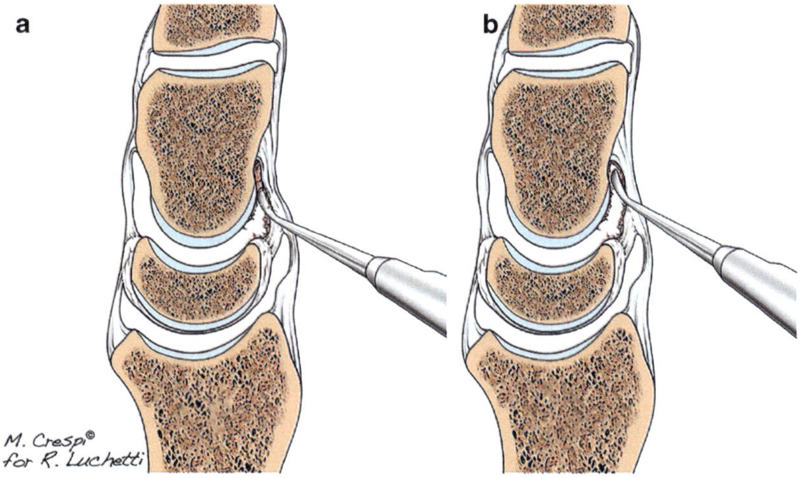

27.4.6.3 Step 3: Volar Capsule Contracture Resection

This step is rarely needed, but in some cases the resection of the hamate-triquetrum (HT) ligament is required to improve the wrist extension and supination. This was first demonstrated in an open technique by Babazadeh et al. [42] (Figs. 27.30a, b and 27.31a, b). They reported that no instability occurs with the resection of HT ligament.

27.4.6.4 Step 4: Step-Off and Bone Resection

Dorsal midcarpal impingement is suspected when wrist extension is limited and painful, with the pain localized to the capitate, with radiographs demonstrating deformity of the dorsal rim of the radius (Fig. 27.1). The degree of chondral damage to the capitate due to impingement may be assessed. After a synovectomy and debridement, a burr is used to remove excess bone from

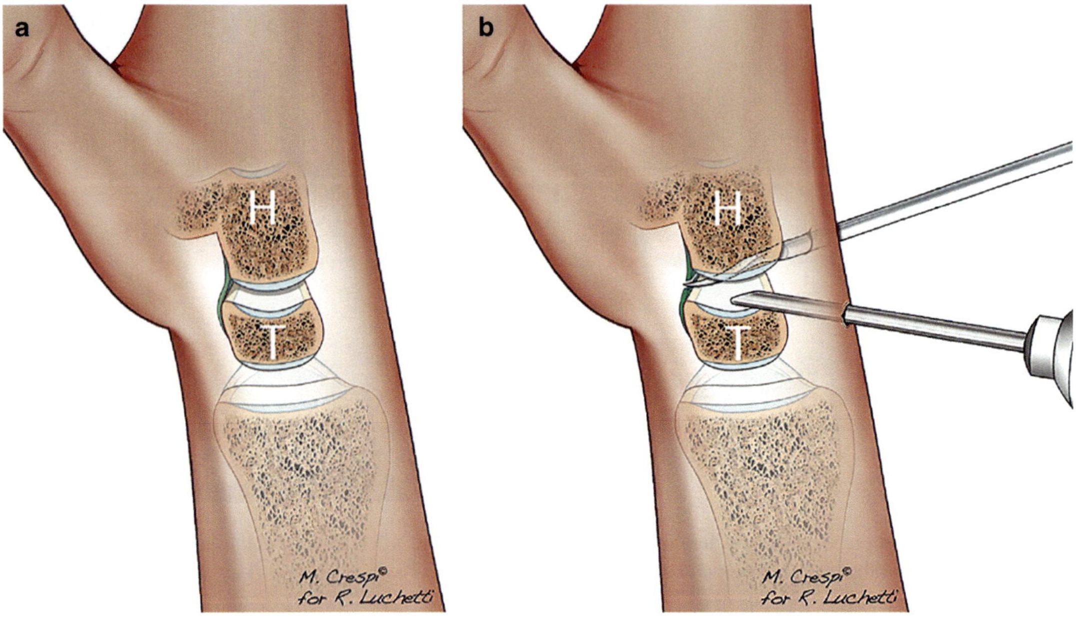

Fig. 27.30 Resection with a small blade or a hook blade of the volar ligament between the hamate (H) and the triquetrum (T) (**a** and **b**)

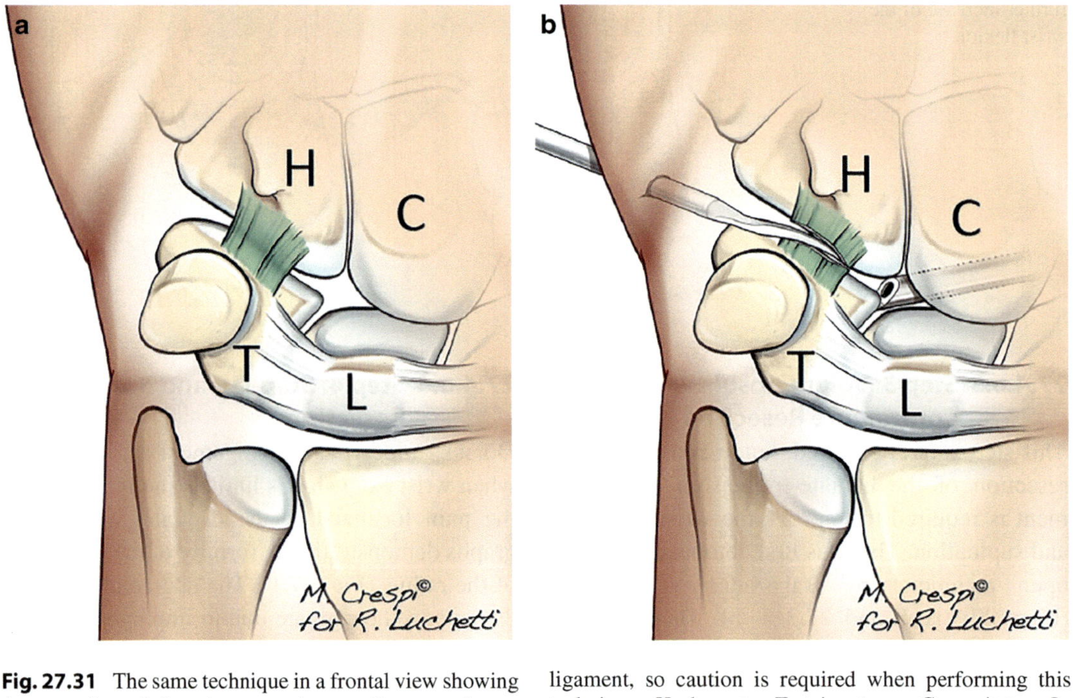

Fig. 27.31 The same technique in a frontal view showing the resection of the triquetrum–hamate ligament (green color). The scope is in the MCU and the hook blade in the TH portal (**a** and **b**). The ulnar nerve is just volar to this ligament, so caution is required when performing this technique. H: hamate; T: triquetrum; C: capitates; L: lunate

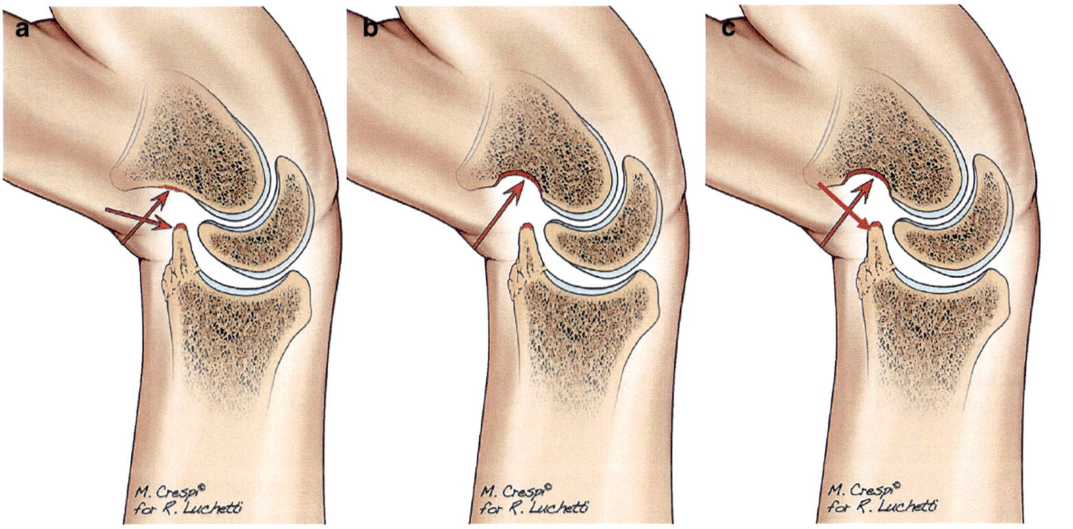

Fig. 27.32 Impaction between the dorsal border of the distal radius and the capitate limiting the complete extension of the wrist (**a**). Improvement of the wrist extension can be obtained through bone grooving of the neck of the capitate (**b**) with a burr or the dorsal lip of the distal radius (**c**)

the dorsum of the neck of the capitate (Fig. 27.32a–c) to facilitate acceptance of the remolded dorsal rim of the distal radius during wrist extension. As alternative or in association, the dorsal border of the distal radius should be resected to improve the extension of the wrist (Fig. 27.32c).

As for the RC procedure, after every step the wrist should be taken off from traction and movement reassessed; if it is sufficient the procedure ends, if not it continues to the next step till movement is satisfying.

27.4.7 Distal Radioulnar Joint

Arthroscopy of the DRUJ has the same setup as of RC and MC joint exploration [31, 43]. The surgeon must choose a traction system that permits prono-supination movements without any limitation. As the joint is narrow, scoping is quite difficult. The authors suggest the use of a wide-angle 1.9 mm videoarthroscope, which may facilitate the exploration and reduce the risk of damaging the articular structures. Even if the joint is small dry arthroscopy is recommended, as in our experience it improves the quality of the view and the evaluation process of the structures. It also has the advantage to permit a hybrid surgery (arthroscopic and open).

27.4.7.1 Indications and Contraindications

The main indication for the procedure is stiffness of the DRUJ with a good articular surface between the sigmoid notch (SN) and ulnar head (UH). Conditions involve the articular surface as: osteochondral lesion, intra-articular or extra-articular malunion of the SN, or the UH should represent a contraindication for the procedure.

The elbow should also be assessed. If the patient has a forearm fracture or radial head fracture, then it may be more appropriate to perform more proximal surgery.

27.4.7.2 Technique

Scoping the DRUJ, requires skills and experience with small joint arthroscopy. In normal conditions, exploring the joint with a decent visualization of the structures is challenging; in a condition of DRUJ, stiffness, capsular contraction, intra-articular fibrosis, and synovitis make this procedure extremely challenging.

The traditional DRUJ portals are on the dorsal aspect of the wrist: proximal (P-DRUJ) and distal (D-DRUJ) DRUJ portals (Figs. 27.33a–c and

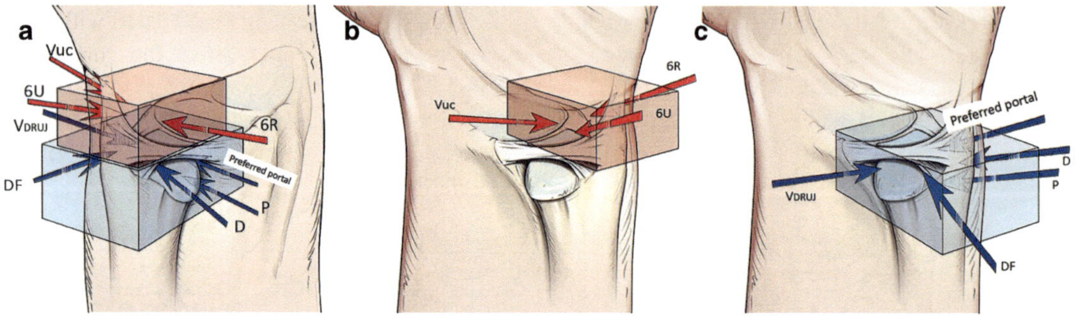

Fig. 27.33 Box concept for arthroscopic approach to the ulnocarpal joint (red box) and distal radioulnar joint (DRUJ) (blue box). Portals of the ulnocarpal joint (red arrows); DRUJ portals (blue arrows). Dorsal and volar view (**a**–**c**). The preferred portal is indicated. (Reproduced with permission from [43])

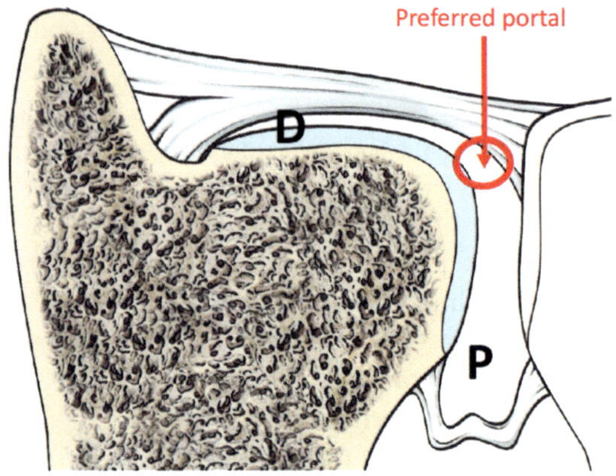

Fig. 27.34 Portals and "preferred portal" to enter into the DRUJ. D: distal portal of the DRUJ; P: proximal portal of the DRUJ. (Reproduced with permission from [43])

27.34). Another two portals have been described: the direct foveal (DF) [44] and the volar-DRUJ portal [45] (Fig. 27.33b, c). The DF portal is immediately under the 6U portal and is used as a working portal about the foveal insertion of the TFCC. The volar-DRUJ portal performed with an inside-out technique is located on the volar aspect of the wrist immediately radial to the edge of the flexor tendons and it is used for scope and instrument introduction.

The authors recommend to begin with a diagnostic arthroscopy using a portal that is at the midpoint between the two traditional dorsal portals (P-DRUJ and D-DRUJ) (Fig. 27.35a–c), in a triangular space that can be defined as the "medial soft corner" and is comprised below the insertion of the TFCC on the radius, at the point where the distal profile of the ulnar head curves to parallel the sigmoid notch. After a 22-gauge needle is inserted to confirm correct portal placement, a longitudinal skin incision is done and a mosquito forceps is used to spread the subcutaneous tissues and penetrate the joint through the dorsal capsule, just below the TFCC and lateral to the ulnar head (Fig. 27.35b). Care should be taken not to damage the Extensor Digiti Minimi, running in the fifth dorsal compartment. The 1.9 mm videoarthroscope is introduced through a cannula with blunt obturator. The videoarthroscope is short enough to be grasped keeping the index finger in constant contact of the skin of the wrist in order to stabilize and control the millimetric movement of the scope within the joint (Fig. 27.36) as for the microsurgery [46]. Wrist supination, when it is possible, allows an easier access to the DRUJ through the dorsal portals

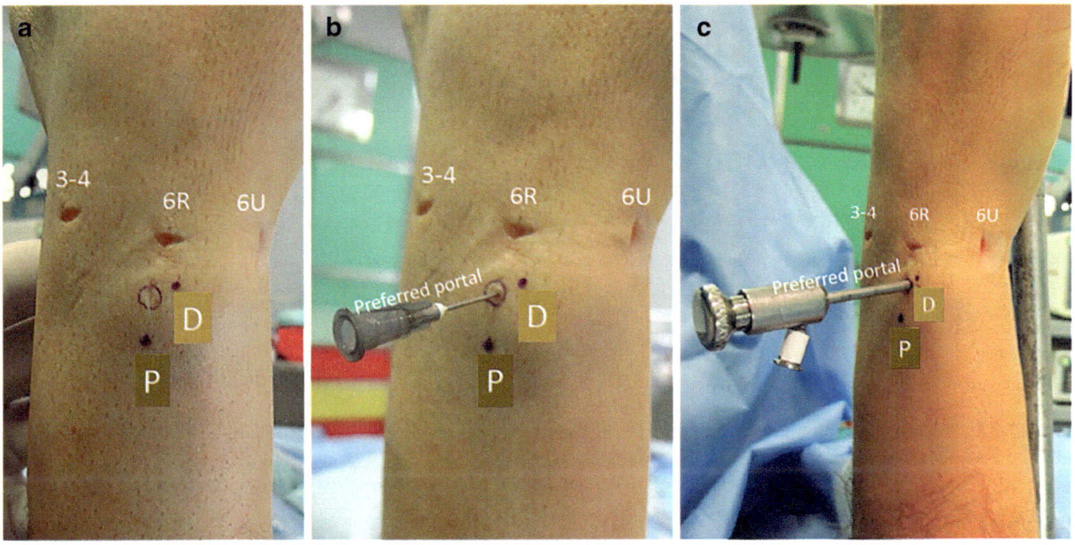

Fig. 27.35 Intraoperative pictures showing the position of the preferred portal (**a**), the technique to identify the correct location using a needle (**b**), and the introduction of the trocar into the DRUJ (**c**)

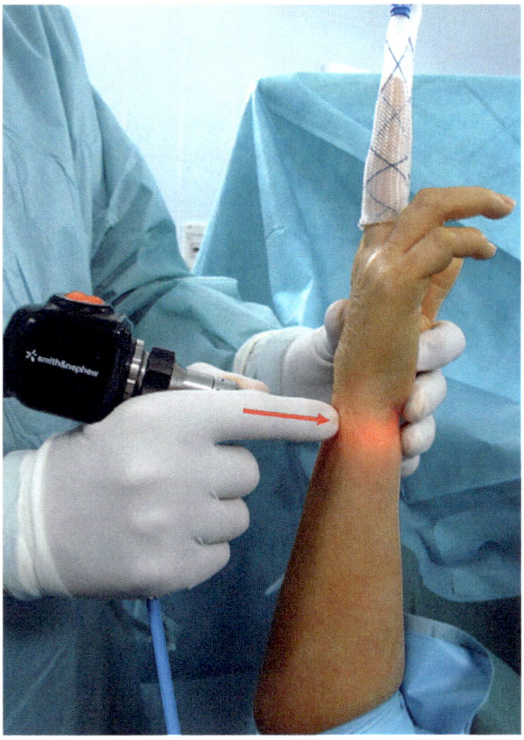

Fig. 27.36 Arthroscope into the DRUJ. Note the handling of the scope (red arrow)

(Fig. 27.37a, b). The internal view between the ulnar head and the TFCC is frequently obscured by fibrosis (Fig. 27.38). In these cases, we suggest introducing a blunt dissector between the TFCC and the ulnar head, and gently dissecting the adhesions [26].

Three different scenarios for the arthroscopic procedure are possible and depend on the integrity of the TFCC.

27.4.8 The Central Disk of the TFCC Is Intact

In this case the DRUJ joint can be visualized only by exploring it directly and DRUJ arthrolysis is required by DRUJ arthroscopy. The joint is difficult to visualize due to fibrotic adhesions and synovitis. Therefore, after performing the modified DRUJ portal the scope is removed and a Freer dissector is introduced through the portal to release the adhesions and create space (Fig. 27.39a, b). The scope is then reinserted; now exploration may be performed. Additionally,

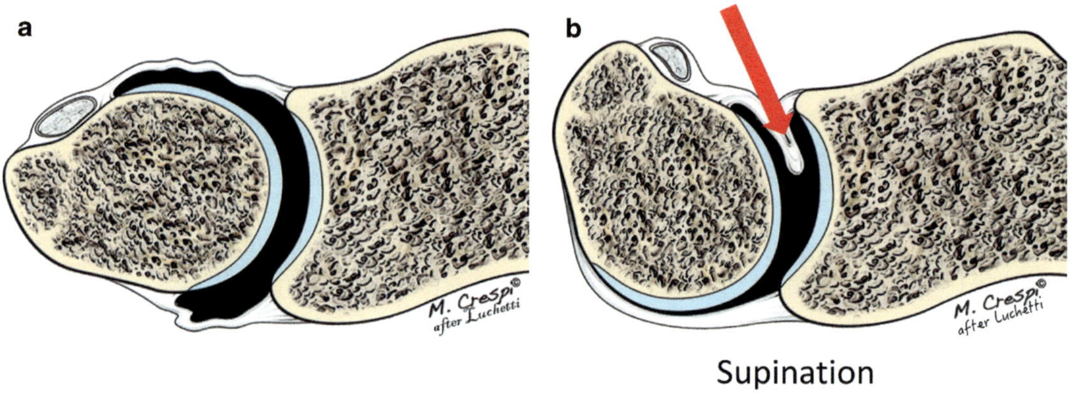

Fig. 27.37 Drawing showing an axial view of the DRUJ in neutral position (**a**) and supination (**b**). Supination is usually the best position to introduce the trocar into the DRUJ (red arrow)

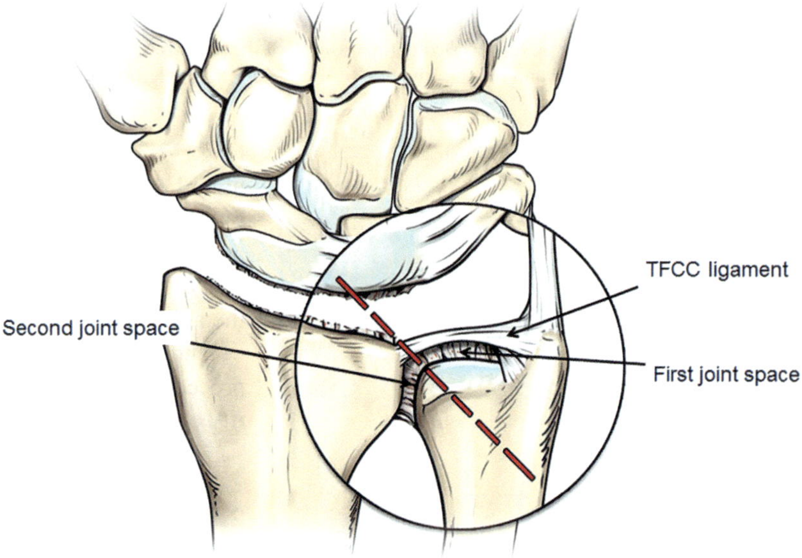

Fig. 27.38 Drawing showing the localization of fibrosis in the DRUJ. This joint is divided in two parts for the sake of the arthroscopic procedure. (Reproduced and modified with permission from [4])

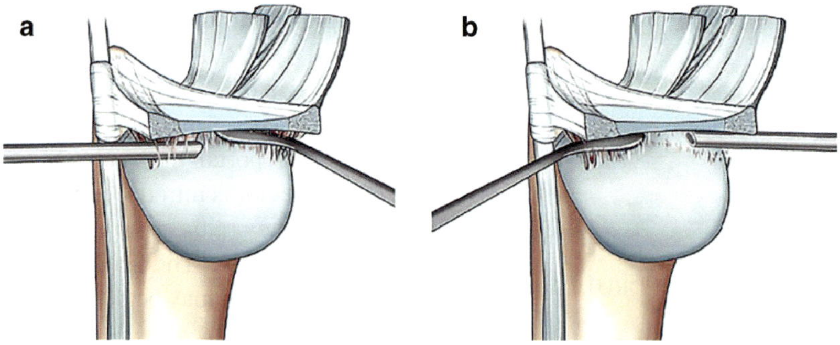

Fig. 27.39 Arthroscopic resection of the adhesions in the distal radioulnar joint. (**a**) Scope in the dorsal portal and periosteal elevator in the palmar portal. (**b**) Scope in palmar portal and dissector in the dorsal portal. Care is required to not damage the foveal insertion of the TFCC. (Reproduced with permission from [26])

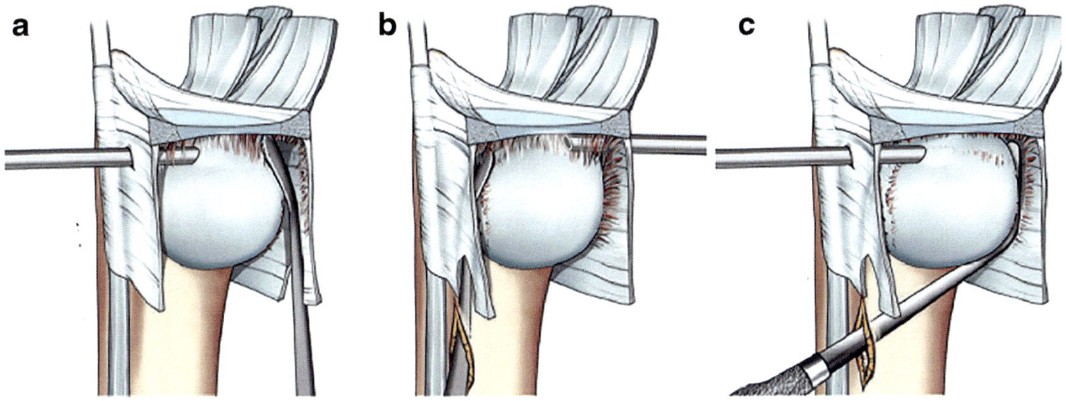

Fig. 27.40 Drawings showing the different approaches on how to use the scope and periosteal elevator to release the adhesions around the ulnar head. (**a**) Scope dorsal, elevator volar palmar DRUJ portal. (**b**) Scope volar, elevator dorsal DRUJ portal. (**C**) Scope in dorsal DRUJ portal, curved elevator proximal dorsal portal. (Reproduced with permission from [26])

a proximal DRUJ portal may be created at the level of the ulnar neck to introduce a periosteal elevator to breakdown any adhesions within the sigmoid notch (Fig. 27.40a, b) or proximal to it. The volar DRUJ portal may be created using an inside-out technique; the Freer dissector may be introduced to release the anterior capsule (Fig. 27.40a). Dorsal and volar portals at this point can be switched. The dorsal capsule is released from the ulnar head ulnarly up to the ECU tendon sheath to complete the arthrolysis. Often, the scope can only see the tip of the periosteal elevator as some other blind maneuvers are required (Fig. 27.39b). Particularly when the periosteal elevator is driven proximally to achieve a complete release, attention must be given to protect the ulnar neurovascular structures palmarly (Fig. 27.40c), and the ECU tendon dorsally. Prono-supination improvement is tested maintaining the wrist in the traction tower.

27.4.9 The Central Disk of the TFCC Is Intact but Perforated by Surgeon

An alternative to the procedure mentioned above is the one described by del Piñal, in which the surgeon with scope in 3–4 and Freer dissector in 6U or 4–5 creates a window in the central disk of the TFCC to reach the DRUJ from RC joint [25]. Moving the periosteal elevator gently over the ulnar head, although in a blind fashion, allows detachment or stretching of the volar and the dorsal capsule restoring motion of the DRUJ (Fig. 27.41a–f).

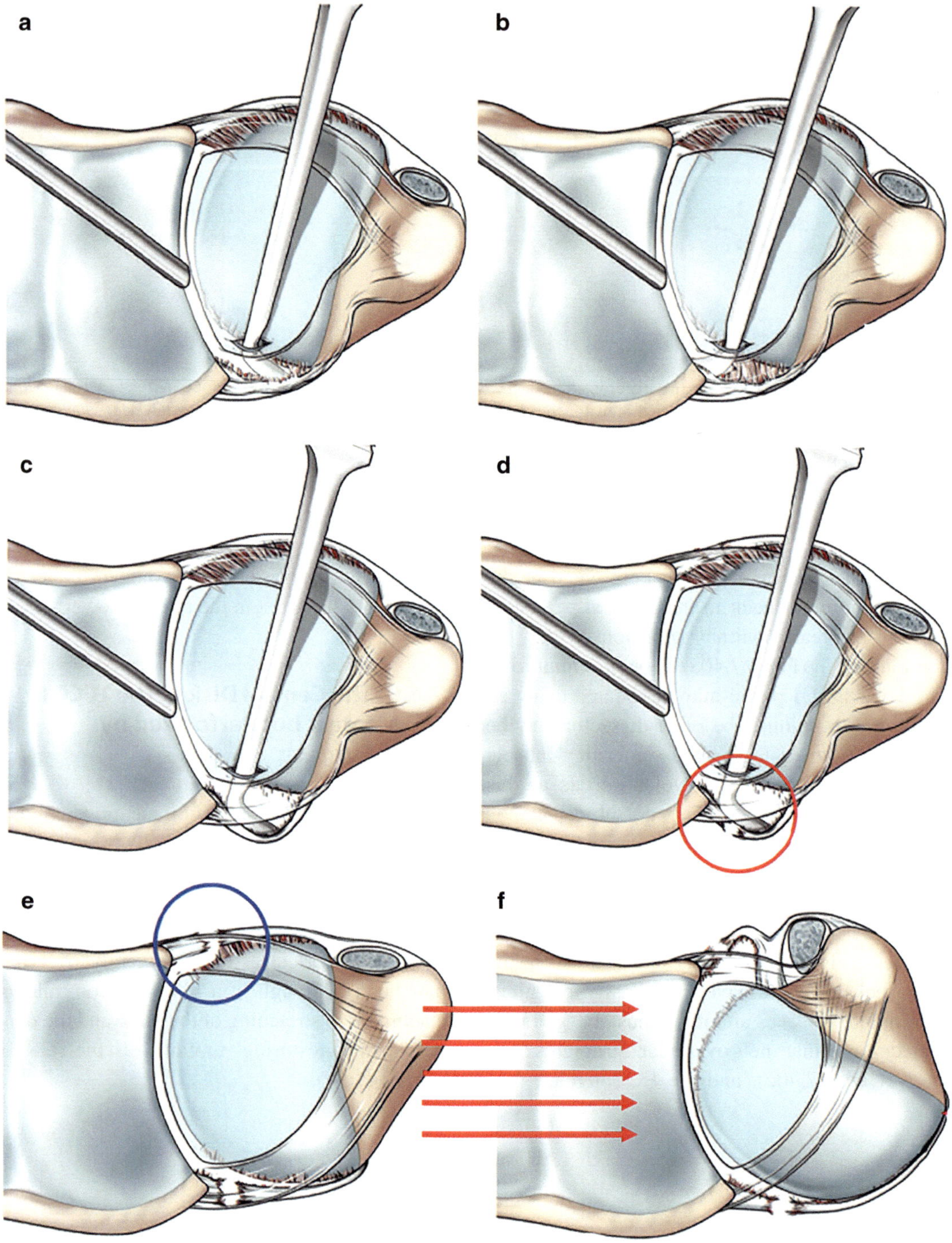

Fig. 27.41 Drawing showing resection of the distal radioulnar joint (DRUJ) adhesions, while maintaining the scope in 3–4 portal and periosteal elevator in 6R portal (according to [25]). Periosteal dissector is introduced into the anterior part of the DRUJ through a mini-incision close to the palmar aspect of the triangular fibrocartilage complex. The adhesions are released with gentle maneuvers with the elevator. (**a** and **b**) Detaching the capsule from the ulna head. Pull maneuver (**c**) of the capsule by periosteal dissector tip ruptures the capsule (**d**) close to the radius (red circle). Same maneuver for the palmar capsule (**e** and **f**) with release of capsular adhesions and capsular tear close to the radius (blue circle). (Reproduced with permission from [26])

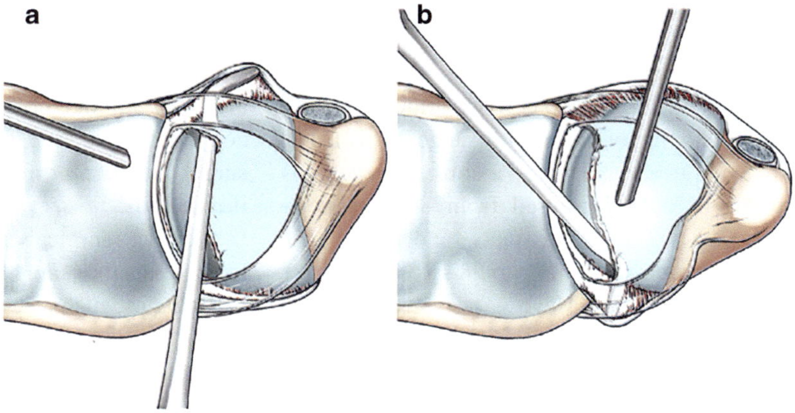

Fig. 27.42 Dissector passing through the TFCC type 1A lesion reachs the volar (**a**) and the dorsal (**b**) capsule providing the detachment of the capsule adherences

27.4.10 The Central Disk of the TFCC Is Absent

This condition facilitates the DRUJ arthrolysis procedure as the procedure can be performed with scope in 3–4 and instruments in 6U or 6R portals. These portals can be switched in between. The DRUJ adhesions are easily removed in this manner with the instruments in RC joint (Fig. 27.42).

27.5 Complications and Management

1. *Osteofibrotic band*: They are thick and dense, often the cause of radio-lunate ankylosis (Fig. 27.12). Unfortunately, this kind of fibrotic bands cannot be treated by arthroscopy as a risk of residual stiffness and patient non-satisfaction is high. Osteochondral lesions are often associated with these conditions.
2. *Extra-articular wrist stiffness due to CRPS*: This is a complex situation in which intra-articular arthroscopic arthrolysis must be associated to an extra-articular release of soft tissues adhesions. The patient who presents with the clinical syndrome of Chronic Reflex Pain Syndrome (CRPS), often has a nerve entrapment [47]. Therefore, the nerve entrapment needs to be diagnosed, and treated. As CRPS is a diagnosis of exclusion, by definition, the nerve entrapment is not CRPS!
3. *Recurrent pain*: Patients may have persistent wrist pain after the procedure. This may indicate an articular pathology that was not diagnosed during the procedure. In other cases pain may develop after the procedure, and may be due to a chronic ligament lesion that now, when the wrist has a better range of motion, has become symptomatic.
4. *Iatrogenic lesions*: Osteochondral or ligament injury may occur during arthroscopic instrumentation, which may present as postoperatively with pain or instability.

27.6 Postoperative Rehabilitation

Rehabilitation is started immediately after surgery [6]. Routine analgesics are used for postoperative pain control. Active and passive pronation–supination and flexion–extension exercises are performed, gradually increasing the passive mobilizing force, under the guidance of a therapist.

Return to work is delayed up to 3 months as per the work requirements of the patient. A volar wrist splint is used for protection while performing heavy activities. Endurance and strengthening exercises using isokinetic and isotonic rehabilitation equipment can be initiated 1 month after surgery under the strict supervision of a physical therapist. The patient protocol is individualized depending on strength/occupational requirements for the individual.

27.7 Clinical Outcome

In 2007, we described the results on 22 patients treated with arthroscopic wrist arthrolysis at a mean follow-up of 28 months (range 9–144) [17]. No complications were identified. Flexion–extension ROM increased from 84° preoperatively to 99° postoperatively and mean grip strength increased from 22 to 28 kg ($P < 0.0001$). The mean modified Mayo wrist score improved from 28 to 79 ($P < 0.0001$), and the mean score on the Disabilities of the Arm, Shoulder and Hand (DASH) questionnaire was 21 points. In the same study we described a method to perform an arthroscopic release of DRUJ contractures by using DRUJ portals. A dissector was introduced into the proximal portal to release the adhesions between the ulnar head and the sigmoid fossa. The prono-supination range increased from 144° to 159° ($P < 0.1$).

27.8 Summary

Wrist arthrolysis is now a common surgical procedure for the treatment of wrist stiffness. The development of the understanding of anatomy, imaging, and more sophisticated arthroscopic techniques has extended the surgical capabilities. As this is an advanced arthroscopic technique, it requires experience and skills in small joint arthroscopy. Arthroscopy allows the surgeon to identify the intra-articular pathology, including visualization and probing of the ligaments and articular cartilage. By combining the clinical history, examination, and advanced imaging, with the arthroscopic findings, we can obtain a better comprehension of patient's condition and causes of pain.

Arthroscopy permits the surgeon to address all of the causes of stiffness, including arthrofibrosis, capsular adhesions, intra-articular septum, and bony impingement. We prefer the dry arthroscopy technique, but it is possible to convert the surgery in open or mini-open (hybrid technique) if required.

Adjunct surgical procedures may be performed at the same time to treat associated pathologies, such as carpal tunnel syndrome and partial or total wrist denervation. This 360° approach improves the surgical morbidity and outcomes, beyond that achieved with open techniques. A review of the published results following arthroscopic wrist arthrolysis is reported in Table 27.3. All series showed a significant improvement in wrist ROM.

Based on our experience, reconstructive procedures that require immobilization should not be simultaneously performed with an arthroscopic arthrolysis. Examples include TFCC tears type 1B or a complete tear of the SL ligament. Unfortunately following arthrolysis, patients with scapholunate tears can have increased postoperative pain. Therefore, careful consideration and discussion with the patient are required before the arthroscopy is performed. If arthrolysis is performed, it is mandatory that the wrist is mobilized and that the patient initiates rehabilitation immediately after an arthroscopic arthrolysis procedure.

It may be seen that an intraoperative increase in wrist flexion–extension ROM is followed by a temporary decrease soon after surgery, but is regained over time [1]. On the contrary, pronation–supination improvement that has been obtained during surgery is almost always maintained postoperatively [1, 6, 17, 18, 20].

Table 27.3 Previous publications

Publications	Cases	Follow-up	Pre-op	Post-op
Pederzini et al. [1]	5	10	44/40	54/60
Osterman and Culp (2000)	20	32	9/15	42/58
Luchetti et al. [6]	19	32	46/38	54/53
Hattori et al. [34]	11	?	29/47	42/56

Note: Follow-up is months. Results are the mean flexion/extension values, measured in degrees
Source: Reproduced and modified with permission from Springer Verlag

DRUJ stiffness may be isolated or in conjunction with RC joint stiffness. When DRUJ stiffness is isolated, ROM recovery after surgery is easier to obtain than when it is associated with RC stiffness, and this improvement of DRUJ motion is maintained.

References

1. Pederzini L, Luchetti R, Montagna G, Alfarano M, Soragni O. Trattamento artroscopico delle rigidità di polso. Il Ginocchio. 1991;XI-XII:1–13.
2. Bain GI, Verhellen R, Pederzini L. Procedure artroscopiche capsulari del polso. In: Pederzini L, editor. Artroscopia di Polso. Milano: Springer; 1999. p. 123–8.
3. Verhellen R, Bain GI. Arthroscopic capsular release for contracture of the wrist. Arthroscopy. 2000;16:106–10.
4. McGuire DT, Luchetti R, Atzei A, Bain GI. Arthroscopic arthrolysis. In: Geissler WB, editor. Wrist and elbow arthroscopy: a practical surgical guide in techniques. New York: Springer; 2015. p. 165–75.
5. Altissimi M, Rinonapoli E. Le rigidità del polso e della mano. Inquadramento clinico, valutazione diagnostica e indicazioni terapeutiche. GIOT (Suppl). 1995;21:187–92.
6. Luchetti R, Atzei A, Mustapha B. Arthroscopic wrist arthrolysis. Atlas. Hand Clin. 2001;6:371–87.
7. af Ekenstam FW. Capsulotomy of the distal radioulnar joint. Scand J Plast Surg. 1988;22:169–71.
8. Marco G, Maurizio C, Riccardo L. Wrist contracture after distal radius fractures. In: Buijze GA, Jupiter JB, Chammas M, editors. Distal radius fractures: evidence-based management. 1st ed. St. Louis: Elsevier; 2020.
9. Bain GI, Clitherow DS. The pathogenesis and classification of shoulder stiffness. In: Itoi E, Arce G, Bain GI, Diercksa RL, Guttmann D, Imhoff AB, Mazzocca AD, Sugaya H, Yoo YS, editors. Shoulder stiffness: current concepts and concerns. Berlin: Springer; 2015. p. 3–19.
10. Warner JJ, Answorth A, Marsh PH, Wong P. Arthroscopic release for chronic, refractory adhesive capsulitis of the shoulder. J Bone Joint Surg. 1995;78A:1808–16.
11. Warner JJ, Allen AA, Marks PH, Wong P. Arthroscopic release of post-operative capsular contracture of the shoulder. J Bone Joint Surg. 1996;79A:1151–8.
12. Watts A, Bain GI. New techniques in elbow arthroscopy. In: Savoie F, Field L, editors. AANA advanced arthroscopy surgical technique: the elbow and the wrist. San Francisco, CA: SLACK Inc; 2010. p. 124–31.
13. Jones GS, Savoie FH. Arthroscopic capsular release of flexion contractures of the elbow. Arthroscopy. 1993;9:277–83.
14. Bain GI, Munt J, Bergman J. Arthroscopic dorsal capsular release in the wrist: a new technique. Tech Hand Upper Extrem Surg. 2008;12:191–4.
15. Bain GI, Munt J, Turner PC. New advances in wrist arthroscopy. Arthroscopy. 2008;24:355–67.
16. Bergman J, Bain GI. Arthroscopic release of wrist contractures. In: Slutsky DJ, Osterman AL, editors. Distal radius fractures and carpal injury: the cutting edge. Philadelphia, PA: Saunders; 2009. p. 503–6.
17. Luchetti R, Atzei A, Fairplay T. Arthroscopic wrist arthrolysis after wrist fracture. Arthroscopy. 2007;23:255–60.
18. Luchetti R, Atzei A. Artrolisi artroscopica nelle rigidità post-traumatiche. In: Luchetti R, Atzei A, editors. Artroscopia di Polso. Mattioli 1885 Editore: Fidenza; 2001. p. 67–71.
19. Luchetti R, Atzei A, Fairplay T. Wrist arthrolysis. In: Geissler WB, editor. Wrist arthroscopy. New York: Springer; 2004. p. 145–54.
20. Luchetti R, Atzei A, Papini-Zorli I. Arthroscopic wrist arthrolysis. Chir Main. 2006;25:S244–53.
21. Luchetti R. The role of arthroscopy in post fracture stiffness. In: del Piñal F, Mathoulin C, Luchetti R, editors. Arthroscopic management of distal radius fractures. Berlin: Springer; 2010. p. 151–73.
22. Osterman AL, Culp RW, Bednar JM. The arthroscopic release of wrist contractures. Scientific Paper Session A1, ASSH Annual Meeting, Boston. NO; 2000.
23. del Piñal F, Garcia-Bernal FJ, Delgado J, Sanmartin M, Regalado J, Cerezal L. Correction of malunited intra-articular distal radius fractures with an inside-out osteotomy technique. J Hand Surg. 2006;31A:1029–34.
24. del Piñal F, Klausmayer M, Thams C, Moralede E, Galindo C. Arthroscopic resection arthrolysis for malunited intra-articular distal radius fractures. J Hand Surg. 2012;37A:2447–55.
25. del Piñal F, Moraleda E, Ruas JS, Rodriguez-Vega A, Studer A. Effectiveness of an arthroscopic technique to correct supination losses of 90° or more. J Hand Surg Am. 2018;43:676.e1–6.
26. Luchetti R, Atzei A. Ulnar pain and pronosupination losses. In: del Piñal F, Haerle M, Krimmer H, editors. Distal radius fractures and carpal instabilities. Stuttgart: Thieme; 2019. p. 255–70.
27. Hanson EC, Wood VE, Thiel AE, Maloney MD, Sauser DD. Adhesive capsulitis of the wrist. Diagnosis and treatment. Clin Orthop Relat Res. 1988;234:51–5.
28. Cerofolini E, Luchetti R, Pederzini L, Soragni O, Colombini R, D'Alimonte P, Romagnoli R. MRI evaluation of triangular fibrocartilage complex tears in the wrist: comparison with arthrography and arthroscopy. J Comput Assist Tomogr. 1990;14:963–7.
29. Zlatkin MB, Chao PC, Osterman AL, Schnall MD, Dalinka MK, Kressel HY. Chronic wrist pain: evaluation with high-resolution MR imaging. Radiology. 1989;173:723–9.
30. Carr R, MacLean S, Slavotinek J, Bain G. Four-dimensional computed tomography scanning for dynamic wrist disorders: prospective

analysis and recommendations for clinical utility. J Wrist Surg. 2019;8(2):161–7. https://doi.org/10.1055/s-0038-1675564.
31. Atzei A, Luchetti R, Sgarbossa A, Carità E, Llusa M. Set-up, portals and normal exploration in wrist arthroscopy. Chir Main. 2006;25:S131–44.
32. Badur N, Luchetti R, Atzei A. Arthroscopic wrist anatomy and setup. In: Geissler WB, editor. Wrist and elbow arthroscopy. A practical surgical guide to techniques. 2nd ed. New York: Springer; 2015. p. 1–27.
33. del Piñal F, Garcìa-Bernal FJ, Pisani D, Regalado J, Ayala H, Studer A. Dry arthroscopy of the wrist. Surgical technique. J Hand Surg. 2007;32A:119–23.
34. Hattori T, Tsunoda K, Watanabe K, Nakao E, Nakamura R. Arthroscopic mobilization for post-traumatic contracture of the wrist. J Jpn Soc Surg Hand. 2004;21:583–6.
35. del Piñal F. Extra-articular distal radius fracture malunions: arthroscopic tips and tricks. In: del Piñal F, editor. Atlas of distal radius fractures. New York: Thieme; 2018. p. 273–81.
36. Doi K, Hattori Y, Otsuka K, Abe Y, Yamamoto H. Intra-articular fractures of the distal aspect of the radius: arthroscopically assisted reduction compared with open reduction and internal fixation. J Bone Joint Surg. 1999;81A:1093–110.
37. Slutsky DJ. Wrist arthroscopy through a volar radial portal. Arthroscopy. 2002;18:624–30.
38. Tham S, Coleman S, Gilpin D. An anterior portal for wrist arthroscopy. Anatomical study and case reports. J Hand Surg. 1999;24B:445–7.
39. Snyder SJ. Diagnostic arthroscopy of the shoulder: normal anatomy and variations. In: Snyder SJ, editor. Shoulder arthroscopy. New York: McGraw-Hill Inc; 1994. p. 23–39.
40. Moritomo H, Murase T, Arimitsu S, Oka K, Yoshikawa H, Sugamoto K. Change in the length of the ulnocarpal ligaments during radiocarpal motion: possible impact on triangular fibrocartilage complex foveal tears. J Hand Surg. 2008;33A:1278–86.
41. Viegas SF, Patterson RM, Eng M, Ward K. Extrinsic wrist ligaments in the pathomechanics of ulnar translation instability. J Hand Surg Am. 1995;20:312–8.
42. Babazadeh S, de la Bellacasa IP, Jamieson RP, Rodriguez-Baeza A, Garcia-Elias M. Anteromedial release for posttraumatic flexion-pronation contracture of the wrist: surgical technique. Tech Hand Up Extrem Surg. 2019;23:170–5.
43. Atzei A, Luchetti R. DRUJ arthroscopy. In: Slutsky DJ, editor. Operative orthopedics of the upper extremity. New York: McGraw Hill; 2014. p. 407–18.
44. Atzei A, Rizzo A, Luchetti R, Fairplay T. Arthroscopic foveal repair of triangular fibrocartilage complex peripheral lesion with distal radioulnar joint instability. Tech Hand Up Extrem Surg. 2008;12:226–35.
45. Slutsky DJ. Distal radioulnar joint arthroscopy and volar ulnar portal. Tech Hand Up Extrem Surg. 2007;11:38–44.
46. Ho PC. Wrist arthroscopy as microsurgery of the joint. Lecture presented at 3rd Course of Arthroscopy and Arthroplasty of the wrist. Verona (Italy), September 28, 2017.
47. del Piñal F. Editorial. I have a dream … reflex sympathetic dystrophy (RSD or Complex Regional Pain Syndrome - CRPS I) does not exist. J Hand Surg Eur Vol. 2013;38(6):595–7. https://doi.org/10.1177/1753193413477058.

28 Wrist Denervation

Margaret Woon Man

28.1 Introduction

Joint stiffness may be caused by prolonged inactivity, a physiological reflex when movement generates pain. Joint denervation is a procedure that eliminates articular pain by destroying its sensory nerves. By abolishing the pain sensation, some movement may be restored.

For wrist denervation, it was first described by Wilhelm [1] in 1959, based on his extensive anatomic studies of the wrist. It can be performed on its own as a buy-time procedure or with other concomitant procedures like soft tissue reconstruction or limited joint arthrodesis. The aim is to achieve of a pain-free wrist, irrespective of the status of the joint and bone.

28.2 Anatomy

In order to denervate the wrist joint, we must first understand the anatomy, that is, the sensory fibers that innervate the joint. Hilton's law defined that for nerves crossing a joint, they yield branches innervating that joint. Wilhelm [1] describes in details on the nerve innervation to the wrist.

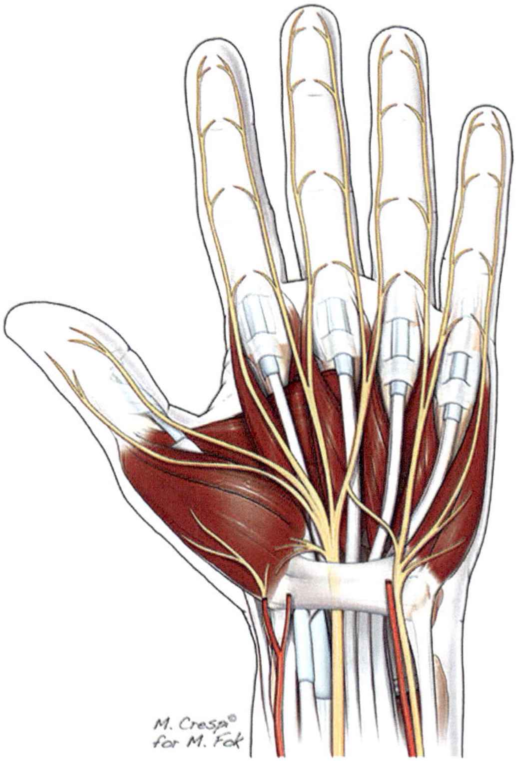

Fig. 28.1 Palmar view of the L wrist and hand showing the nerve distribution

There are numerous nerves that cross the wrist joint and innervate it (Figs. 28.1 and 28.2). In addition, they interconnect with each other, forming a network around the wrist.

M. W. Man (✉)
Department of Orthopaedics and Traumatology, Queen Mary Hospital, The University of Hong Kong, Pok Fu Lam, Hong Kong

L. Pederzini et al. (eds.), *Stiffness of the Elbow, Wrist and Related Pathologies*,
https://doi.org/10.1007/978-3-031-81381-8_28

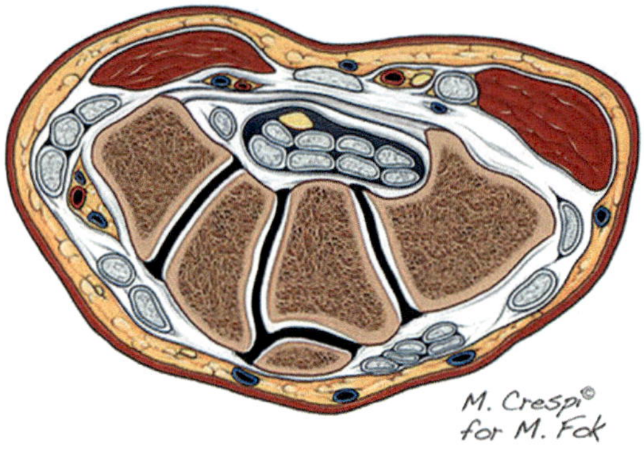

Fig. 28.2 Cross section of L wrist showing nerves with respect to adjacent structures

1. Posterior interosseus nerve (PIN)
2. Superficial radial nerve
3. Antebrachial cutaneous nerve
4. Median nerve
5. Anterior interosseus nerve (AIN)
6. Ulnar nerve
7. Posterior antebrachial cutaneous nerve

28.2.1 Posterior Interosseus Nerve [1]

Terminal branch of PIN runs above the dorsal aspect of the interosseous membrane. Before reaching the distal radius, it sends off a branch to innervate the distal radioulnar joint (DRUJ). It then joins together with the posterior interosseous artery to reach the radiocarpal joint at the base of the fourth extensor compartment. It divides into three to four branches, which supply the radiocarpal, intercarpal, and the second to fifth carpo-metacarpal joints. As a result, it innervates central two-thirds of the dorsal wrist.

PIN sends articular fibers to join (1) the articular branch of *the posterior antebrachial cutaneous nerve* to supply the ulnocarpal joint, and (2) the articular branch of the *superficial radial nerve* and *lateral antebrachial cutaneous nerve* to supply the radial aspect of the radiocarpal joint.

28.2.2 Superficial Radial Nerve [1]

Superficial nerve sends articular branch at the level of the radial styloid process in order to innervate the radiocarpal joint in the proximal part of the anatomic snuffbox. This articular nerve connects with the fibers of *the lateral antebrachial cutaneous nerve* and a branch of *PIN*.

Furthermore, an *articular branch of the first interosseous space* arises from either the first dorsal common digital nerve or from one of its branches at the level of the proximal part of the first interosseous space. It runs along the ulnar side of the first intermetacarpal vein to reach the bases of the first and second metacarpal bone. It then divides into seven branches and anastomoses with the *perforating nerves of the deep branch of the ulnar nerves*.

28.2.3 Lateral Antebrachial Cutaneous Nerve [1]

Lateral antebrachial cutaneous nerve innervates the radial side of the radiocarpal joint. Its articular branch runs along the radial side of the radial artery, before anastomosing with the articular fibers of the *superficial radial nerve* and the *PIN*. A large fiber also runs beneath the radial artery and joins with the articular branches of the *AIN*.

28.2.4 Median Nerve [1]

The articular fiber of the *palmar cutaneous nerve* runs along the palmar aspect of the wrist reaching the radial aspect of the radiocarpal joint. It sends off branches to supply the scapho-trapezial and the trapezio-metacarpal joints. The *recurrent branch of the median nerve*s also makes contribution to the trapezio-metacarpal joint.

28.2.5 Anterior Interosseous Nerve [1]

The articular branch of the AIN arises from the distal border of the pronator quadratus muscle to supply the palmar aspect of the DRUJ and radiocarpal joint. It also innervates the palmar aspect of the intercarpal and the third and fourth carpometacarpal joints. It sends off a branch that anastomoses radially with the *lateral antebrachial cutaneous nerve*, creating an O-shaped network over the scaphoid and lunate bone.

28.2.6 Ulnar Nerve [1]

The *deep motor branch of the ulnar nerve* innervates the ulnocarpal joint. It also sends off *perforating branches* to anastomose with the *PIN* and the *articular branch of the first interosseous space*, forming the intermetacarpal branches. The *dorsal branch of the ulnar nerve* also sends out articular fibers at the level of the ulnar head to innervate the palmar aspect of the ulnocarpal joint.

28.2.7 Posterior Antebrachial Cutaneous Nerve [1]

This short articular nerve branches off the posterior antebrachial cutaneous nerve just proximal to the ulnar head, and travels deep to the extensor carpi ulnaris (ECU) to supply the ulnocarpal joint. It also joins with the articular branches of the *PIN*.

28.2.8 Indications

Patients are indicated for wrist denervation if they are skeletally mature and suffer from wrist pain that is caused by either primary or secondary degenerative changes and is refractory to conservative treatments.

For secondary degenerative arthritis, these include scaphoid non-union and scaphoid non-union advanced collapse, carpal fractures, perilunate fracture dislocations, intra-articular fractures of the distal radius, Kienbock's disease, as well as ligamentous injuries, for example, scapholunate dissociation and scapholunate advance collapse.

While the presence of active infection and acute state of inflammation are contraindicated, post-infective and post-inflammatory arthritis [2] (when the disease is quiescence) are indicated for wrist denervation.

28.2.9 Contraindication

- Patents with complex regional pain syndrome
- Patients with active infection
- Patients suffering from acute state of inflammatory arthritis, e.g., rheumatoid arthritis and gouty arthritis

28.3 Surgical Technique

28.3.1 Preoperative

There are different schools of thoughts on the number of sensory nerves that need to be denervated in order to achieve a pain-free wrist. Some surgeons believe that excision of isolated PIN and AIN at the wrist level is sufficient as these are the major nerves that are responsible for wrist sensation [2–9]. Others believe that additional articular nerves need to be destroyed to achieve a more guaranteed result [1, 10–12]. Temporary lignocaine block to the intended articular nerves has been recommended to evaluate the prognosis in achieving a pain-free wrist [1, 3, 13]. It is noted that a high correlation was found between failure to eliminate pain after preoperative injection and poor outcomes after denervation [3, 6, 14].

Preoperative block can be performed at the following injection points using 1% lignocaine without epinephrine [1]:

Posterior interosseous nerve: above the dorsal periosteum of the distal radius, 3 cm proximal to the radiocarpal joint, centered between the radius and the ulna bone.

Articular branch of the first interosseous space: at the subcutaneous plane, dorsal aspect of the hand between the bases of the first and second metacarpal bone.

Lateral antebrachial cutaneous nerve: at the subfascial plane, 3 cm proximal of the wrist flexion crease, and along the ulnar side of the radial artery.

Superficial radial nerve: at the subcutaneous plane, 4 cm proximal to the radial styloid.

Palmar branch of the median nerve: at the subcutaneous plane, 1 cm proximal of the wrist flexion crease, above the flexor carpi radialis (FCR) tendon.

Anterior interosseous nerve: above the periosteum of the distal radius, 3 cm proximal to the wrist flexion crease at the ulnar aspect of the palmaris longus muscle.

Perforating fibers of the deep branch of the ulnar nerve: dorsal aspect above the first and second intermetacarpal joints.

Dorsal branch of the ulnar nerve: at the subcutaneous plane, ulnar edge of the ulna head.

Posterior antebrachial cutaneous nerve: at the subcutaneous plane, posterior aspect of the ulnar head.

28.3.2 Surgical Procedure

Denervation can be performed under regional or general anesthesia. Pneumatic tourniquet may be applied to create a bloodless field. Wide awake local anesthesia with no tourniquet (WALANT) may also be used.

Different incisions are used to denervate targeted articular nerves (Figs. 28.3 and 28.4) [1, 9]. In cases where all articular nerves are planned to be eliminated, that is, complete denervation, a total of five incisions would be used. Alternatively, incisions are made according to the targeted articular nerves [2, 3, 15]. These incisions may be incorporated with incisions that are used for concomitant procedures.

1. A 3–4 cm dorsal transverse incision 3 cm proximal to the wrist is made. Alternatively, a longitudinal incision can be used, especially if it is combined with other procedures at the dorsal aspect of the wrist (Fig. 28.3).
   (a) For **posterior interosseous nerve** (± **anterior interosseous nerve**).

   The dissection is made between the extensor pollicis longus tendon and the extensor digitorum longus tendons, proximal to the extensor retinaculum. PIN can be identified over the periosteum of the distal radius at the floor of the fourth extensor compartment. It extends proximally to lie adjacent to the interosseous membrane. Excision of 1 cm PIN is performed as far proximal as possible to eliminate the articular fibers to the DRUJ.

   (b) In cases where only anterior and posterior interosseous nerves are planned to be eliminated, a 2 cm longitudinal incision may be made at the distal interosseous membrane [3]. AIN can be identified just beneath the interosseous membrane. An excision of 1–2 cm AIN can then be performed.

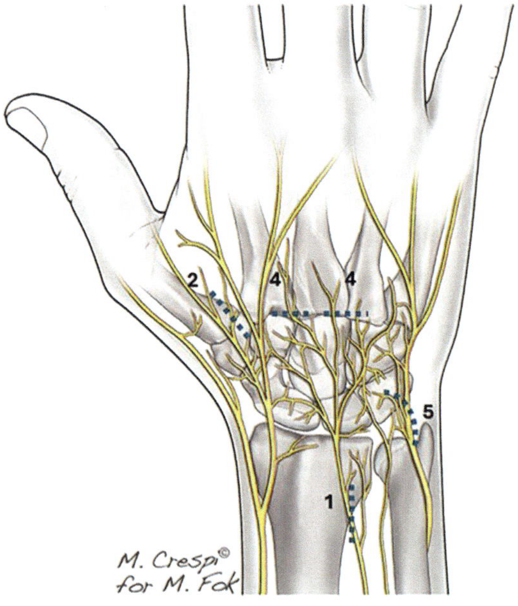

Fig. 28.3 Dorsal view of wrist with different incisions to denervate targeted articular nerves

2. A short longitudinal incision is made dorsally between the bases of first and second metacarpal bones (Fig. 28.3).
   (a) For **articular branch of the first interosseous space**
   The dorsal common digital nerve is first identified before tracing it distally to the articular branch. As it anastomoses with the articular branches of both the lateral antebrachial cutaneous nerve and deep branch of the ulnar nerve, it needs to cut proximally, together with the excision of the distal stump. This can then eliminate the conjoint perforating fibers of the ulnar nerves.
3. A 5 cm curved incision is made at the radial volar aspect of the wrist, from the trapezium to the radial edge of the FCR tendon (Fig. 28.4).
   (a) For **articular branches of the lateral antebrachial cutaneous nerve**
   Radial vessels can be identified after incising the superficial fascia. The main superficial radial nerve and its radiopalmar branches should then be protected. The articular branches of the lateral antebrachial cutaneous nerve run along both sides of the radial artery. A 1 cm resection can be performed by ligating the periarterial tissue, which contains both articular fibers and accompanied venous vessels.
   (b) For **articular branch of the superficial radial nerve**
   This can be done blindly by performing epifascial mobilization of the soft tissue layer in radial and radiodorsal direction until the proximal part of the anatomic snuffbox is exposed.
   (c) For **articular branch of the palmar branch of median nerve**
   This can be done blindly by extending the epifascial mobilization distally in the transverse direction, exposing scaphoid and trapezium.
   (d) For **articular fibers of the anterior interosseous nerve**
   Dissection is made between the radial artery and the FCR tendon, exposing the distal edge of the pronator quadratus muscle. Denervation of the articular nerves is performed by cauterization of the fatty and periosteal tissue up to the radial epiphysis.
4. A 3 cm transverse incision can be made over the dorsal aspect of the base of second to fourth metacarpal base (Fig. 28.3).
   (a) For **perforating branch of the deep branch of the ulnar nerve**
   By incising the superficial fascia and retracting the extensor tendon, the articular nerves can be cut by cauterization of the soft tissue down to the base of second and third metacarpal bone.
5. Curved incision over the dorso-ulnar aspect of the ulnar head, extending up to the hamate distally (Fig. 28.3).
   (a) For **articular fibers of the dorsal branch of the ulnar nerve**
   The main dorsal branch of the ulnar nerve is first identified and traced distally. The articular fibers are cut blindly by epifascial dissection of the soft tissue in the dorso-ulnar and ulnar aspect of the wrist, up to the base of fifth metacarpal bone,

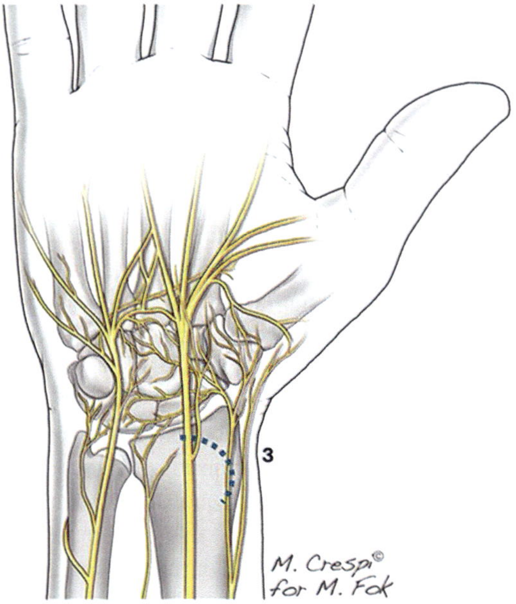

Fig. 28.4 Palmar view of wrist with different incisions to denervate targeted articular nerves

while preserving the sensory fibers of the dorsal branch of the ulnar nerve.

(b) **For articular branch of the posterior antebrachial cutaneous nerve**

This is cut blindly by performing epifascial dissection over the ulnar head, including the dorsal aspect of the DRUJ.

28.3.3 Postoperative Period

Light dressing is applied after skin closure. Fingers, elbow, and shoulder mobilization should be encouraged at the immediate postoperative period. In cases where only wrist denervation is performed, gentle mobilization of wrist is permitted for the first 2 weeks. Strengthening and passive mobilization can be started at the third week. For cases with concomitant procedures, immobilization may be needed, depending on the nature of the additional procedures.

28.4 Tips and Tricks

- Preoperative lignocaine injection can be a good indicator on the outcome of denervation [1]. The persistence of pain noted after injection may suggest poor outcome with wrist denervation only [3, 6].
- Total wrist denervation may not be needed for all cases and do not need to be performed in one setting. Partial wrist denervation may be attempted first in cases of specific area of arthritis [15]; for example, patients with scaphoid non-union advanced collapse II and suffering from radial wrist pain may benefit from selected nerve denervation, that is, AIN and PIN, with or without denervation to the articular branches of lateral antebrachial cutaneous nerve and superficial radial nerve.
- If tourniquet is used, deflation of the tourniquet with good hemostasis is advised before skin closure. This is to prevent hematoma formation.
- Wrist denervation alone is a "buy-time" procedure. Patients need to be aware that degeneration may progress with time and additional procedures may be needed in the future [1, 5, 16, 17].
- Failure to eliminate pain is a possible outcome of wrist denervation. Surgeons should discuss expectations with the patient preoperatively.
- Pain perception may be centralized in patients suffering from long period of wrist pain. Complete elimination of pain by wrist denervation is guarded.
- In cases of severe wrist instabilities or post-traumatic changes of articular surface congruency [1], wrist denervation alone may not be sufficient. Additional procedure in wrist stabilization may be needed.

28.5 Complication

- Sensory nerve damage [1, 14, 17]
- In cases where denervation of articular branch of superficial radial nerve and dorsal branch of ulnar nerve is planned, care must be taken to avoid damage of the sensory branches of superficial radial nerve and dorsal branch of ulnar nerve, thereby affecting the sensation over the snuffbox and dorso-ulnar aspect of the hand, respectively. Neuropraxia, presented as paresthesia, in the affected area may last up to 2–3 months.
- Neuroma [14, 17]
- Neuroma may be formed if sensory branches, together with the articular branches of the intended nerve, are cut [1].
- Bleeding [17]
- Precaution is needed to avoid damage to the radial artery and its branches during the denervation of articular branches of lateral antebrachial cutaneous nerve and superficial radial nerve.
- Charcot joint
- While there is a theoretical possibility of producing a Charcot wrist joint after total wrist denervation, no report is noted in the current literature. It is postulated that it is impossible to denervate the wrist completely due to its complexity of innervation. Studies by Gay et al. [18], Patterson et al. [19], and Rein et al. [20] on the proprioception in patients with

denervated wrist show no difference when compared with healthy wrist joints.

- Complex regional pain syndrome [1, 14, 17]

28.6 Outcomes

The current literature on wrist denervation is mainly case series concerning a heterogenous group of patients with degenerative conditions of the wrist.

For total wrist denervation, Wilhelm [1] presented 48 patients, of which 81% achieved minimal pain at an average follow-up of 1.2 years. Picart et al. [16] also noted 80% pain improvement in 39 patients with a mean follow-up of 56 months. Improvement in grip strength was noted from 60 to 76%.

For partial wrist denervation, Berger [3] and Hofmeister [6] et al. advocated denervation of both AIN and PIN for painful wrist conditions, while Storey et al. [13] preferred denervation of AIN, PIN, and superficial radial nerve. Their reported pain varied from 49 to 80% [6, 7, 13] but the satisfaction rate remained good at 69–85% [7, 13].

Denervation of isolated PIN has also been described in some studies [2, 4, 21, 22]. Riches et al. [21] described a prospective study comparing PIN denervation alone with wrist arthrodesis in rheumatoid arthritis patients. At a mid-term follow-up, that is, 39 months in wrist arthrodesis and 22 months in denervation, pain score, functional outcome, and patient's satisfaction showed no difference between the 2 groups.

For systematic review on isolated PIN denervation [4], up to 88% had a subjective improvement with 89% able to return to work at an average follow-up of 51 months. Yet, the pain recurrence rate was 25.5% at an average follow-up of 12.3 months. In another systematic review of partial wrist innervation [23] including PIN, AIN, or AIN and PIN denervation, while a reduction in pain and functional improvement were noted, additional surgery was required in 24% wrist at an average follow-up of 18 months.

For long-term outcomes, 80% of patients undergoing total wrist denervation [17] had improvement in pain, which was maintained at up to their third postoperative years. The improvement in grip strength was maintained up to 6 years. In general, the pain recurred over time [12, 17] with the median survival rate being 8.8 years. Yet, not all proceeded to have additional surgeries to alleviate pain. By taking revision surgery as the endpoint, the survival was 73.6% of patients at the longest follow-up [12]. Besides, 69–80% were satisfied and would undergo denervation again [12, 24, 25]. Similar findings were noted for long-term result of partial wrist denervation [5]. The overall survival rate decreased over the years, from 85% at 1 year to 57% at 15 years. Also, 31% underwent revision surgery at an average of 26 months postoperatively. It is interesting to note that progressive degeneration was observed radiographically in the long-term follow-up irrespective of the pain status after wrist denervation [1, 5, 16, 17]. This is noted particularly in patents with ligamentous instabilities and joint incongruity, as well as patients who are involved in heavy manual labor [1].

There were no comparative studies comparing different wrist denervation. A systematic review [14] comparing different partial wrist denervation procedures and total wrist denervation showed that both procedures were able to achieve comparable good pain relief and preserved wrist motion. Yet total wrist denervation offers better long-term pain relief with fewer additional surgery (19% vs 4.7%) [26, 27].

For patient selection, Laulan et al. [11] proposed that the best candidates for wrist denervation are patients who are physically inactive or perform light manual work and have good motion ranges and elderly patients. Poor pain relief was noted for heavy manual laborer [11], patients in active military duty [28], patients who had previous wrist surgery [5], patients with poor preoperative range of motion [7], and patients involved in worker's compensation [7]. There was no correlation with age [7, 24], chronicity of symptoms [7], and occupation [6, 7].

28.7 Conclusion

Wrist denervation is a valid option in the management of wrist pain and degenerative conditions. It can be served as a buy-time procedure or an adjunct to concomitant surgery. It enables patients to restore some wrist motion without precluding them from having subsequent revision surgery. Most studies showed promising results in patients with total or partial wrist denervation, especially in the short to medium term. Despite pain may recur and degeneration may progress over time, patient remained satisfied even if pain recurred in the long term.

References

1. Wilhelm A. Denervation of the wrist. Tech Hand Up Extrem Surg. 2001;5:14–30.
2. Peltz TS, Yapp LZ, Elherik FK, Breusch SJ. Patient satisfaction and outcomes of partial wrist denervation in inflammatory arthritis. Clin Rheumatol. 2019;38:2995–3003.
3. BERGER RA. Partial denervation of the wrist. Tech Hand Up Extrem Surg. 1998;2:25–35.
4. Berge DJV, Kusnezov NA, Rubin S, Dagg T, Orr J, Mitchell J, et al. Outcomes following isolated posterior interosseous nerve Neurectomy: a systematic review. Hand. 2017;12:535–40.
5. O'Shaughnessy MA, Wagner ER, Berger RA, Kakar S. Buying time: long-term results of wrist denervation and time to repeat surgery. Hand. 2019;14:602–8.
6. Hofmeister EP, Moran SL, Shin AY. Anterior and posterior interosseous Neurectomy for the treatment of chronic dynamic instability of the wrist. Hand. 2006;1:63–70.
7. Weinstein LP, Berger RA. Analgesic benefit, functional outcome, and patient satisfaction after partial wrist denervation. J Hand Surg. 2002;27:833–9.
8. Patil V, Arenas-Prat J. Radical wrist denervation and preliminary results. Tech Hand Up Extrem Surg. 2016;20:96–8.
9. Ferreres A, Foucher G, Suso S. Extensive denervation of the wrist. Tech Hand Up Extrem Surg. 2002;6:36–41.
10. Ferreres A, Suso S, Foucher G, Ruano D. Wrist denervation: surgical considerations. J Hand Surg Br. 1996;21:16.
11. Laulan J, Marteau E, Bacle G. Wrist osteoarthritis. Orthop Traumatol Surg Res. 2015;101:S1–9.
12. Dellestable A, Cheval D, Kerfant N, Stindel E, Nen DL, Letissier H. Does total wrist denervation give reliable long-term results? Survival curve with an average follow-up of 8.2 years. Orthop Traumatol Surg Res. 2021;107:102967.
13. Storey PA, Lindau T, Jansen V, Woodbridge S, Bainbridge LC, Burke FD. Wrist denervation in isolation: a prospective outcome study with patient selection by wrist blockade. Hand Surg. 2011;16:251–7.
14. Smeraglia F, Basso MA, Famiglietti G, Eckersley R, Bernasconi A, Balato G. Partial wrist denervation versus total wrist denervation: a systematic review of the literature. Hand Surg Rehabil. 2020;39:487–91.
15. Kadiyala RK, Lombardi JM. Denervation of the wrist joint for the management of chronic pain. J Am Acad Orthop Sur. 2017;25:439–47.
16. Picart B, Laborie C, Hulet C, Malherbe M. Total wrist denervation: retrospective study of 39 wrists with 56 months' follow-up. Orthop Traumatol Surg Res. 2019;105:1607–10.
17. Braga-Silva J, Román JA, Padoin AV. Wrist denervation for painful conditions of the wrist. J Hand Surg. 2011;36:961–6.
18. Gay A, Harbst K, Hansen DK, Laskowski ER, Berger RA, Kaufman KR. Effect of partial wrist denervation on wrist kinesthesia: wrist denervation does not impair proprioception. J Hand Surg. 2011;36:1774–9.
19. Patterson RW, Niel MV, Shimko P, Pace C, Seitz WH. Proprioception of the wrist following posterior interosseous sensory Neurectomy. J Hand Surg. 2010;35:52–6.
20. Rein S, Winter J, Kremer T, Siemers F, Range U, Euchner N. Evaluation of proprioception in denervated and healthy wrist joints. J Hand Surg Eur Vol. 2019;45:408–13.
21. Riches PL, Elherik FK, Breusch SJ. Functional and patient-reported outcome of partial wrist denervation versus the Mannerfelt wrist arthrodesis in the rheumatoid wrist. Arch Orthop Trauma Surg. 2014;134:1037–44.
22. Abdelaziz AM, Aldahshan W, El-Sherief FAH, Wahd YESH, Soliman HAG. Posterior interosseous neurectomy alternative for treating chronic wrist pain. J Wrist Surg. 2019;08:198–201.
23. Kadhum M, Riley N, Furniss D. Is partial wrist denervation beneficial in chronic wrist pain? A systematic review. J Plastic Reconstr Aesthet Surg. 2020;73:1790–800.
24. Schweizer A, von Känel O, Kammer E, Meuli-Simmen C. Long-term follow-up evaluation of denervation of the wrist. J Hand Surg. 2006;31:559–64.
25. Fuchsberger T, Boesch CE, Tonagel F, Fischborn T, Schaller HE, Gonser P. Patient-rated long-term results after complete denervation of the wrist. J Plastic Reconstr Aesthet Surg. 2018;71:57–61.
26. Hassebrock JD, Thomas OJ, Breuer LC, Renfree KJ. Midterm patient-reported outcomes in wrist denervation for post-traumatic arthritis. J Hand Surg. 2021;46:1027.e1–6.
27. Ishida O, Tsai TM, Atasoy E. Long-term results of denervation of the wrist joint for chronic wrist pain. J Hand Surg Br. 1993;18:76–80.
28. Sgromolo NM, Cho MS, Gower JT, Rhee PC. Partial wrist denervation for idiopathic dorsal wrist pain in an active duty military population. J Hand Surg. 2018;43:1108–12.

Overview of Wrist Joint Stiffness

29

Margaret Woon Man and Gregory I. Bain

29.1 Introduction

Wrist stiffness can be a result of many different factors. It can be affected by local injuries as well as regional or generalized medical conditions. For local factors, it can be categorized into intra-articular or extra-articular factors. In both cases, capsular structures are frequently involved [1]. In some instances, even minimal injury of the capsule may lead to wrist contracture [2]. Arthrofibrosis may be stimulated by intra-articular and capsular injuries as well as prolonged immobilization, and this can be seen after conservative and surgical treatment. For regional or generalized medical conditions, it can be due to nerve-related disorders [3].

The most common cause of wrist stiffness is triggered by a wrist injury, such as a distal radius fracture, with or without concomitant ligament injuries. The predicable outcomes of these injures are pain, swelling, and deformity. As Colles stated [4], "initially the patient is doomed to endure considerable lameness and stiffness of the limb, accompanied by severe pains on attempting to bend the fingers." However, "at some remote period, the patient will again enjoy perfect freedom in all its motions, completely exempt from pain, but the deformity will remain undiminished."

Thus, the stiffness is thought to be resolved with time. Yet, there are cases wherein the pain and stiffness persist, despite deformity. In the following chapter, we would discuss the possible causes, their assessment and evaluation, and their corresponding management.

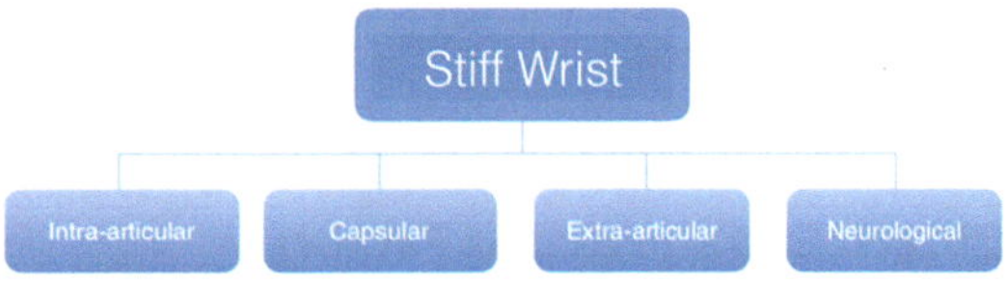

29.2 Classification for Stiff Wrist (Table 29.1)

29.2.1 Intra-articular Factors

- Intra-articular fractures
- Malunion
- Non-union
- Avascular necrosis, e.g., Kienbock's disease, Preiser disease
- Carpal malalignment, e.g., scapholunate dissociation or lunotriquetral dissociation

M. W. Man (✉)
Department of Orthopaedics and Traumatology, Queen Mary Hospital, The University of Hong Kong, Pok Fu Lam, Hong Kong

G. I. Bain
Department of Orthopedic Surgery, Flinders University of South Australia and Flinders Medical Centre, Adelaide, Australia
e-mail: greg@gregbain.com.au

L. Pederzini et al. (eds.), *Stiffness of the Elbow, Wrist and Related Pathologies*,
https://doi.org/10.1007/978-3-031-81381-8_29

Table 29.1 Classification of stiff wrist [20]

Intra-articular (bearings)	**Capsular** (constraints)	**Extra-articular** (motor, cable, levers)	**Neurologic** (control, electrics, sensors)
Articular surface Osteochondral, Defect, degeneration	**Ligaments:** Contracture, calcifications	**Muscles:** Myopathy, Fatty infiltration	**Central:** Behavioral, Dystonia, spasticity
Subchondral Dysplasia, fractures, AVN, degeneration	**Capsule:** Contracture, calcifications	**Tendons and bursa:** Tear, calcifications degeneration, bursitis	**Peripheral:** Ulnar, radial, medial nerve; cutaneous neuritis, or neuropathy
Synovium Inflammatory, Crystal arthroplasty	**Congruity:** Subluxation, dislocation	**Other (external to Joint):** Fracture, malignancy, HO, skin contracture	**Sensory and autonomic:** Charcot joint, CRPS

- Inflammatory disease, e.g., gouty arthritis, rheumatoid arthritis
- Degenerative conditions, e.g., scapholunate advanced collapse (SLAC), scaphoid non-union advanced collapse (SNAC), radiocarpal arthritis

29.2.2 Capsular Factors

- Tearing or bruising of the capsule
- Organization of the hematoma leads to scarring of the capsule onto the adjacent articulation
- Immobilization

29.2.3 Extra-articular Factors

- Skin and subcutaneous soft tissue contracture, e.g., burn, deglove injury
- Tendon/muscle injury or inflammation
- Post-compartment syndrome leading to Volkmann's contracture

29.2.4 Neurological Factors

- General/systematic
  - Spasticity—cerebral palsy, cerebral vascular accident
  - Hypertonic muscles cause a secondary contracture of the joint
  - Myopathies—polio, Duchenne's muscular dystrophy
  - Muscle imbalance—weak muscles struggle to take the joint through the full range of motion, leading to a secondary contracture
  - Extra-pyramidal condition—Parkinson's disease
  - Neuropathies—leprosy
  - Charcot joint
  - Syringomyelia
- Local/Regional—which is usually following trauma or in some cases, iatrogenic incidents
  - Median nerve (refer to below for more detailed discussion)
  - Ulnar nerve

    Distal ulnar fracture, distal radio-ulnar joint injuries, hook of hamate fracture
  - Superficial radial nerve

    K-wire inserted through the anatomical snuff box during distal radius fixation
  - Palmar cutaneous branch of median nerve

    During the flexor carpi radialis approach
  - Dorsal branch of ulnar nerve

    Ulnar styloid fixation or Triangular fibrocartilage complex (TFCC) repair or reconstruction
  - Complex regional pain syndrome (CRPS) (refer to below for more detailed discussion)

29.3 Diagnosis

29.3.1 Presentation

The generalized neuromuscular conditions can usually be diagnosed by assessment of the muscle strength, tone, and coordination. Each condition needs to be assessed on its merit. Intra-articular conditions can usually be confirmed with further imaging like X-ray, computer tomography (CT), and magnetic resonance imaging (MRI). For localized or regional neurological conditions, it is more difficult to differentiate from capsular or extra-articular-related pathologies. This may require detail history, careful examination, and a level of suspicion. To complicate the matters further, wrist stiffness may be caused by a combination of different factors, e.g., a patient who suffers from a distal radius malunion and complex regional pain syndrome, or a patient with open wrist fracture may have intra-articular malalignment, joint contracture, as well as soft tissue scarring. It is important to recognize all the different causes and manage accordingly.

29.3.2 Physical Examination

A detailed generalized neurological examination is beyond the scope of this chapter. This section is mainly focused on hand and wrist.

29.3.3 Inspection

The skin color and turgor, the soft tissue status, and the position in which the hand and wrist are held may give clues on the causes of wrist stiffness.

Local and regional neurological causes like complex regional syndrome may be present with a pale and generalized swollen hand. Lack of sweat and cold in temperature may also be noted.

Intrinsic muscle atrophy may be a cause of ulnar nerve palsy, while a loss of normal finger cascade may be a sign of tendon injuries and imbalance.

Scarring from open injures should also be a tell-tale sign.

29.3.4 Range of Movement (Fig. 29.1)

Apprehension and pain on movement for both finger and wrist joints usually have a neurological element in the contribution of wrist stiffness. The differences in active and passive movement of wrist can help to differentiate intra-articular (including capsular) and extra-articular pathologies. Patients with intra-articular pathologies will have similar active and passive range of movements. The degree of moment does not change with the position of adjacent joints. This contrasts with extra-articular cause of wrist stiffness, of which the range of movement may differ based on the position of adjacent joints. Yet it is important to note that in chronic cases, patients with even extra-articular pathologies may develop secondary joint contracture, which may complicate the presentation.

If neurological causes are suspected, a full neurological examination is needed. This includes the assessment of muscle tone, motor power, and sensation, not just in the limb involved, but also the other parts of the body.

29.3.5 Investigations

X-ray is the first line of investigation to confirm the diagnosis of intra-articular cause of wrist stiffness (Fig. 29.2). Further imaging modalities like computer tomography (CT) and magnetic resonance imaging (MRI) may aid in the diagnoses of intra-articular cause of wrist stiffness, e.g., intra-articular distal radius malunion, scapholunate dissociation, and avascular necrosis of scaphoid. Sometimes ultrasound and MRI may show the soft tissue status, e.g., tendon ruptures or dislocation, as extra-articular pathologies.

In cases of suspected neurological causes, electrophysiological tests are useful to substantiate the diagnosis. In cases of CRPS, patients may not be able to tolerate the test.

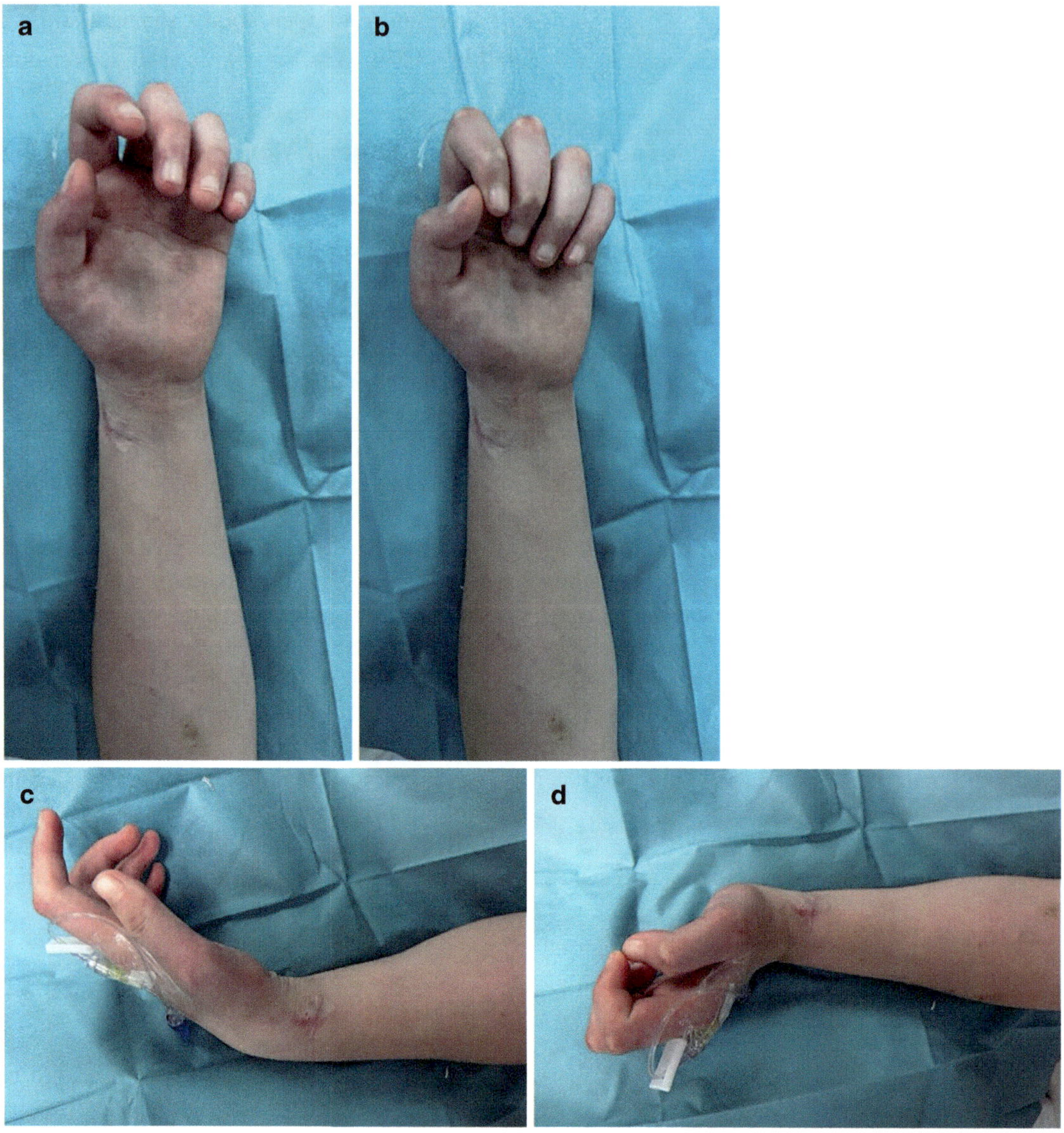

Fig. 29.1 Volkmann's contracture of left upper limb was developed after generalized myositis. The patient was unable to fully extend (**a**) and flex their fingers due to tendon adhesion at the forearm (**b**). Limited wrist range of movement was also noted (**c** and **d**)

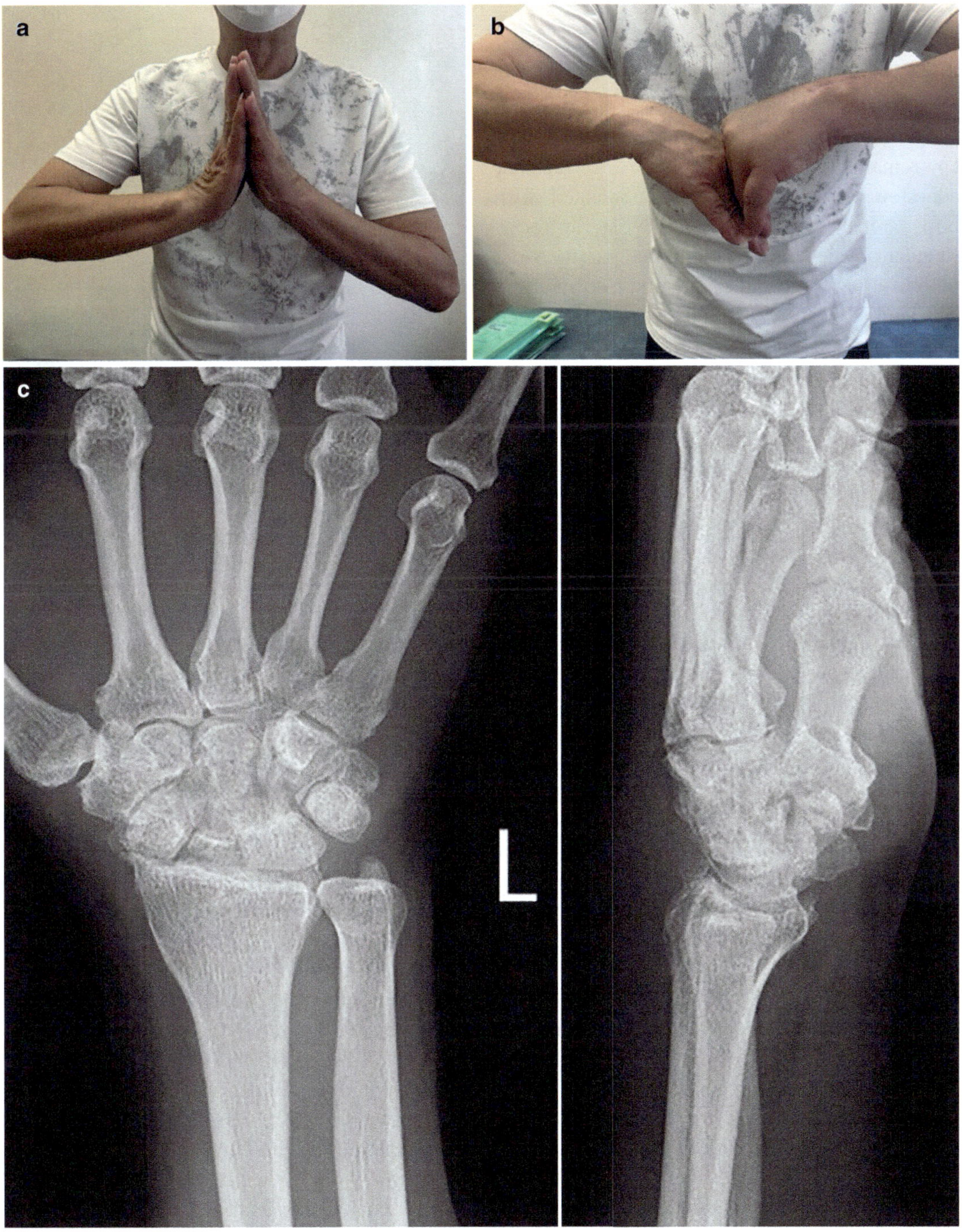

Fig. 29.2 Limited range of movement of left wrist (**a** and **b**) was noted due to SNAC wrist (confirmed by X-ray (**c**))

29.4 Treatment

The management protocol of wrist stiffness is mainly determined by the causes.

For *intra-articular causes*, conservative therapy remains the first line of treatment. Capsular adhesion or scarring is often associated with post-traumatic intra-articular wrist stiffness. Regular physiotherapy with graded passive wrist mobilization could aid in breaking down those adhesion. Progressive splinting by customized splints may also be helpful. In cases where patients experience mechanical pain during mobilization, nerve block may be useful.

In chronic cases, or in cases where conservative therapy has reached its plateau, surgical intervention is indicated. Carpal malalignment due to ligamentous injuries or malunion needs to be corrected [5, 6]. In the presence of degenerative joint diseases, e.g., SNAC wrist or SLAC wrist, salvage procedure including limited carpal fusion or proximal row carpectomy may be offered instead [7]. This can be performed either as an open procedure or an arthroscopic procedure. Neurectomy may be used as an adjunct procedure or a standalone buy-time procedure for painful wrist stiffness (refer to the book chapter: Neurectomy).

For *capsular causes*, as stated above, scaring and adhesion are usually secondary to either intra- or extra-articular causes or both. Splinting and passive graded mobilization may be useful. In static cases, surgical capsular release, either arthroscopic [1, 8] (Fig. 29.3) or open [9], may be beneficial.

For *extra-articular causes*, it is essential to determine whether it is a result of a neurological pathology or a localized soft tissue insult.

Unlike intra-articular wrist causes, stiffness tends to recur if the culprit has not been addressed. Intensive hand therapy including splinting and mobilization exercise should be started as early as possible to prevent the development of secondary capsular scarring and adhesion.

For skin and soft tissue contracture, simple excision and release may be sufficient. Yet, skin graft or even flap coverage may be needed in severe cases, especially when tendons or neurovascular structure are being exposed.

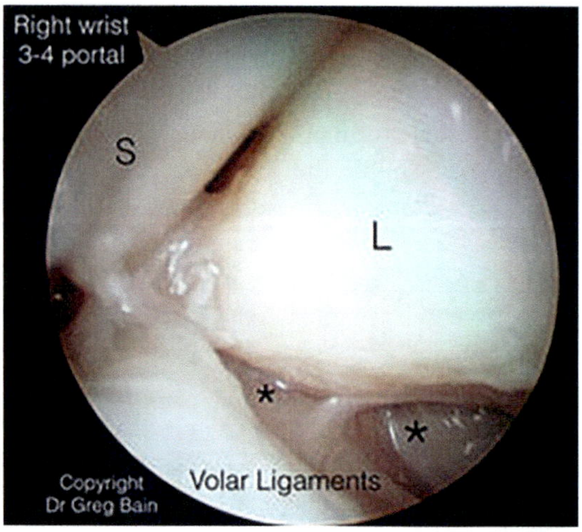

Fig. 29.3 Following a significant wrist injury, the traumatized capsule can heal to the adjacent carpus. The normal capsular recess (*) will be obliterated, and restrict the joint motion. When managing the wrist contracture, the adherent capsule needs to be released from the carpus, and the recess recreated

Tendon repair or reconstruction (if chronic) is needed if tendon is lacerated or ruptured. Tendon adhesion is common in traumatic or inflammatory cases. As such, secondary tenolysis is often indicated when the tendon sheath has been disrupted or the bed is scarred. Post-operative intensive physiotherapy is essential to prevent recurrence.

In cases with neurological causes, especially general or systematic causes, preventative measures like splinting and passive mobilization are the key to prevent stiffness. Depending on the prognosis in recovery, hand and wrist are advised to be put in the safety (reversible) or functional (non-reversible) position. In chronic cases, botulinum toxin injection or systematic muscle relaxant may be useful to reverse the muscle imbalance, especially muscle spasticity. Tenotomy or tendon lengthening may sometimes be indicated.

For local or regional neurological causes, it is usually followed by a traumatic event [10]. This may involve median nerve, ulnar nerve, or cutaneous nerves, or it may be a controversial condition namely complex regional pain syndrome (CRPS). High index of suspicion is needed for most instances. Nerve release may be indicated.

29.5 Median Nerve (Acute Carpal Tunnel Syndrome)

This is an acute form of median nerve entrapment at the wrist. Unlike the typical (chronic) carpal tunnel syndrome we come across every day, which is presented with paresthesia, worse with activity and night-time, this is acute median neuritis, presented with pain and paresthesia [11].

The median nerve involved is at either the carpal tunnel or just distal forearm level. It can be caused by (1) compression (from displaced distal radius fracture, perilunate dislocation, bone fragment in carpal tunnel, a tight plaster cast), (2) traction (from hyper-extension injury of the wrist), (3) crush injury, or (4) neuroma (from stab injury or iatrogenic partial laceration associated with carpal tunnel release).

The presentation is mainly burning, severe pain at the hand and wrist region, together with swelling and paresthesia of the fingers. The pain may be worse at night and may be partially relieved by elevating their hand and making a fist. The finger and wrist movement will be limited due to the swelling of the soft tissue, which restricts flexion, but also the pain that discourages the patient from moving the finger.

On physical examination, there will be swelling and deformity from the trauma. While the maximal tenderness is at the site of injury, the patient may be apprehensive and would complain of diffuse pain at the hand and wrist. Sensory and motor deficit may also be less defined in the median nerve distribution.

This is a clinical diagnosis. High index of suspicion is essential. Investigations like radiographs, computer tomography (CT), and magnetic resonance imaging (MRI) are mainly used to delineate the cause of the acute median neuritis. Nerve conduction study is often not tolerated due to pain. MRI with IV gadolinium may be useful as it reveals the hyperemia of the nerve.

For management, surgical decompression of the median nerve remains the crucial step, together with the address of the pathology, e.g., reduction of fracture fragment. Yet, it is essential to give adequate analgesic, and to collaborate with the hand therapist for perioperative treatment including: edema control, splinting, and mobilization exercise. Unfortunately, many of these cases may be diagnosed as CRPS, by medical/non-medical individuals who are not trained in hand surgery.

29.6 Is it Complex Regional Pain Syndrome (CRPS)?

This is a diagnosis by exclusion and its entity remains controversial among pain specialists, physicians, and surgeons. It is a chronic pain condition that is usually followed by a traumatic incident (can be a fracture or a minor sprain) and is characterized by spontaneous and evoked regional pain that is disproportionate in magnitude or duration to the typical course of pain after similar tissue trauma [10]. The most important aspect of the diagnosis of CRPS is that it is a diagnosis of exclusion. Therefore, to be diagnosed with CRPS, it requires a detailed assessment, by an experienced individual trained in the assessment of disorders of the hand.

Even in severe cases, it is difficult to distinguish due to the presence of the prominent autonomic and inflammatory changes in the affected limb. These changes can be a typical response to disuse, and acute neurological compress. The case demonstrated in Fig. 29.4 had a provisional diagnosis of CRPS after a suspensoplasty. The

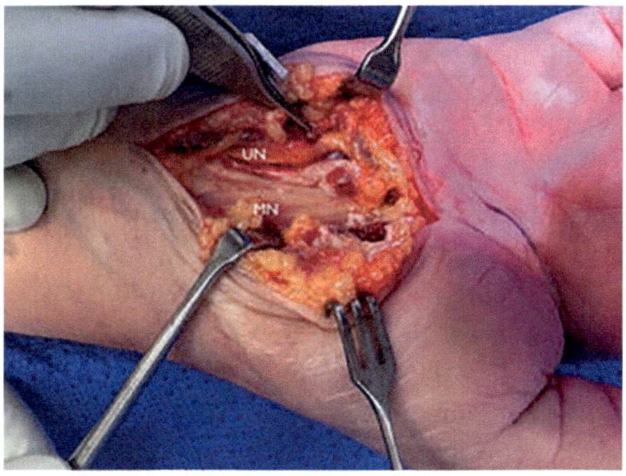

Fig. 29.4 Open ulnar nerve release in a patient who was thought to have CRPS. The forceps point to the narrowed ulnar nerve. Release of the ulnar nerve, relieved the patient's disabling pain

patient was significantly disabled with pain, mainly on the ulnar side of the wrist. The patient had pain over the entire wrist/hand. Taking a history was difficult due to the level of pain, but after allowing the patient to vent their distress regarding the pain, the patient could describe the burning numbness on the ulnar side of the hand. The hand was swollen, and the patient had difficulty in mobilizing the fingers and the wrist.

An open ulnar nerve and median nerve release was performed. The ulnar nerve had an obvious constriction that was released. When the flexor retinaculum was released, fluid was seen to be draining out of the hand into the forearm. Following the surgery, the patient was instructed to keep the hand elevated and mobilize the fingers.

There are a few very important points for this case.

The patient had significant improvement after the surgical release. The diagnosis is difficult, and best made by a trained hand surgeon. The classic pain description of CRPS is of severe pain, which is characteristic of acute nerve entrapment. The signs also are the same. A pain specialist is the best person to manage the patient, but only after anatomical/pathological assessment and diagnosis has been complete. The diagnosis is ulnar nerve entrapment, not CRPS. If the treatment continued to be pain management, then the rehabilitation would have been prolonged, and the patient denied surgical release of the ulnar nerve.

But there are a few important points that we have learnt from the pain specialists. Due to the extensive research into pain, it is known that the proximal arm and spine become sensitized, which reinforces the neurological pathways. Also, there is central sensitization due to the effects of the pain. The pain medications, especially the narcotics, have a profound effect on the patient. This becomes much more complex if there is litigation, worker's compensation, loss of work, and breakdown of relationships. This is a perfect storm for mental health disorders. The greater majority of this can be prevented by an early accurate assessment.

There may be extreme hyperalgesia, allodynia, pallor, cold, sweat, edema, and altered patterns of hair skin or nail growth. There may be a decrease in movement and strength, tremor, and dystonia. As a result, it affects activities of daily living and ability to function.

CRPS is a clinical diagnosis. Objective tests like thermography, triple phase bone scan, quantitative sudomotor axon reflex test, or a trial of sympathetic ganglion block are not diagnostic and not specific to CRPS. While Harden et al. proposed the use of Budapest Criteria (Table 29.2), in 2007 [12], which involved the presence of four criteria, there are debates on whether most of the patients are just suffering from acute carpal tunnel syndrome (as described above) [11, 13]. The lack of complete understanding regarding the pathophysiology of CRPS

Table 29.2 Budapest Criteria for complex regional pain syndrome

1. Continuing pain disproportionate to any inciting event
2. At a minimum, one symptom must be reported in at least three of the four following categories:
    - Sensory: Hyperesthesia or allodynia
    - Vasomotor: Temperature asymmetry, skin color changes, or skin color asymmetry
    - Sudomotor/edema: Edema, sweating changes, or sweating asymmetry
    - Motor/trophic: Decreased range of motion (ROM), motor dysfunction (e.g., weakness, tremor, and dystonia), or trophic changes (e.g., hair, nail, and skin)
3. Patients must display at least one sign at the time of evaluation in at least two of the following categories:
    - Sensory: Evidence of hyperalgesia (to pinprick) or allodynia (to light touch, temperature sensation, deep somatic pressure, or joint movement)
    - Vasomotor: Evidence of temperature asymmetry (>1 °C), skin color changes, or asymmetry
    - Sudomotor/edema: Evidence of edema, sweating changes, or sweating asymmetry
    - Motor/trophic: Evidence of decreased ROM, motor dysfunction (e.g., weakness, tremor, and dystonia), or trophic changes (e.g., hair, nail, and skin)
4. No other diagnosis better explains the signs and symptoms

Reproduced with permission from Ref. [12]

adds to the challenge [10]. In reality, there may be some acute carpal tunnel syndrome that is being misdiagnosed as complex regional pain syndrome [11].

Prevention is the key to success. High index of suspicion is needed to prevent the development of an acute/subacute episode into a chronic painful condition [14]. There remains lack of good evidence (randomized controlled trials) to guide treatment protocols. Multidisciplinary team approach is recommended. Some efficacy is noted on CRPS that is functionally focused, centering around physical and occupational therapy designed to normalize the use of the affected limb and mitigate problems related to disuse [15, 16]. These include mirror therapy and graded motor imagery [17]. The use of medications like bisphosphonates, subanesthetic ketamine, free radical scavengers (topical dimethylsulfoxide, oral N-acetylcysteine, or oral vitamin C for prevention), and corticosteroids has shown low efficacy [18]. Analgesic antidepressants, anticonvulsants, and transdermal lidocaine are thought to be effective clinically, although their efficacy in CRPS has not been evaluated adequately in randomized controlled trials. A recent Cochrane review suggests that sympathetic blocks are probably ineffective [19].

29.7 Conclusion

The causes of wrist stiffness vary and are often multifactorial. Yet, it is essential to delineate all the factors leading to wrist stiffness and tackle them accordingly. This chapter provides an overview on how to identify the causes of wrist stiffness and highlights two of the controversial localized neurological conditions of wrist stiffness. Early diagnosis is beneficial. Preventative measures are often essential to prevent cases to become chronic conditions. Apart from surgical intervention for specific cases, therapy remains a crucial part to the initial management as well as perioperative period.

References

1. Verhellen R, Bain GI. Arthroscopic capsular release for contracture of the wrist: a new technique. Arthroscopy. 2000;16:106–10.
2. McGuire DT, Luchetti R, Atzei A, Bain GI. Wrist and elbow arthroscopy with selected open procedures. Cham: Springer; 2021. p. 321–33.
3. Bain GI, Clitherow HDS. The pathogenesis and classification of shoulder stiffness. In: Itoi E, et al., editors. Shoulder stiffness. Berlin, Heidelberg: Springer; 2015. https://doi.org/10.1007/978-3-662-46370-3_1.
4. Colles A. On the fracture of the carpal extremity of the radius. N Engl J Med. 1814;3:368–72.
5. Doarn M, Xu B, Winterton M, Fernandez JJ, Cohen MS, Wysocki RW. Carpal joint malalignment with distal radius Malunion and factors in correction after distal radius osteotomy. J Hand Surg Glob Online. 2023;5:722.
6. Fok MWM, Fernandez DL, Maniglio M. Carpal instability nondissociative following acute wrist fractures. J Hand Surg. 2020;45:662.e1–662.e10.
7. Dacho AK, Baumeister S, Germann G, Sauerbier M. Comparison of proximal row carpectomy and midcarpal arthrodesis for the treatment of scaphoid nonunion advanced collapse (SNAC-wrist) and scapholunate advanced collapse (SLAC-wrist) in stage II. J Plast Reconstr Aesthet Surg. 2006;61:1210–8.
8. Luchetti R, Atzei A, Fairplay T. Arthroscopic wrist arthrolysis after wrist fracture. Arthroscopy. 2005;23:255–60.
9. Kamal RN, Ruch DS. Volar capsular release after distal radius fractures. J Hand Surg. 2017;42:1034.e1–6.
10. Bruehl S. Complex regional pain syndrome. BMJ. 2015;351:h2730.
11. Piñal FD. Outcomes of carpal tunnel release in complex regional pain syndrome/reflex sympathetic dystrophy/Sudeck disease patients. Plast Reconstr Surg. 2022;150:93–101.
12. Harden RN, Bruehl S, Stanton-Hicks M, Wilson PR. Proposed new diagnostic criteria for complex regional pain syndrome. Pain Med. 2007;8:326–31.
13. del Piñal F. Editorial*: I have a dream … reflex sympathetic dystrophy (RSD or complex regional pain syndrome - CRPS I) does not exist. J Hand Surg Eur Vol. 2013;38:595–7.
14. Bean DJ, Johnson MH, Kydd RR. The outcome of complex regional pain syndrome type 1: a systematic review. J Pain. 2014;15:677–90.
15. Smart KM, Ferraro MC, Wand BM, O'Connell NE. Physiotherapy for pain and disability in adults with complex regional pain syndrome (CRPS) types I and II. Cochrane Database Syst Rev. 2022;5:CD010853.
16. Shafiee E, MacDermid J, Packham T, Walton D, Grewal R, Farzad M. The effectiveness of

rehabilitation interventions on pain and disability for complex regional pain syndrome. Clin J Pain. 2023;39:91–105.

17. Shafiee E, MacDermid J, Packham T, Grewal R, Farzad M, Bobos P, et al. Rehabilitation interventions for complex regional pain syndrome: an overview of systematic reviews. Clin J Pain. 2023;39:473–83.
18. Perez RS, Zollinger PE, Dijkstra PU, Thomassen-Hilgersom IL, Zuurmond WW, Rosenbrand KC, et al. Evidence based guidelines for complex regional pain syndrome type 1. BMC Neurol. 2010;10:20.
19. Ferraro MC, Cashin AG, Wand BM, Smart KM, Berryman C, Marston L, et al. Interventions for treating pain and disability in adults with complex regional pain syndrome- an overview of systematic reviews. Cochrane Database Syst Rev. 2023;2023:CD009416.
20. Bain GI, Kuberakani K, Luchetti R, Atzei A. Arthroscopy and endoscopy of the elbow, wrist and hand, surgical anatomy and techniques. Cham: Springer; 2021. p. 953–62.

30 Complications of Wrist Stiffness and Their Treatment

Andrew Y. H. Chin and Camelia Qian Ying

30.1 Introduction

Wrist stiffness is a significant and disabling complication following wrist surgery. The functional ranges of movement of the wrist are between 40° of flexion, 40° of extension [1], 10° of radial deviation, and 15° of ulnar deviation [2]. The normal range of motion of the forearm is 80° of pronation and supination. Reduction in ranges of movement of the wrist can lead to significant functional limitation. However, there is a lack of consensus on the diagnostic criteria for post-operative wrist stiffness. This in turn limits the reporting of its prevalence.

The cause of post-operative wrist stiffness is often multifactorial, but usually stimulated by intra-articular and capsular injuries, then compounded by immobilisation. Not infrequently, extra-capsular inflammation and fibrosis, such as tendon and burn injuries, also result in wrist stiffness. This chapter seeks to explore the causes and pathophysiology of post-operative wrist stiffness as well as its treatment options.

30.2 Pathophysiology of Post-operative Wrist Stiffness

The pathophysiology of post-operative wrist stiffness is intricate [3]. It involves the disruption of cellular growth, differentiation and death, as well as tissue homeostasis and organisation, eventually leading to uninhibited proliferation of fibroconnective tissue [4] (Fig. 30.1). Histologically, arthrofibrosis is characterised by the production of excessive extracellular matrix in a joint [5]. The fibrotic scar tissue, composed primarily of collagen, leads to stiffness and loss of range of movement, ultimately compromising on the patient's ability to perform functional tasks.

Recent research on the pathophysiology and cellular process of arthrofibrosis continues to shed light on this complex process, leading to some authors to further differentiate arthrofibrosis into two subtypes [6]—active and residual—to better explain role of inflammatory cytokines in the development of wrist pain and stiffness.

A. Y. H. Chin (✉) · C. Q. Ying
Department of Hand and Reconstructive Microsurgery, Singapore General Hospital, Singapore, Singapore

L. Pederzini et al. (eds.), *Stiffness of the Elbow, Wrist and Related Pathologies*, https://doi.org/10.1007/978-3-031-81381-8_30

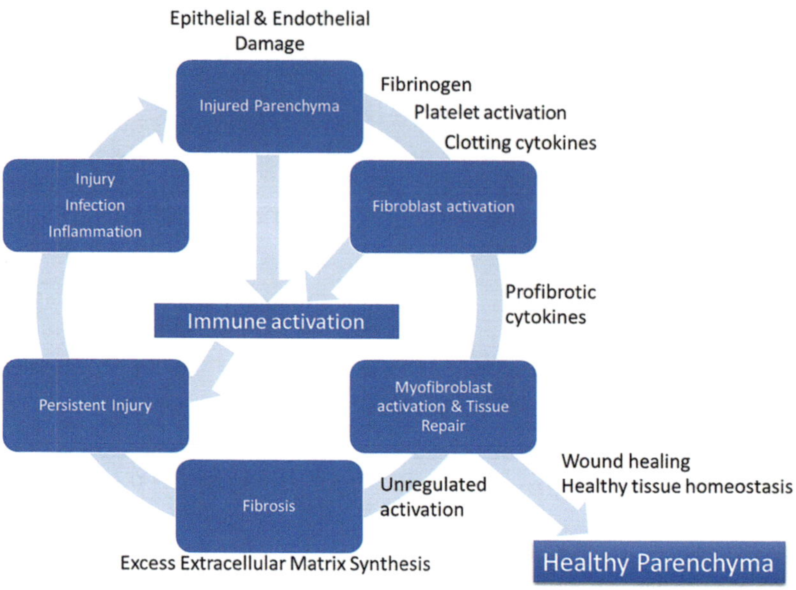

Fig. 30.1 Summary of biological reaction and cascade leading to dysregulation and excessive fibrosis. (Source: Blessing et al. [4])

30.3 Patho-Anatomy of Post-operative Wrist Stiffness

The wrist capsule is a special structure that is particularly prone to contracture. Range of movement at the wrist is a composite movement of three intercalated joints. In determining the aetiology of wrist stiffness, the location of causative factors (i.e. intra-articular, capsular, extra-articular and/or neurological) as well as the joint involved (i.e. midcarpal, radiocarpal and/or distal radioulnar joint [DRUJ]) could be examined. This is summarised in Fig. 30.2.

Wrist stiffness can also be classified based on the ISAKOS classification (Table 30.1). Lee et al. [7] have similarly classified causes of wrist arthrofibrosis based on the location of the pathology, broadly classifying the aetiology into intrinsic adhesions (i.e. radiocarpal joint, midcarpal joint, distal radioulnar joint [DRUJ] or combination) vis-à-vis extrinsic capsular fibrosis (i.e. dorsal, palmar, DRUJ or combination).

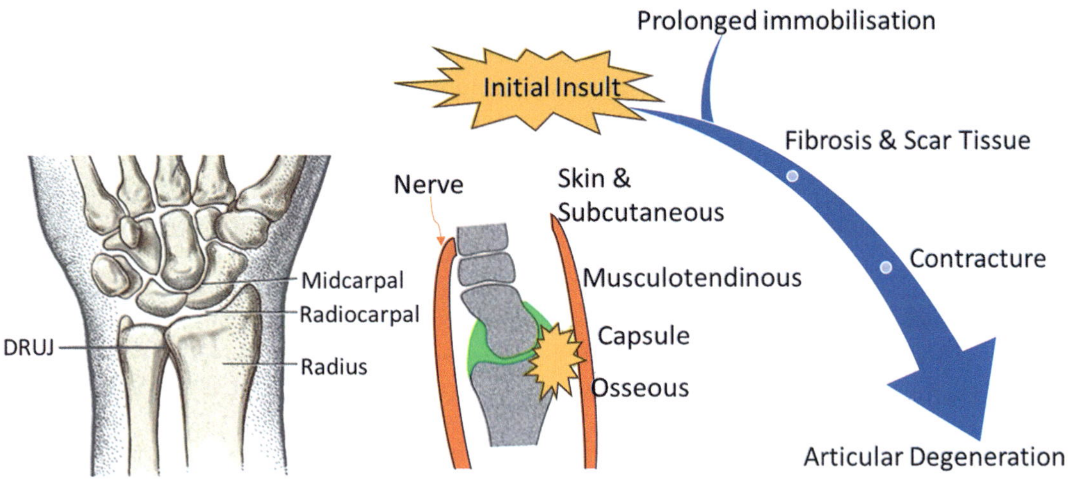

Fig. 30.2 Representation of the wrist joint with emphasis on the midcarpal, radiocarpal, and distal radioulnar joints where pathologies resulting in wrist stiffness commonly occur. The cascade of reactions resulting in post-operative wrist stiffness starts with injury, exacerbated by excessive immobilisation, resulting in fibrosis and scar tissue, wrist joint contracture, and ultimately leading to articular degeneration

Table 30.1 Patho-anatomical classification of joint stiffness, developed by ISAKOS Upper Extremity Committee

Intra-articular (bearings)	Capsular (constraints)	Extra-articular (motor, cable, levers)	Neurological (control, electrics, sensors)
Articular surface Osteochondral defect Degeneration *Subchondral* Dysplasia, fracture AVN, degeneration *Synovium* Inflammatory Crystalopathy	*Labrum and ligaments* Deficient Tear *Capsule* Patulous capsule Capsulitis, contracture *Congruity* Subluxation Dislocation	*Muscles* Myopathy Fatty infiltration *Tendons and bursa* Tear, calcification degeneration, bursitis *Other (external to shoulder)* Fracture, malignancy, HO Skin contracture	*Central* Behavioural, dyskinesia, Dystonia *UMN and LMN* Spasticity Flaccid paralysis *Sensory and autonomic* Charcot joint Chronic regional pain

30.4 Wrist Stiffness in Distal Radius Fracture or Ligament Repair and Reconstruction

Despite an understanding of the pathogenesis of wrist stiffness, early mobilisation might not be possible due to a myriad of reasons. This includes surgical factors such as unstable fracture fixation or ligamentous reconstruction and infection, and patient factors such as poor motivation. All these inevitably lead to wrist stiffness. There however remains no conclusive evidence pointing to the ideal duration of immobilisation [8, 9] or forearm position during immobilisation [10]. Pain is almost always present with articular rigidity [11].

Incorrect or incomplete reduction of intra-articular distal radius fracture has often been cited as the commonest cause of post-operative wrist stiffness [12]. Following distal radius fracture, two conditions often lead to painful arc of movement: (1) capsular contracture with intra-articular adhesions, and (2) radiocarpal impingement caused either by fracture malunion of the distal radius dorsal rim, or increased volar tilt of the distal radius articular surface. Both conditions are not mutually exclusive and should be treated if present.

While literature on post-operative wrist stiffness is scarce, current clinical practice often suggest the need for treatment of wrist stiffness should there be persistent pain or swelling, restricted ranges of movement or a plateauing of improvement in ranges of movement after a 6-month trial of intensive physiotherapy [7].

30.5 Preventing Wrist Stiffness with Oedema Control and Early Mobilisation

The initial post-operative biological response of the wrist is the setting in of oedema, which typically begins within 3 days. Oedema control and controlled mobilisation are essential to achieve good post-operative outcome. During the proliferative phase post-surgery, fibrin is deposited at the surgical site and adhesions form between the various structures in the joint. As such, early motion therapy and control of post-operative oedema is paramount in reducing adhesion formation and preventing wrist stiffness.

Early motion therapy should be a conscientious deliberate effort. The prerequisite for early motion therapy is a stable fracture fixation. Another crucial factor is to avoid unnecessary loading on the fracture fixation or ligament reconstruction site, for which mutual understanding and good cooperation with a hand therapist are essential to achieve adequate mobilisation without unnecessary loading. A case in point would be that of excessive contraction of the flexor muscles, which may cause unnecessary loading of the fracture fixation and ligament reconstruction site, potentially jeopardising the surgical fixation. Hand therapist should also warn patient against the usage of small stress ball or similar-sized object for grip strengthening to avoid excessive flexor contraction during the initial stages of fracture or ligament healing.

Forearm position also plays an important role during early motion therapy. During wrist flexion–extension movement, the summed peak wrist extensor forces are significantly lesser with the forearm in the supinated position than with the forearm in the neutral position during active rotation [13]. Hence to reduce the deforming forces on the carpal or distal radius fracture site, hand therapy rehabilitation should begin with the forearm in supination wherein the wrist tendon forces are the least. Following this, progressive resistive exercises with the use of orthotics or Canadian table may help to remodel connective tissue and improve the passive ranges of movement.

30.6 Assessment of Wrist Stiffness

Evaluation of post-operative wrist stiffness begins with a thorough history and physical examination. Patients commonly present with a plateau in improvement after 6 months of intensive post-operative therapy. Ranges of wrist movement across the three axes (namely flexion–extension, radial–ulnar deviation, and pronosupination) should be accurately recorded. The presence of pain and quality of endpoints should be noted as well.

Careful physical examination should be performed to ascertain the pathological structures involved. This includes a meticulous examination of the midcarpal, radiocarpal and DRUJ. Treatment of post-operative stiffness can then be directed towards the afflicted structure. While DRUJ stiffness results in limitation of pronosupination, movement at the radiocarpal and midcarpal joints might be difficult to distinguish from one another. Anaesthetic blocks of the posterior interosseous nerve, anterior interosseous nerve and/or ulnar nerve can help to ascertain whether limitations in range of movement are secondary to pain or mechanical pathology [7].

Advanced imaging, such as magnetic resonance imaging or computed tomography, may help to reveal pathologies that limit the ranges of movement at the wrist. These include failure of fracture fixation or ligament reconstruction, as well as loss of reduction of distal radius fracture. Articular surface degeneration may be apparent in severe cases, for which salvage procedures, such as wrist denervation, arthrodesis or arthroplasty, may be considered in managing such post-traumatic osteoarthrosis.

30.7 Treatment of Wrist Stiffness

Conservative management involving aggressive rehabilitation of the wrist remains the first line of treatment for post-operative stiffness (Figs. 30.3 and 30.4). This involves good pain control, strategic use of splints and diligent physiotherapy. Adequate pain management is paramount in breaking the vicious cycle between pain and stiffness, whereby pain is both a precipitating and aggravating factor of wrist stiffness (Fig. 30.5).

Signs of nerve dysfunction should also be carefully examined as concomitant nerve involvement, such as median nerve compression or intra-operative injury to the cutaneous nerve, could be present. Incidence of complex regional pain syndrome (CRPS) following distal radius fractures has been reported up to 37% [14]. Hence, patients presenting with wrist pain and stiffness following distal radius fracture should also be assessed for CRPS and treated accordingly [15] (Table 30.2). Wrist manipulation under anaesthesia may be used to aid rehabilitation of post-operative wrist stiffness. However, the associated risk of iatrogenic injuries, such as torn ligaments and fractures, should be counselled to such patients.

Should stiffness persist despite extensive wrist rehabilitation, surgical arthrolysis could be offered. There is however, no common consensus on the optimal duration of wrist rehabilitation prior to consideration of such surgical intervention.

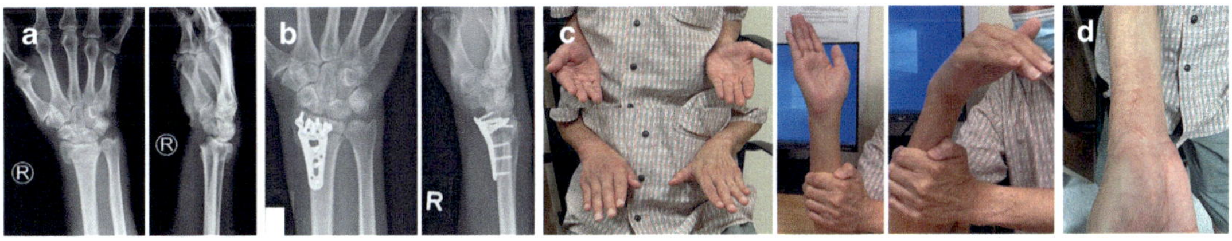

Fig. 30.3 Case illustration of post-operative wrist stiffness treated successfully in early stages of recovery, following fixation for (**a**) displaced distal radius fracture that was (**b**) treated with open reduction and volar plating. With early mobilisation and oedema control, good ranges of motion were attained (**c**) at 5 weeks post-operatively, with (**d**) well-healed scar

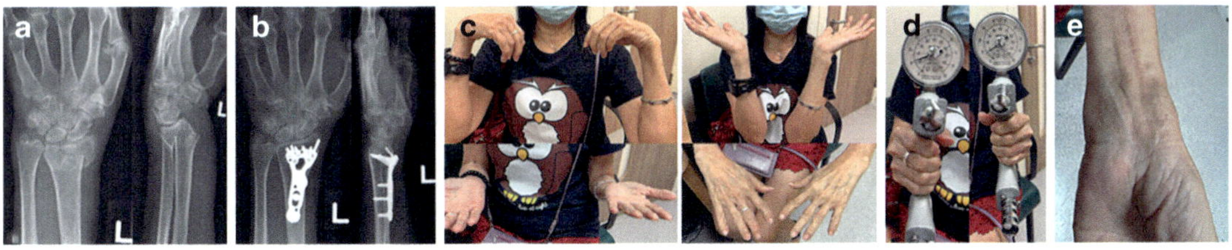

Fig. 30.4 A case of post-operative wrist stiffness resolving with conservative treatment, with (**a**) pre-operative radiographs and (**b**) post-operative radiographs. Post-operatively, patient developed significant wrist stiffness that was treated with aggressive rehabilitation following fracture union. At 2 years post-operatively, patient was satisfied with (**c**) improved range of motion, (**d**) comparable grip strength, and (**e**) well-healed scar

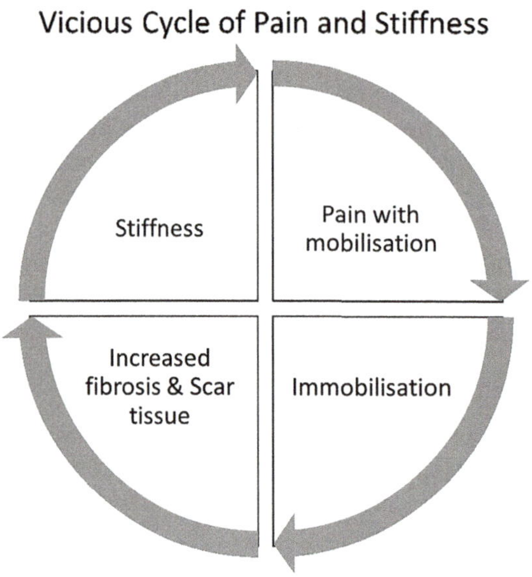

Fig. 30.5 Without good pain management, patients are understandably more apprehensive towards mobilisation, leading to prolonged periods of inactivity, increased fibrosis, and ultimately wrist stiffness

30.8 Wrist Arthrolysis: Open or Arthroscopic

Surgical arthrolysis can be performed via open or arthroscopic technique. There is however no clear superiority between the two techniques [16], and the decision to proceed with either rests on the surgeon's expertise and clinical judgement. In our opinion, open arthrolysis is useful in addressing extra-articular causes of wrist stiffness such as tendon adhesions, while arthroscopic arthrolysis is preferred when addressing intra-articular or capsular pathologies.

Intra-operative pre- and post-procedure ranges of movement should be documented and improvements noted.

Open arthrolysis and capsulotomies provide direct visualisation and the opportunity to address factors causing wrist stiffness, starting from releasing extra-capsular soft tissues to treating

Table 30.2 Detailing the commonly accepted diagnostic criteria [15] for complex regional pain syndrome (CRPS) with highlights on decreased range of movement as a crucial symptom and sign for the diagnosis of CRPS

Proposed clinical diagnostic criteria for CRPS
General definition of the syndrome:
CRPS describes an array of painful conditions that are characterized by a continuing (spontaneous and/or evoked) regional pain that is seemingly disproportionate in time or degree to the usual course of any known trauma or other lesion. The pain is regional (not in a specific nerve territory or dermatome) and usually has a distal predominance of abnormal sensory, motor, sudomotor, vasomotor, and/or trophic findings. The syndrome shows variable progression over time
To make the *clinical* diagnosis, the following criteria must be met:
1. Continuing pain, which is disproportionate to any inciting event
2. Must report at least one symptom in *three of the four* following categories:
Sensory: Reports of hyperesthesia and/or allodynia
Vasomotor: Reports of temperature asymmetry and/or skin color changes and/or skin color asymmetry
Sudomotor/Edema: Reports of edema and/or sweating changes and/or sweating asymmetry
Motor/Trophic: Reports of decreased range of motion and/or motor dysfunction (weakness, tremor, dystonia) and/or trophic changes (hair, nail, skin)
3. Must display at least one sign **at time of evaluation** in *two or more* of the following categories:
Sensory: Evidence of hyperalgesia (to pinprick) and/or allodynia (to light touch and/or temperature sensation and/or deep somatic pressure and/or joint movement)
Vasomotor: Evidence of temperature asymmetry (>1 °C) and/or skin color changes and/or asymmetry
Sudomotor/Edema: Evidence of edema and/or sweating changes and/or sweating asymmetry
Motor/Trophic: Evidence of decreased range of motion and/or motor dysfunction (weakness, tremor, dystonia) and/or trophic changes (hair, nail, skin)
4. There is no other diagnosis that better explains the signs and symptoms
For *research* purposes, diagnostic decision rule should be at least one symptom ***in all four*** symptom categories and at least one sign (observed at evaluation) in two or more sign categories.

Source: Reproduced with permission from Harden et al. [15].

intra-articular pathologies. Additional procedures such as removal of implants, carpal tunnel release and wrist denervation may also be performed during the same procedure. A case in point would be wrist stiffness following distal radius fixation whereby it may be beneficial to remove the surgical implant if there is evidence of tendon irritation from a distally positioned volar plate with flexor tendon adhesions [17]. Nonetheless, it is also imperative to be cognisant that open procedures carry a potential for greater tissue damage leading to adhesions, pain, oedema and recurrent stiffness. Excessive capsular release may also lead to wrist joint instability.

Arthroscopic arthrolysis aims to minimise collateral damage to soft tissues and has been shown to produce promising results in patients with capsular contracture without bony deformities, especially where the articular surfaces are congruent. General contraindications to arthroscopy include active infection and soft tissue pathology affecting portal entry points, as well as altered anatomy. Visual field may be obscured by fibrosis, adhesions and synovitis, and hence the surgeon's expertise and experience are necessary to avert secondary damage.

30.9 Open Arthrolysis

The surgical approach for open wrist arthrolysis is dependent on site of expected pathology as well as any previous surgical intervention. In wrist stiffness characterised by restricted wrist flexion, a dorsal approach to the wrist is employed. This involves a longitudinal skin incision and dorsal capsulotomy. If limitations in passive flexion persists after the dorsal release, following up with a volar approach to the wrist may be necessary. The aforementioned dorsal approach can also be used to address wrist stiffness following scapholunate ligament reconstruction.

For patients with limited wrist extension or requiring removal of volar plate used in previous distal radius fracture fixation, a volar approach to the wrist is recommended. When median nerve entrapment or pathology is also suspected, an extended carpal tunnel incision may be required. The radiocarpal joint is carefully examined, and any motion-restricting scar tissue is incised [18].

DRUJ capsulectomy can markedly improve the range of forearm rotation [19]. The usage of either dorsal or volar approach is dependent on the extent of pronosupination limitations [20]. In patients with significant pronation limitations, the DRUJ capsule can be approached dorsally via the floor of the fifth compartment. In patients with significant loss of supination, the volar approach can be performed through the interval between the ulnar neurovascular bundle and the flexor carpi ulnaris tendon. During the procedure, careful release of causative extra-capsular factors while preserving the triangular fibrocartilage complex is key. Capsular resection of the DRUJ capsule in the direction parallel to the radioulnar ligament can then be performed. Intra-articular adhesions can be lysed with a Freer elevator. Good clinical outcomes with high long-term patient satisfaction have been reported [21].

30.10 Arthroscopic Wrist Arthrolysis

Arthroscopic wrist arthrolysis is our preferred treatment of choice, especially in cases where additional procedures are not required. With the rise in popularity of wrist arthroscopy, a plethora of arthroscopic wrist arthrolysis techniques with good clinical outcomes have been described [22]. In a standard wrist dry arthroscopy, 3–4 portal is used as the main viewing portal for the radiocarpal joint, which is examined before proceeding to inspect the midcarpal joint via the radial and ulnar midcarpal portals [23]. 1–2 and 6R portals are commonly used as the working portals for the resection of fibrous tissue within the radiocarpal joint. As fibrosis of ulnocarpal joint is uncommon, resection of fibrotic bands within radiocarpal joints is usually sufficient to improve range of movement of the wrist [24].

Nonetheless, should restricted range of movement of the wrist persist despite resection of intra-capsular fibrotic bands within the radiocarpal joint, volar and dorsal capsule resections can also be performed arthroscopically to address capsular causes of wrist stiffness [25]. We recommend starting with the volar capsule and ligaments, which are immediately seen on insertion of the arthroscope through the dorsal arthroscopy portals, before proceeding to resect the dorsal capsule [23]. Sections of the volar capsule that can be released to improve wrist range of movement include the radioscaphocapitate ligament, short and long radiolunate ligaments, and radioscapholunate ligament [24]. Care should, however, be taken to preserve the ulnotriquetral and ulnolunate ligaments [24].

The dorsal capsule can be released from the sigmoid notch to the radial styloid, with caution taken to preserve the dorsal ulnar ligament complex. In principle, volar ulnar ligament and dorsal ulnar ligament complex should be protected and preserved to avoid inadvertent ulnar translation of the carpus [26]. Passive range of movement should be assessed intermittently before proceeding to further releases to avoid excessive resections. In addition, avoiding damage to surrounding tendons during capsular resection is also imperative, with Bain et al. [27] ingeniously describing the use of intra-capsular nylon tape to retract the extensor tendons.

Small articular incongruences, such as those seen in malunited distal radius fractures, can be addressed arthroscopically with the use of burrs [24]. This is commonly employed in small articular steps less than 1 mm, as well as in dorsal radiocarpal impingement where the dorsal rim of the distal radius is resected. Should there be limited changes in passive range of movement of the wrist following radiocarpal arthrolysis, a midcarpal arthroscopy is useful to examine for and address pathological causes such as adhesions. Cartilage degeneration between the capitate and hamate should be noted and taken into consideration for future treatments.

In patients with limited forearm rotation, DRUJ arthroscopy is a clinically rewarding but technically challenging procedure, partly due to the difficulty in inserting the arthroscope through the designated DRUJ portals due to fibrosis. Visualisation of the joint structure is often aided with the introduction of fluid to expand the joint. Once adequate visualisation is achieved, fibrosis can be addressed with the use of an aggressive resector. Both the volar and dorsal capsules can be resected to improve forearm rotation as well. Arthroscopic DRUJ arthrolysis carries a steep learning curve, especially when there is no central TFCC perforation, and conversion into open DRUJ surgery may be necessary when difficulty is encountered.

30.11 Post-operative Rehabilitation

Wrist rehabilitation should be commenced immediately after surgery starting with passive range of movement exercises [24]. Hand therapists should work closely with patients to ensure that intra-operative gains in ranges of movement of the wrist are not lost to inadequate mobilisation efforts. Long-acting wrist block or pain pump indwelling catheter regional block [7] may be used to achieve adequate pain relief during immediate post-operative period.

Good clinical outcomes have been reported post arthrolysis, with similar and satisfactory results reported in both arthroscopic and open procedures [16].

30.12 Conclusion

Post-operative wrist stiffness is a debilitating complication. Its pathogenesis is multifactorial, but largely contributed by immobilisation. In cases of persistent post-operative wrist stiffness despite aggressive rehabilitation, wrist manipulation under anaesthesia may be trialled. Surgical arthrolysis generally produces satisfactory clinical results and can be offered. Post-operative rehabilitation following arthrolysis is crucial in maintaining intra-operative gains in the ranges of movement of the wrist.

References

1. Ryu JY, Cooney WP 3rd, Askew LJ, An KN, Chao EY. Functional ranges of motion of the wrist joint. J Hand Surg Am. 1991;16(3):409–19.
2. Palmer AK, Werner FW, Murphy D, Glisson R. Functional wrist motion: a biomechanical study. J Hand Surg Am. 1985;10(1):39–46.
3. McAlister I, Sems SA. Arthrofibrosis after periarticular fracture fixation. Orthop Clin North Am. 2016;47(2):345–55.
4. Blessing WA, Williamson AK, Kirsch JR, Grinstaff MW. The prognosis of arthrofibroses: prevalence, clinical shortcomings, and future prospects. Trends Pharmacol Sci. 2021;42(5):398–415.
5. Lee DR, Therrien E, Song BM, Camp CL, Krych AJ, Stuart MJ, et al. Arthrofibrosis nightmares: prevention and management strategies. Sports Med Arthrosc Rev. 2022;30(1):29–41.
6. Usher KM, Zhu S, Mavropalias G, Carrino JA, Zhao J, Xu J. Pathological mechanisms and therapeutic outlooks for arthrofibrosis. Bone Res. 2019;7:9.
7. Lee SK, Gargano F, Hausman MR. Wrist arthrofibrosis. Hand Clin. 2006;22(4):529–38. abstract vii
8. Handoll HH, Elliott J. Rehabilitation for distal radial fractures in adults. Cochrane Database Syst Rev. 2015;2015(9):CD003324.
9. van Delft EAK, van Bruggen SGJ, van Stralen KJ, Bloemers FW, Sosef NL, Schep NWL, et al. Four weeks versus six weeks of immobilization in a cast following closed reduction for displaced distal radial fractures in adult patients: a multicentre randomized controlled trial. Bone Joint J. 2023;105-B(9):993–9.
10. Jamnik AA, Pirkle S, Chacon J, Xiao AX, Wagner ER, Gottschalk MB. The effect of immobilization position on functional outcomes and complications associated with the conservative treatment of distal radius fractures: a systematic review. J Hand Surg Glob Online. 2022;4(1):25–31.
11. Luchetti R, Bain G, Morse L, McGuire D. Arthroscopic Arthrolysis. In: Randelli P, Dejour D, van Dijk CN, Denti M, Seil R, editors. Arthroscopy: basic to advanced. Berlin: Springer; 2016. p. 935–51.
12. Gabl M, Arora R, Klauser AS, Schmidle G. Characteristics of secondary arthrofibrosis after intra-articular distal radius fracture. Arch Orthop Trauma Surg. 2016;136(8):1181–8.
13. Farr LD, Werner FW, McGrattan ML, Zwerling SR, Harley BJ. Wrist tendon forces with respect to forearm rotation. J Hand Surg Am. 2013;38(1):35–9.
14. Mathews AL, Chung KC. Management of complications of distal radius fractures. Hand Clin. 2015;31(2):205–15.
15. Harden RN, Bruehl S, Stanton-Hicks M, Wilson PR. Proposed new diagnostic criteria for complex regional pain syndrome. Pain Med. 2007;8(4):326–31.
16. Guidi M, Luchetti R, Besmens I, Rothenfluh E, Calcagni M. Wrist Arthrolysis: a systematic review of open and arthroscopic techniques. J Wrist Surg. 2021;10(6):543–50.
17. Snoddy MC, An TJ, Hooe BS, Kay HF, Lee DH, Pappas ND. Incidence and reasons for hardware removal following operative fixation of distal radius fractures. J Hand Surg Am. 2015;40(3):505–7.
18. Kamal RN, Ruch DS. Volar capsular release after distal radius fractures. The Journal of Hand Surgery. 2017;42(12):1034.e1. e6
19. Kleinman WB, Graham TJ. The distal radioulnar joint capsule: clinical anatomy and role in posttraumatic limitation of forearm rotation. J Hand Surg Am. 1998;23(4):588–99.
20. Kleinman WB. DRUJ contracture release. Tech Hand Up Extrem Surg. 1999;3(1):13–22.
21. Kooi K, Shoji MM, Jupiter JB, Chen NC, Garg R. DRUJ capsular release for forearm rotational limitation: surgical technique and case series. Hand (NY). 2023; https://doi.org/10.1177/15589447231207911.
22. Luchetti R, Atzei A, Fairplay T. Arthroscopic wrist arthrolysis after wrist fracture. Arthroscopy. 2007;23(3):255–60.
23. Luchetti R, Bain G, Morse L, McGuire D. Arthroscopic arthrolysis. Arthroscopy: basic to advanced; 2016. p. 935–51.
24. Bain GI, Kuberakani K, Luchetti R, Atzei A. Arthroscopic Arthrolysis of the wrist. In: Bhatia DN, Bain GI, Poehling GG, Graves BR, editors. Arthroscopy and endoscopy of the elbow, wrist and hand: surgical anatomy and techniques. Cham: Springer; 2022. p. 953–62.
25. Verhellen R, Bain GI. Arthroscopic capsular release for contracture of the wrist: a new technique. Arthroscopy. 2000;16(1):106–10.
26. Viegas SF, Patterson RM, Ward K. Extrinsic wrist ligaments in the pathomechanics of ulnar translation instability. J Hand Surg Am. 1995;20(2):312–8.
27. Bain GI, Munt J, Turner PC, Bergman J. Arthroscopic dorsal capsular release in the wrist: a new technique. Tech Hand Up Extrem Surg. 2008;12(3):191–4.

Joint Replacement Arthroplasty for the Stiff Wrist

31

Guillaume Herzberg, Lyliane Ly, Marion Burnier, and Michel Boeckstyns

31.1 Introduction

Wrist stiffness associated with pancarpal destruction may be an indication for joint replacement arthroplasty only if there is significant pain. Wrist stiffness without pain is not an indication for joint replacement [1, 2]. This chapter will focus on the currently available arthroplasty options to treat incapacitating painful stiff wrists with pancarpal destruction in patients with rheumatoid arthritis (RA) (Fig. 31.1) or osteoarthritis (OA) (Fig. 31.2). The new European medical devices regulation (MDR) recently led to the withdrawal of several total wrist arthroplasties (TWAs). Although RA patients' functional needs are very different from those of OA patients, the arthroplasty options are the same. However, the indications may still be influenced by the nature of disease and the functional needs of the patient.

Due to the MDR, the current TWA options include only two fourth-generation total wrist arthroplasties (Remotion TWA and Motec TWA). We will include into the discussion the pyrocarbon implant interposition arthroplasty (Amandys) since it represents also a replacement arthroplasty.

The aim of this article was to consider the expected results of those three commercially available implants with focus on range of motion (ROM) outcomes, especially active wrist extension since it is a key parameter for providing a functional hand grip. We will also mention the published complications of each of these implants.

G. Herzberg (✉)
Clinique Parc Lyon, Val Ouest Lyon, Lyon, France

L. Ly
Hopital Herriot, Lyon, France

M. Burnier
Medipole Villeurbanne, Villeurbanne, France

M. Boeckstyns
Capio Private Hospital Hellerup, Copenhagen, Denmark

L. Pederzini et al. (eds.), *Stiffness of the Elbow, Wrist and Related Pathologies*, https://doi.org/10.1007/978-3-031-81381-8_31

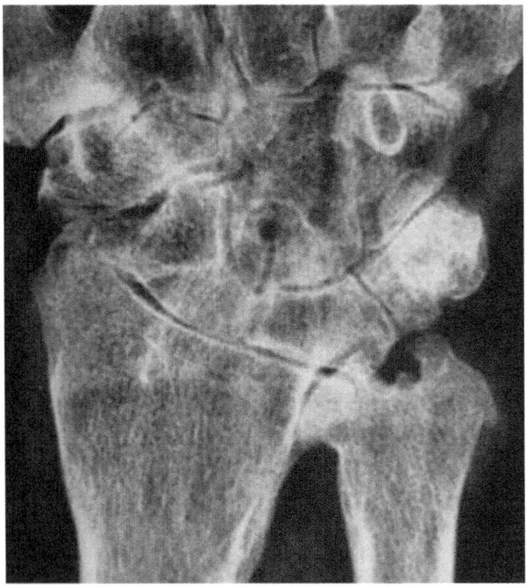

Fig. 31.1 Example of pancarpal wrist destruction in a rheumatoid patient

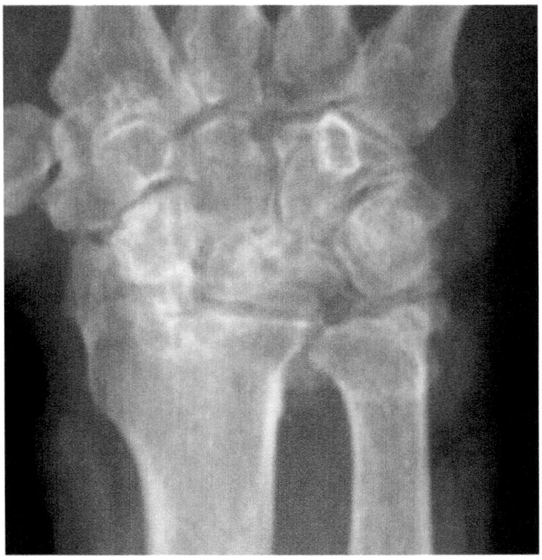

Fig. 31.2 Example of pancarpal wrist destruction in a non-rheumatoid patient. This was the spontaneous evolution of a neglected perilunate injury

31.2 Current Wrist Motion, Outcomes, and Complications After Remotion TWA

In a multicenter study [2] gathering 215 Remotion TWAs at a mean follow-up of 4 years, there were 129 rheumatoid arthritis (RA) patients and 86 non-rheumatoid (non-RA) patients. Wrist pain improved dramatically (average gain of 51 points on a 100-point visual analog scale [VAS]). Patient satisfaction was high. However, there was no significant gain in terms of active ROM. In RA patients, the comparison of pre- and postoperative active ROM showed very little improvement (mean postoperative active wrist extension 29°, average gain +2°). In non-RA patients, at a mean follow-up of 4 years, the comparison of pre- and postoperative active ROM showed a slight decrease (mean active wrist extension 36°, average loss −4°). These changes between pre- and postoperative wrist active extension were non-significant. In terms of complications, the authors found a revision rate of 5% and 6% in RA and non-RA patients, respectively. Radiological loosening with implant migration was observed in 4% and 3% in RA and non-RA patients, respectively. Overall, the incidence of signs of periprosthetic loosening was 12% and 18% in RA and non-RA patients, respectively. The survival rate with failure defined as implant revision was 96% and 92% at 4-year follow-up in RA and non-RA patients, respectively.

Boeckstyns and Herzberg [3] reviewed 44 consecutive Remotion (22 RA, 22 non-RA) implanted in 2 specialized surgical centers. The authors specifically focused on periprosthetic osteolysis (PPO) (Fig. 31.3). They found high incidences of 36% of periprosthetic radiolucency at the radial side and 16% at the carpal side, regardless of the primary diagnosis of RA versus non-RA. The PPO seemed to stabilize in most patients after 1–3 years.

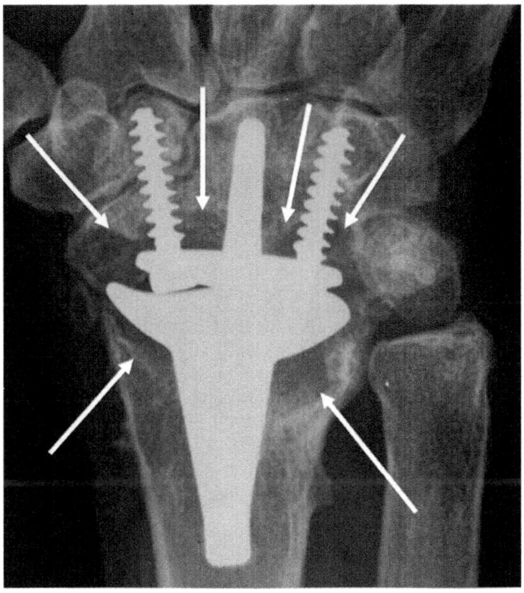

Fig. 31.3 Example of periprosthetic osteolysis after Remotion total wrist arthroplasty

Honecker et al. [4] reviewed 19 RA cases at a mean follow-up of 6 years. The QuickDASH score improved significantly (gain of 19 points). However, the average gain was only +11° in active wrist extension (postoperative wrist extension 44°). The authors observed 39% of radial periprosthetic loosening and 26% of carpal periprosthetic loosening. The average survival rate was 69% at 8-year follow-up.

Fischer et al. [5] prospectively reviewed at 10 years of follow-up 69 Remotion TWA in 57 RA and 12 non-RA patients. There was a significant improvement of VAS pain scores. However, in both RA and non-RA patients, the comparison of pre- and postoperative active ROM showed little improvement (mean postoperative active wrist extension gain +5°). Severe radiological loosening, defined as extensive osteolysis affecting both the radial and the carpal component, was found in 10% of the cases. With revision as final end-point, the 10-year Remotion implant survival was 94%.

31.3 Current Wrist Motion, Outcomes, and Complications After Motec TWA

Reigstad [6] first reported in 2012 the outcomes of a series of 30 patients with SLAC/SNAC 3 or 4 wrists operated on with a Motec TWA. Although the distribution of stages 3 versus 4 was not mentioned, previous surgery had been performed in 73% of the cases. At 5 years of follow-up, wrist pain improved significantly (average gain of 3.1 points in radial wrist pain at activity with remaining pain at 4.3, average gain of 4.2 points in ulnar wrist pain at activity with remaining pain at 0.5). Although the results in terms of active wrist extension were not specifically addressed, a 20° improvement of active wrist motion at follow-up was noted. In terms of complications, revision surgery was performed in 23% of the wrists (Fig. 31.4). Focal PPO developed in 10% at the radial side and 7% at the carpal side at follow-up. The 6-year estimated survival rate was 93%.

Giwa et al. [7] reviewed 25 Motec implants (20 non-RA, 5 RA patients) at a mean follow-up of 4 years. The QuickDASH score improved dramatically (gain of 37 points). Although the results in terms of active wrist extension were not specifically addressed, a 34° improvement of active wrist motion at follow-up was noted. Sixteen percent of the implants had to be revised. Periprosthetic loosening was not specifically addressed.

Reigstad [8] reviewed 56 non-RA patients operated on with a Motec implant at a mean follow-up of 8 years. The QuickDASH score improved significantly (gain of 15 points). Although the results in terms of active wrist extension were not specifically addressed, a 29° improvement of total active wrist motion at follow-up was noted. A total of 13 wrists (23%) sustained additional surgeries and 8 wrists (14%) had revision surgery. Radiological examination revealed 2 loose but not revised implants and 23

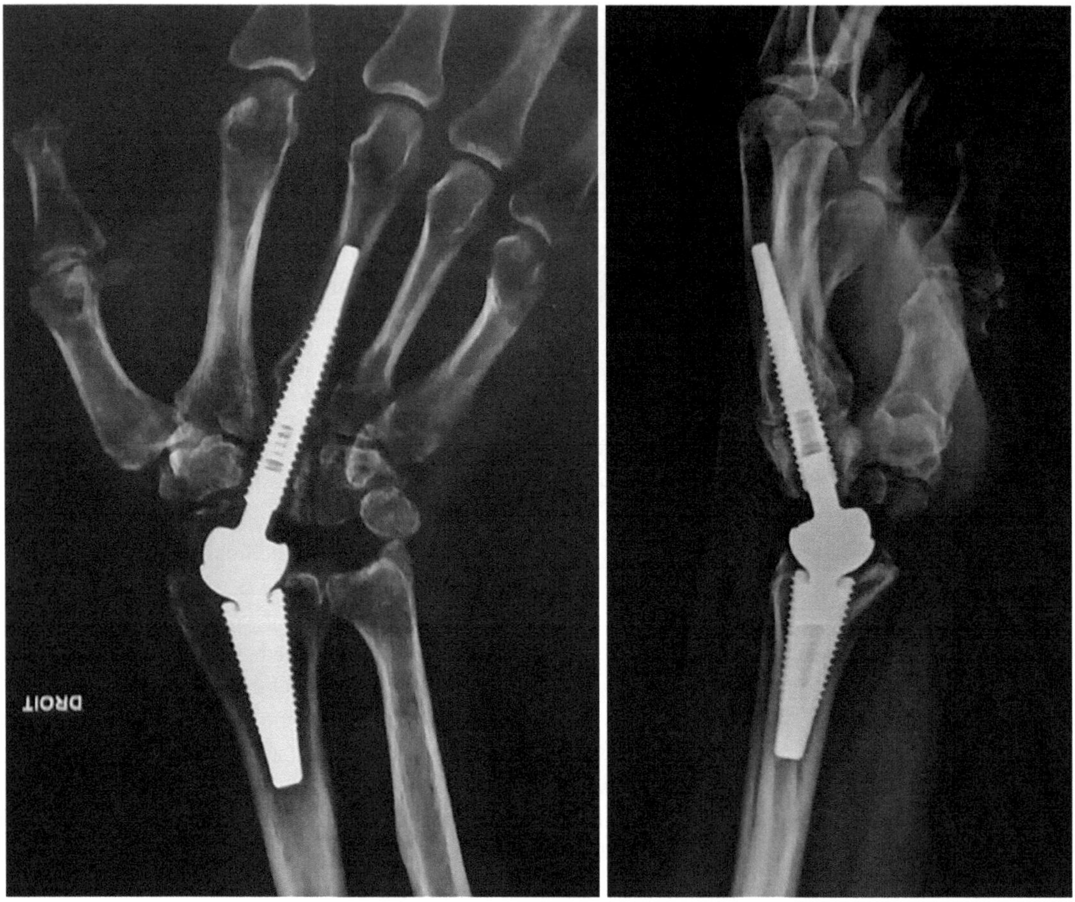

Fig. 31.4 Postoperative radiograph of a patient with fixed ulnar and extension wrist deformity after Motec total wrist arthroplasty

periprosthetic osteolysis (a total of 45% of major or minor periprosthetic osteolysis). The 10-year survival rate of the implants was 86% for revision for any cause.

Holm-Glad [9] prospectively compared the short-term outcomes (2 years) of 20 Remotion and 20 Motec TWA in non-RA patients. They noted a similar and significant improvement of QuickDASH scores in both series (gain of 22 points after Remotion, 24 points after Motec). Although the results in terms of active wrist extension were not specifically addressed, a 4° improvement of active wrist motion at follow-up was noted after Remotion whereas a 31° improvement of active wrist motion at follow-up was noted after Motec implantation. PPO was observed in 17 Remotion (85%) and 15 Motec (75%). At 2-year follow-up, the revision rate was 10% after Remotion and 15% after Motec.

Redfern et al. [10] specifically analyzed the complication rates and modes of failure in Motec TWA in a retrospective multicenter analysis of 171 cases at a mean follow-up of 5.8 years. The revision rate was 8%. Failure of osseointegration was the most common complication. Problems with soft tissue balancing, impingement-related osteolysis, bony impingement, and metacarpal fracture were found to be the other causes of failure in this large series.

31.4 Current Wrist Motion Outcomes and Complications After Amandys Pyrocarbon Interposition Wrist Arthroplasty

Lestienne and Bellemère [11] retrospectively reviewed 28 pyrocarbon Amandys interposition arthroplasties at a mean follow-up of 5 years for patients with RA. There was no major *preoperative* carpal subluxation in any of the cases in this series. Wrist pain improved significantly (average gain of 4 points on a 10-point visual analog scale). The gains in QuickDASH and PRWE scores were 26 and 37 points, respectively. However, there was no significant gain in terms of active wrist extension. The comparison of pre- and postoperative active wrist extension showed very little improvement (mean postoperative active wrist extension 33°, average gain +3°). No implant had to be removed (Fig. 31.5). There was no implant subsidence. In terms of complications, the authors mentioned a revision in four (14%) of the cases. There were four implant subluxations of which three sustained revision for reposition and palmar capsular reinforcement. No implant had to be removed (Fig. 31.6).

Marie et al. [12] retrospectively reviewed 21 Amandys implants (19 non-RA, 2 RA) at a mean follow-up of 41 months. The preoperative clinical status was not available. Residual wrist pain was 3.1/10 points. The result in terms of active wrist extension was 33°, which was similar to the results by Lestienne and Bellemère [11].

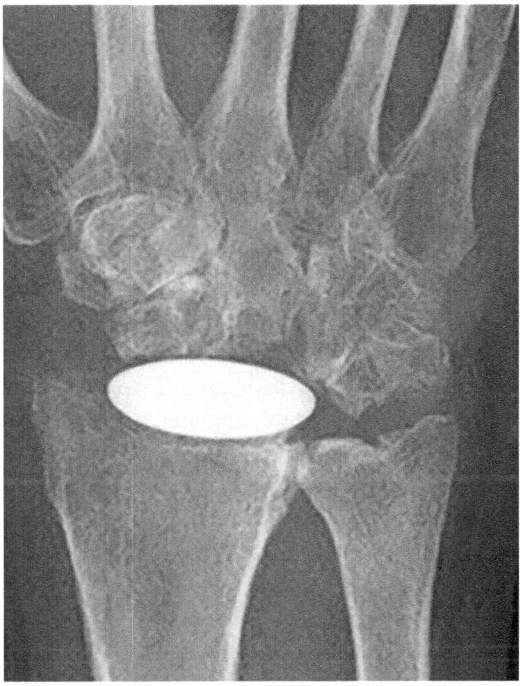

Fig. 31.5 Satisfactory postoperative position of an Amandys pyrocarbon interposition implant

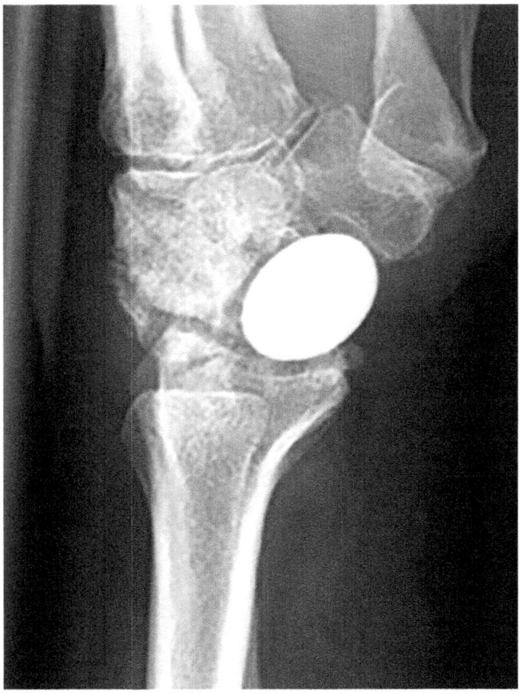

Fig. 31.6 Volarly dislocated Amandys implant

31.5 Conclusion

The review of these papers confirms the fact that TWA or interposition pyrocarbon should not be performed for wrist stiffness without pain. The active wrist extension improvement after all these procedures is very limited, insignificant after Remotion and Amandys procedures, and modest after Motec procedure. The main indication for TWA is incapacitating wrist pain in completely destroyed wrists. Since there is a significant complication rate with revision after TWA and interposition pyrocarbon implants, a shared decision-making has to be made for each patient regarding the option of a motion-preserving procedure versus total wrist arthrodesis. A weakness of this review is that there only exists a paucity of unbiased long-term reports of the most recent implants. Several reports are authored or co-authored by surgeons who are closely involved in the development or production of the prostheses and many series include small numbers only with rather short observation periods.

References

1. Boeckstyns MEH, Herzberg G, Sorensen AI, Axelsson P, Kroner K, Liverneaux P, et al. Can TWA be an option in the treatment of the severely destroyed post traumatic wrist? J Wrist Surg. 2013;2(4):324–9.
2. Herzberg G, Boeckstyns MEH, Sorensen AI, Axelsson P, Kroener K, Liverneaux P, et al. "Remotion" total wrist arthroplasty: preliminary results of a prospective international multicenter study of 215 cases. J Wrist Surg. 2012;1(1):17–21.
3. Boeckstyns MEH, Herzberg G. Periprosthetic osteolysis after total wrist arthroplasty. J Wrist Surg. 2014;3(2):101–6.
4. Honecker S, Facca S, Liverneaux P. Survival rate on a 10 year follow up of TWA implants: a 23 patients case series. J Wrist Surg. 2019;8(1):24.
5. Fischer P, Sagerfors M, Pettersson K. Total wrist arthroplasty: a 10-year follow up. J Hand Surg Am. 2020;45(8):780.
6. Reigstad O. Promising one to six year results with the Motec wrist arthroplasty in patients with post traumatic OA. J Bone Joint Surg (Br). 2012;94B(11):1540–5.
7. Giwa L, Siddiqui A, Packer G. Motec wrist arthroplasty: 4 years of promising results. J Hand Surg Asian Pac Vol. 2018;23(3):364–8.
8. Reigstad O. Five to 10-year prospective follow-up of wrist arthroplasty in 56 nonrheumatoid patients. J Hand Surg Am. 2017;42(10):788–96.
9. Holm-Glad T, Reigstad O. A randomized controlled trial comparing two. Modern total wrist arthroplasties. Bone Joint J. 2023;104-B(10):1132–41.
10. Redfern JAI, Mehta N, Farnebo S, McGuire D, Solomons M, Thorvaldson T, et al. Complication rates and modes of short and medium-term failure in Motec total wrist arthroplasty: an international cohort study. J Hand Surg Eur Vol. 2024;49(1):27–33.
11. Lestienne V, Bellemère P. Results of interposition ARP with the Amandys pyrocarbon implant in RA wrists. Hand Surg Rehabil. 2021;40(5):579.
12. Marie C, Forli A, Corcella D. Clinical, functional and radiological results of the Amandys. Hand Surg Rehabil. 2021;40(4):420.

32 Open and Arthroscopic Procedures for Pronation–Supination Contracture

Toshiyasu Nakamura

32.1 Pronation–Supination Contracture

Pronation–supination contracture indicates loss of forearm rotation, either pronation or supination or both. Loss of pronation can be compensated by shoulder abduction, while loss of supination cannot be compensated with any motion because of the interference of humeral adduction by the body itself, thus indicating severe restriction in the activity of daily life.

32.2 Kinematics of Pronation–Supination Motion

There are several factors controlling forearm pronosupination, which are classified as static factors and dynamic factors. Static factors are (1) bone configuration [1], (2) position of rotation axis [2, 3], and (3) soft tissue restraints. Soft tissue restraints for pronation–supination movement are the triangular fibrocartilage complex (TFCC) or radioulnar ligament (RUL) [4], joint capsule of the distal radioulnar joint (DRUJ) [5], the annular ligament in the proximal radioulnar joint (PRUJ) [6], and interosseous membrane (IOM) [7–11]. Dynamic factors are (1) muscles, including the extensor carpi ulnaris (ECU) and the pronator quadratus (PQ) [8, 10], supinator, and pronator teres (PT), and (2) direction of the motion, pronating or supinating. The PT and PQ are important muscles for pronation and biceps and supinator are for supination. All of static and dynamic factors can be affected in pronation–supination contracture, while main cause of the contractures are soft tissues.

T. Nakamura (✉)
Department of Orthopaedic Surgery, School of Medicine, International University of Health and Welfare, Tokyo, Japan
e-mail: toshiyasu@ae.em-net.ne.jp

32.3 Pathology of Pronation–Supination Disorders

32.3.1 Incongruity of Bony Configuration

Malunion of both the radius and ulna or malunion of the radius introduces loss of pronation–supination range (Fig. 32.1a). Malunion of the ulnar shaft has little effect for pronation–supination. Curvature of the radius is very important to rotate over the ulna during forearm rotation, and malunited radial shaft can impinge to the ulna to indicate mechanical loss of rotation. Bronstein et al. [12, 13] described that a dorsal tilt to 30° and radial translation to 10 mm led to no significant restriction in forearm pronosupination range, while a 5 mm ulnar translation deformity resulted in a mean 23% loss of pronation range and radial

L. Pederzini et al. (eds.), *Stiffness of the Elbow, Wrist and Related Pathologies*,
https://doi.org/10.1007/978-3-031-81381-8_32

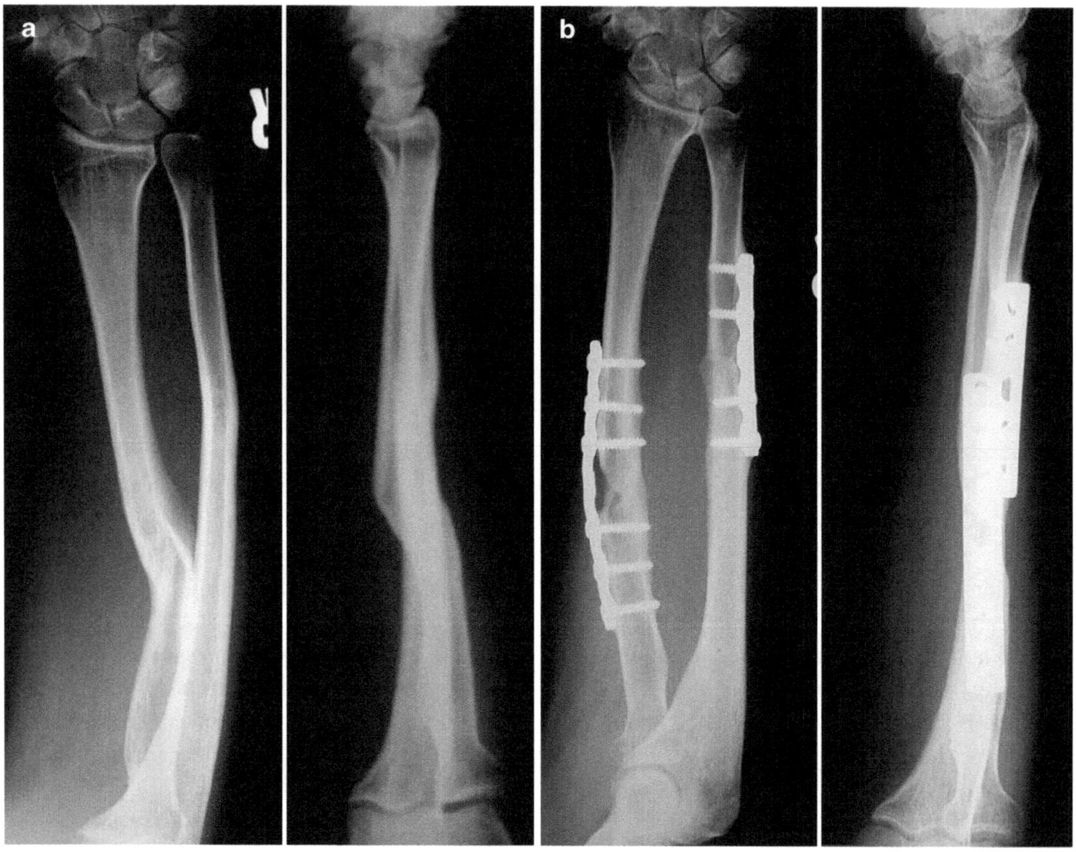

Fig. 32.1 (**a**) Posteroanterior (PA; left) and lateral (right) preoperative radiographs of malunited radius and ulna indicating severe loss of pronation of 40° and supination of 0°. (**b**) Posteroanterior (right) and lateral (left) radiographs of corrected osteotomy with iliac bone graft showing almost normal bone configuration of the forearm. Patient indicated 60° of pronation and 60° of supination at the final follow-up

shortening of 10 mm reduced forearm pronation by 47% and supination by 29% [1].

32.3.2 Malposition of the Rotation Axis

When the DRUJ dislocation or subluxation occurs, the ulnar head tends to displace dorsally and the avulsed RUL locates volary. After healing process of the RUL occurs, it tends to reattach to the volar part of the fovea due to dorsal subluxation of the ulnar head. In this scenario, the dorsal subluxated ulnar head restricts forearm supination severely.

32.3.3 Malalignment of the DRUJ

Malalignment of either the ulnar head or sigmoid notch of the radius or both after intra-articular fracture can be a cause of loss of forearm rotation range (Fig. 32.2).

32.3.4 Soft Tissue Problem

The pronation–supination contracture is mainly caused by shortening of surrounding soft tissue of the DRUJ, such as the TFCC, capsule [5], and distal side of the interosseous membrane (IOM) (so-called membranous part) [14]. After trauma,

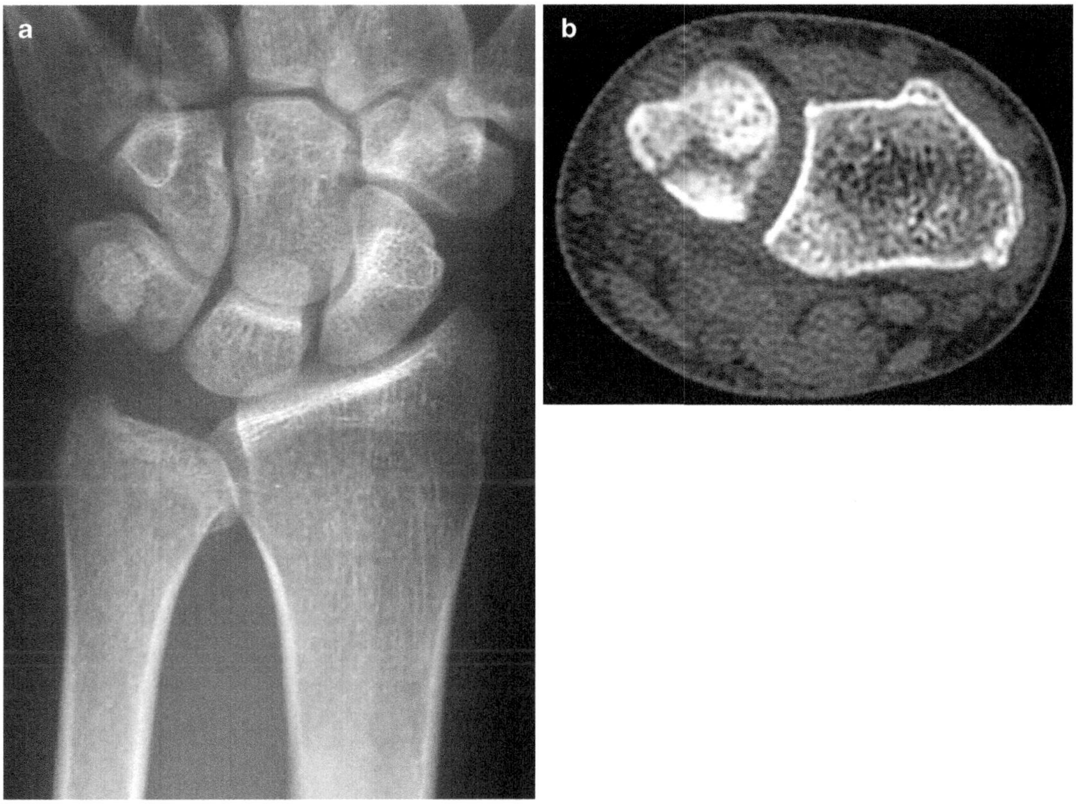

Fig. 32.2 (**a**) PA radiograph of fracture of the ulnar head indicating loss of pronosupination. (**b**) Axial computed tomography (CT) indicates malalignment of the ulnar head articulation with respect to the sigmoid notch of the radius

minor hematoma or ligament rupture can cause shrinkage of collagen fibers to shorten the length of the ligament, capsule, or other soft tissue. Soft tissue contracture of the annular ligament or PRUJ also indicates loss of forearm rotation.

32.3.5 Dynamic Factors

Contracture of the muscles may cause severe restriction of the forearm range, such as the biceps brachii, supinator, or pronator quadratus. Contracture of the biceps or supinator may show loss of pronation and contracture of the pronator quadratus may show loss of supination. Direction of motion may not have so much influences on range of pronosupination.

32.3.6 Other Causes

Heterotopic ossification around the PRUJ can also cause pronation–supination contracture [6]. Contracture after tumor resection with aggressive proliferation of scar tissue also causes restriction of forearm rotation [14].

The DRUJ locking is a new entity of loss of forearm supination [15, 16]. The ulnar head entrapped by the longitudinal tear in the RUL or by the flap of the triangular fibrocartilage indicates blocking of palmar translation of the ulnar head, demonstrating locking. Pronation is possible.

32.4 Diagnosis of Pronation–Supination Contracture

Diagnosis of pronation–supination is easy. Just simply patient cannot either pronate or supinate or both. Radiographs and computed tomography (CT) can only demonstrate malunion of the radius or ulna, or dislocation (subluxation) of the DRUJ or PRUJ [17, 18]. Magnetic resonance imaging (MRI) shows soft tissue problems including TFCC lesions, malposition of the TFCC attachment after trauma, or contracture of the IOM [10, 11]. However, true cause of the contracture may be difficult to be determined.

32.5 Treatment Options for Pronosupination Contracture

32.5.1 Reduction and Fixation of the Bony Configuration

For malunion of the radius and ulna or isolated radial malunion, correction of the radius and ulnar shaft with/without bone grafting is recommended [1, 19]. Synthes Low Contact- Locking Compression Plate (LC-LCP) plate or 2.7 mm LCP plate is an adequate fixation device for correction osteotomy (Fig. 32.2). After correction osteotomy of the radius and ulna, soft tissue release at the DRUJ capsule may be needed for complete recovery of pronation–supination range of motion (ROM).

32.5.2 Reduction of Malpositioned Rotation Axis

Malposition of the rotation axis is mainly caused by malposition of the RUL or TFCC at the fovea. Once the RUL is detached from the fovea, ulnar head tends to subluxate in dorsal direction and the RUL is healed to volar site from the original attachment at the fovea. In this situation, the RUL is sectioned once, then is reattached to the correct position of the fovea (always central attaching lesion of the RUL) to correct the ulnar head subluxation and to resume the rotation axis.

32.5.3 Rotation Osteotomy of the Radius and/or Ulna

Rotation osteotomy induces recovery of forearm rotation range in forearm rotational contracture. Hutchinson et al. [19] described that rotational osteotomy of both forearm bones can create approximately 100° of correction when performed at the proximal ulna followed by the distal radius. If less rotation is needed then the distal radius osteotomy alone can provide approximately 60° of correction, while correction of the ulnar rotation has minimum effect. However, author's preference is rotational corrective osteotomy of the ulna, when the bony configuration is nearly normal with release of soft tissue at the DRUJ. Wedge-type corrective osteotomy of the ulna also helps to resume rotation axis. Dorsal subluxation of the ulnar head is reduced to the normal position after wedge osteotomy (Fig. 32.3). Additional soft tissue release of the joint capsule is sometimes necessary.

32.5.4 Soft Tissue Release

If the bony configuration of the radius and ulna or rotation axis is normal, pronation–supination contracture may be due to the soft tissue. Sequential sectioning of the soft tissue can increase the rotation range of the forearm [20, 21]. Last sectioning has always a great impact to increase the pronation–supination range. Bert and Linscheid [21] described that sectioning of the soft tissues started as follows: (1) quadrate ligament; (2) IOM; (3) DRUJ capsule; and (4) TFCC. Author's preference is starting from: (1) dorsal DRUJ capsule; (2) membranous part of the IOM; (3) TFCC; and (4) tendinous part of the IOM (Figs. 32.4 and 32.5). DRUJ joint capsule is normally released from dorsal aspect (Fig. 32.6), while additional capsule release from palmar aspect may be necessary in some cases. If there is DRUJ instability after complete sectioning of the soft tissue, the TFCC should be reattached to the central lesion of the fovea.

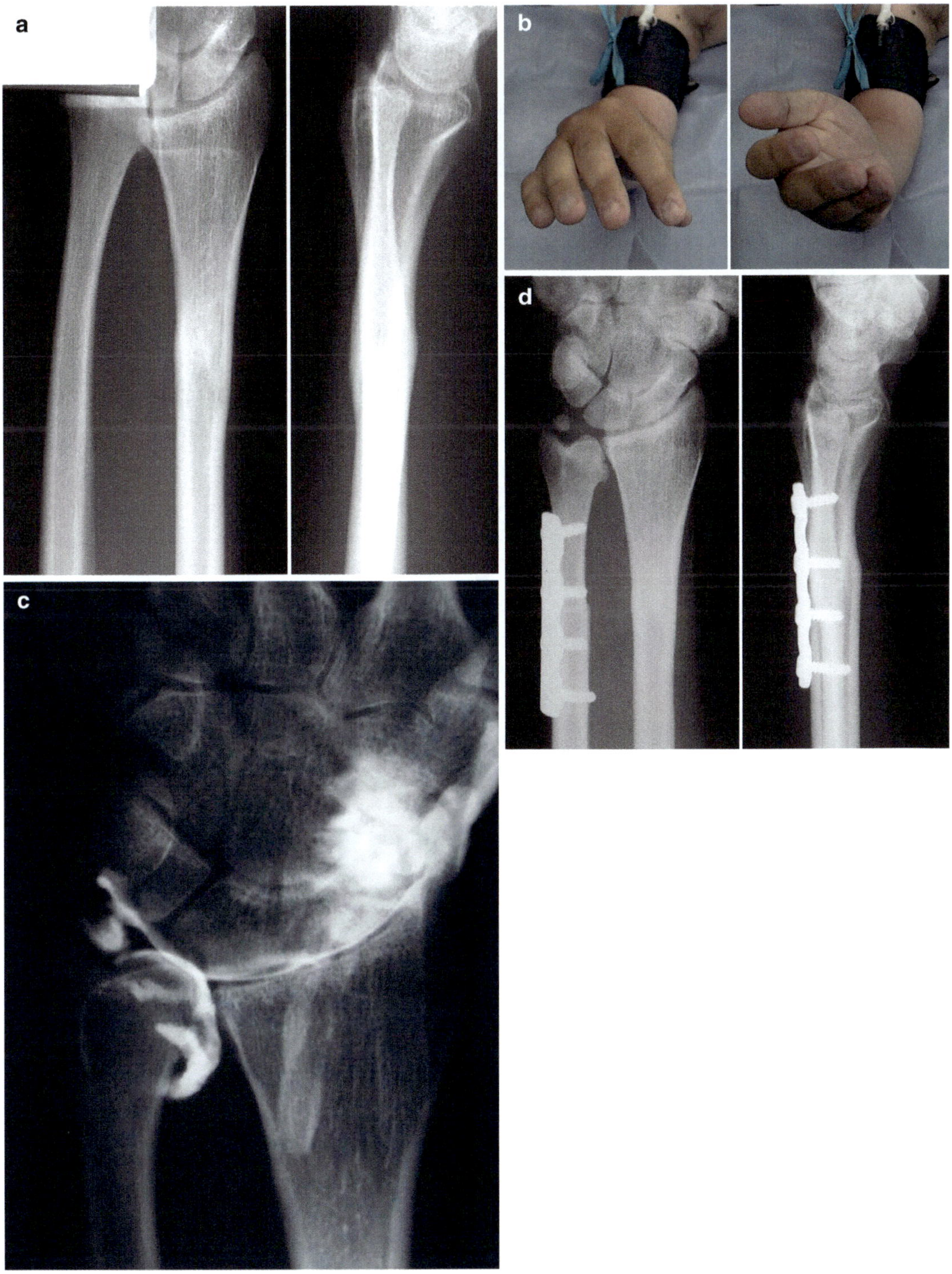

Fig. 32.3 (**a**) The case indicates minor malunion of the radius with dorsally subluxated ulnar head and with 3 mm positive ulnar variance. This case seems a chronic Galeazzi fracture. (**b**) Preoperative pronation range was 70° (left) and supination 0° (right). (**c**) Arthrogram indicates overlapping of the ulnar head to the TFCC. (**d**) Wedge-type shortening corrective osteotomy of the ulna may resume the DRUJ articulation and rotation axis. In this case, release of the volar DRUJ capsule was added to achieve 90° of pronation and 80° of supination

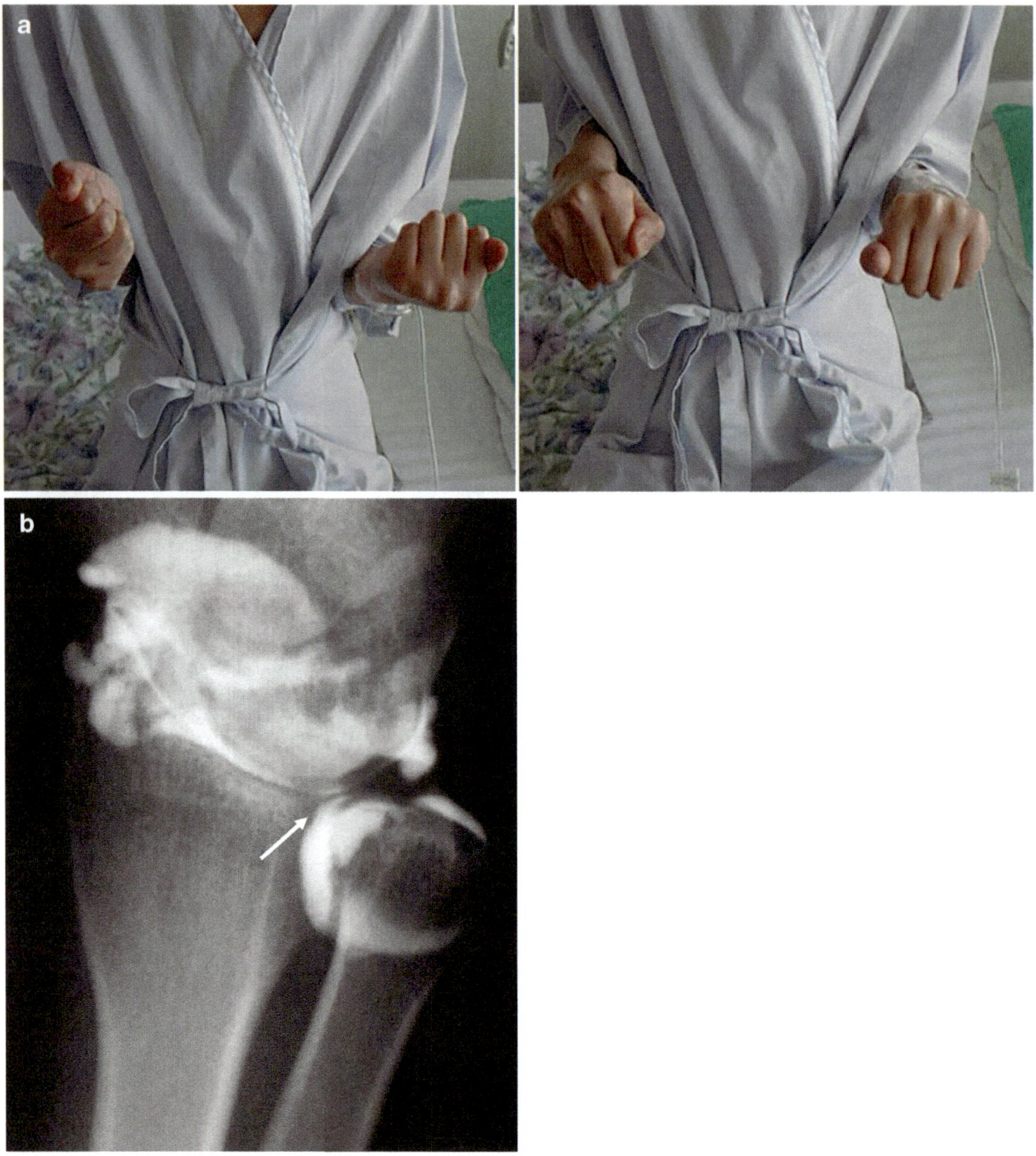

Fig. 32.4 (**a**) DRUJ locking case in her right wrist indicating loss of supination (left) with full pronation (right). (**b**) Arthrogram demonstrates overlapping of the TFCC onto the ulnar head (white arrow)

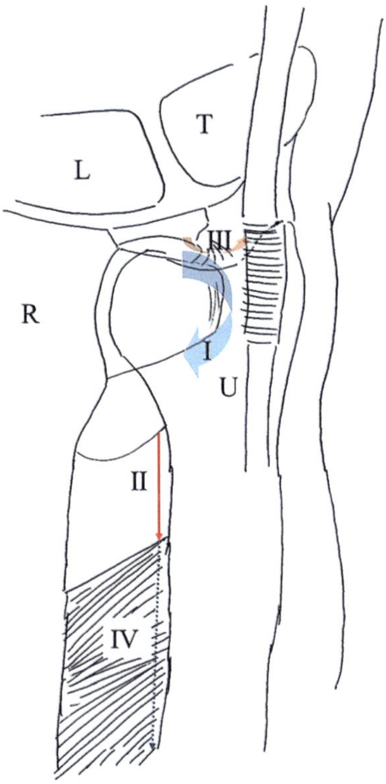

Fig. 32.5 Schematic illustration of release of the soft tissue around the DRUJ. I: DRUJ capsule; II: Membranous portion of the IOM; III: foveal lesion of the TFCC; IV: tendinous portion of the IOM (interosseous ligament; IOL). Author normally sections the soft tissue in pronation–supination contracture cases in this order

32.5.5 Reduction and Fixation of the Malunited Ulna Styloid Process

In chronic Galeazzi fracture dislocation, malunion of the ulnar styloid may lead to loss of pronation–supination after reduction and fixation of the malunion of the radial shaft. The ulnar styloid process is one of the attaching areas of the RUL as well as the fovea. Malunion of the ulnar styloid indicates abnormal tension inside the TFCC. In such case, corrective osteotomy and fixation of the ulnar styloid process to the original position induce normal pronosupination range, while an additional reattachment of the RUL to the fovea may be necessary in some cases.

32.5.6 Reduction of DRUJ Locking

Arthroscopic or open reduction was successful to reduce DRUJ locking. Patients with positive ulnar variance require additional ulnar shortening to the neutral ulnar variance avoiding recurrence of locking [15, 16].

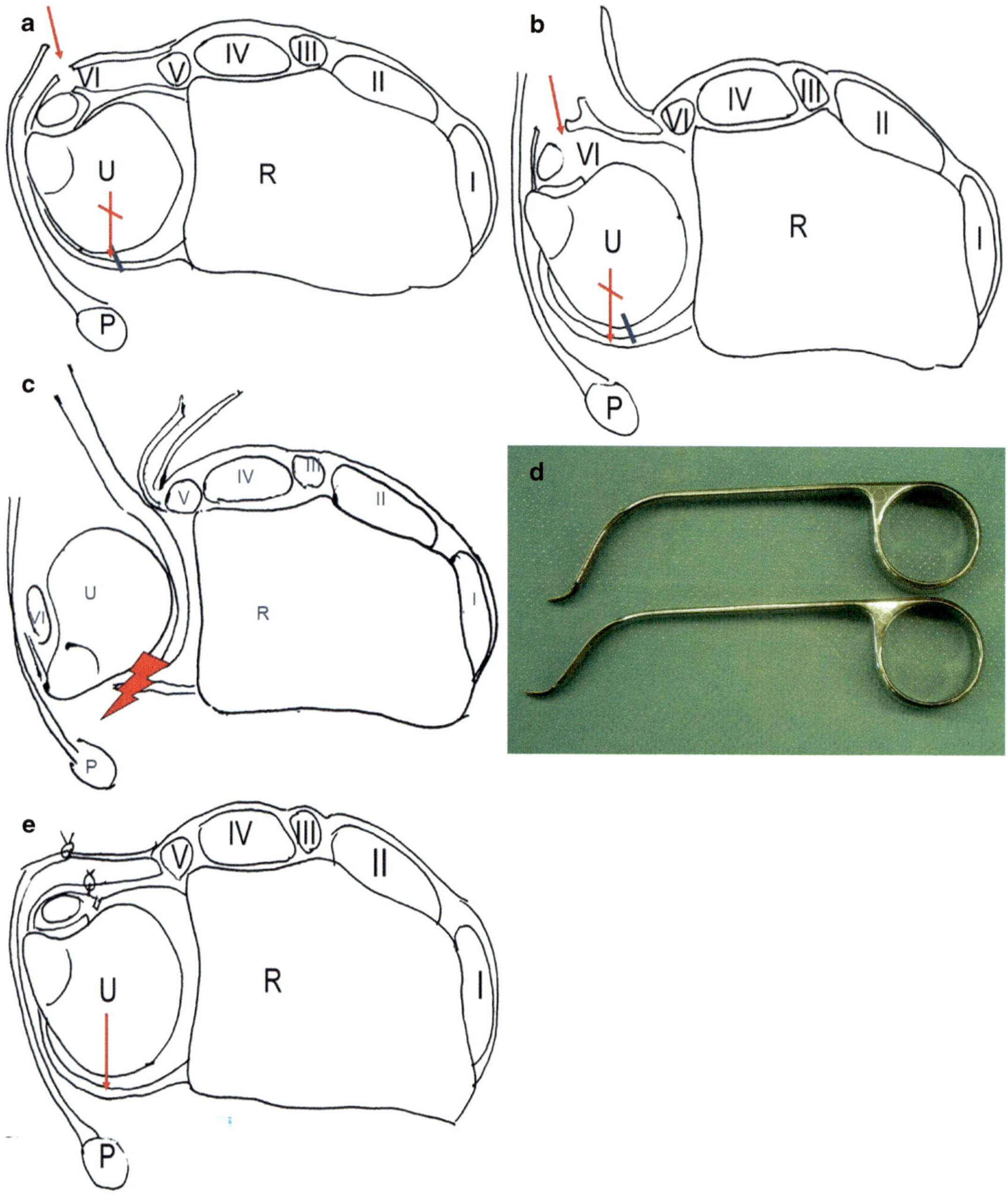

Fig. 32.6 Schematic illustration of DRUJ joint capsule release (axial plane). (**a**) Opening of the sixth compartment. (**b**) Release of the dorsal capsule from the ulna. (**c**) Release of the volar DRUJ capsule from dorsal aspect. (**d**) Special designed elevator. Two types of elevator with different diameter of releasing part. (**e**) After release, the fibro-osseous band of the sixth compartment and extensor retinaculum are repaired

References

1. Schemitsch EH, Richards RR. The effect of malunion on functional outcome after plate fixation of fractures of both bones of the forearm in adults. J Bone Joint Surg Am. 1992;74(7):1168–78.
2. Nakamura T, Yabe Y, Horiuchi Y, Yamazaki N. In vivo motion analysis of forearm rotation utilizing magnetic resonance imaging. Clin Biomech. 1999;14(5):315–20. https://doi.org/10.1016/s0268-0033(98)90091-2.
3. Nakamura T, Yabe Y, Horiuchi Y. A biomechanical analysis of pronation-supination of the forearm using magnetic resonance imaging: dynamic changes of the interosseous membrane of the forearm during pronation-supination. Nihon Seikeigeka Gakkai Zasshi. 1994;68(1):14–25. (in Japanese)
4. Nakamura T, Yabe Y, Horiuchi Y. Functional anatomy of the triangular fibrocartilage complex. J Hand Surg Br. 1996;21(4):571–86. https://doi.org/10.1016/s0266-7681(96)80135-5.
5. Kleinman WB, Graham TJ. The distal radioulnar joint capsule: clinical anatomy and role in posttraumatic limitation of forearm rotation. J Hand Surg Am. 1998 Jul;23(4):588–99. https://doi.org/10.1016/S0363-5023(98)80043-9.
6. Vasileiadis GI, Ramazanian T, Kamaci S, Bachman DR, Park SE, Thaveepunsan S, Fitzsimmons JS, O'Driscoll SW. Loss of pronation-supination in patients with heterotopic ossification around the elbow. J Shoulder Elb Surg. 2019;28(7):1406–10. https://doi.org/10.1016/j.jse.2018.10.029.
7. Nakamura T, Yabe Y, Horiuchi Y. Functional anatomy of the interosseous membrane of the forearm—dynamic changes during rotation. Hand Surg. 1999;4(1):67–73. https://doi.org/10.1142/s0218810499000034.
8. Nakamura T, Yabe Y, Horiuchi Y. In vivo MR study of dynamic changes in the interosseous membrane of the forearm during rotation. J Hand Surg. 1999;24(2):245–8. https://doi.org/10.1054/jhsb.1998.0185.
9. Nakamura T, Yabe Y, Horiuchi Y. Normal kinematics of the interosseous membrane during forearm pronation-supination; a three dimensional study. Hand Surg. 2000;5(1):1–20. https://doi.org/10.1142/s0218810400000077.
10. Nakamura T, Yabe Y, Horiuchi Y, Yamazaki N. Three-dimensional magnetic resonance imaging of the interosseous membrane of forearm: a new method using fuzzy reasoning. Magn Reson Imag. 1999;17(3):463–70. https://doi.org/10.1016/s0730-725x(98)00183-0.
11. Nakamura T, Yabe Y, Horiuchi Y, Seki T, Yamazaki N. Normal kinematics of the interosseous membrane during forearm pronation-supination. A three dimensional MRI study. Hand Surg. 2000;5(1):1–10. https://doi.org/10.1142/s0218810400000077.
12. Bronstein A, Heaton D, Tencer AF, Trumble TE. Distal radius malunion and forearm rotation: a cadaveric study. J Wrist Surg. 2014;3(1):7–11. https://doi.org/10.1055/s-0034-1365826.
13. Bronstein AJ, Trumble TE, Tencer AF. The effects of distal radius fracture malalignment on forearm rotation: a cadaveric study. J Hand Surg Am. 1997;22(2):258–63. https://doi.org/10.1016/S0363-5023(97)80160-8.
14. Okamoto S, Nakamura T, Yamabe E, Takayama S, Toyama Y. Pronation contracture of the forearm due to iatrogenic scar formation on the membranous portion of the forearm interosseous membrane: a case report. J Hand Surg Br. 2006;31B(4):397-400, 2006. https://doi.org/10.1016/j.jhsb.2006.03.173.
15. Suzuki T, Nakamura T, Tanino Y, Obara Y, Yoshikawa Y, Iwamoto T. Acute blocking of forearm supination secondary to tearing of the triangular fibrocartilage complex. J Hand Surg Eur. 2020;45(9):939–44. https://doi.org/10.1177/1753193420926104.
16. Takahashi Y, Nakamura T, Sato K, Toyama Y. Subluxation of the palmar radioulnar ligament as a cause of blocked forearm supination: a case of DRUJ locking. J Wrist Surg. 2013;2(1):83–8. https://doi.org/10.1055/s-0032-1333065.
17. Mino DE, Palmer AK, Levinsohn EM. The role of radiography and computerized tomography in the diagnosis of subluxation and dislocation of the distal radioulnar joint. J Hand Surg Am. 1983;8(1):23–31. https://doi.org/10.1016/s0363-5023(83)80046-x.
18. Mino DE, Palmer AK, Levinsohn EM. Radiography and computerized tomography in the diagnosis of incongruity of the distal radioulnar joint. J Bone Joint Surg Am. 1985;67(2):247–52.
19. Hutchinson DT, Wang AA, Ryssman D, Brown MA. Both-bone forearm osteotomy for supination contracture: a cadaver model. J Hand Surg Am. 2006;31(6):968–72. https://doi.org/10.1016/j.jhsa.2006.01.010.
20. Guidi M, Luchetti R, Besmens I, Rothenfluh E, Calcagni M. Wrist arthrolysis: a systematic review of open and arthroscopic techniques. J Wrist Surg. 2021;10(6):544–50. https://doi.org/10.1055/s-0041-1726291.
21. Bert JM, Linscheid RL, McElfresh EC. Rotatory contracture of the forearm. J Bone Joint Surg Am. 1980;62(7):1163–8.

GPSR Compliance

The European Union's (EU) General Product Safety Regulation (GPSR) is a set of rules that requires consumer products to be safe and our obligations to ensure this.

If you have any concerns about our products, you can contact us on ProductSafety@springernature.com

In case Publisher is established outside the EU, the EU authorized representative is:

Springer Nature Customer Service Center GmbH
Europaplatz 3
69115 Heidelberg, Germany

Batch number: 10732799

Printed by Printforce, the Netherlands